ANTISEPSIS, DISINFECTION, AND STERILIZATION

ANTISEPSIS, DISINFECTION, AND STERILIZATION

TYPES, ACTION, AND RESISTANCE

GERALD E. McDONNELL

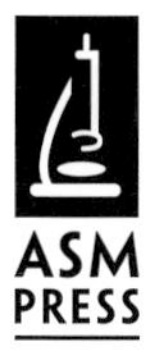

ASM PRESS

Washington, DC

Library of Congress Cataloging-in-Publication Data

Names: McDonnell, Gerald E., author.
Title: Antisepsis, disinfection, and sterilization / Gerald E. McDonnell.
Description: Second edition. | Washington, DC : ASM Press, [2017] | Includes index.
Identifiers: LCCN 2017015076 | ISBN 9781555819675 (hardcover)
Subjects: LCSH: Sterilization. | Asepsis and antisepsis. | Disinfection and disinfectants.
Classification: LCC QR69.S75 M33 2017 | DDC 614.4/8–dc23 LC record available at https://lccn.loc.gov/2017015076

Printed in Canada

10 9 8 7 6 5 4 3 2 1

Address editorial correspondence to
ASM Press, 1752 N St., N.W.,
Washington, DC 20036-2904, USA

Send orders to ASM Press, P.O. Box 605, Herndon, VA 20172, USA
Phone: 800-546-2416; 703-661-1593
Fax: 703-661-1501
E-mail: books@asmusa.org
Online: http://www.asmscience.org

ACKNOWLEDGMENTS

I greatly appreciate the many colleagues and friends who reviewed selected chapters of this book, as well as my wife, Lesley, for her encouragement.

GERALD E. MCDONNELL
Basking Ridge, New Jersey
USA

CONTENTS

PREFACE

The control of microorganisms and microbial growth is an important consideration in medical, veterinary, dental, industrial, pharmaceutical, environmental, and food processing settings. This book has been developed to provide a basic understanding of the various chemical and physical antisepsis, disinfection, and sterilization methods used for infection prevention and contamination control. Disinfection and sterilization technologies are used for the control of microorganisms on surfaces, in products, or in air, while antisepsis is particularly associated with microbial reduction on the skin or mucous membranes. Many of these applications have been used over many years and continue to play important roles in our daily lives, including the provision of safe drinking water, production and preservation of products, laboratory safety, food safety, sterilization of medical devices, and disinfection of critical surfaces. The benefits of microbial control have been appreciated since ancient times—for example, in the use of heating, salts, and metals for preservation and wound treatment—despite the absence in those times of any pure understanding of microbiology. Over the last 160 years, we have gained a greater appreciation of microorganisms and their roles in contamination and infection. In parallel, various chemical and physical antisepsis, disinfection, and sterilization methods have been developed and are widely used to render surfaces and products safe for use. Despite these advancements, microbial control issues continue to challenge us. Notable examples include controlling the risk of virus transmission in outbreaks of Zika virus, Ebola virus, and noroviruses; medical device contamination associated with health care outbreaks of infection (such as with flexible endoscopes); the emerging concerns with unique infectious agents (such as prions or other transmissible proteinaceous agents); and the continuing concern of anti-infective (including antibiotic)-resistant microorganisms in hospitals and the general community. As our knowledge increases in microbiology, so does our understanding of the novel ways that microorganisms can present with mechanisms of surviving the many broad-spectrum contamination control technology that we use, including chemical and physical disinfection and sterilization methods.

As a background to this subject, a brief introduction to microbiology is provided, to include the various types of microorganisms in their major classes. This section also provides the definitions of some key terms widely used in the area, the overall resistance profiles of microorganisms to inactivation, and the variety of methods that are used to test the effectiveness and optimize the use of antimicrobial products and processes.

Disinfection and sterilization can be generally considered as either based on chemical or physical antimicrobial technologies. Chemicals include various types of aldehydes, halogens, and oxidizing agents, while physical processes include the use of heat, filtration, and radiation. For each general group, the various types of technologies are discussed, along with their applications, spectra of activity, advantages, and disadvantages, and a brief description of their modes of action. A wider range of methods is used for disinfection and antisepsis applications. Many of these are required to reduce the number of microorganisms, or even the number of certain types of microorganisms, to an acceptable level. In contrast, only a limited number of technologies are utilized for sterilization, which has the ultimate goal of rendering a surface, area, or substance free of all viable microbial contamination. For this reason, disinfection and sterilization methods are considered separately, with a specific chapter dedicated to the various antimicrobials used as antiseptics and in antisepsis applications.

The current understanding of the mechanisms of action on microorganisms is considered in chapter 7. It is important to note that the modes of action of these technologies are generally nonspecific and distinct from the more specific mechanisms of action described for anti-infective agents, such as antibiotics and antiviral agents. Most biocides demonstrate a wider range of antimicrobial activity, generally corresponding to nonspecific and varied modes of action. The mechanisms of action of biocides are considered in four general categories: oxidizing agents, cross-linking agents, agents that act by transfer of energy, and other structure-disrupting agents. Despite these general mechanisms, some biocides have been shown to have primary targets similar to those of certain antibiotics, and a better understanding of their mechanisms of action is of interest in the development of the next generation of anti-infectives and/or optimized antimicrobial processes.

Microorganisms demonstrate various natural (intrinsic) and acquired mechanisms to resist the antimicrobial effects of chemical and physical processes. These mechanisms are discussed in further detail in chapter 8 and are important to consider in order to ensure the safe and effective use of these technologies. This topic, and the impact of microbial resistance, has been particularly well published in the use of widely used anti-infectives (notably antibiotic-resistant bacteria like methicillin-resistant *Staphylococcus* and carbapenem-resistant *Enterobacteriaceae*), but similar and distinct mechanisms in microbial resistance to more broad-spectrum antimicrobial products and processes have been described. Biocide resistance in bacteria has been studied in greater detail since the publication of the first edition of this book, with many examples of intrinsic and acquired mechanisms of resistance. Intrinsic mechanisms include biofilm formation, development of dormant endospores, and the accumulation of resistance mechanisms in extremophiles. Acquired resistance mechanisms due to mutations and the acquisition of transposons and/or plasmids, not unlike those described for antibiotics, have also been described in more detail. Although many of these mechanisms allow for the tolerance in the presence of antimicrobial chemicals at normally inhibitory levels, other mechanisms have been shown to dramatically change the response of some microorganisms to biocides and to enable them to survive highly toxic conditions. Further advances have also been made in our understanding of specific mechanisms of resistance in other microorganisms such as viruses, prions, fungi, and protozoa.

Overall, it is intended that this book will give a basic understanding of and reference for the various types, modes of action, and mechanisms of resistance of antiseptics, disinfectants, and sterilization processes for students of microbiology, chemistry, infection prevention, contamination control, public health, and industrial applications. A greater understanding and appreciation of these technologies will continue to ensure their long-term safe and effective use in contamination and infection prevention.

ABOUT THE AUTHOR

Gerald E. McDonnell received a B.Sc. degree in medical laboratory sciences from the University of Ulster (1989) and a Ph.D. in microbial genetics at the Department of Genetics, Trinity College, University of Dublin (1992). His graduate work involved studies on the control of gene expression in *Bacillus subtilis*. He spent 3 years at the Mycobacterial Research Laboratories, Colorado State University, investigating the mechanisms of antibiotic resistance and cell wall biosynthesis in mycobacteria. In 1995 he joined the St. Louis, Mo., operations of ConvaTec, a division of Bristol-Myers Squibb, as a group leader in microbiology in the research and development of skin care, hard surface disinfection, and cleaning chemistries. He worked for STERIS Corporation for 19 years in the USA and in Europe on the development, research, and support of infection and contamination prevention products and services in health care and industrial applications, with a particular focus on cleaning, antisepsis, disinfection, and sterilization. Dr. McDonnell is currently the senior director for sterility assurance for DePuySynthes, a Johnson & Johnson company, and a member of the Johnson & Johnson Sterility Assurance leadership team. He serves as the global technical leader in the areas of microbiology and contamination control including sterilization, aseptic technique, reprocessing, microbiology, and cleanliness requirements. His basic research interests include infection prevention, decontamination microbiology, emerging pathogens, and modes of action and resistance to biocides. His work also includes the development and implementation of international and national guidance and standards in cleaning, disinfection, and sterilization. He has over 180 publications, 22 patents and is a frequent presenter on various aspects of his work internationally.

INTRODUCTION

1

1.1 GENERAL INTRODUCTION

Microbiology is the study of microscopic organisms (microorganisms). Microorganisms play important roles in our lives, both for our benefit as well as to our detriment. Of primary consideration are those microorganisms that cause diseases under a variety of circumstances. Other issues include the economic aspects associated with microbial contamination such as food spoilage, plant infections, and surface damage. The control of microorganisms is therefore an important concern, in preventing contamination as well as removing or reducing it when it occurs. A variety of physical and chemical methods are used for these purposes in antisepsis, disinfection, and sterilization applications. Disinfection and sterilization are used for the control of microorganisms on surfaces, in liquids, or in areas, while antisepsis is particularly associated with microbial reduction on the skin or mucous membranes. These antimicrobial applications can include skin washing, wound treatment, product preservation, food and water disinfection, surface disinfection, and product sterilization. Many of these processes have been used historically, being described in ancient texts before we had any true understanding of the nature of microorganisms. Despite this, it is only in the past 160 years, as our knowledge and understanding of microbiology have expanded, that the impact of antiseptics, disinfectants, and sterilization has been truly appreciated. Their utilization has played and continues to play an important role in significantly reducing the incidence of infectious diseases, including gastroenteritis, health care-acquired infections, and pneumonia. Today microorganisms continue to be a significant cause of morbidity, mortality, and economic loss. We continue to be challenged with the identification of new strains of microorganisms such as antibiotic-resistant *Enterobacteriaceae* (e.g., strains of *Escherichia coli* and *Klebsiella pneumoniae*), *Clostridium difficile*, viruses (e.g., Ebola, influenza, Zika virus, coronaviruses, and parvoviruses), protozoa such as *Acanthamoeba* and their internal communities of microorganisms, and proteinaceous infectious agents (such as prions).

Antimicrobial (or biocidal) processes include many types of physical and chemical methods. Physical processes include heat (e.g., steam or incineration) and radiation (e.g., UV or γ radiation). A wide range of chemicals such as aldehydes, halogens, and phenolics are also used due to their potent antimicrobial activities. The choice and use of these processes depend on the required application. For example, many aggressive chemicals or high-temperature processes can be used on various hard surfaces (such as medical devices) but would not be acceptable for use as antiseptics on the skin. Therefore, there are two primary considerations in the choice of an antimicrobial process: the effectiveness against target microorganisms (antimicrobial efficacy) and safety. Safety can include damage to the person or material on which the process is being used (e.g., tissue damage, toxicity, or material compatibility), as well those using the process. Further considerations can include the environmental impact, undesired odors, and product-specific concerns (e.g., changes in the taste or stability of foods).

There is no perfect biocide for any application, but the desired attributes include the following:

- Activity against a wide range, if not all, microorganisms
- Rapid activity
- Efficacy in the presence of contaminating organic and inorganic materials, which can inhibit the activity of the biocide
- Low or no toxicity, irritancy, mutagenicity (may cause genetic mutations), and carcinogenicity (may cause cancer)
- Can be used safely
- Lack of damage to target surfaces or liquids (material compatibility)
- Lack of unwanted or toxic residues (biocompatibility)
- Stability, yet ability to be naturally degraded in the environment
- Environmental friendliness

The advantages and disadvantages of using particular antimicrobials should be considered in deciding their suitability for any given application.

This book describes the major widely used antiseptic, disinfectant, and sterilization methodologies. For the purpose of introduction, this chapter gives a brief description of the various types of target microorganisms, as well as a discussion of some key considerations in biocidal applications including the evaluation of efficacy, formulation effects, and the importance of surface cleaning. Chapters 2 and 3 describe the various types of physical and chemical biocides, including filtration, which is not a true antimicrobial process but is widely used in the disinfection and sterilization of liquids and gases. For each biocide group the various types, applications, spectrum of antimicrobial activity, advantages, disadvantages, and mode of action are given. Chapter 4 addresses the particular use of biocides as antiseptics and antiseptic applications. Chapters 5 and 6 discuss various types of physical and chemical sterilization methods, which are distinct from disinfection applications. Chapter 7 addresses the current understanding of the mechanisms of biocidal action on microorganisms. In most cases, the modes of action of biocides are general and distinct from the more specific mechanisms described for anti-infective agents such as antibiotics. Biocide mechanisms are considered in four general groups with similar modes of action: oxidizing agents, cross-linking agents, action by transfer of energy, and other structure-disrupting agents. Finally, chapter 8 introduces the impact of microbial resistance to biocides. This topic has been particularly studied in bacteria, and a discussion of the various intrinsic and acquired mechanisms of resistance is provided. Further, known mechanisms of resistance in viruses, prions, fungi, and other eukaryotes are also described.

1.2 DEFINITIONS

Many of the terms and definitions associated with the use of biocides can vary regionally, in their regulatory (or legal) use, in the scientific literature, and in common usage. This can often lead to confusion and misunderstanding. Despite some attempts to harmonize the use and definition of some of these terms, there is often no standardized consensus internationally. For the purpose of this book, the following terms and definitions are used and, where possible, are consistent with international consensus documents.

Aerobe (adj., *aerobic*): A microorganism that requires oxygen for metabolism. Can be obligate (requiring oxygen), facultative (can grow in the presence or absence of oxygen), and microaerophilic (requiring lower concentrations of oxygen than normally present in air).

Anaerobe (adj., *anaerobic*): A microorganism that does not require oxygen for metabolism. Can be obligate (requiring the absence of oxygen) or facultative (able to grow in the presence or absence of oxygen).

Antibiotic: A substance (or drug) that kills or inhibits the growth of bacteria. This definition has also been applied to substances that affect other microorganisms, such as fungi. Originally, antibiotics were discovered as substances that were produced by one type of microorganism (fungi in particular) that selectively inhibited the growth of another microorganism (bacteria in particular). Many antibiotics are now synthetically produced.

Anti-infective: A substance (or drug) capable of killing microorganisms or inhibiting their growth, in particular, pathogenic microorganisms. This term is used to encompass drugs that specifically act on certain types of microorganisms including antibacterials (antibiotics), antifungals, antivirals, and antiprotozoal agents. For the purpose of discussion in this book, the term "anti-infective" will be used to describe a drug used to treat specific infections within animals, plants, and humans. This is in contrast to biocides or biocidal processes, which are considered to be broad-spectrum antimicrobials that are used on inanimate surfaces or the skin and mucous membranes. The differentiation between anti-infectives and biocides is further considered in chapter 7, section 7.1.

Antimicrobial: A process or product that is effective at killing microorganisms. This can vary depending on the process or product and the target microorganism (e.g., antibacterial or antifungal). Antimicrobial agents can include physical and chemical methods.

Antisepsis (noun and adj., *antiseptic*): Destruction or inhibition of microorganisms in or on living tissue, e.g., on the skin. An antiseptic is a biocidal product used on the skin.

Aseptic (noun, *asepsis*): Free of, or using methods to keep free of, microorganisms.

Aseptic processing: The act of handling materials in a controlled environment, in which the air supply, materials, equipment, and personnel are regulated to control microbial and particulate contamination within acceptable levels.

Bioburden: The population of viable microorganisms on or in a product or surface.

Biocide: A chemical or physical agent that typically inactivates a broad spectrum of microorganisms. Chemical biocides include hydrogen peroxide and phenolics, while physical biocides include heat or radiation. Biocides are generally broad-spectrum, in contrast to anti-infectives, which have a narrower range of antimicrobial activity (see chapter 7, section 7.1).

Biocompatibility: The condition of being compatible with living tissue or a living system by not being toxic, injurious, or causing an immunological reaction. Hazards can range from short-term (e.g., acute toxicity, irritation, or hemolysis) to long-term reactions (e.g., sensitization, genotoxicity, or carcinogenicity).

Biofilm: A community of microorganisms (either single or multiple species) developed on or associated with a surface.

Biological indicator: Test system containing viable microorganisms providing a defined resistance to a specified antimicrobial process (such as disinfection or sterilization).

-cidal: Suffix indicating lethal activity against a group of microorganisms (e.g.,

sporicidal means the ability to kill bacterial spores, and bactericidal means having the ability to kill bacteria). Compare to *-static*.

Chemical indicator: Test system that reveals change in one or more predefined process variables based on a chemical or physical change resulting from exposure to a process (e.g., temperature during thermal disinfection or sterilization).

Cleaning: Removal of contaminants (often referred to as "soil" or "contamination") from a surface to the extent necessary for further processing or for an intended use. In this respect, contaminants can include microorganisms as well as other extraneous materials (e.g., blood, tissues, dust, manufacturing process residues, etc.). In practice, a "clean" surface is defined as being visually free of soil and quantified as below specified levels of analytes (such as protein or other specific components of contamination).

Decontamination: Physical and/or chemical means to render a surface or item safe for handling, use, or disposal. Decontamination can refer to chemical and biological (including microbiological) removal and/or inactivation of those materials. The term "biocontamination" is often used to refer specifically to the removal/inactivation of viable particles such as microorganisms to an acceptable level. Surface decontamination is generally a combination of cleaning (contamination removal) and an antimicrobial process (disinfection or sterilization).

Deinfestation: The removal or destruction of microorganisms (e.g., insects).

Depyrogenation: The inactivation (or removal) of pyrogenic substances (pyrogens) on a surface or in a liquid.

Detergent: A surface-active agent (or surfactant) that can emulsify oils and hold dirt in suspension; generally used for cleaning, where "detergents" can refer to cleaning products containing specific surfactants.

Disinfection (noun, *disinfectant*): Antimicrobial process to remove, destroy, or deactivate microorganisms on surfaces or in liquids to a level previously specified for its intended use. Disinfection is often considered as a reduction of the numbers and types of viable microorganisms (or "bioburden") but may not be assumed to render the surface or liquid free from viable microbial contamination (in contrast to sterilization). Disinfection processes or disinfectants may be effective against many types of microorganisms, with the notable exception of bacterial spores, which are considered the most resistant types of microorganisms to disinfection and sterilization. Chemical disinfectants or disinfection processes are often subdivided into high-level, intermediate, and low-level (depending on the product claims and regulatory requirements in different parts of the world). High-level disinfectants are considered effective against all microbial pathogens, with the exception of large numbers of bacterial spores. These products are typically sporicidal over longer exposure times. Intermediate-level disinfectants are effective against mycobacteria, vegetative bacteria, most viruses, and fungi, but not necessarily bacterial or some fungal spores. Low-level disinfectants are typically effective against most bacteria, some (in particular, enveloped) viruses, and some fungi, but not mycobacteria or bacterial spores. Other definitions can be used to describe specific types of disinfection processes such as antisepsis, fumigation, sanitization, and pasteurization.

D value (or *D_{10} value*): Time (or dose) required to achieve inactivation of 90% (or 1 $\log_{10}$ unit) of a population of a given test microorganism under stated conditions.

Endotoxin: Any of a class of toxins (or pyrogens) present in a microorganism but released only on cell disintegration. Endotoxins are the lipopolysaccharide component of the cell wall of Gram-negative bacteria that elicits a variety of inflammatory responses in animals and humans.

Exotoxin: Any of a class of toxins produced and secreted from a microorganism.

Formulation: Combination of chemical ingredients, including active (e.g., a biocide) and other ingredients, into a product for its intended use (e.g., preserved products, antiseptics, and chemical disinfectants).

Fumigation: Delivery of an antimicrobial process (gas or liquid) indirectly to the internal surface of an enclosed area. An example is fogging, which is the indirect application of a liquid disinfection into to a given area.

Germ: A general term referring to a microorganism.

Germicidal (noun, *germicide*): The ability to kill microorganisms. In some countries (such as in the United States), this definition specifically refers to bactericidal activity against certain types of bacteria only.

Germination: The initiation of vegetative growth in a dormant spore.

Hydrophilic (*polar*): Able to attract and absorb water ("water-loving"). Similar to lipophobic ("lipid-hating"; avoiding lipid).

Hydrophobic (*non-polar*): Having the properties of repelling and not absorbing water ("water-hating"). Similar to lipophilic ("lipid-loving"; having an affinity for lipid).

Inactivation: Loss of the ability of microorganisms to grow and/or multiply.

Minimum effective concentration (*MEC*): The lowest concentration of a chemical or product, used in a specified process, that achieves a claimed activity.

Minimum recommended concentration (*MRC*): The lowest concentration of a chemical or product specified by the equipment manufacturer for use in a process.

Parasite: An organism able to live on and cause damage to another organism.

Pathogen: A disease-causing microorganism.

Pasteurization: The antimicrobial reduction, usually by heat, of microorganisms that can be harmful or cause product spoilage. "Pasteurization" is a term widely used for moist heat disinfection, including in foods and liquids.

Preservation: The prevention of the multiplication of microorganisms.

Pyrogen: A substance that can cause a rise in body temperature, including exotoxins and endotoxins.

Reference microorganism: Microbial strain obtained from a recognized culture collection.

Resistance: The inability of an anti-infective or biocide to be effective against target microorganisms. See *tolerance*.

Safety data sheet (*SDS*): Document specifying the properties of a substance or product, its potential hazardous effects for humans and the environment, and the precautions necessary to handle and dispose of the substance safely. Traditionally referred to as an MSDS (material safety data sheet).

SAL (*sterility assurance level*): Probability of a single viable microorganism occurring on an item after sterilization, expressed as the negative exponent to the base 10.

Sanitization: The removal or inactivation of microorganisms that pose a threat to public health.

Secondary metabolites: Various products produced by microorganisms at the end of exponential growth or during stationary phase.

Soil: Natural or artificial contamination on a device or surface following its use or simulated use.

Sporulation: The process of spore development in microorganisms.

-static: Suffix indicating the ability to inhibit the growth of a group of microorganisms (e.g., bacteriostatic means having activity

to inhibit the growth of vegetative bacteria, and fungistatic means to inhibit the growth of fungi). Compare to *-cidal*.

Sterile (noun, *sterility*): Free from viable microorganisms.

Sterile barrier system: Packaging that prevents the ingress of microorganisms following a sterilization process, thereby preserving the sterile state.

Sterilization: Defined process used to render a surface or product free from viable microorganisms. Note that terminal sterilization is a process by which a product is sterilized within a sterile barrier system that preserves the sterile state following the process (e.g., during storage or transportation).

Sterilizer: Equipment designed to achieve sterilization.

Sterilizing agent: Physical or chemical agent (or combination of agents) that has sufficient microbicidal activity to achieve sterility under defined conditions.

Tolerance: A decreased effect of an anti-infective or biocide against a target microorganism, requiring increased concentration or other modification to be effective. Compare to *resistance*.

Validation: A documented procedure for obtaining, recording, and interpreting the results required to establish that a process will consistently yield product complying with predetermined specifications.

Verification: Confirmation through the provision of objective evidence that specified requirements have been fulfilled.

Viable: Alive and able to reproduce.

1.3 GENERAL MICROBIOLOGY

1.3.1 Introduction

Microbiology is the study of microscopic organisms, which include multicellular forms (helminths), cellular forms (including eukaryotes and prokaryotes), and noncellular forms (e.g., viruses) (Table 1.1).

Microorganisms play a large part in our daily lives, both for our benefit and to our detriment (Table 1.2). Many of these benefits have been well described, while others are still being explored; for example, the complex roles of microorganisms in microbiomes (communities of microorganisms in particular environments) are a particular area of recent research because of their impacts in healthy and diseased situations. The use of antiseptics, disinfectants, and sterilization methods is essential to the control of the growth, multiplication, and transfer of microorganisms to reduce detrimental effects. A particular example is reducing the impact of pathogenic, or disease-causing, microorganisms that can cause a variety of infections and stresses in humans, plants, and animals. Further considerations include the control of product contamination or spoilage, including that of foodstuffs and pharmaceutical drugs, which can have significant commercial consequences.

1.3.2 Eukaryotes and Prokaryotes

Eukaryotes and prokaryotes in their basic structures consist of single discrete cells. Cells are the basic units of life for these microorganisms, as well as the building blocks for multicellular organisms—helminths, plants, and animals. Eukaryotes and prokaryotes are distinguished based on their microscopic structure; prokaryotes are considered to be much smaller and less compartmentalized in their structure, while eukaryotes are larger and more compartmentalized (Table 1.3). Eukaryotic cells include fungi, protozoa, algae, and human and plant cells. Prokaryotes include a diverse variety of eubacteria and archaea. Viruses are structurally distinct and considered separately, because they do not possess the mechanisms for self-replication and depend on cells, in which they grow and multiply, for survival.

1.3.3 Eukaryotes

1.3.3.1 Multicellular Eukaryotes. Multicellular eukaryotes can include microscopic (or indeed macroscopic) arthropods and helminths (or worms). These are essentially

TABLE 1.1 Examples of various types of microorganisms

Microorganism	Typical structures[a]	Size(μm)	Nucleic acid	Cell wall
Prions	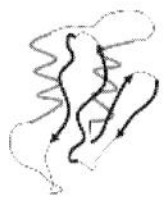	<0.01	None	No
Viruses	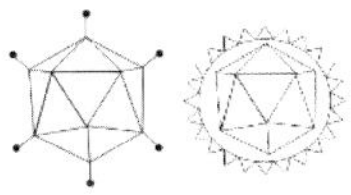	0.01–0.4	DNA or RNA	No Envelop may be present
Chlamydia/rickettsia	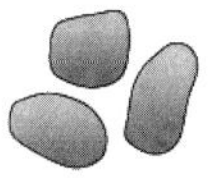	0.3	DNA	Minimal or simple cell wall
Mycoplasma	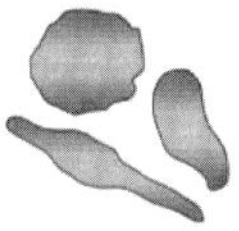	0.1–0.3	DNA	No
Bacteria	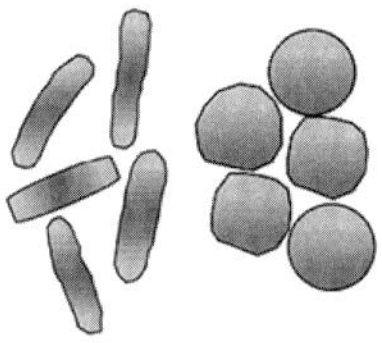	0.3–0.8	DNA	Yes
Fungi	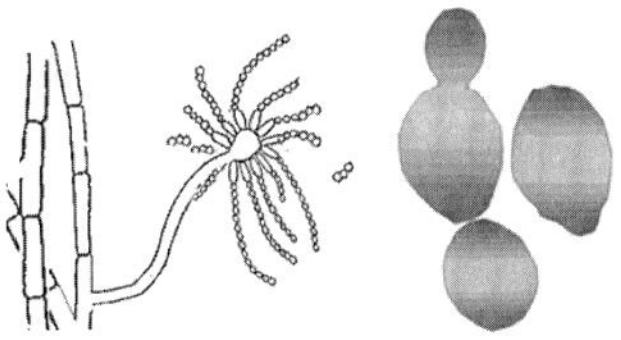	Yeast: 8–10 Fungi: >0.5 (wide), >5 (long)	DNA	Yes
Algae	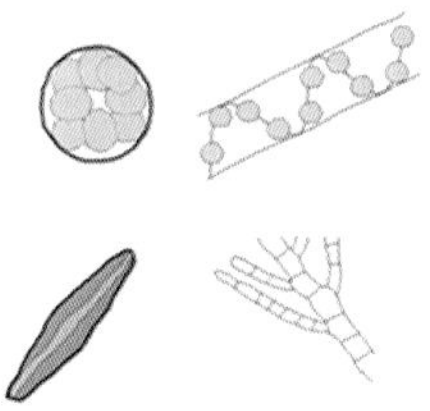	1–>1,000	DNA	Yes/No (Some)
Protozoa	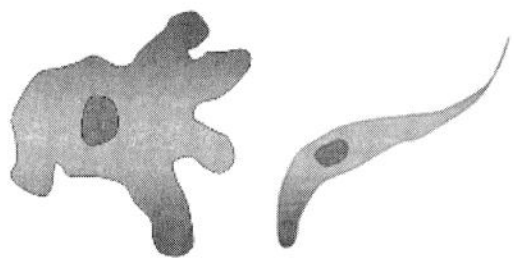	10–200	DNA	No
Helminths	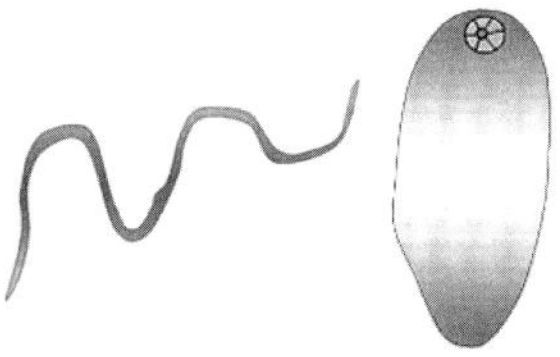	>1,000	DNA	N/A[b]

[a]Not to scale; simplified structures shown. In addition, the basic structures of microorganisms can vary considerably based on their type, environmental conditions, and growth (or life cycle) phase.

[b]N/A, not applicable.

TABLE 1.2 Some advantages and disadvantages of microorganisms

Advantages	Examples
Food and beverage production	*Saccharomyces cerevisiae*: bread and beer production
	Saccharomyces ellipsoideus: wine fermentation
Antibiotic production	*Bacillus licheniformis*: bacitracin
	Penicillium chrysogenum: penicillin
Vitamin metabolism	*Pseudomonas* spp.: vitamin B12 production
	Escherichia spp.: vitamin K synthesis in the gut
Genetic engineering	*Agrobacterium tumefaciens*: plasmids used for generating transgenic plants (e.g., herbicide or pathogen resistance)
Disease prevention	*Bacteroides, Enterococcus* spp.: prevent pathogen colonization of the intestinal tract
Bioremediation	*Desulfotomaculum* spp.: arsenic detoxification
Gut microbiomes	Communities of microbes involved with disease resistance, nutrient uptake, and immune system interactions
Disadvantages	**Examples**
Animal/human diseases	*Mycobacterium* spp.: tuberculosis
	HIV virus: AIDS
	Plasmodium spp.: malaria
Plant diseases	*Phytophora*: potato blight
	Corynebacterium: vegetable infections
Surface damage	*Pseuodomonas* spp.: biofilm development and surface corrosion
Food spoilage	*Rhizopus*: bread mold
	Streptococcus: milk souring
Allergic reactions	Fungal spores, including *Stachybotrys* and *Aspergillus*
General product contamination	Bacterial and fungal spores, including *Bacillus*

composed of eukaryotic cells that are specialized into various organs and structures. Arthropods are not considered further here, but some introduction is given to parasitic helminths. Helminths are a diverse group of multicellular parasites and can be further classified as nematodes (roundworms) and platyhelminths (flatworms). Over 20,000 species of nematodes have been defined, although it is estimated that 10 to 100 times this number possibly exist. The flatworms can be further separated into trematodes (flukes) and cestodes (tapeworms). Many helminths can be free-living in water environments (in particular, the roundworms), but most are parasitic in nature. Some of the key diseases caused by helminths are summarized in Table 1.4. Helminths reproduce sexually and have a typical associated life cycle (Fig. 1.1).

Externally, the adult forms (including worms and flukes) are protected by a rigid, proteinaceous (collagen) cuticle, which can resist the effects of biocidal processes; however, parasitic forms do not survive in the environment without their respective hosts (including in some cases intermediate hosts). Further, during their respective life cycles they produce dormant structures (such as ova [eggs] or cysts) that can survive harsh environmental conditions. Little work has been published on the detailed structure of these eggs/cysts or their relative resistance to biocides, but microscopically they are diverse, consisting of various proteins and carbohydrates and having a variety of thicknesses (see chapter 8, section 8.11).

1.3.3.2 Fungi. Fungi are eukaryotic cells, many of which can reproduce asexually (by cell division) or sexually (by the production of spores). A limited number of fungi are implicated in plant and animal diseases (mycosis), but fungi are also widely used for bioremediation/biodegradation, product fermentation (beer, wine, and bread), and the production of biochemical products (e.g, antibiotics, enzymes, and vitamins). Due to their ubiquitous nature, they are often implicated in spoilage and as general contaminants. They are chemo-heterotrophs (requiring organic nutrition), and many are saprophytes (living off

TABLE 1.3 Comparison of general prokaryotic and eukaryotic structures[a]

Structure	Prokaryotes	Eukaryotes
Basic structure	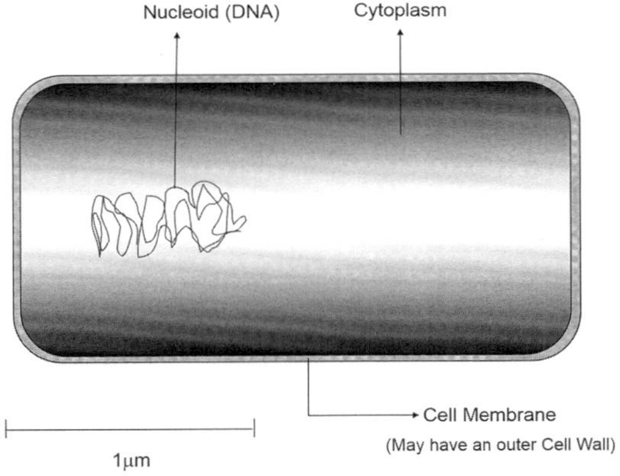 Nucleoid (DNA); Cytoplasm; Cell Membrane (May have an outer Cell Wall); 1µm	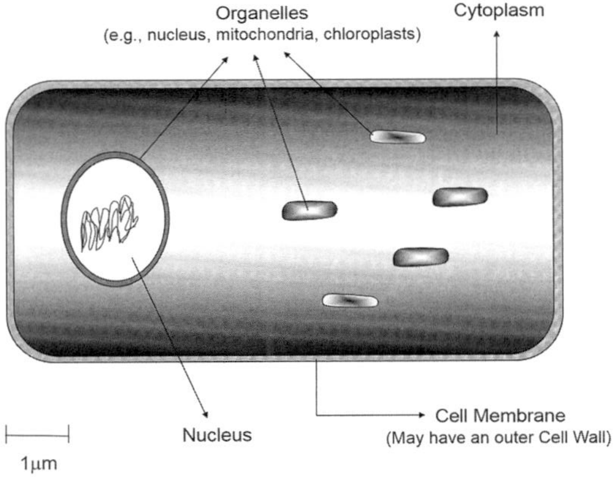 Organelles (e.g., nucleus, mitochondria, chloroplasts); Cytoplasm; Nucleus; Cell Membrane (May have an outer Cell Wall); 1µm
Cytoplasmic membrane	+	+
Organelles, e.g., chloroplasts, mitochondria	–	+
Nucleus, defined by a membrane	–	+
Ribosomes	70S	80S
Cell wall	+/–	+/–

[a]Structural differences vary depending on the microorganism. For example, some prokaryotes (e.g., mycoplasmas) and eukaryotes (animal cells) do not have a cell wall.

TABLE 1.4 Helminths associated with disease

Species	Disease	Comments
Nematodes (roundworms)		
Wuchereria bancrofti	Elephantiasis (blood or lymphatic system blockage)	Transferred via mosquitoes; can grow up to 10 cm long
Onchocerca volvulus	River blindness	Transferred via black flies
Ascaris lumbricoides	Generally asymptomatic but can develop ascariasis (pneumonitis and intestinal obstruction)	From contaminated water, food, or direct surface contact; worms can grow up to 30 cm long
Enterobius vermicularis	Pinworms; dysentery, intestinal blockage	From contaminated water, food, or direct surface contact; worms are ~1 cm
Cestodes (tapeworms)		
Taenia saginata	Generally asymptomatic but can cause mild intestinal complications (including abdominal pain and diarrhea)	Contaminated meat; worms can be very long (>100 cm)
Trematodes (flukes)		
Fasciola hepatia	Can be asymptomatic, with complications including liver abscesses	Contaminated grasses; snails are intermediate hosts
Schistosoma spp.	Schistomiasis; can cause many complications due to growth in the bloodstream and body tissues	Water contamination; snails are intermediate hosts

Nematodes image: Image courtesy of CDC-PHIL/Dr. Mae Melvin, 1974 (ID#1448), with permission; Cestodes image: Image courtesy of CDC-PHIL, 1986 (ID#5260), with permission; Trematodes image: Image courtesy of CDC-PHIL/Dr. Shirley Maddison, 1973 (ID#11193), with permission.

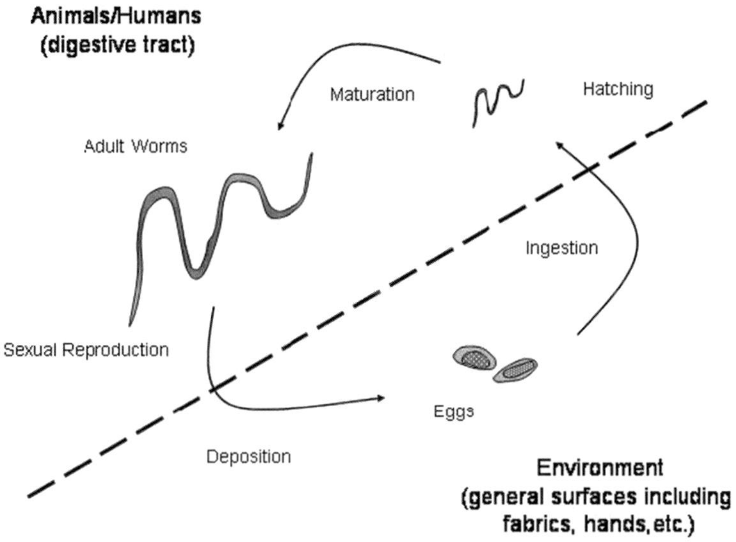

Animals/Humans (digestive tract)

Maturation

Hatching

Adult Worms

Ingestion

Sexual Reproduction

Eggs

Deposition

Environment (general surfaces including fabrics, hands, etc.)

FIGURE 1.1 A typical helminth life cycle (example: *Enterobius vermicularis*).

dead organic matter), acquiring their food by absorption. Fungi are generally classified as being filamentous (molds) or unicellular in their microscopic structures (Fig. 1.2).

Filamentous fungi multiply by cell division, but cells do not separate to form long tubular structures known as hyphae (singular, hypha). The further development and branching of hyphae lead to the development of a mass of fungal growth on a surface known as a mycelium (plural, mycelia). Mycelia can often grow to such an extent that they are clearly visible to the naked eye (e.g., mold growth on bread). Fragments of hyphae can break off and allow development of further mycelia. As the mycelia develop, a variety of fruiting bodies or other structures are formed, which contain spores. Fungal spores can be present in a variety of shapes and sizes, being produced asexually and/or sexually. The various molecular structures of fungal spores have not been studied in detail. In general, most are surrounded by a rigid wall

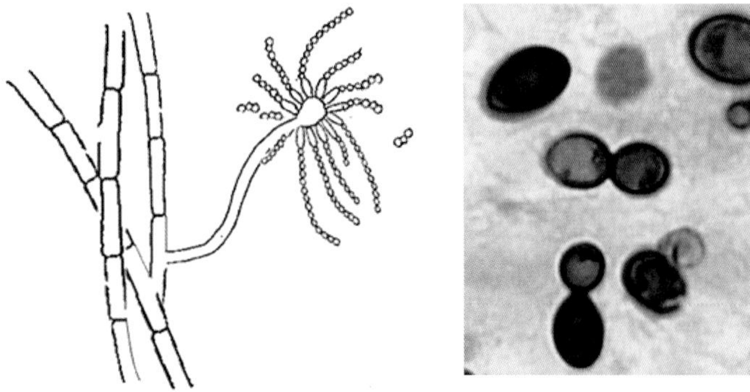

FIGURE 1.2 Typical fungal structures. On the left, filamentous fungus (molds). Hyphae are shown as long lines of unseparated cells, with the development of a fruiting body with attached spores. On the right, typical unicellular fungal (yeast) cells. Cells are generally polymorphic. In two cases, budding cells are shown. Image on right courtesy of CDC-PHIL/Dr. Libero Ajello, 1972 (ID#4219), with permission.

distinguished by its low water content and low metabolic activity and can contain various lipids, pigments, and nutrient reserves. Fungal spore structures are further discussed in chapter 8, section 8.10.

Unicellular fungi (yeasts) do not generally form hyphae and produce growth that appears similar to bacteria (section 1.3.4.1). Asexual reproduction of yeasts can occur by binary fission (e.g., in *Schizosaccharomyces*), similar to bacteria, or by budding directly from the parent cell (e.g., in *Saccharomyces* [Fig. 1.2]). In addition, some fungi are dimorphic, growing as either unicellular or hyphal (or pseudohyphal) forms. Examples of common fungi types are given in Table 1.5.

The fungal protoplasm is surrounded by a rigid cell envelope consisting of the plasma membrane, periplasmic space, and outer cell wall (Fig. 1.3).

Although some details of the structure and function of the yeast cell envelopes of *Saccharomyces cerevisiae* and *Candida albicans* have been studied, much less is known about the range of other fungi structures. The plasma membrane is a lipid bilayer, similar in gross structure to bacterial membranes (section 1.3.4.1) but also including some unique sterols such as ergosterol and zymosterol. The membrane may also contain many types of integral proteins that are involved in processes such as cell wall synthesis and solute/molecule transport. Examples include various chitin and glucan synthases. Between the membrane and outer cell wall is an area known as the periplasm that can contain various mannoproteins, including enzymes such as invertase and acid phosphatase, which play a role in substrate uptake by the cell. The cell wall is a cross-linked, modular structure that varies in structure between different mold and yeast types. It is a major component of the cell, typically ranging from 15 to 25% of the whole structure and consisting of ~80 to 90% polysaccharide. The basic structure consists of chitin (~5 to 10% of the cell wall) or, in some cases, cellulose fibrils within an amorphous matrix of various polysaccharide glucans with associated proteins and lipids. Chitin is a polysaccharide of acetylglucosamine and gives the cell wall rigidity. In yeasts, the chitin fibrils are normally located toward the inner surface of the cell membrane, associated with various mannans and the cell membrane itself; however, only some species such as *C. albicans*, have chitin, while others do not. The outer layers of the cell wall are pri-

TABLE 1.5 Examples of common fungi

Type	Example	Comments
Filamentous	*Trichophyton mentagrophytes*	Dermatophytes, causing superficial infections on the outer layers of skin, hair, and nails, e.g., ringworm (tinea) or athlete's foot
	Aspergillus niger *Aspergillus fumigatus*	Ubiquitious in nature and often isolated as microbial contaminants. Rare cause of ear infections (otitis) and pulmonary disease (aspergillosis) in immunocompromised individuals. Also used in the bioremediation of tannins and for the bioproduction of citric acid.
	Phytophthora infestans	Potato blight, a plant disease
	Penicillium chrysogenum *Penicillium roquefortii*	Ubiquitous in nature and often isolated as microbial contaminants (e.g., as a bread mold). Rarely identified as pathogenic and usually in the immunocompromised. Some strains used for the production of penicillin and cheese.
Unicellular	*Cryptococcus neoformans*	Ubiquitous but can cause meningitis or pulmonary infections (cryptococcosis; valley fever)
	Saccharomyces cerevisiae	Used for wine and beer production
Dimorphic	*Candida albicans*	Widely found as a commensal, including as part of normal human flora, but can cause candidiasis in immunocompromised patients (e.g., thrush and in some cases septicemia)
	Histoplasma capsulatum	Histoplasmosis, a rare pulmonary disease similar to tuberculosis

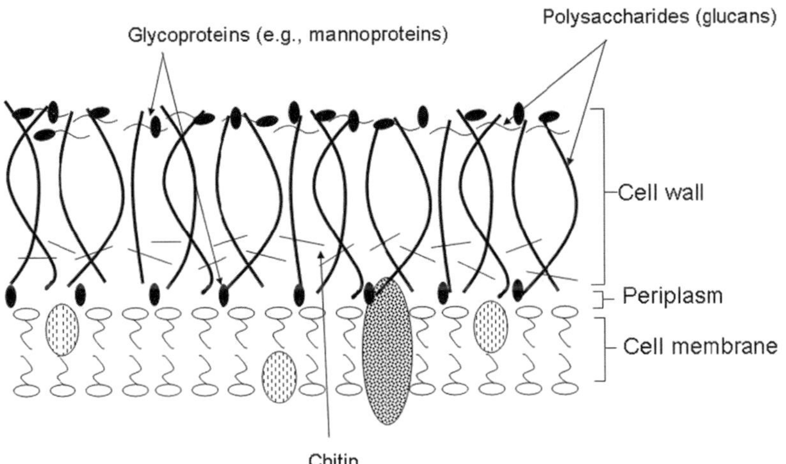

FIGURE 1.3 Simplified fungal cell envelope. The cross-linked cell wall is associated with the inner cell membrane. The cell wall usually consists of the innermost fibrils of chitin or cellulose, with outer layers of amorphous, cross-linked glucans.

marily composed of β-1,3- and β-1,6-glucan fibrils, with various associated proteins, mannoproteins, and lipids. In some cases, such as with the ascomycetes, a defined protein layer has been described between the outer glucans and inner chitin fibrils. Overall, fungal cell walls are predominantly (80 to 90%) composed of polysaccharides. The various mold cell walls have a similar, but overall more rigid, structure than those of yeasts.

The cell wall acts as a barrier for the action of many biocides, and for this reason, fungi are considered relatively resistant to many antimicrobial processes compared to most bacteria. Some fungi (e.g., *Cryptococcus*) also produce a capsule structure external to the cell wall, which can act as an additional barrier. Further, fungal spores are generally more resistant than vegetative cells to biocides and heat, but not to the same extent as bacterial spores. Fungal spores have been described as being more resistant to some radiation methods, as is observed when they are exposed to UV light.

1.3.3.3 Algae. Algae are a diverse group of microorganisms that can be found as single, free-living cells but also as colonies, including multicellular filaments. Algae are phototrophs and therefore derive their energy by photosynthesis (light-mediated energy biosynthesis). Photosynthesis is conducted within special cytoplasmic organelles (chloroplasts) that contain light-sensitive pigments known as chlorophylls. Some bacteria and plants also use photosynthesis. Their major habitats for algae are in water (marine or freshwater), and they are commonly encountered as colorful slimes on the water surface, particularly on polluted water. Examples include chlorophyta ("green algae"; e.g., *Chlamydomonas*), rhodophyta ("red algae"), and dinoflagellata (e.g., *Gonyaulax*). Some species produce toxins, which can be lethal to fish and other marine life, as well as causing generally mild effects (headaches and respiratory problems) in humans. Structurally, algae cells are typical eukaryotes. Cell wall structures vary considerably, including the presence of cellulose-, chitin-, and silica-based structures modified by polysaccharides and peptides.

1.3.3.4 Protozoa. Protozoa are one of the most abundant groups of life in the world. Over 60,000 species have been described, but estimates of the total variety that exist are much higher. They are single-celled eukaryotes, but unlike fungi, in their vegetative form they lack a cell wall. They can be found in a variety of ecosystems, including water, soil, and as parasites in animals and plants. They are generally mobile and can be classified based on their respective modes of movement and microscopic morphologies (Table 1.6).

Similar to helminths, protozoa can produce multiple forms during their respective life cycles, including vegetative forms such as trophozoites and sporozoites, as well as dormant forms known as oocysts and cysts. Oocysts/cysts can survive for extended periods of time in the environment and can demonstrate particular resistance to chemical disinfection methods (Fig. 1.4). Of particular note, various types of bacteria and viruses have been found to be present, or even multiply, in different strains of amoeba. This may protect them from the effects of biocides, particularly when included in dormant forms of amoeba. Most amoebas and flagellates reproduce asexually, while the human parasitic sporozoans are capable of both asexual and sexual reproduction.

1.3.4 Prokaryotes

Prokaryotes are a diverse group of microorganisms that show some similarities in their basic structure but can also be very distinct. They are typically single-celled, range in size from ~0.1 to 10 μm, and unlike eukaryotes, their nucleic acid is free (not membrane-bound) in the cytoplasm (Table 1.3). They can be considered as two general groups, the archaea and eubacteria.

1.3.4.1 Eubacteria. Eubacteria (or bacteria) can be subdivided into those that contain cell walls and those that do not. The cell wall-free types are known as the mycoplasmas (or mollicutes). Mycoplasmas are a distinct group of prokaryotes that contain a small genome and are surrounded by a unique cell membrane structure. Unlike other bacteria, they lack a cell wall. The surface structure of a typical mycoplasma cell is shown in Fig. 1.5.

The cytoplasm is surrounded by a lipid bilayer consisting of phospholipids. Phospholipids are molecules that consist of fatty acids linked to glycerol and then, via a phosphate group, to an alcohol. Essentially, these molecules form the basic structure of the cell membranes of most bacteria (with the exception of archaea [see section 1.3.4.2]). They contain a hydrophilic end (alcohol end) and a hydrophobic end (fatty acids) which associate to form two layers (known as a bilayer) consisting of an inner hydrophobic core and an outer hydrophilic surface. Mycoplasmas are unique as prokaryotes because they can also contain other lipids (sterols such as cholesterol) associated in the lipid core of the membrane; sterols are usually only present in eukaryotes and add rigidity to the cell membrane, which confers greater resistance to extracellular factors than typical bacterial cell membranes do. Proteins are also present, spanning the membrane or associated with just the membrane surface. Glycolipids (polysaccharides linked to surface lipids) have also been reported on cell surfaces, and they are believed to be involved in cell attachment. The reduced genome size is presumably linked to the lack of cell wall metabolism and other biosynthetic pathways (e.g., purine metabolism) that are required for other bacteria. Overall, because mycoplasmas have no cell wall, they are pleomorphic (multishaped) (Table 1.1). Mycoplasmas can be commensals or pathogens of plants, humans, and animals (Table 1.7). They are frequently implicated contaminants in laboratory cell cultures and as a cause of atypical pneumonia (*Mycoplasma pneumoniae*) and have also been implicated in certain chronic diseases such as chronic fatigue syndrome and rheumatoid arthritis. The lack of a protective cell wall may make mycoplasmas more sensitive to drying, heat, and some biocides compared to other bacteria, but they can still demonstrate remarkable persistence in certain environments. Other bacteria (as discussed below) that typically present with a cell wall can also be present as cell wall-free forms and are referred to as L or cell wall-deficient forms. These forms have been described in artificial culture media and on histological examination of infected tissues. They are speculated to be stationary or dormant forms that can circumvent host defense mechanisms.

TABLE 1.6 Classification of protozoa, based on their motility mechanisms and microscopic morphologies

Classification and organism	Disease(s)	Comments
	Flagellates (motility by flagella)	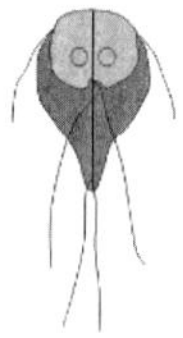
Giardia lamblia	Giardiasis, including dysentery	Trophozoites (~20 μm; shown above) produce cysts, which can survive water chlorination under some concentrations
Trypanosoma gambiense	Sleeping sickness	Transferred by tsetse flies
Leishmania donovani	Leishmaniasis (kala azar)	Transferred by sandflies
	Amebas (motility by flowing cytoplasm, "pseudopodia")	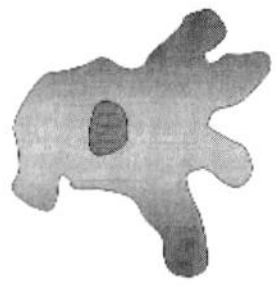
Entamoeba histolytica	Amebiasis, including dysentery and liver abscesses	Trophozoites reproduce asexually by binary division and can produce cysts which can be transferred in contaminated food or water (surviving for up to 5 weeks at room temperature)
Acanthamoeba castellanii	Eye infections, associated with contaminated contact lenses	Commonly found free-living in water, with two life cycle stages (trophozoites and cysts)
	Ciliates (motility using cilia)	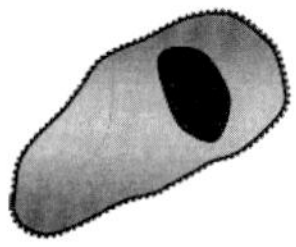
Paramecium spp.	Dysentery	Trophozoite has two types of nuclei and can be up to 60 μm in length
Balantidium coli	Dysentery	Trophozoites can measure up to 150 μm, with transmission via cyst-contaminated meat
	Sporozoans/apicomplexans (no specific motility extensions used)	
	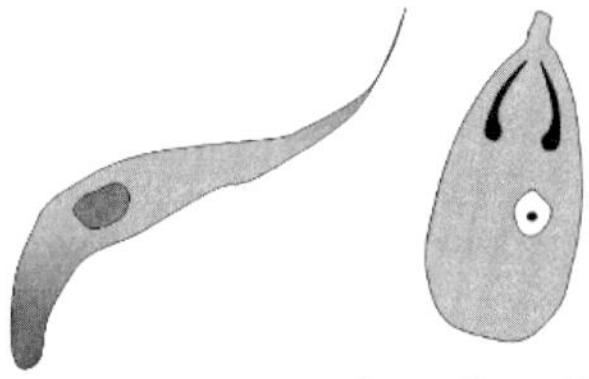	
Plasmodium falciparum	Malaria	Complicated life cycle; sporozoites transferred to humans by female mosquitoes
Cryptosporidium parvum	Severe diarrhea	Oocysts have marked resistance to biocides, surviving in water. When ingested, they hatch to release sporozoites. These forms invade cells of the intestine, can reproduce asexually through two generations, and then produce oocysts by sexual reproduction
Toxoplasma gondii	Toxoplasmosis	Oocysts are formed in the intestine of cats and transferred to other animals

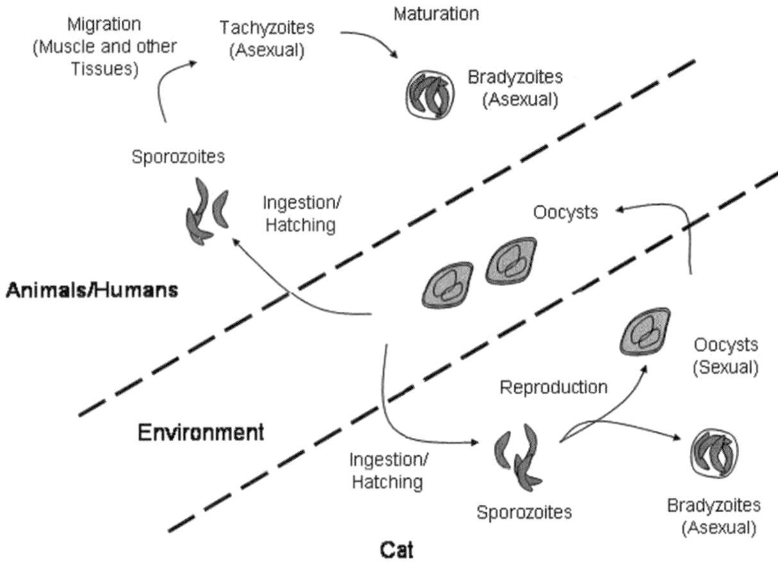

FIGURE 1.4 Life cycle of *Toxoplasma gondii*.

Examples of described cell wall-deficient forms of bacteria are *Helicobacter*, *Mycobacterium*, *Pseudomonas*, and *Brucella*. Some are suspected of being involved in autoimmune diseases such as rheumatoid arthritis (*Propionibacterium acnes*) and multiple sclerosis (*Borrelia mylophora*).

Bacteria that contain cell walls can be simply classified based on their cell morphology and general reaction to a staining method, known as the Gram stain. The Gram stain is used to differentiate between two types of cell wall structures: Gram positive (+) and Gram negative (–). Microscopic examination of stained preparations allows further differentiation based on their shape (Table 1.8). However, this is an oversimplification, because bacteria vary widely in their morphologies and staining characteristics; many other methods are used for further differentiation including oxygen requirements, growth characteristics, lipid composition, immunoassays, and more recent molecular techniques.

The basic structure of cell wall-containing bacteria consists of an outer cell wall and an inner cell membrane surrounding the internal cytoplasm (Fig. 1.6). The cell surface can also contain additional structures such as pili, flagella, and capsules, depending on the bacterial species and its growth conditions.

The cell membrane is similar to that described for mycoplasma and consists of a phos-

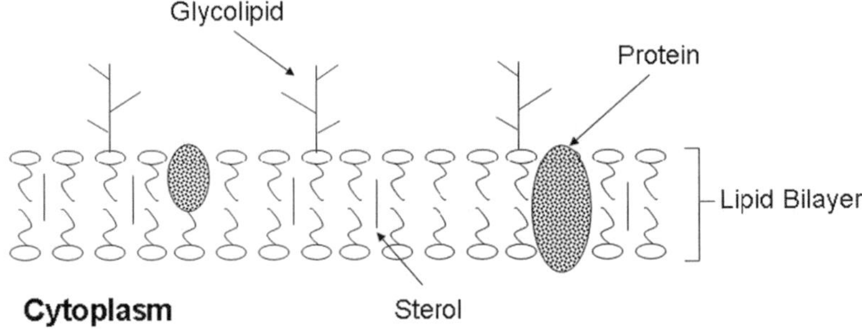

FIGURE 1.5 Simple representation of a mycoplasma cell surface structure.

TABLE 1.7 Examples of pathogenic mycoplasmas

Type	Examples	Significance
Spiroplasma	*Spiroplasma citri*	Plant pathogens, insect parasites
Ureaplasma	*Ureaplasma urealyticum*	Human parasite, genital tract diseases
Mycoplasma	*Mycoplasma genitalium, M. pneumoniae*	Urethritis, atypical pneumonia

pholipid bilayer (without sterols) and associated proteins. Membrane proteins can be at the interface with the cytoplasm, embedded within the membrane, and/or associated with the external cell wall of the cell. Examples are some lipoproteins (proteins with lipid groups attached), in which the lipid component allows anchoring to the membrane. The overall structure is fluid but serves as a barrier to contain the cytoplasm and restrict access of nutrients/ions in and out of the cell. Membrane proteins play a vital part in many cellular activities, including transport mechanisms, enzymatic reactions, cell signaling, energy generation, and cell wall synthesis. For these reasons, damage to the cell membrane can render bacteria nonviable. The cell wall structures are less similar and can be considered as three basic types: Gram-positive, Gram-negative, and mycobacterial cell walls (Fig. 1.7). Mycobacteria (not to be confused

TABLE 1.8 General differentiation of bacteria types based on their microscopic morphology and reaction to Gram staining

Bacterial structure	Shape	Examples
Cocci		Gram positive: *Staphylococcus, Streptococcus* Gram negative: *Neisseria, Veillonella*
Bacilli (rods)		Gram positive: *Bacillus, Listeria* Gram negative: *Escherichia, Pseudomonas*
Spirals		Gram negative: *Treponema, Borrelia*
Pleomorphic		Gram negative: *Bacteroides* Cell wall-free bacteria, e.g., *Mycoplasma*

Cocci image: Image courtesy of CDC-PHIL/Medical Illustrator/James Archer, 2013 (ID#16879), with permission; Bacilli Rods image: Image courtesy of CDC-PHIL/National Institute of Allergy and Infectious Diseases (NIAID), 2002 (ID#18160), with permission; Spirals Treponema, Borrelia image: Image courtesy of CDC-PHIL/Susan Lindsley, 1972 (ID#14969), with permission; Pleomorphic mycoplasma image: Image courtesy of CDC-PHIL/Dr. E. Arum/Dr. N. Jacobs, 1974 (ID#11021), with permission.

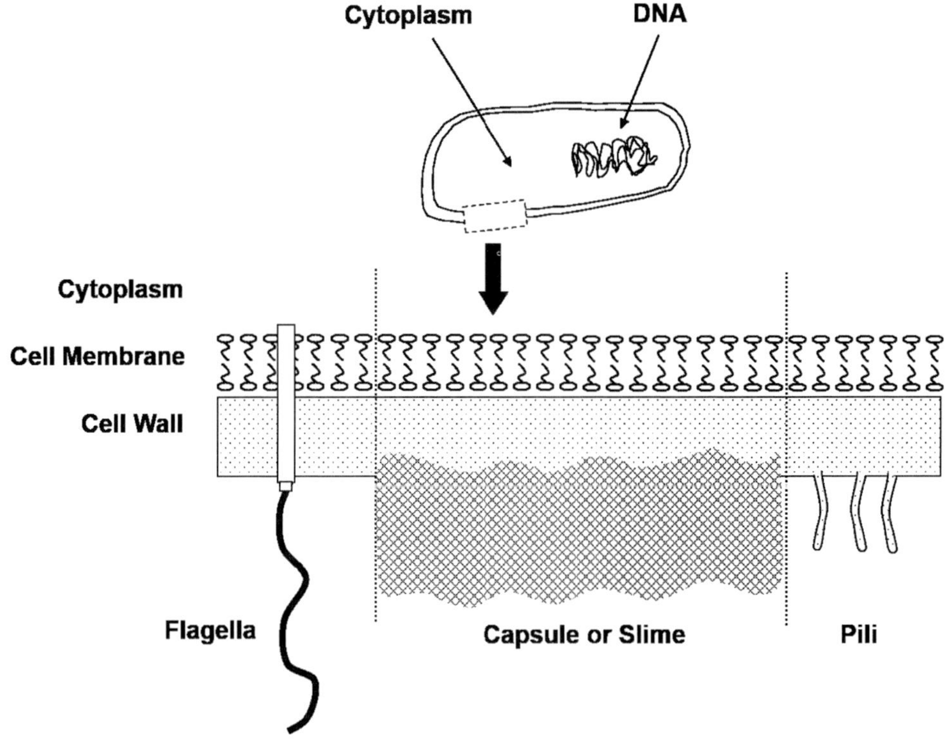

FIGURE 1.6 Basic structure of a bacterial cell, showing the cell surface in greater detail.

with the cell wall-free mycoplasmas) are considered separately due to their unique cell wall structures. The cell wall can play an important role in the resistance of bacteria to disinfection (chapter 8).

A key component of all bacterial cell walls is peptidoglycan, which is a polysaccharide (a polymer of sugar units) of two repeating sugars, *N*-acetylglucosamine and *N*-acetylmuramic acid, linked by β-1,4 glycosidic (sugar-sugar) bonds (Fig. 1.8). The *N*-acetylmuramic acids have attached tetrapeptides (peptides of 4 amino acids), which are composed of amino acids such as L-alanine, D-alanine, D-glutamic acid, and lysine (typically in Gram-positive bacteria) or diaminopimelic acid (usually in Gram-negative bacteria). These tetrapeptides cross-link the polysaccharide layers. The exact structure, extent of cross-linking, and thickness of the peptidoglycan vary among bacteria. For example, *E. coli* (Gram-negative) tetrapeptides consist of L-alanine, D-glutamic acid, diaminopimelic acid, and D-alanine, and the peptidoglycan is only a minor component of the cell wall (~10%), which is loosely cross-linked. In contrast, the *Staphylococcus aureus* peptidoglycan has lysine instead of diaminopimelic acid in the tetrapeptide but is also indirectly linked to an adjacent tetrapeptide by a 5-amino-acid (glycine) bridge. The peptidoglycan makes up ~90% of the staphylococcal cell wall and is highly cross-linked. It is the dense nature of peptidoglycan in the Gram-positive cell walls that allows for differentiation in the Gram stain. Some archaea have been found to have a similar but distinct peptidoglycan structure present in their cell walls (section 1.3.4.2).

Overall, the basic structure of a Gram-positive bacterium cell wall consists of peptidoglycan; however, other proteins and polysaccharides have been described and can be specific to different bacterial species. These include polysaccharides (e.g., the A, B, and C streptococcal polysaccharides), teichoic acids,

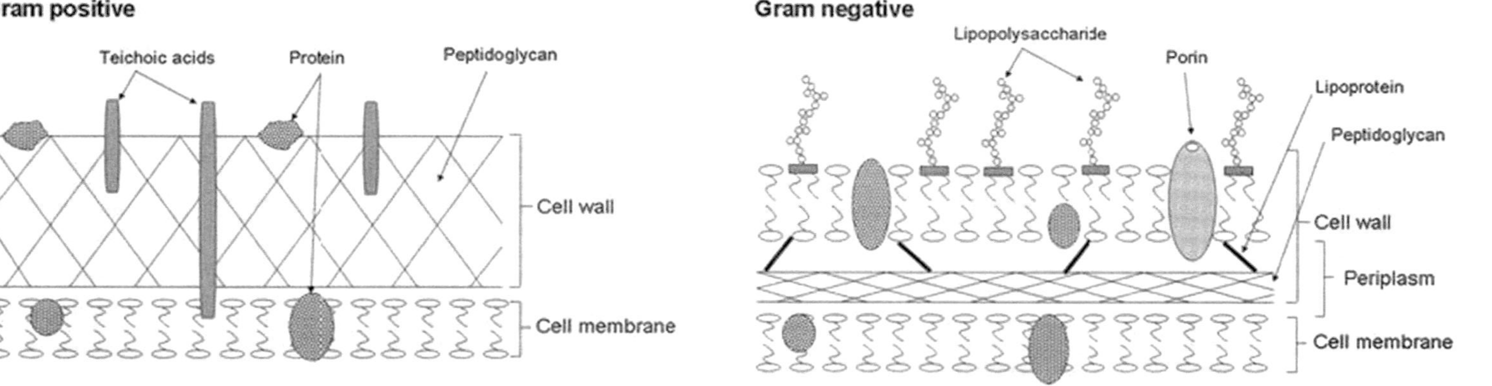

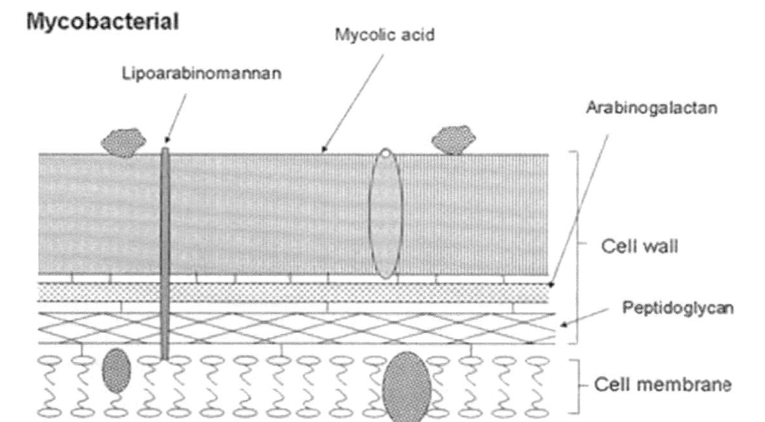

FIGURE 1.7 Bacterial cell wall structures. The cell membrane is a similar structure in all types. Gram-positive bacteria have a large peptidoglycan layer (shown as crossed lines) with associated polysaccharides and proteins. Gram-negative bacteria have a smaller peptidoglycan layer linked to an outer membrane. The mycobacterial cell has a series of covalently linked layers, including the peptidoglycan-, arabinogalactan- and mycolic acid-containing components.

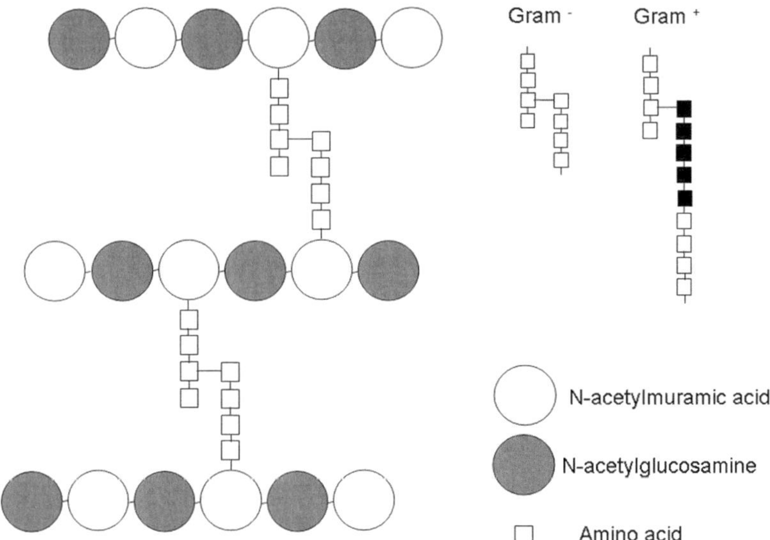

FIGURE 1.8 Basic structure of peptidoglycan. Polysaccharides of repeating sugars are cross-linked by peptide bridges. Two different types of peptide bridges, which have been described in Gram-positive and Gram-negative bacterial cell walls, are shown.

and teichuronic acids. The teichoic acids are found in the cell walls of many Gram-positive bacteria, including *Bacillus*, *Staphylococcus*, and *Lactobacillus*. They are polysaccharides based on ribitol or glycerol, with attached sugars and amino acids, and are covalently linked to peptidoglycan. Some may also be bound to the cell membrane and are known as lipoteichoic acids. Other polysaccharides include the teichuronic acids (e.g., in *Bacillus*), which are also linked to peptidoglycan. Proteins and enzymes are also found attached to the peptidoglycan or otherwise associated with the cell wall; they may be involved in certain functions such as the interaction with host tissues, peptidoglycan turnover, cell division, and nutrient acquisition. Finally, the actinomycetes typically stain Gram positive, but with different types of cell wall structures. Structurally, they resemble fungi, can form hyphae, and produce spores (sporophores) by filament fragmentation; however, the nucleic acid is free in the cytoplasm, and the filaments and cell sizes are much smaller than in eukaryotic fungi (section 1.3.2). *Nocardia*, as an example, has a tripartite cell wall structure similar to mycobacteria (see below), while *Streptomyces* has a more typical Gram-positive bacterial cell wall structure consisting of an external peptidoglycan but also contains a major portion of fatty acids. Table 1.9 gives some common examples of Gram-positive bacteria.

In general, the cell wall in Gram-negative bacteria has a minor peptidoglycan layer directly bound to an external outer membrane by lipoproteins (Fig. 1.7). The area between the inner and outer membranes is known as the periplasm. The periplasm can contain a variety of proteins involved in cellular metabolism or interactions with the extracellular environment. The outer membrane is essentially similar to the inner, cytoplasmic membrane, with a lipid bilayer and associated, integral proteins. But the lipid bilayer is unique, with phospholipids only associated with the internal part of the membrane and the external part made up of glycolipids and lipopolysaccharides (LPSs). LPS contains a lipid portion (known as lipid A) which forms part of the external surface of the outer membrane, linked to a polysaccharide (containing a core and O-polymer of sugars); the types of fatty acids and sugars that make up

LPS structures vary between Gram-negative species. LPSs, in particular the lipid A portions, are also known as endotoxins, which are pyrogenic and play a role in bacterial infections (see section 1.3.7). Similar to the inner membrane, proteins can be found associated through or at the periplasmic or external surface of the outer membrane. An important group of integral proteins are the porins, which form channels to allow for the transport of molecules through the outer membrane. Some common examples of Gram-negative bacteria are given in Table 1.10.

Some unique Gram-negative, obligate intracellular bacteria have been identified that were previously thought to be viral in nature, including the chlamydias and rickettsias. Rickettsias are small bacteria with a simple cell wall structure, similar to Gram-negative bacteria, and are pleomorphic in shape (ranging from rods to cocci). Most are transferred to humans by arthropods (e.g., ticks and lice). Typical diseases include typhus (*Rickettsia prowazekii* and *Rickettsia typhi*) and Q-fever (*Coxiella burnetii*). The chlamydias are also small obligate parasites. They are therefore difficult to isolate *in vitro*, requiring cell culturing, and typically stain as Gram-negative coccoid bacteria. They are a serious cause of urogenital infections (*Chlamydia trachomatis*) and pneumonia (*Chlamydophila pneumoniae* and *Chlamydophila psittaci*). Chlamydia cell wall structure is unique; similar to the Gram-negative cell wall, it contains an inner and outer membrane and LPS but does not appear to have a peptidoglycan layer. As obligate parasites, their cells are often considered relatively sensitive to heat, drying, and biocides.

Figure 1.6 shows that other structures can be present on the surface of bacteria. Of particular interest in the consideration of biocidal processes are external barriers that can protect the cell from its environment. Many bacteria produce an external layer of high-molecular-weight polysaccharides, as well as associated lipids and protein, which is referred to as a glycocalyx. This can be a simple, loosely associated slime layer or a more rigid, thicker, and firmly attached capsule structure. Capsules can range in structure and size, typically from one half to five times the cell diameter thickness. Glycocalyx production plays an important role in the development of bacterial biofilms, which are a further intrinsic resistance mechanism (chapter 8, section 8.3.8). Glycocalyx structures are found in both Gram-positive and Gram-negative bacteria. Examples are *Streptococcus mutans* (in dental plaque), *S. pneumoniae* (in nasopharyngeal colonization), and *E. coli* (enteropathogenic strains which attach to epithelial cells in the intestine). In addition to direct cell protection, they can also play roles in pathogenesis, bacterial attachment to surfaces, and preventing drying of the cell. Other bacteria (including archaea) produce an S-layer, similar to polysaccharide capsules, which is composed of protein and glycoproteins to form an external crystalline structure; an example is the external surface of *Bacillus anthracis*, which produces an S-layer consisting of two protein types that is itself covered by a unique protein (poly-D-glutamic acid) capsule layer.

Bacteria can also have a variety of other proteinaceous cell surface appendages, including pili, fimbriae, and flagella (Fig. 1.6). For example, flagella filaments are composed primarily of flagellin protein subunits and have other proteins that interact with the cell membrane/wall structure. Flagella are specifically involved with bacterial motility. Fimbriae and pili play an important role in surface, including cell surface, interactions.

Another cell wall structure that deserves separate consideration is the mycobacterial cell wall (Fig. 1.7). Mycobacteria are aerobic, slow-growing rod-shaped bacteria (for example, *Mycobacterium tuberculosis* [Fig. 1.9]), which typically stain Gram positive and can be further differentiated by the acid-fast stain (staining with fuchsin, which resists acid/alcohol decolorization) due to its unique hydrophobic cell wall structure.

This mycobacterial cell wall structure presents a strong permeability barrier and is responsible for the higher level of resistance to antibiotics and biocides compared to other

TABLE 1.9 Examples of Gram-positive bacteria

General type	Key characteristics	Examples	Significance
Gram-positive cocci	Diverse group of Gram-positive cocci, non-sporeformers	*Enterococcus faecalis*, *Enterococcus faecium*	Widely distributed in soil, water, and animals. Normal flora in lower gastrointestinal tract. Often identified as causing urinary tract diseases and wound infections. Vancomycin-resistant strains are a concern in hospital-acquired infections.
		Lactococcus	Found in plant and dairy products; can cause food spoilage
		Staphylococcus epidermidis, *Staphylococcus aureus*	Common human/animal parasites. *S. epidermidis* is usually found on the skin/mucous membranes. *S. aureus* is commonly identified as a pathogen, including skin, wound, gastrointestinal, and lower respiratory tract diseases. Methicillin-resistant *S. aureus* strains are a leading cause of hospital-acquired wound infections.
		Streptococcus pyogenes, *Streptococcus pneumoniae*	Common human/animal pathogens. *S. pyogenes* and *S. pneumoniae* are both associated with upper and lower respiratory tract diseases, including pharyngitis (sore throat), pneumonia, and scarlet fever. *S. pyogenes* can also cause a wide variety of other diseases, including skin/soft tissue infections (e.g., cellulitis).
Endospore-forming rods/cocci	Rods or cocci that form dormant, heat-resistant endospores; can be aerobic or anaerobic	*Geobacillus*	*Geobacillus stearothermophilus* spores are widely regarded as the most resistant to heat and other sterilization methods; used as biological indicators of sterilization efficacy
		Bacillus	Aerobic, rod-shaped bacteria; various strains also used as biological indicators for chemical sterilization processes (e.g., *Bacillus atrophaeus*, formally known as *Bacillus subtilis* for ethylene oxide sterilization). Some strains are pathogenic, including *Bacillus cereus* (food poisoning) and *Bacillus anthracis* (anthrax in animals/humans). Widely distributed and often identified as environmental contaminants.

		Clostridium	Anaerobic, rod-shaped bacteria; widely distributed, including in soil and water. Some species form part of the normal flora of the human intestine (e.g., *Clostridium difficile*, but it is also a leading cause of hospital-acquired diarrhea). Others can cause wound infections (including *Clostridium perfringens* and *Clostridium tetani*, the cause of tetanus) and food poisoning (e.g., *Clostridium botulinum*).
Regular, nonsporulating rods	Rods, but also other regular forms	*Lactobacillus*	Used in the preparation of fermented dairy products such as yogurt
		Listeria	Widely distributed; *Listeria monocytogenes* is a leading cause of food-borne illness, which can cause meningitis and septicemia.
Irregular, nonsporulating rods	Rods, but form irregular shapes	*Corynebacterium*	Often isolated as human/animal pathogens, in particular on skin and mucous membranes. *Corynebacterium diphtheriae* causes an upper respiratory tract infection with systemic effects (diphtheria) (see Table 1.11).
		Propionibacterium	*Propionibacterium acnes* is a leading cause of skin acne. Some strains can be found as contaminants in dairy products.
Other Gram-positive bacteria	Mycobacteria: rods	*Mycobacterium*	See Table 1.11.
	Actinomycetes: pleomorphic, including the production of hyphae in appearance similar to fungi	*Nocardia*	Widely distributed; some are opportunistic pathogens (see Table 1.11).
		Streptomyces	Some strains produce antibiotics (e.g., streptomycin) and form spores; widely distributed; some pathogenic, including plant pathogens.

TABLE 1.10 Examples of Gram-negative bacteria

General type	Key characteristics	Examples	Significance
Spirochetes	Thin, helical/spiral-shaped	*Borrelia*	Cause many types of tick-borne diseases in animals, humans, and birds (e.g., *Borrelia burgdorferi*, implicated in Lyme disease)
		Treponema	Human and animal diseases; *Treponema pallidum* causes syphilis, a persistent sexually transmitted disease
Helical/vibroid	Usually mobile, vibroid-shaped	*Campylobacter*	*Campylobacter jejuni* causes gastroenteritis
		Helicobacter	*Helicobacter pylori* causes peptic ulcers due to gastritis
Aerobic/microaerophilic rods/cocci	Diverse group of rods or cocci that use oxygen for growth	*Acetobacter*	Food spoilage and fermentation
		Acinetobacter	*Acinetobacter baumannii* is a common opportunistic pathogen in wounds (especially hospital-acquired infections), associated with prolonged survival in the environment and antibiotic resistance profiles
		Bordetella	*Bordetella pertussis* causes whooping cough, a respiratory disease
		Legionella	Associated with water or moist environments. *Legionella pneumophila* causes a form of pneumonia known as Legionnaires' disease.
		Neisseria	Most strains nonpathogenic and found on mucous membranes. *Neisseria gonorrhoeae* causes the sexually transmitted disease gonorrhoea, and *Neisseria meningitidis* can cause meningitis in young adults.
		Pseudomonas/ *Burkholderia*	Common environmental contaminants in water and soil. Some strains are plant pathogens. *Pseudomonas aeruginosa* and *Burkholderia cepacia* are frequently implicated in hospital-acquired infections, usually associated with proliferation in moist environments and water lines. Pseudomonads can cause biofilm fouling in industrial water lines.

Facultative anaerobes	Rod-shaped; can grow in the presence or absence of oxygen	*Enterobacteriaceae*	
		Erwinia	Plant saprophytes and pathogens
		Escherichia	*E. coli* is the most prevalent microorganism in the lower intestinal tract and a common cause of intestinal and urinary tract infections. It is also widely used as a cloning host in molecular biology
		Salmonella	Leading cause of gastroenteritis, mostly food- and waterborne; examples include *Salmonella enterica* serovar Typhi (causing typhoid fever) and *S. enterica* serovar Typhimurium (causing gastroenteritis and enteric fever)
		Yersinia	Zoonotic infections; *Yersinia pestis* causes plague
		Vibrionaceae	Gastrointestinal diseases, including cholera (*Vibrio cholerae*) and food poisoning (*Vibrio parahaemolyticus*)
		Vibrio	
		Pasteurellaceae	Commonly found in the upper respiratory tract of humans and some animals
		Haemophilus	*Haemophilus influenzae* is a leading cause of meningitis in children
		Pasteurella	Can cause septicemia in animals and humans
Other Gram-negative bacteria	Various shapes and growth requirements	*Bacteroides*	Anaerobic rods; commonly found in the intestine and opportunistic pathogens in wounds
		Veillonella	Anaerobic cocci; human/animal parasites
		Rickettsia/Chlamydia/Chlamydophila	Obligate intracellular pathogens, causing typhus, Rocky Mountain spotted fever, and sexually transmitted diseases
		Cyanobacteria	Free-living in water, photosynthetic; can be unicellular or filamentous
		Myxobacteria	Waterborne bacteria which are motile by a gliding mechanism
		Leptothrix	Polluted water-associated, sheathed, filamentous bacteria

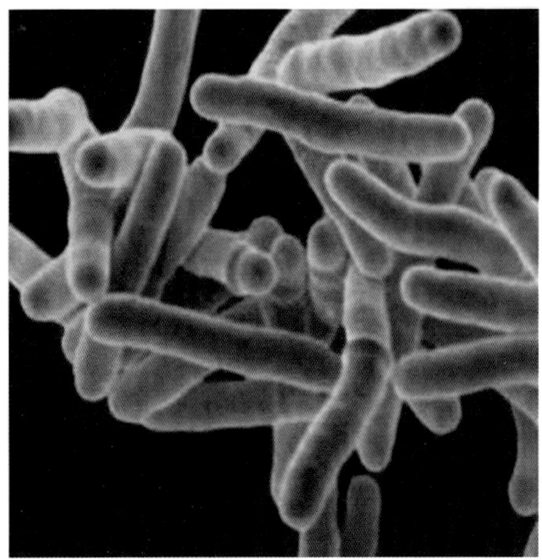

FIGURE 1.9 Cells of *M. tuberculosis*. Courtesy of Clifton Barry, NIAID.

bacteria. The cell membrane is similar to that described in other bacteria, which can be linked to the cell wall by glycolipids. The cell wall has a three-layer structure, consisting of a peptidoglycan layer external to the cell membrane, which is covalently linked to a specific polysaccharide (known as arabinogalactan), and an external mycolic acid layer. The peptidoglycan is similar to that in other bacteria, but *N*-acetylmuramic acid is replaced with *N*-glycoylmuramic and cross-linked by 3- and 4-amino acid peptides. Arabinogalactan is a polysaccharide of arabinose and galactose. The mycolic acids are attached to arabinose residues of the arabinogalactan and are some of the longest known fatty acids in nature. In mycobacteria they typically range in carbon length from C_{60} to C_{90} and can make up >50% of the cell weight. In addition, the mycobacterial cell wall can contain a variety of proteins (including enzymes), short-chained fatty acids, waxes, and LPS. Examples in some mycobacteria are the LPS lipoarabinomannan, which plays a role in host interactions during *M. tuberculosis* infections, and porin proteins, with a function in molecule transport similar to that seen in the outer membrane of Gram-negative bacteria. In some disease-causing mycobacteria these may also form an external capsule containing enzymes and adherence factors that play a role in mycobacterial pathogenesis. Similar cell wall structures have been identified in other bacteria, including the actinomycetes (e.g., *Nocardia*) and Gram-positive rods (*Corynebacterium*) with notable shorter-chained mycolic acids of C_{46-60} and C_{22-32}, respectively, and in some cases no mycolic acids (as in *Amycolatopsis*). Examples of bacteria with mycobacteria-like cell wall structures are given in Table 1.11.

1.3.4.2 Archaea. Archaea are prokaryotic but are phylogenetically distinct from eubacteria. They are a diverse group that has not been widely studied due to difficulties in culturing them from various environments. They are considered briefly here because many have been isolated from severe environments that are typically biocidal to other microorganisms, and they offer some interesting if not rare examples of microbial resistance mechanisms (chapter 8, sections 8.3.9 and 8.3.10). It should be noted that bacteria and other microorganisms can survive and even multiply over a quite wide range of conditions, including temperatures, pH, and the presence or absence of oxygen (aerobic or anaerobic). Those that grow under extremes of these conditions are referred to in combining form as -philes; for example, thermophiles (or thermophilic microorganisms) can survive at higher temperatures, psychrophiles grow in colder environments, halophiles survive extreme salt conditions, and acidophiles or alkaliphiles are found in low or high pH environments, respectively (see further discussion in chapter 8, section 8.3.10). In general, the archaea are found under extreme conditions within these ranges. For this reason, they are often referred to as extremophiles and can be considered as four general groups: thermophiles (survive extreme high or low temperatures), halophiles (survive extreme high-salt concentrations), methanogens (survive unique anaerobic conditions), and barophiles (survive under high hydrostatic pressure). Examples are given in Table 1.12.

It should be noted that in many cases these extreme conditions are actually required for the growth of archaea. For example, *Pyrococcus* cells have an optimum growth temperature of ~100° C and require at least 70°C for growth. Further,

TABLE 1.11 Cell wall structures in mycobacteria and other related organisms

General type	Key characteristics	Examples	Significance
Mycobacteria	Slow- to very slow-growing, acid-fast, generally Gram-positive, aerobic, rod-shaped but also pleomorphic/filamentous	*Mycobacterium*	
		Slowly growing (weeks to months)	
		M. tuberculosis/ *Mycobacterium bovis*	Cause tuberculosis, a respiratory tract disease, in humans and animals
		Mycobacterium leprae	Causes leprosy, a skin and nerve disease
		Mycobacterium avium	Ubiquitous in nature, including water, dust, and soil; can cause disease in poultry, swine, and immunocompromised humans
		Rapidly growing (3–7 days)	Can be found as water contaminants and have been identified in persistent infections and pseudoinfections; some strains show unusual resistance to some biocides (e.g., aldehydes)
		Mycobacterium chelonae/ *Mycobacterium gordonae*	Identified in a variety of immunocompromised patient infections, including wound infections
		Mycobacterium fortuitum	
Actinomycetes	Filamentous Gram-negative, pleomorphic	*Nocardia*	Widely distributed, including in soil; some pathogenic, including *Nocardia asteroides* in pulmonary and systemic infections in humans
Irregular rods	Irregular rods, Gram-positive	*Corynebacterium*	Obligate parasites on skin/mucous membranes; pathogenic strains include *Corynebacterium diphtheriae*

halobacteria such as *Halobacterium* require a minimum salt level of 1.5 M for growth.

Structurally, the archaea are similar to eubacteria (Table 1.3), but they present with diverse cellular mechanisms that allow survival under extreme conditions. Overall, they have unique lipids (generally shorter-chained fatty acids) in their cell membranes, but also different polysaccharides and/or proteins in their cell walls that differ from eubacteria. It is interesting to note that, similar to the mycoplasma (section 1.3.4.1), some archaea have no associated cell wall. Examples are *Thermoplasma* spp. that contain a thick, unique cell membrane, which allows for the growth and metabolism of this genus (chapter 8, section 8.3.10). The cell

TABLE 1.12 Examples of extremophile archaea

Type	Description	Habitat examples	Typical conditions	Examples
Halophiles	Grow under high-saline conditions	Salt or soda lakes	9–32% NaCl	*Halobacterium* *Natronobacterium*
Thermophiles	Grow at high temperatures and some under extreme acidic or basic conditions	Hydrothermal vents, hot springs	50–110°C	*Sulfolobus* *Thermococcus* *Pyrococcus*
Methanogens	Strict anaerobes which produce methane (CH_4) gas from CO_2 and other substrates	Sediments, bovine rumens (anaerobic digesters)	Strict anaerobic, H_2 and CO_2 used for CH_4 production	*Methanobacterium* *Methanospirillium*
Barophiles (or piezophiles)	Grow optimally at high hydrostatic pressure	Deep sea	Low temperature (2–3°C) and high pressure (>100 kPa, e.g., 20–100 MPa)	*Methanococcus*

membrane contains a unique LPS, consisting of mannose/glucose polysaccharide attached to lipid molecules and glycoproteins, that gives the membrane greater rigidity and temperature resistance. Some archaea have a surface structure similar to eubacteria, with a cell membrane bounded by a cell wall. The cell wall may contain a polysaccharide similar to peptidoglycan, called pseudopeptidoglycan, with alternating *N*-acetylglucosamine and *N*-acetylalosaminuronic acid. Others do not have peptidoglycan but have a cell wall made up of proteins and polysaccharides. Examples are the halophilic *Halobacterium*, which contains a salt-stabilized glycoprotein cell wall. Other strains (such as *Pyrococcus* spp.) produce an external proteinaceous layer, similar to bacterial capsules (chapter 8, section 8.3.7) which are known as S-layers. In many methanogens, S-layers consisting of a crystalline structure of proteins may be found.

1.3.5 Viruses

Structurally, viruses are simple forms of life consisting of a nucleic acid surrounded by protein and, in some cases, a lipid envelope. They are much smaller than bacteria (<0.5 μm) and are obligate intracellular parasites, which depend on host cells, including prokaryotes and eukaryotes, for replication. They can be classified by a variety of methods, including their size, structure, presence or absence of a lipid-containing envelope, type of nucleic acid, diseases they cause, and cell type they infect. When considering the activity of biocidal processes, viruses can be classified as being nonenveloped ("naked") or enveloped (Fig. 1.10).

Nonenveloped viruses consist of a nucleic acid surrounded by a protein-based capsid and are considered hydrophilic. Enveloped viruses have a similar basic structure but also contain an external lipid bilayer envelope, which can include proteins (typically glycoproteins, proteins with linked carbohydrate groups). Central to all viral structures is the nucleocapsid, consisting of the nucleic acid (which can be single- or double-stranded DNA or RNA) protected by a protein capsid (Fig. 1.10). The capsid is made of individual capsomeres, which can

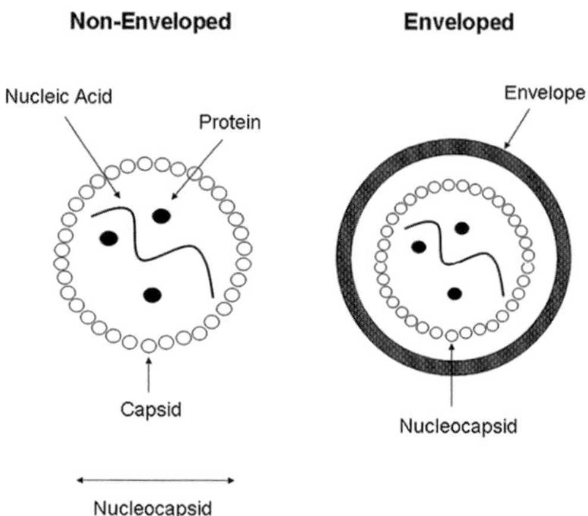

FIGURE 1.10 Basic viral structures.

consist of single or multiple protein types. Parvoviruses are examples of nonenveloped viruses, consisting of ~50% DNA and 50% protein. The capsid in these viruses is composed of three proteins, the structure of which is an important factor in their instrinsic resistance to disinfection. In addition to their core capsid structures, certain viruses can contain proteins within the capsid, associated with the capsid structure or externally within an outer envelope. These associated proteins often play a role in the infection or replication of the virus particle in a susceptible host. An example is the adenoviruses, which are nonenveloped DNA viruses with a capsid containing 252 capsomeres of at least 10 different proteins, which are involved in viral structure, cell binding, and penetration; in addition, they have slender glycoproteins projecting from the capsid.

Enveloped viruses are more complicated in their structure. Herpesviruses, for example, have an inner core consisting of DNA wound around a proteinaceous scaffold and surrounded by a capsid of 162 capsomeres, a protein-filled tegument, and an outer lipophilic envelope containing numerous glycoproteins and an evenly dispersed surface spike structure (Table 1.13). Another group is the enveloped orthomyxoviruses (including influenza viruses), which contain two major surface proteins associated with the envelope that are

TABLE 1.13 Viral families with examples of classifications

Viral family	Structure	Size (nm)	Envelope	Nucleic acid	Examples
Parvoviridae		18–26	No	DNA	Mouse parvovirus Parvovirus B19
Flaviviridae		40–50	Yes	RNA	Ebola Marburg
Adenoviridae		70–90	No	DNA	Adenovirus serotypes
Retroviridae		90–120	Yes	RNA	HIV-1
Herpesviridae		180–200	Yes	RNA	Epstein-Barr virus Herpes simplex
Poxviridae		250–400	Yes	DNA	Monkeypox Variola (smallpox)

involved in virus infectivity: hemagglutinins and neuraminidases. Hemagglutinins facilitate the viruses binding to target host cells, and neuraminidases are particularly involved in the further replication and release of virions from cells. Viruses may have additional proteins associated with their viral nucleic acid including nucleic acid polymerases; for example, retroviruses are RNA viruses that contain reverse transcriptases that allow the generation of DNA from the viral RNA molecule, which is subsequently transcribed and translated to produce viral proteins in the host cell.

Based on these basic viral structures, a variety of virus families that vary in shape and composition have been described. Examples of these are given in Table 1.13, but this list is not complete. For example, there are at least 20 families of viruses that are of medical importance and that vary in size, shape, and chemical composition; additional viral families have been described for plants, fungi, protozoa, and bacteria.

Viruses are dependent on host cells for survival and multiplication. Despite the range of viruses described, viral infection occurs in a similar series of steps: attachment, penetration, synthesis of biomolecules, assembly, and release (Fig. 1.11). The first stage is attachment of the virus to the cell surface. This is mediated by specific proteins on the capsid or envelope surface that specifically interact with molecules on the cell surface known as receptors. Receptors can be cell membrane or cell wall proteins, lipids, carbohydrates, and even combinations of these. Therefore, the presence of specific receptors on the cell surface determines sensitivity or resistance to virus infection. Examples of receptors include the HIV receptor CD4 protein on the surface of human

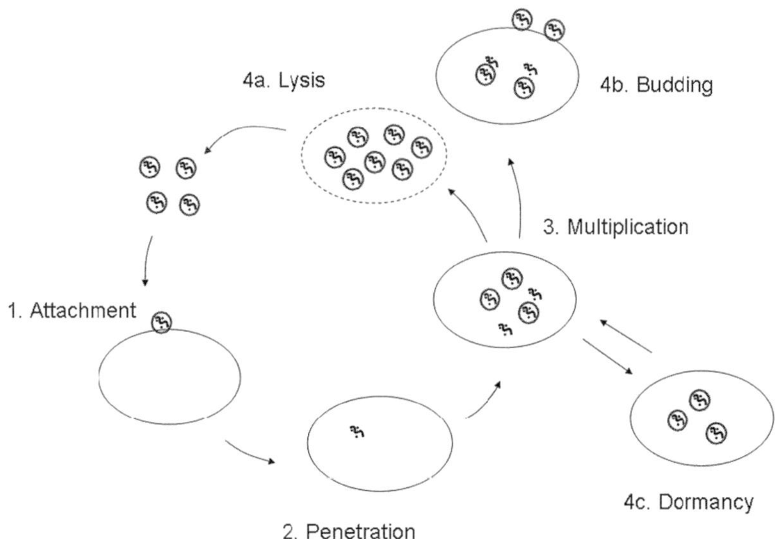

FIGURE 1.11 Typical viral life cycle. Stages include **(1)** attachment, **(2)** penetration into the cell, and **(3)** multiplication. Depending on the virus type, viral particles can be released by cell lysis **(4a)** or by budding **(4b)**; alternatively, the virus can remain dormant in the cell **(4c)**.

T cells and the binding of influenza to sialic acid, a carbohydrate linked to a cell membrane protein.

The next stage is penetration of the virus into the target cell, which can occur by different mechanisms. The nucleocapsid or nucleic acid, as the source genetic material that encodes the viral structure, can be injected or released in the cell. Similarly, the whole virus can be endocytosed into the cell or in the case of some enveloped viruses by fusion with the cell membrane, which is subsequently uncoated to allow for nucleic acid release. Endocytosis is typical for penetration of many vertebrate viruses. As mentioned above, some enzymes that are associated with the virus capsid are required for viral multiplication (e.g., reverse transcriptase in retroviruses such as HIV) and are released into the target cell. In some viruses, the nucleic acid is modified (e.g., by methylation) to protect it from damage (by cell-based nucleases) when free in the host cell. Once the cell is infected, the virus uses the available cell metabolic processes to replicate its nucleic acid and allow for the synthesis of specific viral proteins during the multiplication stage. Multiplication depends on the transcription and translation of viral mRNA. For DNA viruses this can be achieved by use of existing host enzymes such as DNA-dependent RNA polymerases; for RNA viruses this may require specific viral proteins.

An example already mentioned is the use of reverse transcriptase in retroviral multiplication, which generates DNA from a single-stranded RNA viral template. The viral proteins that are subsequently produced can be involved in the multiplication process (e.g., viral replication) or as structural parts of the virus. If viral multiplication continues, the cell will eventually burst or lyse to release the viral particles (Fig. 1.11, 4a); an example occurs in poliovirus infection. Lysing, however, does not occur with all viruses. A further mechanism of virus release is by budding from the cell surface, which creates persistent infection in a cell. Examples include influenza and HIV; it should be noted that both of these are enveloped viruses and that the viral envelope is formed around the viral nucleocapsid during the budding release from the cell surface. Some viruses can remain dormant in their host cells, referred to as latent infections, which can reactivate at a later stage to cause disease. During dormancy, the virus may not affect the normal cellular functions. Examples of latent viral infections include the varicella-zoster virus, which can remain dormant in neurons; varicella-zoster virus can cause chickenpox, commonly in children, and can reactivate to cause shingles, which is more prevalent in adults. In some cases, the presence of the virus may also trigger the uncontrolled growth of cells leading to the development of cancers. Strong associations of viruses in cancers include papillomaviruses in skin/cervical cancer and some herpesviruses in lymphomas and carcinomas.

Viruses have been identified as the cause of a variety of plant, human, and animal diseases including respiratory, sexually transmitted, neurological, and dermatological diseases (Table 1.14). The traditional difficulty in isolation and identification of viruses limits their study; however, it is thought that many more

TABLE 1.14 Examples of viral diseases

Family/virus	Disease or note
***Parvoviridae* (DNA, nonenveloped)**	
Human parvovirus B19	Erythema infectiosum (fifth disease)
Minute virus of mice	Cell line contamination, oncolysis
***Papovaviridae* (DNA, nonenveloped)**	
Human papillomavirus	Cervical cancer, genital warts
***Picornaviridae* (RNA, nonenveloped)**	
Poliovirus	Poliomyelitis
Rhinoviruses	Common cold
Coxsackie A-16	Foot-and-mouth disease (FMD)
***Retroviridae* (RNA, enveloped)**	
Human immunodeficiency virus (HIV-1)	Acquired immunodeficiency syndrome (AIDS)
HTLV-1	Human T-cell leukemia
***Orthomyxoviridae* (RNA, enveloped)**	
Influenza A, B, C	Influenza, pharyngitis
***Hepadnaviridae* (DNA, enveloped)**	
Hepatitis B virus	Hepatitis
***Poxviridae* (DNA, enveloped)**	
Variola	Smallpox
Vaccinia	Smallpox vaccine
***Rhabdoviridae* (RNA, enveloped)**	
Rabies virus	Rabies, paralysis
Vesicular stomatitis	Similar to FMD, flu-like
***Coronaviridae* (RNA, enveloped)**	
Human coronavirus	Severe acute respiratory syndrome (SARS), colds
Mouse hepatitis virus	Wasting syndrome
***Herpesviridae* (DNA, enveloped)**	
Herpesvirus (HSV-I, HSV-2)	Conjunctivitis, gingivostomatitis, genital herpes, meningitis
Varicella-zoster virus	Chickenpox/shingles

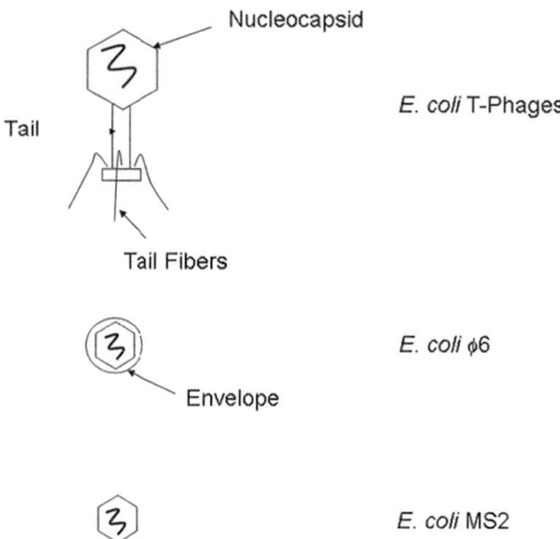

FIGURE 1.12 *E. coli* bacteriophages. The T phages are complex DNA viruses; MS2 and ϕ6 are RNA viruses, with ϕ6 being enveloped.

viruses remain to be identified and implicated in diseases by developing molecular biology, culturing, and electron microscopy techniques.

Separate families of plant viruses have also been described including tobamoviruses (nonenveloped RNA viruses; e.g., tomato-tobacco mosaic virus is a significant agricultural/horticultural concern because it infects vegetables, flowers, and weeds, leading to leaf, flower, and fruit damage), *Comoviridae* (nonenveloped RNA viruses), and *Geminiviridae* (nonenveloped DNA viruses). Viruses that infect fungi (e.g., the nonenveloped RNA viruses barnavirus and chryovirus) and bacteria (bacteriophages) (Fig. 1.12) have also been described.

Bacteriophages (commonly known as phages) are mostly DNA viruses (e.g., the T3, T7, and lambda [λ] phages are *E. coli* viruses), although some RNA viruses have been described (e.g., nonenveloped MS2 and enveloped ϕ6 *E. coli* phages). Although most phages are similar to viruses in their need to replicate in their bacterial hosts, some types only bind to target bacteria and cause cell lysis but do not inject their nucleic acid for replication purposes. Bacteriophages have been studied for many years as genetic engineering tools, but they have other practical applications, including uses in typing bacteria, in bacteria detection, as indicators of fecal contamination in water, and in limited medical applications (such as pathogen-specific antibacterials). *Lactobacillus* phages are a significant contamination concern in the dairy industry. Their sensitivity to inactivation can vary depending on the structure, which can include both enveloped and nonenveloped forms. Many phages are considered to be as resistant to biocides as are other animal or plant viruses and are therefore used to investigate biocidal activity (e.g., MS2 phage) and modes of action. They can be routinely cultured and purified in most bacteriology laboratories.

Two other groups of infectious agents are also considered viruses but are unique in their morphology. The first are viroids, which are devoid of protein and appear to consist of naked RNA molecules. The second are proposed to be devoid of a nucleic acid and are termed "prions"; these are discussed in further detail in section 1.3.6. To date, viroids are known to infect only higher plants and have been identified as the cause of a number of crop diseases. Examples include the potato spindle tuber virus, coconut cadang-cadang virus, and tomato apical stunt virus. They consist of small, circular RNA sequences that range in size from 246 to 375 nucleotides. It is interesting to note that their sequences do not encode proteins and that they are dependent on the host for replication in the cell nucleus. Although at first it would seem that these agents would not survive well in the environment, their structures are somewhat protected by forming double-stranded portions (by base pairing) within their circular, single-stranded structure. Although no human viroids have been identified, hepatitis D (delta) virus is similar to a viroid and is known as a satellite virus. A satellite virus is an agent that consists of a nucleic acid and depends on the coinfection of a host with another virus, which is required for its replication. In all effects, hepatitis delta appears to be a defective transmissible pathogen that is dependent on hepatitis B virus infection. It consists of a circular RNA molecule

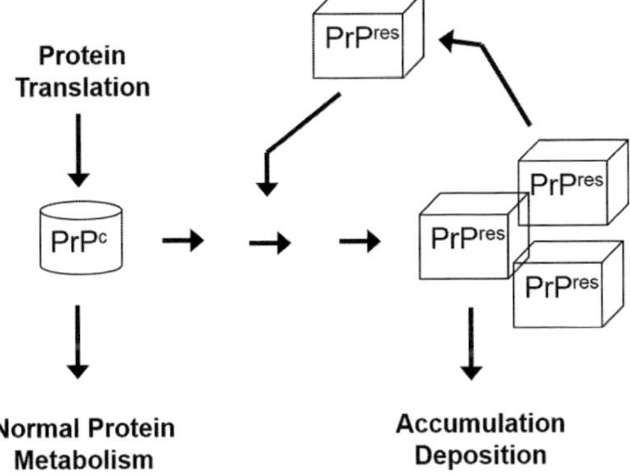

FIGURE 1.13 Theory of prions as infectious proteins. PrP^c is the normal form of the protein, and PrP^{res} is the abnormal form.

(~1,680 bp), but unlike a true viroid it does encode a capsid protein. The virus consists of a nucleocapsid of 60 proteins surrounding the RNA molecule and an external envelope of lipid and hepatitis B surface antigens.

1.3.6 Prions

Prions are unique infectious agents that are composed exclusively of protein and do not appear to have unique, associated nucleic acid. The protein in question is a normal cellular protein (cellular prion protein, PrP^C) that is expressed in many body tissues (particularly in the brain) and in vertebrates, including humans and animals. Proteins are produced in cells as chains of amino acids (known as their primary structures), which then fold into higher-order structures (e.g., secondary and tertiary structures). It is these forms that allow proteins to function in their biological roles, such as in the various cell structures and functions (e.g., as enzymes). Like other cellular proteins, PrP^C is manufactured by the cell, assumes its normal structure, and can be subsequently broken down by normal cellular processes (Fig. 1.13). The exact function (or functions) of the PrP^C protein is unknown, but it is a eukaryotic cell membrane-associated glycoprotein and may be involved in copper metabolism or other functions.

However, PrP^c appears to be able to change its conformational secondary and tertiary structure into insoluble, infectious forms (known as PrP^{Sc} and also as PrP^{res}). The conformational change to PrP^{res} renders the protein structure highly resistant to normal cellular degradative processes, leading to accumulation and cell damage or death, with particular consequences to neural tissues. More specifically, an insoluble portion of the protein (PrP^{27-30}, a 27- to 30-kDa protein) accumulates to form amyloid deposits in the brain. Therefore, the protein primary structure does not specifically change, but the protein secondary/tertiary structure is radically altered to give an overall greater proportion of β-sheets over α-helices in the folded protein structure (Fig. 1.14). What specifically triggers this reaction is currently unknown; PrP^{res} itself has been shown to be involved in this transition but may also require other, yet unidentified factors.

Prions are the causative agents in a group of diseases known as transmissible spongiform encephalopathies. Animal (scrapie in sheep and bovine spongiform encephalopathy in cattle) and human (Creutzfeld-Jakob disease [CJD] and variant CJD) diseases have been particularly well described. Some forms of the disease are known to be inherited, e.g., familial CJD (~10% of CJD cases) and Gerstmann-

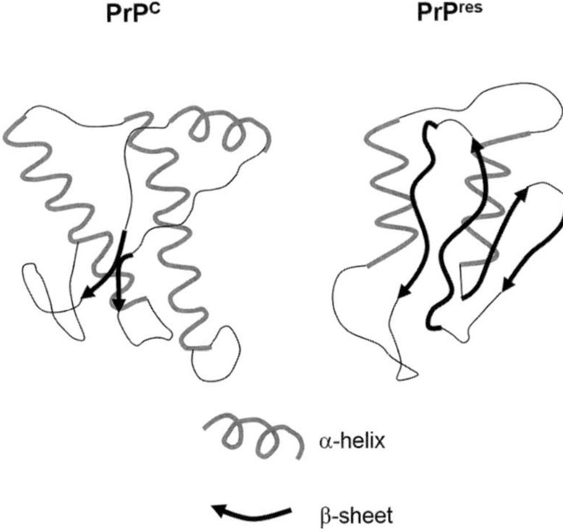

FIGURE 1.14 A representation of the proposed secondary structure changes in the two forms of the prion protein, PrP.

Sträussler-Scheinker syndrome, which is associated with modifications in the PrP-encoding gene. Human diseases are considered very rare; for example, CJD is the most common known human transmissible spongiform encephalopathy, with an approximate rate of 1 to 3 cases per 1,000,000 population being reported in most countries. Animal diseases are often considered more widespread; for example, scrapie is estimated to affect 4 to 8% of sheep. Prions have been shown to be transferred in contaminated tissues (including infected foods, neural tissues, and blood) and on the surfaces of contaminated instruments (surgical devices used in neurosurgical procedures). Zoonotic transmission to humans has been reported, with the cattle bovine spongiform encephalopathy now widely accepted as the source of variant CJD in humans. Finally, some researchers have speculated that other diseases that are associated with the deposition of protein (for example, the neurodegenerative diseases Parkinson's and Alzheimer's) could also be associated with similar transmissible agents; these reports, however, remain to be substantiated.

1.3.7 Toxins

Toxins are microbial substances that are able to induce damage to host cells, an immunogenic/allergic response, and/or fever. Fever is an abnormal increase in body temperature often associated with acute microbial infections. As toxins are released from the microorganism, either during normal cell metabolism or on cell death, they can have dramatic effects on a susceptible host away from the actual site of infection or microbial growth. In some cases, the toxins can remain present despite the removal or inactivation of the source microorganism. Although many toxins may be inactivated by biocidal processes used to control microorganisms, in some cases toxins are con-

TABLE 1.15 Examples of bacterial, fungal, and algal toxins

Microorganism	Toxin	Effects/disease
Bacterial exotoxins		
C. jejuni	Enterotoxin, cytotoxin	Food-borne illness; cell toxicity
C. botulinum	Neurotoxins	Paralysis (relaxed muscles); botulism
Clostridium tetani	Neurotoxin	Paralysis (tensed muscles); tetanus
E. coli (some enteropathogenic strains)	Enterotoxins	Food poisoning, including diarrhea
B. anthracis	Three-protein component toxin (protective antigen, lethal factor, and edema factor)	Anthrax
V. cholerae	Enterotoxin	Cholera
C. diphtheriae	Two-protein component toxin	Diphtheria
Bacterial endotoxins		
E. coli, Shigella, Salmonella	Endotoxin	Fever, diarrhea, inflammation
Fungal toxins		
Aspergillus flavus	Aflatoxins	Hepatic disease and known carcinogens; often associated with contaminated foods and feeds
Penicillium rubrum	Rubratoxins	Liver and kidney toxicity; often associated with contaminated foods and feeds
Stachybotrys spp.	Mycotoxins (e.g., trichothecenes)	Respiratory effects, headaches, flu-like illness, allergic reactions; associated with water-damaged buildings
Algal toxins		
Gonyaulax	Saxitoxins	Food-borne illness (associated with shellfish)
Microcystis	Hepatoxins	Liver damage; associated with contaminated water

sidered highly heat and/or chemical resistant. Examples are Gram-negative bacteria endotoxins, and they require special consideration to reduce their risks in medical applications.

Toxins are potent poisons and are important factors in the pathogenic nature of bacteria, fungi, and algae (Table 1.15).

Many toxins are macromolecules, in particular, proteins, polysaccharides, and LPSs, but can also include chemical toxins, as in the case of many fungal and algal toxins. They can be classified in various ways including their site of activity (e.g., neurotoxins, affecting neural tissue, and enterotoxins, affecting the small intestine), their structures, and their mechanism of action.

Bacterial toxins are categorized as exotoxins when they are actively produced and released from the bacterial cell during growth and as endotoxins when they are a normal part of the cell wall structure but are toxic when released following damage to the cell wall or on cell death.

The most widely studied bacterial exotoxins are proteins (ranging in size from ~50 to -1,000 kDa) which are released from actively growing Gram-positive and Gram-negative bacteria. As proteins, they are generally heat-sensitive, although some have been shown to survive heat treatment processes. Many exotoxins are potent poisons at relatively low concentrations and are important virulence factors in bacterial diseases such as anthrax, tetanus, cholera, and food poisoning. Their toxic effects can include cell damage (AB toxins), cell lysis (cytotoxic toxins), and inflammatory responses (superantigen toxins). Examples of exotoxins and their effects on host cells are given in Table 1.16.

By definition, endotoxins can be any cell-bound toxin that is released on cell damage or cell death, although this term is generally used to refer to the LPS component of the cell wall of Gram-negative bacteria, including *E. coli*, *Salmonella*, *Shigella*, and *Pseudomonas* (section 1.3.4.1; Fig. 1.7). LPS contains a lipid portion (known as lipid A) that forms part of the external surface of the outer membrane, which is linked to a polysaccharide (containing a core and *O*-polymer of sugars) extending to the outside of the cell (Fig. 1.15). The exact fatty acid and sugar structures of LPS vary between Gram-negative species. In general, the polysaccharide can contain various types of sugars, and the lipid A portion consists of fatty acids attached to a disaccharide of *N*-acetylglucosamine phosphate.

Endotoxins can have a variety of biological activities when introduced directly into the blood and are therefore an important consideration in various pharmaceutical, medical device, and water purification applications. LPS is pyrogenic (fever-causing) and induces an inflammatory response, which can lead

TABLE 1.16 Examples of bacterial exotoxins and their clinical effects

Type	Example	Microorganism	Effects
AB toxins Two-component toxins which cause cell damage	Diphtheria toxin	*C. diphtheriae*	Inhibition of protein synthesis
	Tetanus and botulism toxins	*C. tetani*, *C. botulinum*	Neurotoxins; block neurotransmitters
	Cholera toxin	*V. cholerae*	Enterotoxin; secretion of fluids from small intestine
Cytotoxic toxins Cause cell lysis	α, β, γ toxins	*C. perfringens*	Cell lysis, including damage to cell membrane
	α toxin	*S. aureus*	Cell lysis
Superantigen toxins Cause an immunological response and inflammation	Toxic shock syndrome (TSS) toxin	*S. aureus*	Septic shock
	Erythrogenic toxin	*S. pyogenes*	Scarlet fever rash

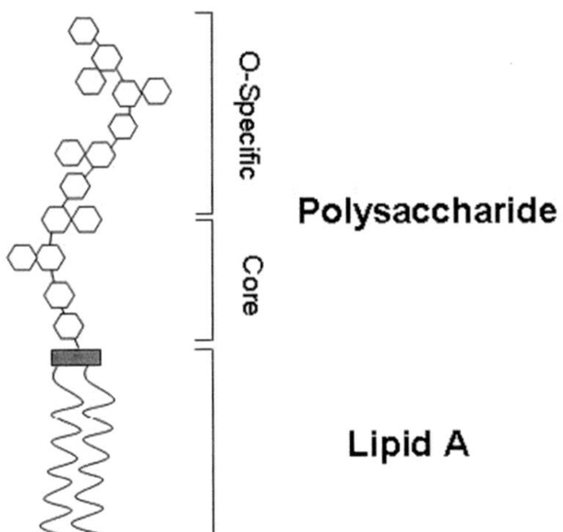

FIGURE 1.15 The general structure of LPS, a bacterial endotoxin.

to septic shock, diarrhea, and under some circumstances, death. The polysaccharide component is considered responsible for fever and inflammation, while the lipid A component is linked to the toxicity effect on host cells. Overall, the toxic effects of LPS are considered less of a concern than exotoxins, but this will depend on the dose. Endotoxins are notably resistant to heat, including to moist heat sterilization (see chapter 5, section 5.2), but can be neutralized by dry heat in depyrogenation processes (see section 5.3).

Mycotoxins are produced by fungi, in particular, molds such as *Aspergillus*, *Fusarium*, *Stachybotrys*, *Penicillium*, and *Chaetomium*. They are usually produced during the late exponential/stationary phase of growth and, like other fungal secondary metabolites (like antibiotics), provide competitive advantages to the microorganism in its environment. They can be associated with the active vegetative molds, their spores, or the area surrounding mold growth. Most of these toxins are chemical in nature, and they include aflatoxins, ochratoxins, trichothecenes, and gliotoxins; an example of the structure of a fungal aflatoxin is given in Fig. 1.16.

Mycotoxins also have multiple effects on host cells, including membrane damage, cell death, and free radical-associated damage. Aflatoxins have been particularly reported in food and feed (grain) contamination and have been shown to be carcinogenic. Some fungal cell wall components (e.g., β-1-3 glucan) are also considered toxins and can cause allergic reactions, including coughing and other respiratory effects.

Many algae produce toxins, which are often associated with contaminated water. These include hepatoxins (in particular, from blue-green algae), neurotoxins, cytotoxins, and endotoxins (similar to Gram-negative bacteria, as LPS structures from the outer membrane of the algal cell wall).

1.4 GENERAL CONSIDERATIONS

1.4.1 Microbial Resistance

Different types of microorganisms vary in their response to antiseptics, disinfectants, and sterilization processes. This is hardly surprising in view of their different cellular structures, composition, and physiology (section 1.3). Traditionally, microbial susceptibility to biocides has been classified based on these differences (Fig. 1.17). Bacterial spores are generally considered the most resistant organisms to biocides, although prions have shown unique resistance to many traditional physical and chemical processes (chapter 8, section 8.9). It is important to note that this general classification system should only be considered as a guide to antimicrobial activity and can vary depending on the specific biocide being used, as well as its formulation or process conditions. For example, while the resistance profile shown in Fig. 1.17 may be considered representative for some heat-based processes, some fungal spores

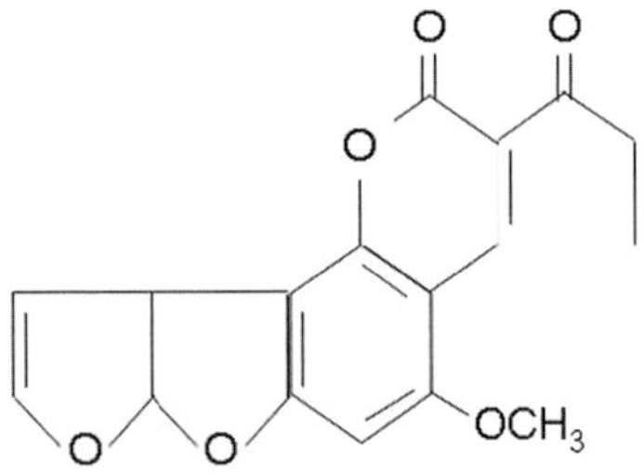

FIGURE 1.16 Typical fungal aflatoxin structure.

	Microorganism	Examples
More Resistant	Prions	Scrapie, Creutzfeld-Jakob disease, Chronic wasting disease
↑	Bacterial Spores	*Bacillus, Geobacillus, Clostridium*
	Protozoal Oocysts	*Cryptosporidium*
	Helminth Eggs	*Ascaris, Enterobius*
	Mycobacteria	*Mycobacterium tuberculosis, M. terrae, M. chelonae*
	Small, Non-Enveloped Viruses	Poliovirus, Parvoviruses, Papilloma viruses
	Protozoal Cysts	*Giardia, Acanthamoeba*
	Fungal Spores	*Aspergillus, Penicillium*
	Gram negative bacteria	*Pseudomonas, Providencia, Escherichia*
	Vegetative Fungi and Algae	*Aspergillus, Trichophyton, Candida, Chlamydomonas*
	Vegetative Helminths and Protozoa	*Ascaris, Cryptosporidium, Giardia*
	Large, non-enveloped viruses	Adenoviruses, Rotaviruses
	Gram positive bacteria	*Staphylococcus, Streptococcus, Enterococcus*
Less Resistant	Enveloped viruses	HIV, Hepatitis B virus, Herpes Simplex virus

FIGURE 1.17 General microbial resistance to biocides and biocidal processes. This classification can vary depending on the biocide or biocidal process under consideration.

and certain types of bacteria can demonstrate greater resistance to radiation methods than can bacterial spores, although some types of protozoan oocysts are relatively sensitive to heat but resistant to chemical disinfectant with known sporicidal activity. Extremophiles can also show atypical resistance patterns to various biocides under investigation (chapter 8, section 8.3.10). The mechanisms of resistance of microorganisms to biocides are considered in more detail in chapter 8.

The resistance of a microorganism also depends on direct contact with the biocide and is affected by many other associated variables including the following:

- The specific microbial strain and culture conditions used for growth of the microorganism. In some cases, strains recently isolated from environmental sources may show greater resistance profiles but lose this profile during culturing under laboratory conditions.
- The growth phase of a microbial culture (e.g., population on a surface, exponential- versus stationary-phase growth).
- The type of contaminated surface and/or medium (e.g., water, pharmaceutical preparation, plastic, metals, paper, etc.).
- Presence of organic or inorganic soils often associated with microbial contamination that can interfere with the biocidal action.
- Presence within its normal environmental conditions, e.g., within a biofilm (see chapter 8, section 8.3.8).

A range of microorganisms can be chosen to establish the broad-spectrum activity of an

TABLE 1.17 Examples of surrogate microorganisms used to test and verify the antimicrobial activity of biocide products and processes

Efficacy claim	Surrogate	Example of use
Sporicidal	*B. atrophaeus*, *B. cereus*, *Clostridium sporogenes*	General disinfectant and sterilant testing; sterility assurance testing for sterilization processes
Fungicidal	*T. mentagrophytes*, *A. niger*, *C. albicans*	General disinfectant testing
Bactericidal	*S. aureus*, *P. aeruginosa*, *Salmonella choleraesuis*, *Enterococcus hirae*, *E. coli*, *Serratia marcescens*	General antiseptic and disinfectant testing
Virucidal	Poliovirus, adenovirus, herpesvirus, bacteriophages (e.g., *Lactococcus* phage F7/2)	General antiseptic and disinfectant testing
Mycobactericidal	*M. bovis*, *M. terrae*, *M. smegmatis*	High-level disinfectant
Oocysticidal	*C. parvum*	General disinfectant testing

antimicrobial product or process depending on the required or desired application. For example, a true sterilizing agent should be expected to be effective against viruses, fungi, protozoa, mycobacteria, and other bacteria, including bacterial spores. Bacteria (including spores), fungi, mycobacteria, and to a lesser extent viruses are most commonly used as test microorganisms to establish antimicrobial activity expectations. Considering the multitude of microorganisms and applications, it is common to use surrogates as test organisms to establish the spectrum of efficacy of a product/process or the antimicrobial activity against a class of microorganisms (Table 1.17).

Despite the acceptance of these surrogates, in some cases the specific test organisms found in a given environment (the natural bioburden) are used, or are required to be used, to verify the claimed antimicrobial activity.

1.4.2 Evaluation of Efficacy

The antimicrobial activity of a biocide or biocidal process can be investigated using a variety of methods ranging from simple laboratory tests to evaluation under actual use conditions. These tests are not only important in the investigation of biocides and the development of products and processes but are also the basis for the regulatory clearance, labeling, and use of antiseptics, disinfectants, and sterilization processes worldwide. Tests and requirements can vary considerably, and there are currently no standardized requirements that apply to all situations worldwide. Many country-specific regulatory requirements specify particular test methods to verify antimicrobial activity, but these also vary for the particular application (e.g., medical, dental, agricultural, water disinfection, or industrial), type of biocide/process, and use of the formulation/process (e.g., preservation, antisepsis, disinfection, or sterilization).

1.4.2.1 Suspension Testing. Suspension tests are widely used under laboratory conditions in the development, verification, and registration of biocidal products. The simplest test is the determination of a minimum inhibitory concentration (MIC)—the lowest concentration of a chemical biocide that inhibits the growth of a test organism—which is similarly used in the evaluation of antibiotic activity against bacteria. A series of biocide dilutions (usually in growth media specific for the test organism) are inoculated with a known concentration of the microorganism and then incubated to determine the MIC. This method is useful for evaluating the potential effectiveness of biocides against a wide range of vegetative organisms such as bacteria and fungi and in the development of effective liquid product preservation. MICs are limited, because many biocides also react with organic and inorganic constituents of the growth media used during these tests and are therefore not available for activity against the test organism; examples of these include oxidizing agents, halogens, and aldehydes. Because biocide MICs are generally at relatively low levels, they have limited use in demonstrating the various formulation effects that can enhance the efficacy of an antiseptic or disinfectant. Similar to MIC determination, the minimum microbicidal concentration (e.g., minimum bactericidal concentration) can be determined by exposing the test organism to biocide or biocidal product dilutions for a fixed time and then determining at what concentration no growth is observed. These tests can be useful research tools but are not widely used to evaluate the true activity of biocidal products or processes and can even be misleading.

Time-kill, or *D*-value, determinations are used to study the effect of biocides over time. In these tests' simplest form, the test organism at a known concentration is exposed to a product or process and samples are removed over time to determine the concentration of test organisms remaining (Fig. 1.18). An important consideration in these tests (as for any microbicidal test) is to stop the activity of the biocide at a required exposure time, which is referred to as neutralization. Neutralization in the investigation of physical biocidal processes can be relatively straightforward, such as by cooling in heat-based studies and directly removing a radiation source. With chemical biocides, neutralization can be by physical removal (the most obvious method being filtration), dilution, or chemical sequestration/inactivation. Filtration is achieved by passing the sample through a 0.1-to 0.4-μ filter, trapping the organism (usually bacteria or fungi), and allowing the biocide to pass through into the filtrate. Chemical neutralizers include sodium thiosulfate (for some oxidizing agents and halogens), Tween/lecithin (for quaternary ammonium compounds [QACs] and chlorhexidine), and sodium sulfite or glycine (for glutaraldehyde). It is important to demonstrate that no inhibitory substances, including the neutralizer itself or reaction between the biocide and neutralizer, are present or formed that could inhibit the potential growth of the test organism. For example, chlorhexidine has specific affinity for certain filter materials,

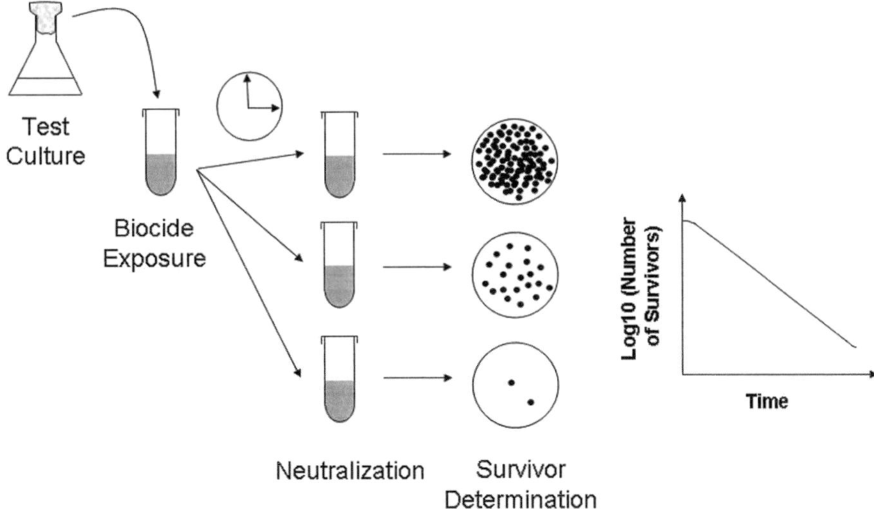

FIGURE 1.18 A typical time-kill or *D*-value determination. A known concentration of the test culture is exposed to the biocide (in this case a chemical solution), samples are withdrawn at various times, they are neutralized, and the population of survivors is determined by incubation on growth media. The actual exposure can be conducted at various temperatures, in the presence/absence of test soils, or other test conditions.

which can subsequently inhibit the growth of the test organism on incubation of the filter on growth media. It is therefore important that positive, negative, and neutralization growth controls be included to ensure correct interpretation of results.

Following exposure and neutralization of the biocide, the survivor population can be determined qualitatively or quantitatively. Quantitative methods determine the number of survivors by direct enumeration, e.g., by plating onto growth agar for bacteria and fungi (as shown in Fig. 1.18). The data from this analysis can be plotted as a time/log reduction relationship (Fig. 1.19).

From this plot the decimal reduction time or *D* value can be calculated; it is defined as the time (or for radiation methods, the dose) required to achieve inactivation of 90% (or 1 $\log_{10}$ unit) of a population of a given test microorganism under stated conditions (e.g., temperature, radiation dose, exposure to a chemical) (Fig. 1.19). It is usual for the average *D* value to be determined as the negative

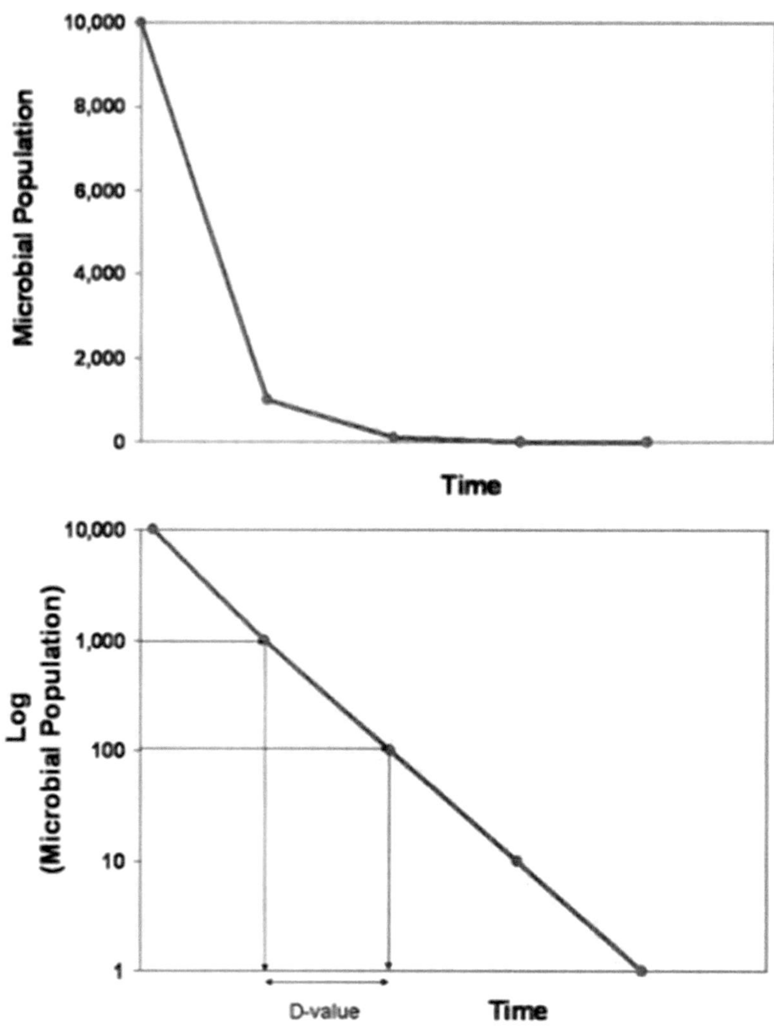

FIGURE 1.19 Determination of the *D* value on microbial exposure to a biocide.

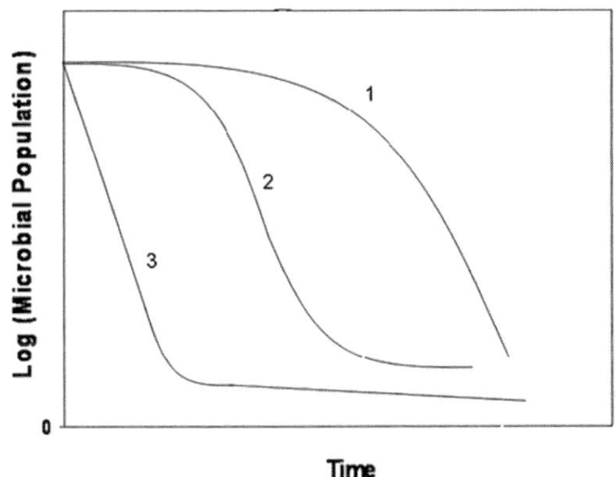

FIGURE 1.20 Typical survivor curves on biocide exposure. Curve 1 is concave downward, curve 2 is sigmoidal, and curve 3 is concave upward.

reciprocal of the slope (m) of the plotted relationship (-1/slope):

$$m = \Delta \log \mathrm{N} \, \Delta \mathrm{T}$$

$$D \, \text{value} = -1/\mathrm{m}$$

where Δ logN is the change in $\log_{10}$ microbial population, ΔT is the change in time/dose, and m is the slope of the survivor curve.

Graphical presentation of the microbial response to a biocide over time can also be useful for analysis of the biocide-microbial population interaction. Although the data presented in Fig. 1.19 demonstrate a linear relationship, typical biocide survivor curves are often found to be nonlinear (examples are shown in Fig. 1.20). Practically, these data can have many interpretations. For example, curve 1 suggests an initial lag phase in biocidal activity that can be due to factors such as chemical penetration into target microorganisms or limited access of the biocide to the microbial population, such as by the presence of interfering soils or microbial clumping. Curve 3 may be indicative of insufficient biocide concentration or the presence of a microbial subpopulation (or mixed population) with greater resistance to the biocide. Curve 2 may indicate a combination of the effects described for both previous data sets.

Qualitative methods determine the simple presence or absence of growth in a sample, although the data from this analysis can be used to estimate the actual population present by serial dilution if it is accepted that the microbial population is randomly distributed (e.g., not clumped) (Fig. 1.21).

By serial dilution of the initial sample (in Fig. 1.21 using 10-fold dilutions) in growth media and monitoring of microbial growth, the highest dilution demonstrating growth must have contained ≤10 viable cells and can be used to estimate the most probable number in the initial sample. This analysis is also referred to as "fraction-negative" determination.

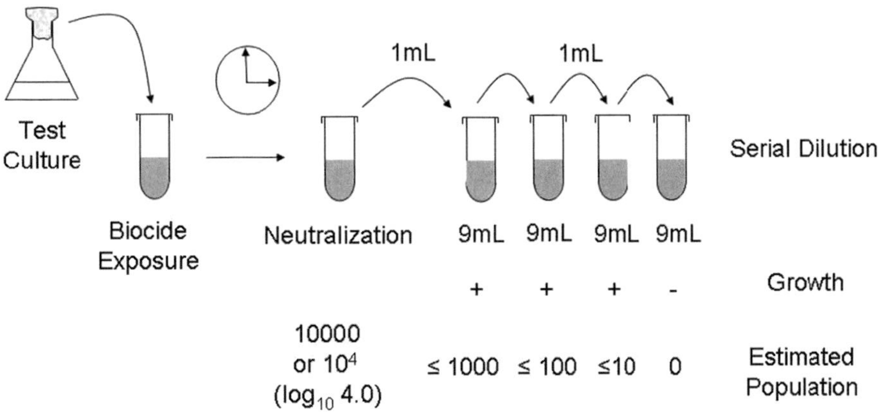

FIGURE 1.21 Qualitative and semiquantitative population determination.

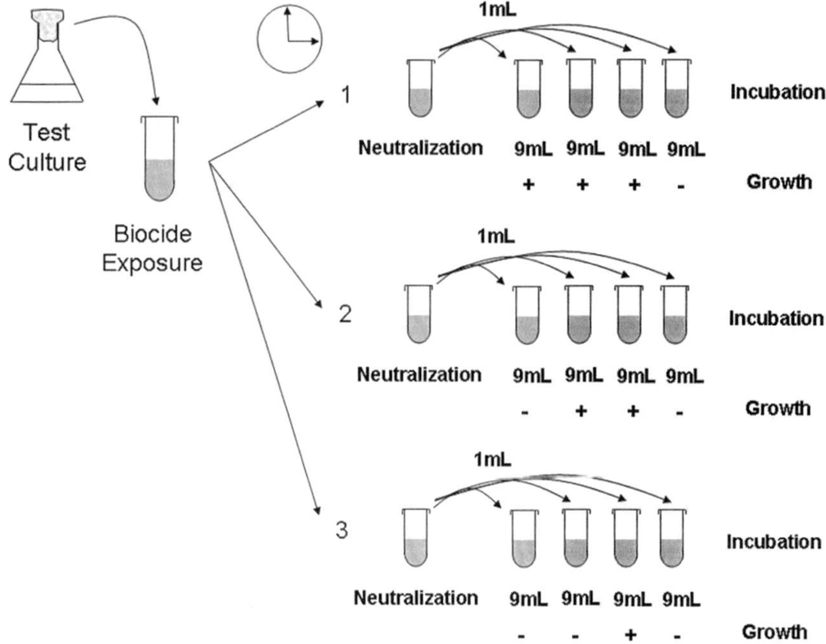

FIGURE 1.22 *D*-value estimation using most probable number estimations.

In certain situations, these methods can be used to estimate *D* values (a representation of a test is shown in Fig. 1.22).

In this case, the fraction of observed growth or no growth can be used to estimate the number of survivors in the sample at a specific exposure time. Different mathematical equations are used, for example, the Halvorson-Ziegler equation:

$$N_t = 2.303 \log_{10} (n/r)$$

where N_t is the population at time *t*, *n* is the number tested, and *r* is the number sterile.

Therefore, if we take the example from Fig. 1.22, we can generate the following table:

Time	n	r	n/r	N_t
1	4	1	4	1.4
2	4	2	2	0.7
3	4	3	1.3	0.3

From this analysis, the *D* value can be estimated by plotting (as described previously) or using mathematical equations such as the Stumbo-Murphy-Cochran equation:

$$D \text{ value at exposure time or dose } (t)$$

$$= t/(\log_{10} N_0 - \log_{10} N_t)$$

where *t* is the exposure time, N_0 is the initial microbial population, and N_t is the population at exposure time *t*.

Clearly, fraction-negative methods are relatively restrictive, but they are typically used in combination with direct-enumeration methods to estimate the number of survivors in the quantal range (10^2 to 10^{-2} CFU/ml range) of a survivor curve (see section 1.4.3). They are also widely used in the estimation of microbial populations on biological indicators (see section 1.4.2.3).

The effects of various types of physical and chemical exposure conditions can be tested using suspension methods. Physical effects can include the impact of temperature or mixing, while chemical effects include the biocide concentration or dilution, formulation type, and

TABLE 1.18 Examples of standardized suspension tests

Reference[a]	Title	Summary
AOAC official method 955.11	Testing disinfectants against *Salmonella* Typhi (includes phenol coefficient method)	Tests the bactericidal activity in comparison to known concentrations of phenol (also used to standardize test cultures). Using *Salmonella* Typhi, *S. aureus*, and *P. aeruginosa*
ASTM E1052-11	Standard test method for efficacy of antimicrobial agents against viruses in suspension	Guidelines on testing of the virucidal activity of a product in suspension
ASTM E1891-10	Standard guide for determination of a survival curve for antimicrobial agents against selected microorganisms and calculation of a *D*-value and concentration coefficient	Guidelines on the determination of survival curves and calculation of *D* values
USP ⟨51⟩	Antimicrobial effectiveness testing	To confirm the preservative effectiveness in a formulated product by inoculation of *S. aureus*, *E. coli*, *P. aeruginosa*, *C. albicans*, and *A. niger*; determines that a product does not promote but prevents microbial growth over time
EN 1040	Chemical disinfectants and antiseptics. Quantitative suspension test for the evaluation of basic bactericidal activity of chemical disinfectants and antiseptics. Test method and requirements (phase 1)	Testing for the basic bactericidal efficacy of a disinfectant or antiseptic using *P. aeruginosa* and *S. aureus*; required to observe $\geq 10^5$ log reduction in 60 s
EN 1650	Chemical disinfectants and antiseptics. Quantitative suspension test for evaluation of fungicidal activity of chemical disinfectants and antiseptics used in food, industrial, domestic, and institutional areas. Test method and requirements (phase 2, step 1)	Testing for fungicidal activity of a disinfectant or antiseptic using *C. albicans* and *A. niger* in the presence of hard water (if dilution required) and organic soil (albumin, skimmed milk, and other components); required to observe $\geq 10^4$ log reduction in 15 min
EN 13610	Chemical disinfectants. Quantitative suspension test for the evaluation of virucidal activity against bacteriophages of chemical disinfectants used in food and industrial areas. Test method and requirements (phase 2, step 1)	Testing for virucidal activity using *Lactococcus lactis* F7/2 bacteriophage; required to show $\geq 10^4$ log reduction in 15 min

[a]AOAC, Association of Official Analytical Chemists; ASTM, American Society for Testing and Materials; USP, United States Pharmacopeia; EN, European Norm, from CEN (European Committee for Standardization).

the impact of interfering substances, including organic (e.g., serum, blood) and inorganic (e.g., heavy metals, hard water) soils. These effects are often important considerations in the practical use of the biocidal product or process. Examples of some standardized suspension tests are given in Table 1.18.

1.4.2.2 Surface Testing. Surface tests are used to verify the antimicrobial activity of a product or process on a test surface. This is an important consideration in the use of many surface antiseptics, disinfectants, and sterilization processes. Tests can be considered to belong to three types: carrier tests, simulated-use tests, and in-use tests (see section 1.4.2.3).

In the carrier method, the test microorganism is inoculated onto a defined carrier material, in the presence or absence of interfering soils, and is then exposed to the biocidal process or product. The carrier material can simply consist of a coupon (a defined piece) of any test surface (including paper, stainless steel, glass, or plastic). It may also be a defined test carrier; for example, stainless steel and porcelain penicylinders are widely used in the United States to test the surface-disinfectant efficacies of products. For antiseptic testing, sections of *ex vivo* skin have been used as test surfaces. Following exposure, the test coupons are retrieved (with neutralization if required) and tested for the survival of the test microorganism. This can also be performed qualitatively (by immersion into growth media and incubation, followed by observation of growth or no growth) or quantitatively (by elution of the test culture and direct enumeration or fraction negative determination as described in section 1.4.2.1). Examples of various types of standardized carrier tests are given in Table 1.19. Some of the most widely used carrier tests are defined biological and chemical indicators for various sterilization process tests, which are described in more detail in section 1.4.2.3.

Simulated-use tests are also laboratory-based; an artificial inoculum is applied to a surface to simulate the actual use of the product or process in a typical application. Examples include the use of an artificial inoculum onto the skin or onto various surfaces, such as medical devices. It is important to validate these test methods, including the inoculation, neutralization, and recovery steps, to ensure that they are reproducible and reliable. As well as direct application of the test culture to a surface, in some situations the microbial culture can be inoculated onto a carrier or inserted into the test equipment at a worst-case location (e.g., in the internal channel of a lumened device), exposed to the product or process, and recovered for evaluation. Recovery methods can include elution, swabbing, air filtering, and contact plates. Examples of various simulative-use test guidelines and standards are given in Table 1.20.

TABLE 1.19 Examples of standardized carrier tests

Reference[a]	Title	Summary
AOAC official methods 991.47, 991.48, 991.49	Hard surface carrier test	Bactericidal activity of disinfectant/sterilants against *P. aeruginosa*, *S. aureus*, and *S. choleraesuis* quantitatively inoculated onto glass penicylinders. Carriers tested for growth/no growth following exposure
AOAC official method 965.12	Tuberculocidal activity of disinfectants	Porcelain penicylinders contaminated with *M. bovis* and exposed to the product; carriers tested for growth/no growth following exposure
AOAC official method 966.04	Sporicidal test method	*C. sporogenes* and *B. subtilis* cultures (including spores) dried onto porcelain penicylinders and suture loop carriers; exposed to the test disinfectant/sterilant for the required time and incubated to detect presence/absence of growth
ASTM E1053-11	Standard test method to assess virucidal activity of chemicals intended for disinfection of inanimate, nonporous environmental surfaces	Guidelines on testing of the virucidal activity of a product on an inanimate surface
ASTM E2111-12	Standard quantitative carrier test method to evaluate the bactericidal, fungicidal, mycobactericidal and sporicidal potencies of liquid chemicals	Carrier (glass vials) test for the potency of liquid disinfectants against bacteria and fungi
EN 13697	Chemical disinfectants and antiseptics. Quantitative non-porous surface test for the evaluation of bactericidal and/or fungicidal activity of chemical disinfectants used in food, industrial, domestic and institutional areas. Test method and requirements without mechanical action (phase 2, step 2)	Various bacteria (e.g., *P. aeruginosa* and *E. hirae*) and fungi (*C. albicans* and *A. niger*) inoculated onto stainless steel discs in the presence/absence of interfering soil and exposed to the test disinfectant/antiseptic. Demonstrate a $\geq 10^4$ reduction of bacteria in 5 min and $\geq 10^3$ reduction of fungi in 15 min

[a]AOAC, Association of Official Analytical Chemists; ASTM, American Society for Testing and Materials; EN, European Norm, from the CEN (European Committee for Standardization).

TABLE 1.20 Examples of simulated-use and/or in-use tests and/or guidelines. Simulated testing uses an artificial inoculum and in-use testing uses the normal bioburden present on a surface or device

Reference[a]	Title	Summary
ASTM E1837-96	Standard test method to determine efficacy of disinfection processes for reusable medical devices (simulated use test)	Simulated-use testing for the effectiveness of a disinfection process for reprocessing reusable medical devices using bacteria, viruses, and/or fungi
ISO 11737-1	Sterilization of medical devices - microbiological methods - part 1: determination of a population of microorganisms on products	In-use testing guidelines on the estimation of the population of viable microorganisms (or bioburden) on a medical device
ISO 11737-2	Sterilization of medical devices - microbiological methods - part 2: tests of sterility performed in the definition, validation and maintenance of a sterilization process	Sterility testing criteria for medical devices that have been exposed to treatment with a sterilizing agent under reduced conditions from those used for routine sterilization
ISO 14698-1	Clean rooms and associated controlled environments - biocontamination control - part 1: general principles and methods	Testing guidelines on the assessment and control of biocontamination within a clean room environment
WHO	Guidelines for drinking-water quality	Guidelines on the microbial and chemical safety of drinking water, including water testing methods for monitoring water disinfection efficacy
ASTM E1174-06	Standard test method for evaluation of healthcare personnel hand-wash formulations	Simulative test of the activity of an antiseptic on the hands using an artificial inoculum of *S. marcescens*
ASTM E1173-15	Standard test method of a evaluation of a preoperative, precatheterization, or preinjection skin preparations	In-use test for the activity of an antiseptic to reduce the resident microbial flora of the skin

[a]ISO, International Standards Organization; ASTM, American Society for Testing and Materials; WHO, World Health Organization.

1.4.2.3 In-Use Testing. In-use testing is done to test a product or process under the actual conditions of use. Such tests are recommended to verify the effectiveness of antimicrobial methods during their development (to meet specific registration and labeling criteria) and/or to actively monitor the success or failure of such methods over time in specific applications. Typical examples include:

- Routine microbial sampling of environmental surfaces (e.g., food contact surfaces or clean room benchtops) before and/or after disinfection using recovery methods such as swabbing, contact agar plates, or elution
- Periodic air sampling in clean rooms or other controlled environments (see section 2.5)
- Routine analysis of sterile manufactured pharmaceuticals or preserved cosmetics
- Skin antisepsis testing, by sampling the normal flora of the skin (or if artificially inoculated with a test bacterial suspension) to determine the effectiveness of antiseptics compared to untreated controls
- Estimation of the number and types of microorganisms on medical devices before or after a full or partial disinfection or sterilization process

Such tests are used to estimate the associated bioburden or sterility (i.e., lack of detectable microorganisms) in these various applications. "Bioburden" is defined as the population of viable microorganisms on or in a product, surface, or area. The sources of bioburden in or on a product can include manufacturing materials, people handling the product, and the environment in which the product is manufactured or handled. Bioburden-based methods are usually performed in three steps: removal (if appropriate, from a surface), culturing (specific for the types of microorganisms that may be present, such as bacteria and fungi on environmental-exposed surfaces), and enumeration (to determine the estimated bioburden and allow for further identification). As for other tests, it is important to validate these steps to ensure that they are reproducible and reliable. Bioburden-based methods are widely used in establishing the effectiveness of medical device disinfection and sterilization processes, as well as the periodic verification that they remain effective over time. Typical culturing methods used in medical device sterilization assessments of bioburden or sterility are tryptic soya agar at 30 to 35°C for 3 to 7 days (for facultative and aerobic, nonfastidious bacteria) and sabourand dextrose agar at 20 to 25°C for 5 to 7 days (for yeasts and molds).

1.4.2.4 Biological, Chemical, and Other Indicators. Indicators are routinely used to check the effectiveness of various cleaning, disinfection, and sterilization processes. These include biological, chemical, and other (e.g., mechanical) indicators.

Biological indicators (commonly known as BIs) consist of a standardized population of microorganisms inoculated onto a carrier material or a test solution (Fig. 1.23). They are particularly widely used in the monitoring and validation of sterilization processes, being defined as test systems containing viable microorganisms providing a defined resistance to specified processes (e.g., heat or ethylene oxide sterilization). Bacterial endospores are commonly used as test microorganisms because they are generally nonpathogenic, stable and demonstrate high resistance to various sterilization processes (Table 1.21). Defined bacterial strains, obtained from standard culture collections (e.g., the American Type Culture Collection, ATCC) are widely used for these purposes. The intrinsic resistance of the inoculated spore population can vary depending on the culturing methods used and other variables. Therefore, to standardize the use of biological indicators, manufacturers test each batch of indicators to determine the population and the relative resistance to a given sterilization process (e.g., *D*-value determination at 121°C with saturated steam or at 55°C, 800 mg/liter ethylene oxide and 70% relative humidity for ethylene oxide). Depending on the application, other microorganisms may be used but to a much lesser extent.

The carrier can consist of any material, with typical examples including paper, stainless steel, glass, and plastics. In its true definition, a biological indicator consists of the inoculated coupon placed into a "primary pack," which can be a protective envelop or pouch, or into an assembled vial/ampoule (Fig. 1.23). In their simplest form, biological indicators can be

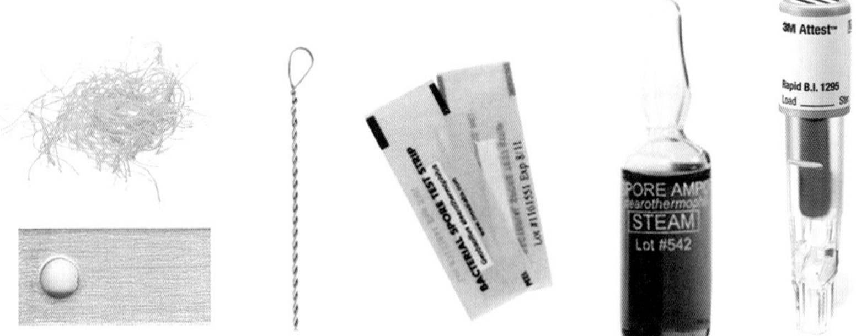

FIGURE 1.23 Example of biological indicators, including (from left to right) simple inoculated thread, coupons and wires, paper in sealed pouches (center), and two examples of self-contained biological indicators (with a rapid-read example on the far right). Far right image courtesy of 3M Health Care, with permission.

TABLE 1.21 Bacterial endospore species used to monitor and validate sterilization processes

Sterilization process	Biological indicator
Moist heat	*G. stearothermophilus*
Dry heat	*B. atrophaeus*
Ethylene oxide	*B. atrophaeus*
Low-temperature steam formaldehyde	*G. stearothermophilus*
Hydrogen peroxide vapor	*G. stearothermophilus*

naked or present within a protective envelope, and following exposure to a given sterilization process, the inoculated coupon is aseptically removed from its pack and incubated in a specified growth media to determine the presence or absence of spore viability. Due to the release of acid (dipicolinic acid; chapter 8, section 8.3.11) on germination and outgrowth of the spores, pH indicator dyes can be used in the growth media to indicate the presence of viability before visual growth (turbidity in the test media) is observed. To minimize aseptic handling, self-contained biological indicators that can include the test microorganism directly in growth media or on an inoculated carrier within a vial containing a sealed ampoule of growth media have also been developed (Fig. 1.23). In the latter case, following exposure, the media ampoule is broken to allow for incubation without direct handling of the coupon. Additional "rapid-read" biological indicators have become widely available in recent years that can detect the presence or absence of growth without the need for traditionally longer incubation times. One example detects the presence of certain endospore enzymes (e.g., α-D-glucosidase) whose heat destruction correlates with the loss of viability of the spore; the presence of enzyme activity can be detected fluorimetrically and can give a rapid indication of spore viability (usually within 1 to 4 hours). These indicators may be further incubated to demonstrate the presence or absence of growth, as for traditional biological indicators. Various standards that define the requirements for and use of biological indicators are given in Table 1.22.

Chemical indicators are based on a chemical change (e.g., color change, melting, or another visual change) on exposure to a given disin-

TABLE 1.22 Examples of biological indicator standards

Reference[a]	Title	Summary
ISO 11138-1	Sterilization of health care products - biological indicators - part 1: general requirements	General requirements for production, labeling, test methods, and performance characteristics of biological indicator systems to be used in the validation and routine monitoring of sterilization processes
ISO 11138-2	Sterilization of health care products - biological indicators - part 2: biological indicators for ethylene oxide sterilization processes	Specific requirements for biological indicators used for ethylene oxide sterilization including test organism and performance criteria
ISO 11138-3	Sterilization of health care products - biological indicators - part 3: biological indicators for moist heat sterilization processes	Specific requirements for biological indicators used for moist heat (steam) sterilization including test organism and performance criteria
ISO 14161	Sterilization of health care products - biological indicators - guidance for the selection, use and interpretation of results	Guidance for the selection, use, and interpretation of results with biological indicators when used in the development, validation, and routine monitoring of sterilization processes
USP 31 ⟨55⟩	Biological indicators - resistance performance tests	Testing on the resistance and population of biological indicators
EP 7.0, 5.1.2	Biological indicators of sterilization	Requirements for biological indicators including population and resistance

[a]ISO, International Standards Organization; EN, European Norm, from the CEN (European Committee for Standardization); USP, United States Pharmacopoeia; EP, European Pharmacopoeia.

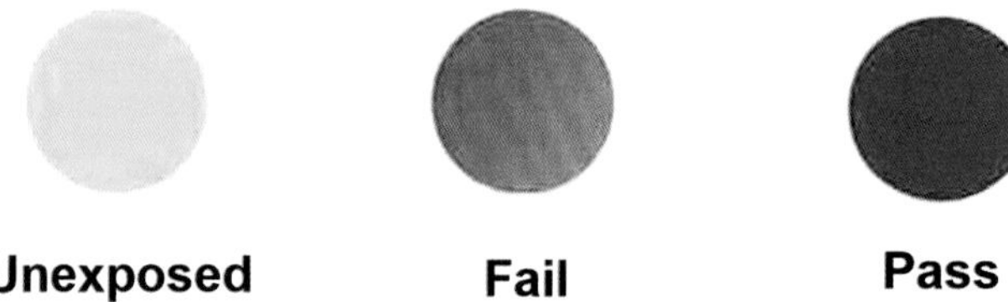

FIGURE 1.24 Example of a chemical indicator color change.

fectant or sterilization process (Fig. 1.24). They can range from simple process indicators that indicate exposure to a given process parameter (e.g., exposure to heat, but not necessarily at the right temperature or for the right time) to more specific integrating or emulating indicators, which change color only on exposure to multiple variables (e.g., temperature and time for steam sterilization and concentration, time, temperature, and humidity for ethylene oxide sterilization). They can be classified in various ways, and an example is given in Table 1.23.

Chemical indicators are widely used because they give an instant result and in some cases (as in the case of some integrators) can be correlated to a biological indicator result. Applications include specific direct parameters that are required for disinfection or sterilization (e.g., verification of the presence of minimal concentration of a biocidal formulation prior to use or that a range of conditions have been met in a sterilizer) but also other indirect variables that are important to the efficacy of the process (e.g., Bowie-Dick tests are used to confirm the adequate removal of air in prevacuum type steam sterilizers [chapter 5, section 5.2]). Dosimeters are specific types of chemical indicators used to measure ionizing radiation doses (see section 5.4), both for human protection as well as for estimating the dose provided to a load during a radiation sterilization process. Examples of various standards that define the requirements for and use of chemical indicators are given in Table 1.24.

Other miscellaneous indicators include mechanical gauges or sensors for indicating temperature, concentration, pressure, time, pH, etc., which are used to monitor various physical parameters during a given process. Mechanical indicators play an important role in the para-

TABLE 1.23 An example of the classification of chemical indicators (in accordance with ISO 11140-1)

Classification	Type	Description
Class 1	Process indicators	Indicate exposure to minimal process conditions; used to differentiate exposed to unexposed items (e.g., autoclave tape)
Class 2	Indicators for use in specific tests	Indicate that a specific process is obtained which is linked to the sterilization process (e.g., a Bowie-Dick test indicates the adequate removal of air from a prevacuum steam sterilizer)
Class 3	Single-parameter indicators	Indicate a change on exposure to one critical process parameter (e.g., concentration of a biocide or a specific temperature)
Class 4	Multiparameter indicators	Indicate a change on exposure to at least two critical process parameters
Class 5	Integrating indicators	Indicate a change on exposure to all the critical process parameters. These indicators are typically equivalent to, or can exceed, the performance requirements for specific biological indicators defined for a given process
Class 6	Emulating indicators	Indicate a change on exposure to all the critical process parameters for full, specified sterilization Processes (e.g., ethylene oxide sterilization with temperature, gas concentration, relative humidity, and defined sterilization time)

TABLE 1.24 Examples of chemical indicator standards

Reference[a]	Title	Summary
ISO 15882	Chemical indicators - guidance on the selection, use, and interpretation of results	Guidance for the selection, use, and interpretation of results of chemical indicators used in process definition, validation, and routine monitoring and control of sterilization processes
ISO 11140-1	Sterilization of health care products - chemical indicators - part 1: general requirements	General requirements for production, labeling, test methods, and performance characteristics of chemical indicators to be used in the validation and routine monitoring of sterilization processes
ISO 11140-3	Sterilization of health care products - chemical indicators - part 3: class 2 indicators for steam penetration test sheets	Specific requirements for class 2 steam penetration test indicators
ISO 18472	Sterilization of health care products - biological and chemical indicators - test equipment	Requirements for test equipment to be used to test chemical and biological indicators used in sterilization processes
ISO/ASTM 52628	Standard practice for dosimetry in radiation processing	Requirements for measuring absorbed dose during radiation sterilization

[a]ISO, International Standards Organization; EN, European Norm, from the CEN (European Committee for Standardization); ANSI/AAMI, American National Standards Institute/Association for the Advancement of Medical Instrumentation.

metric release of a product or process as an alternative to the use of chemical and biological indicators for routine monitoring of sterilization processes (see above, this section). Other examples include cleaning indicators that use artificial test soils inoculated onto a surface to test (generally by visual inspection) physical removal during a cleaning process or cycle.

1.4.2.5 Parametric Control. The concept of parametric control (or release) as a method to verify the effectiveness of a biocidal process is based on the understanding of all the key physical parameters that can affect its success or failure. Although theoretically this could be applied to any disinfection or sterilization process, it is generally restricted to well-characterized sterilization methods including steam, dry heat, ethylene oxide, and ionizing radiation. An example can be given with steam sterilization. The efficacy of steam is affected by the temperature and time, but also by the presence of air (see chapter 5, section 5.2). These parameters are reasonably well understood and can be physically measured (using mechanical indicators [see section 1.4.2.3]) to ensure that the correct conditions have been met during a given steam sterilization cycle. In addition to monitoring these conditions, a series of in-process tests and controls are conducted that provide further assurance that the sterilization process has been efficient. Similarly, thermal (moist heat) disinfection can be ensured by monitoring time-temperature relationships (see chapter 2, section 2.2). However, the concern with parametric release as an alternative to biological monitoring is in the control of other variables that can affect the effectiveness of the process. In the example of steam, this can include the quality of the steam (section 5.2), variations in the load being sterilized, and in the case of reusable devices, if the cleaning process has been sufficient prior to sterilization (section 1.4.8). Despite these concerns, parametric controlled processes have been successfully adopted in many industrial and medical applications. Disinfection and sterilization processes are also routinely tested and monitored using mechanical indicators, in combination with chemical and/or biological indicators.

1.4.2.6 Microscopy and Other Techniques. Other methods can be used to evaluate the efficacies of biocidal processes and products. These are generally used due to restrictions on the cultivation of various microorganisms under laboratory conditions. Microscopy or other detection (biochemical and genetic) methods for the presence of microbial contaminants have been used; however, these methods can identify the presence of an organism but may not necessarily detect its actual viability. A specific example of the use of microscopy is in the determination of viability of protozoan (oo)cysts or helminth eggs. In the case of protozoa, the viability of cysts can be determined *in vitro* by suspension in a specific medium and under controlled conditions (including temperature) to cause cysts to excyst and release their vegetative forms (section 1.3.3.4); this can be monitored microscopically and is considered a reasonable indication of cyst viability. Cell culture methods (using mammalian cells) have also been developed to determine cyst viability and are also widely used to culture viruses and some bacteria. In many of these cases, *in vitro* methods are not sufficiently developed to determine microbial viability, and the use of *in vivo* (animal) models is required. An example of this is with prions (section 1.3.6), which are proposed infectious proteins; although the biochemical detection of the protein can be used as an initial (yet unreliable) indication of inactivation, and cell culture assays have been described, *in vivo* infectivity models are unfortunately preferred to confirm activity against these unusual agents.

1.4.3 Disinfection versus Sterilization

In the consideration of biocides and biocidal processes there is an important distinction to be made between disinfection and sterilization. Disinfection is the reduction of the number of viable microorganisms to a level previously specified as appropriate for the surface or product's intended further handling or use; however, "safe to handle" does not necessarily mean that all microorganisms are killed or removed, and different levels of disinfection can be defined including pasteurization, sanitization, and high-, intermediate-, or low-level disinfection (see chapters 2 and 3). In contrast, sterilization is defined as a validated process used to render a surface or product free from viable organisms, or "sterile." This includes physical (e.g., heat and radiation [chapter 5]) and chemical (e.g., ethylene oxide gas [chapter 6]) processes. Disinfection efficacy can be demonstrated using various surface and suspension tests (section 1.4.2), many of which are specified to meet local requirements for product registration and labeling (e.g., in the United States with Food and Drug Administration- or Environmental Protection Agency [EPA]-registered disinfectants). Sterilization processes require investigations that are more detailed. These include an analysis of the sterilizing agent itself and the definition of the use of the agent in a standardized sterilization process for specific applications.

Characterization of any sterilizing agent should include:

- Definition of the sterilization agent (e.g., generation, stability, physical chemistry, and safety)
- Detailed antimicrobial studies (see below)
- Identification of the variables that can affect the antimicrobial activity of the agent, including temperature, humidity, time, distribution, penetration, and (for some applications) the presence of soil

The sterilization process should be shown to be effective against a broad range of microorganisms including bacteria, mycobacteria, viruses, fungi, protozoa, and bacterial spores. From this analysis, specific resistant microorganisms (usually bacterial spores [see section 1.4.2.3]) are chosen to establish the mathematical relationship on exposure to the sterilizing agent. This can be determined using the various suspension and surface tests (direct enumeration and fraction negative) specified in section 1.4.2) and by plotting the number of microbial survivors on exposure to the sterilizing agent over time (Fig. 1.25).

This analysis allows the determination of the probability that a microorganism will survive the sterilization process when the microbial reduction has been shown to be predictable (linear). Because it is difficult to confirm by testing that sterility has been achieved in a given process, the concept of the mathematical probability of having a survivor is used and

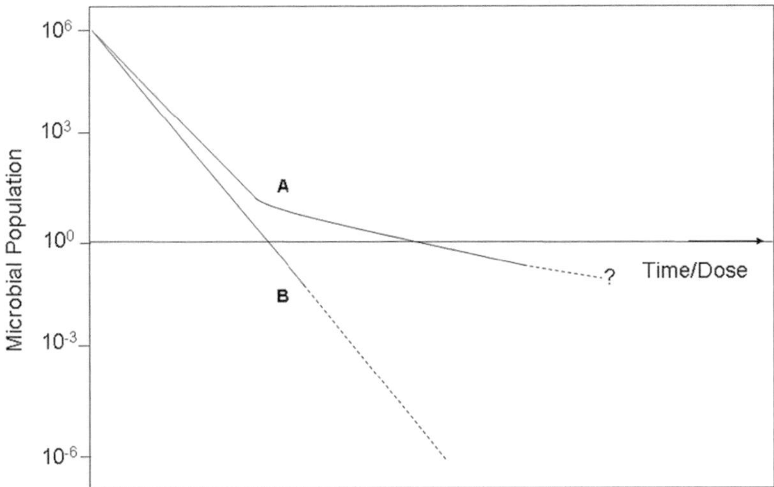

FIGURE 1.25 The rate of microbial inactivation on exposure to sterilization processes. In this case, the test microorganism (generally bacterial spores) at a starting population of 10^6 is exposed to the sterilizing agent under two conditions (A and B). The number of microorganisms can be determined over the contact time with or dose of the antimicrobial using a combination of direct enumeration and fraction negative methods (solid lines). Note that the microbial population (y axis) is plotted in a $\log_{10}$ scale. In process A, "tailing" is observed which may not allow the extrapolation of the kill curve to a defined probability of survival (known as a sterility assurance level, SAL). In process B, the kill curve is linear, allowing extrapolation (dotted line) to an SAL of 10^{-6}.

defined as the sterility assurance level (SAL). The SAL can be defined as the probability of survival of a single viable microorganism after a sterilization process (generally expressed as 10^{-n}). For example, it is common in health care sterilization applications to use an SAL of 10^{-6}, implying a <1 in a million chance that an item may be contaminated. Note that the lower the SAL, the greater the assurance of sterility (e.g., an SAL of 10^{-6} has a greater assurance of sterility than an SAL of 10^{-3}). Remember that sterility is an absolute term defined as the state of being free from viable microorganisms (or sterile). It is therefore not correct to state that a product exposed to a given sterilization process is more or less sterile, although the assurance of sterilization can be greater or less. If we consider the example in Fig. 1.25, if the product had a starting population of the test microorganism at 1×10^6 (6.0 $\log_{10}$), then a 6 $\log_{10}$ reduction would theoretically leave 1 (0 $\log_{10}$) remaining. A 7 $\log_{10}$ reduction would therefore be 0.1 (-1 $\log_{10}$), a 9 $\log_{10}$ reduction would be 0.001 (-3 $\log_{10}$), and a 12 $\log_{10}$ reduction would be 0.000001 (-6 $\log_{10}$); all of these may be considered sterile, but the SAL is lower (10^{-6} compared to 10^{-3} or 10^{-1}) and gives greater mathematical assurance that an organism could survive.

When the sterilizing agent conditions are understood experimentally, they can then be applied in actual sterilization processes, which include specific loads for treatment (such as packaged liquids and devices) in equipment that is used to provide and control the required conditions (e.g., steam sterilizers or radiation exposure chambers; chapters 5 and 6). These processes are also required to be tested to ensure that the minimum sterilizing conditions previously determined to be effective are met within the load. Two basic methods are recommended: overkill and bioburden-based methods. Overkill methods are widely used because they assume a worst-case scenario, such as in the sterilization of single-use and reusable devices. With these methods, a known population of a test microorganism (generally a resistant bacterial spore strain inoculated directly into or onto a product, or indirectly using a biological indicator [see section 1.4.2.4]) is placed at worst-case locations within the load. The minimum time or dose to give complete kill of the test microorganism is determined, typically based on previous analysis of the sterilization process being used. This time/dose is then at least doubled to give a conservative sterilization cycle. A typical overkill method is shown in Fig. 1.25B, using a starting population of 10^6 and being extrapolated, based on previous analysis, to provide an SAL of 10^{-6}. These methods are widely used in the validation of heat and gaseous sterilization processes. Bioburden-based methods are based on a knowledge of the population and resistance of microorganisms present on or in a product; similarly, the reduction of the natural bioburden over the exposure time or dose is determined and extrapolated to give the minimum conditions for the required SAL. Such methods are widely used in the validation of radiation sterilization processes. In some cases, these methods can be combined in the validation of sterilization processes for a specific application.

1.4.4 Choosing a Process or Product

At least two factors should be considered in the choice of any biocidal process or product for a given application: antimicrobial efficacy and safety. For antimicrobial efficacy, the requirements and choice of a biocide for a preservation application (generally being used for bacteriostatic and fungistatic activity) will vary from that of a sterilization process that should render a product sterile and free from microbial contamination. The spectrum of antimicrobial activities for various physical and chemical biocides is considered further in chapters 2 to 6. The choice of biocidal treatment will depend on the risks associated with the level and type of contamination on the surface or in a given product. An example of a risk-based approach is the Spaulding classification system for guidance on reusable devices. These devices are designed for repeated use in many medical, dental, and veterinary applications (e.g., surgery and diagnostics). The Spaulding classification defines these devices as being critical, semicritical, or noncritical based on the risk of transmitting an infection from one patient to another. Critical devices demonstrate the greatest risk because they are introduced directly into the body, contacting the bloodstream or other normally sterile areas of the body. Examples include surgical instrumentation. Due to the risks associated with contamination, it is recommended that critical devices be cleaned and then sterilized between patient uses. Cleaning (or the removal of gross contamination such as tissues, blood, and other body fluids) is required in these and other risk categories, because these materials' presence can reduce or even compromise the effectiveness of the antimicrobial process (see section 1.4.8). Semicritical devices present a lower risk because they may contact intact mucous membranes or nonintact skin during use. Examples include various types of probes or flexible endoscopes used for noninvasive procedures. In these cases, a minimum requirement for cleaning and high-level disinfection is typically recommended, although sterilization is always preferred. High-level disinfectants are considered effective against all microbial pathogens, with the exception of large numbers of bacterial spores. Finally, noncritical devices present the lowest risk of transmission of infection, e.g., they contact intact skin only and at a minimum should be cleaned but are often recommended to be treated with intermediate or low-level disinfectants. Examples may include blood-pressure cuffs, stethoscopes, and miscellaneous patient ward equipment. A similar risk assessment can be used in the choice of any antiseptic, disinfectant, or sterilization process for a given application. In some situations, such as in microbiological research laboratories, the choice of disinfection processes used may be dictated by specific pathogens being handled in these areas or in reducing the risk of cross-contamination during laboratory procedures.

Safety aspects can include hazards in the use of the product, residues that remain on or in a treated product following application, environmental concerns, and the reactivity on mixing with other agents. For this reason, liquid and gaseous biocides are usually provided with safety data sheets that contain information regarding ingredients, hazards, first aid measures, personnel protection, stability/reactivity, toxicology, and ecological (e.g., bioaccumulation) concerns. For automated processes, these details should also be provided with equipment manuals and are often specified in various guidelines and standards. These safety aspects should be reviewed and considered prior to the use of a biocidal product or process. In many countries or regions, the specific use of certain biocides may be restricted due to certain health and environmental concerns.

A particular safety concern is compatibility with the surface or product (material compatibility) to reduce the risk of unexpected damage. Material compatibility may be defined as the suitability of a biocidal product or process to be used on or in a surface or solution without causing unacceptable interactions, damage, or other undesirable effects. It is for this reason that a restricted number of biocides are used on foods or on the skin (as antiseptics [chapter 4]). A wider range of biocides are used on hard surfaces but also vary in compatibility (e.g., some heat-based processes cannot be used for temperature-sensitive surfaces or products). For some applications, biocompatibility may also need to be considered, such as in the use of disinfected or sterilized devices and instruments. Biocompatibility in these cases would consider the risk of an adverse reaction if the biocide remained on a surface and its impact on contact with living tissue or a living system (e.g., toxicity, injury, immune-reactivity, or mutagenicity). In addition to the direct toxicity of biocide residuals, a further consideration can be the impact of the biocide on the surface to create additional toxic substances.

Further considerations in choosing a biocidal product or process depend on the specific application and include reproducibility, ease of use, cycle or application time, costs, national or international guidelines and standards (which are further considered in section 1.4.5), and specific regulatory requirements.

1.4.5 Guidelines and Standards

Various guidelines and standards are available that assist in the choice, use, testing, and validation of biocidal processes and products (examples of these are given in Table 1.25). These include international, country-specific, and even regional requirements, many of which are mandatory for the use of the product or process in certain countries.

1.4.6 Formulation Effects

Unlike many therapeutic antimicrobials (e.g., antibiotics), most biocides are provided in formulation with other ingredients as products. "Formulation" may be defined as the combination of ingredients, including active (biocides) and inert ingredients, into a product for its intended use (e.g., cosmetics, antiseptics, and disinfectants). Other (or excipient) ingredients can include water, nonaqueous solvents, emulsifiers, chelating agents, and corrosion inhibitors. The functions of these ingredients are summarized in Table 1.26.

The formulation of a biocide can be a complex task to ensure the optimization of antimicrobial efficacy, compatibility, required characteristics, and aesthetics of a final product. The first consideration is the choice of the biocide itself, which has an optimal range of concentration, pH, temperature, solubility, stability, and spectrum of activity. It is also clear that the desired performance attributes of the product also need to be considered during its formulation (e.g., the effect of water quality if the product is diluted prior to use, compatibility with surfaces, improved antimicrobial activity in combination with other biocides or excipients). These considerations allow the choice of various formulation ingredients (Table 1.26). The basic components of many formulations are water and other solvents (such as alcohols); although many biocides and other excipients are soluble (ionic or hydrophilic)

TABLE 1.25 Examples of guidelines, standards, and requirements for antisepsis, disinfection, and sterilization

Reference[a]	Title	Summary
Standards		
ISO 14937	Sterilization of health care products - general requirements for characterization of a sterilizing agent and the development, validation and routine control of a sterilization process	Basic requirements for any sterilization process, including characterization of the sterilizing agent and validation of specific sterilization processes
ISO 11137-1	Sterilization of health care products - requirements for the development, validation and routine control of a sterilization process for medical devices - radiation - part 1: requirements	Requirements and tests for radiation sterilization processes including the use of radionucleotides, X rays, and electron beams
EN 285	Sterilization: steam sterilizers. Large sterilizers	Requirements and tests for large steam sterilizers primarily used in health care facilities
ISO 13408-1	Aseptic processing of health care products - part 1: general requirements	Requirements and guidance on the validation and control of aseptically processed health care products in clean rooms and barrier isolator systems
Guidelines		
PDA technical report 11	Sterilization of parenterals by gamma radiation	General information on the development and validation of γ radiation sterilization of parenteral drug preparations
CDC-HICPAC	Guideline for disinfection and sterilization in health care facilities, 2008	Recommendations on methods for cleaning, disinfection, and sterilization of patient care medical devices and the health care environment
APIC	Guideline for hand washing and hand antisepsis in health-care settings	Guidelines on the type and use of various antiseptics in health care applications
WHO/CDS/CSR/LYO/2003.4	Laboratory biosafety manual	Codes of practice for the safe handling of pathogenic microorganisms in laboratories
Requirements		
U.S. FDA CDRH Guidance for Industry and Reviewers	Submission and review of sterility information in premarket notification (510(k)) submissions for devices labeled as sterile	Guidance on the requirements for the registration of devices labeled as sterile that are subject to industrial terminal sterilization processes in the United States
EU 528/2012	Biocidal products regulation	Requirements for the use of biocidal products in the European Union, including disinfectant and preservative safety and efficacy
TGA, TGO ⟨54⟩	Therapeutic goods order no. 54 - standard for disinfectants and sterilants	Guidelines for the registration or listing of disinfectants and sterilants in Australia
EPA, DIS-TSS 01	Disinfectants for use on hard surfaces	Efficacy data requirements for the registration of disinfectants for use on hard surfaces with the U.S. EPA

[a]ISO, International Standards Organization; EN, European Norm, from the CEN (European Committee for Standardization); APIC, Association for Professionals in Infection Control and Epidemiology (United States); U.S. EPA, U.S. Environmental Protection Agency; U.S. FDA CDRH, U.S. Food and Drug Administration, Center for Devices and Radiological Health; CDC-HICPAC, U.S. Centers for Disease Control and Prevention Healthcare Infection Control Practices Advisory Committee; EU: European Union; TGA, Therapeutic Goods Administration, Australia.

in water, many are insoluble (hydrophobic). Biocides are therefore often mixed with emulsifiers, including soaps and detergents, to increase their solubility or dispersion in a formulation. Emulsifiers form micelles, which are aggregated units of surface-active molecules (Fig. 1.26). Soaps are water-soluble salts or fatty acids, which are made by reactions of fats and/or oils with an alkali (e.g., sodium hydroxide). Detergents are mixtures of surfac-

TABLE 1.26 Various constituents of formulated biocidal product

Ingredient	Purpose	Examples
Biocide	Antimicrobial or preservative activity	Quaternary ammonium compounds, phenolics, biguanides
Solvent	Substance (usually liquid) that is capable of dissolving other substances, with water being the most common; used for dissolution and dilution of the biocide and other ingredients	Deionized water, isopropanol, propylene glycol, urea
Emulsifiers/ surfactants	Ingredients (including surfactants) that allow for the formation of stable mixtures ("emulsions") of water- and oil-soluble ingredients. Surfactants (surface acting agents) can also be used as emulsifiers, but also to reduce surface tension, improve wettability on a surface, disperse contaminants, and inhibit foam formation	Sodium lauryl sulfate, potassium laurate, lecithin, nonionic and other surfactants (see chapter 3, section 3.16)
Thickeners	Used to increase the viscosity of a formulation	Polyethylene glycol, polysaccharides such as pectin, gums, and alginates
Chelating agents or sequestrants	Bind metals (such as calcium and magnesium) and inhibit their precipitation; water softening and prevention of mineral deposition	Ethylenediamine, EDTA, EGTA
Alkali or acid	pH stabilization. Alkalis are used as builders to optimize the activity of surfactants, including emulsification of soils. Acids are also used to prevent mineral deposition and for water softening	Alkalis: NaOH, KOH, silicates. Acids: acetic acid, citric acid, phosphoric acid
Buffer	Maintaining the pH over time and increasing alkalinity	Disodium phosphate
Corrosion inhibitors	Reducing corrosion rates and protecting the surface of metals	Nitrates, phosphates, molybdates, ethanolamine
Others	Aesthetic qualities	Colors and fragrances

tants, which are defined as surface-active agents. Surfactant molecules act as low concentrations to change the properties of liquid at its surface or interfaces with a surface. This increases the wettability of the liquid, by breaking its surface tension or the force that holds the surface molecules together and allowing it to spread over a surface better. Surfactants are further defined as nonionic (no charge), anionic (negatively charged), cationic (positively charged), and amphotheric (positively and negatively charged), and many possess antimicrobial activity (chapter 3, section 3.16). Surfactants form micelles (Fig. 1.26) which are useful for the solubilization, dispersion, or emulsification of incompatible materials, as well as aiding in cleaning processes by removal and dispersion of hydrophobic soils from a surface.

Other formulation ingredients, including thickeners, buffers, chelating agents, and fragrances, allow for the further optimization of the stability, efficacy, aesthetics, and compatibility of the product. Due to the variety of ingredients that can be present in a given formulation, the preservative and/or antimicrobial activity can vary considerably. For this reason, those using formulated products should pay close attention to the instructions (or labeling) given for the intended use, including shelf life, application, dilution (if required), contact time for antimicrobial efficacy, spectrum of activity, safety, and compatibility.

1.4.7 Process Effects

Just as the antimicrobial activity of a biocidal product can vary depending on various formulation effects, various process conditions can have a significant impact. These include variables such as temperature, humidity, pressure, time, and biocide concentration. Important process

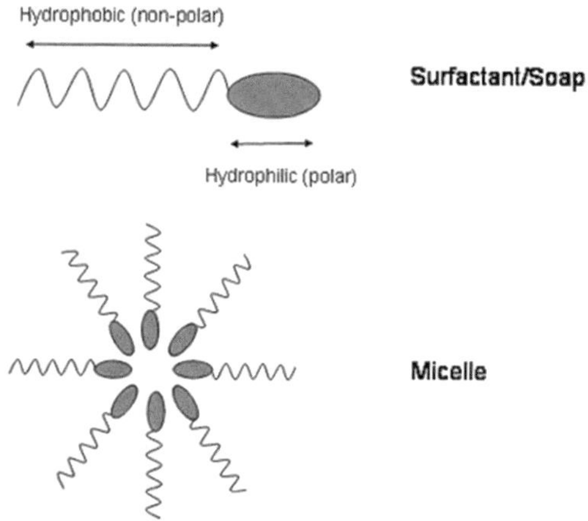

FIGURE 1.26 Basic structures of surfactants/soaps and micelles (a water-in-oil micelle is shown).

variables in various disinfection and sterilization techniques are given in Table 1.27. These are discussed in further detail in chapters 2, 5, and 6.

The activity of a biocide is usually greater as the contact time, temperature, or concentration increases. The effect of contact time is often demonstrated by studying the loss of microbial viability over time, for example, *D*-value determinations (section 1.4.2.1). Some biocidal applications are required to be rapid in action due to their practical use, as in the case of hand-washing or surface disinfection. In contrast, preservative applications are required to control microbial growth within a product over a longer exposure time or within a given shelf life. Temperature itself can be a reliable method of disinfection and sterilization, dependent on the contact time and temperature for a given application (chapter 2, section 2.2). In most cases, the activities of chemical biocides are also increased as the temperature increases; however, in the case of higher temperatures, increased degradation can also be observed depending on the biocide type and temperature conditions. Various materials or applications may also be restricted to lower temperature exposure conditions, for example, in the case of thermosensitive materials or due to safety concerns.

Antimicrobial activity is also greater as the concentration of biocide is increased, but it varies depending on the biocide and its application. A notable example is with alcohols, for which less bacteriocidal activity is observed at concentrations greater than 90% alcohol in water, and the optimal range is 60 to 80%; efficacy is dramatically less at lower concentrations. Further, despite the alcohol concentration, little to no efficacy has been reported against bacterial spores. The optimization of biocide concentration is an important consideration in various disinfection and sterilization processes. Higher biocide concentrations can lead to unwanted effects, including material incompatibility and safety risks, in particular with gas-based applications. In the case of liquid applications, as discussed in section 1.4.6, the efficacy of a biocide can be dramatically enhanced or reduced by various formulation effects that should also be appreciated. These effects include pH (for biocide efficacy and stability), the chemical quality of the water, and the presence of excipients such as surfactants.

The control of relative humidity is an important consideration for most gaseous chem-

TABLE 1.27 Examples of process variables in various disinfection and sterilization techniques

Biocidal process	Variables
Steam (moist heat)	Temperature, time, pressure, quality of steam (including saturation), biocide penetration
Ethylene oxide	Formulation, temperature, humidity, biocide concentration, pressure, time, biocide penetration
Liquid peracetic acid	Formulation, temperature, biocide concentration, time, biocide penetration (e.g., directed flow)
Hydrogen peroxide gas	Temperature, biocide concentration, time, humidity, biocide penetration (vacuum or directed flow)
Radiation	Radiation dose, penetration, exposure time

ical biocidal processes, including ethylene oxide and formaldehyde. Other effects can include the state of the biocide (in liquid or gaseous form) and its delivery (to ensure that all sites are contacted). Many physical and chemical sterilization processes are conducted under vacuum (e.g., ethylene oxide and hydrogen peroxide gas systems), in vacuum/pressure cycles (e.g., steam), or under specific directed flow conditions (with liquids and gases) to optimize the penetration of the biocide to all contact sites within a given load.

1.4.8 The Importance of Cleaning

Cleaning is the removal of contamination from an item to the extent necessary for its further processing or its intended subsequent use. In many applications it is important to ensure the removal of residuals following the use of a reusable surface, for example, to prevent cross-contamination between pharmaceutical manufacturing batches, to reduce the level of bioburden on the surface, and particularly, to ensure that a subsequent biocidal process can be effective. Various surfaces that require routine cleaning including manufacturing vessels, equipment, or areas; food handling surfaces; and reusable medical, veterinary, and dental devices. The presence of various organic (including lipids, proteins, and carbohydrates) and/or inorganic (including various heavy metals such as calcium and iron) soils on these surfaces can often dramatically interfere with the activity of a biocide.

Cleaning is generally achieved by a combination of physical and chemical processes. Physical methods include simple immersion, manual cleaning (brushing and wiping), and automated cleaning. Automated cleaning includes the use of washers (or washer-disinfectors [Fig. 1.27]) and clean-in-place systems. Clean-in-place systems are integrated into manufacturing equipment (such as reaction vessels), which can be automatically cleaned without disassembly. Automated washing machines allow for the placement of items into the washing chamber for exposure to a cleaning process. They can be used for washing only or as washer-disinfectors, which are used to clean and disinfect (using heat and/or chemicals) devices and other articles. They can consist of single- or multiple-chamber washers and provide physical cleaning by agitation, directed flow, spraying, and ultrasonics (where the items are immersed and exposed to sound waves that aid in the physical removal of soil).

Chemical cleaning is achieved using various types of cleaning chemistries (Fig. 1.28). Similar to the formulation of biocides (section

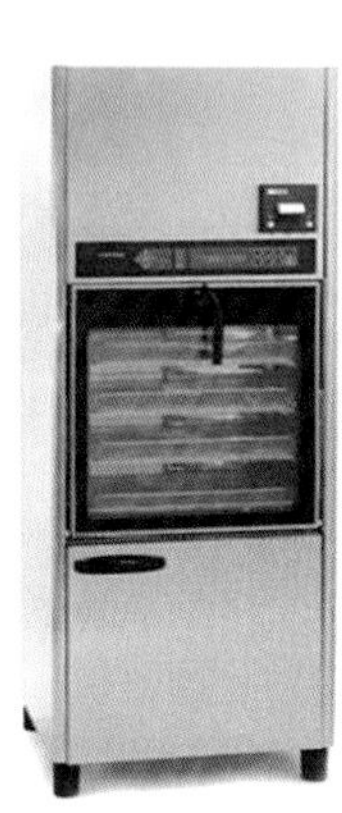

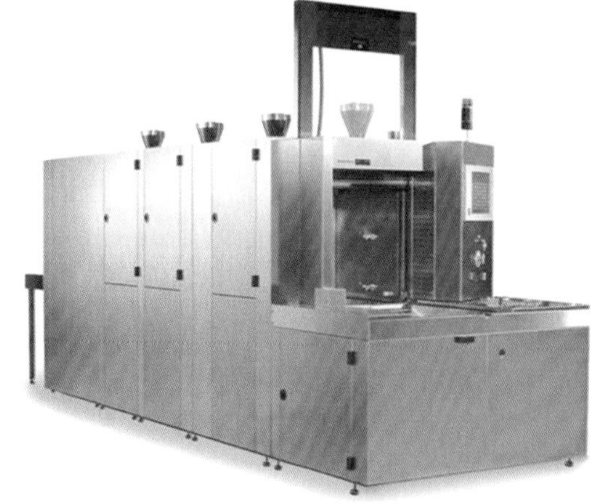

FIGURE 1.27 Examples of single-chamber (left) and multiple-chamber (right) washer-disinfector machines. Washer-disinfectors come in a variety of shapes and sizes depending on their required use. Images courtesy of STERIS, and ©2017 Getinge AB, with permission.

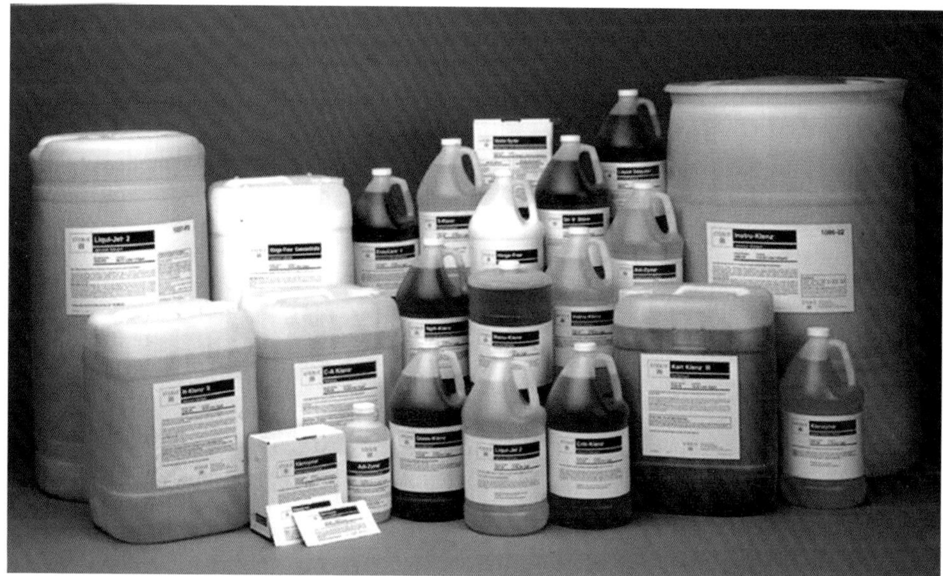

FIGURE 1.28 Various types of cleaning chemistries. Image courtesy of STERIS, with permission.

1.4.6), cleaning formulations can contain a variety of components that aid in the chemical removal of soils from a surface (Table 1.28). Cleaning chemistries can be classified into various types, including enzymatics and nonenzymatics. Enzymatic formulations contain active enzymes that degrade various organic soil components over time, including lipases (lipids and oils), proteases (proteins), and amylases (starch and other carbohydrates). Nonenzymatic formulations can be further subclassified into neutral, acidic, or alkaline cleaning formulations. Acid cleaners are particularly used for the removal of scale and

TABLE 1.28 Various components of cleaning formulations

Ingredient	Purpose
Solvent, including water	A substance (usually liquid) that is capable of dissolving other substances, water being the most common; are also used for solubilization of various soil components
Emulsifiers/surfactants	Ingredients (including surfactants) that allow for the formation of stable mixtures (emulsions) of water- and oil-soluble ingredients. Surfactants (surface-acting agents) can also be used as emulsifiers, but also to reduce surface tension, improve wettability on a surface, disperse contaminants, and inhibit foam formation
Chelating agents or sequestrants	Binding metals (such as calcium and magnesium) and inhibiting their precipitation; water softening and prevention of mineral deposition
Enzymes	Digestion of soil components, including proteases (protein digestion), lipases (lipid/oil digestion), and amylases (carbohydrate such as starch, digestion)
Alkali	Physical removal and breakdown of organic materials such as proteins; pH stabilization; used as builders to optimize the activity of surfactants, including emulsification of soils and degradation of proteins
Acid	Physical removal and breakdown of inorganic material deposits such as scale (calcium carbonate) or pharmaceutical drugs; pH stabilization; also used to prevent and remove mineral deposits and for water softening
Dispersants	Suspending solids
Corrosion inhibitors	Reducing corrosion rates and protecting the surface of metals
Others	Aesthetic qualities, such as perfumes and colors, and biocides such as preservatives

TABLE 1.29 Examples of common water contaminants and their consequences

Contaminant	Examples	Concerns
Inorganic salts	Hardness (dissolved compounds of calcium and magnesium)	Inhibits activity of cleaners and biocidal products; can also cause the buildup of scaling over time or spotting on a surface
	Heavy metals (metallic elements with high atomic weights, e.g., iron, chromium, copper, and lead)	Can inhibit the activity of cleaners and biocidal products; cause damage to some surfaces (e.g., corrosion); in some cases, toxic and bioaccumulative
Organic matter	Trihalomethanes	Toxic chlorine disinfection by-products
	Proteins, lipids, polysaccharides	Can leave harmful residues, including protein toxins and endotoxins (LPS [section 1.3.7]); also reduce the effectiveness of biocides
Biocides	Chlorine, bromine	Can cause corrosion and rusting on surfaces (in particular, when carried in steam)
Microorganisms	*Pseudomonas*, *Salmonella*, and *Cryptosporidium* oocysts	Biofilm formation and biofouling; deposition onto surfaces or products and cross-contamination; infection
Dissolved gases	CO_2, Cl_2, and O_2	Can cause corrosion and rusting (in particular, when carried in steam); noncondensable gases such as CO_2 and O_2 can inhibit the penetration of steam in sterilization processes

mineral deposits, while alkaline cleaners are particularly effective at removing and degrading protein-based soils. Neutral cleaners, depending on their formulations, usually have the widest compatibility with various types of surfaces. In some applications, simpler cleaning chemistries that are employed include alcohol wipes and high-quality water (such as water-for-injection [chapter 5, section 5.2]).

The choice of physical and chemical cleaning processes depends on the types and level of soils that are present on a surface. The overall efficacy and efficiency of these processes can be optimized for a given application by consideration of the cleaning contact time, chemical concentration, temperature, and efficiencies of physical effects.

1.4.9 Water Quality

Water is an important component in many antiseptic, disinfectant, and sterilization applications. Typical uses of water include:

- Biocidal-product formulation (as a solvent)
- Biocidal-product dilution on use (e.g., antiseptics and disinfectants)
- Cleaning alone or in combination with cleaning formulations, prior to disinfection or sterilization
- Pharmaceutical-product preparation (e.g., dilution for injection)
- Rinsing to remove residuals following cleaning or disinfection
- As a disinfectant (moist heat) or sterilization agent (steam)
- Humidification as part of the sterilization processes (e.g., ethylene oxide and formaldehyde)

In addition to these applications, water itself can be a source of microbial contamination. Examples include *Cryptosporidium* and *Giardia*; Gram-negative bacterial pathogens such as *E. coli*, *Legionella*, and *Vibrio*; and toxins such as endotoxins. Various biocidal products and processes are used to render water safe for its intended uses. The most important of these are halogens (such as chlorine and bromine [chapter 3, section 3.11]), oxidizing agents (such as chlorine dioxide and ozone [section 3.13]), moist heat (boiling and steam distillation [chapter 2, section 2.2, and chapter 5, section 5.2]), irradiation (such as UV treatment [section 2.4]), and filtration (for physical removal [section 2.5]).

Water can include various dissolved and suspended contaminants, many of which have negative effects on antiseptic, disinfectant, and sterilization applications (Table 1.29).

Overall, the quality of water used for a particular application will vary. Various qualities include:

- Potable water (water that is considered safe for human consumption, which in many countries is tap water)
- Pretreated water (e.g., softened to remove hardness due to calcium/magnesium ions)
- Disinfected (e.g., UV radiation; chapter 2, section 2.4)
- Filtered to remove gross particulates or pretreated to remove contaminants (e.g., with activated carbon or sodium bisulfite to remove chlorine)
- Sterile filtered water (to physically remove microorganisms; section 2.5)
- Purified water (e.g., by reverse osmosis, deionization, and distillation; section 2.5 and chapter 5, section 5.2)

In some applications, the quality of water required is specified to include microbiological and chemical limits, which should be considered to ensure the safety and effectiveness of biocidal products and processes.

PHYSICAL DISINFECTION

2

2.1 INTRODUCTION

Disinfection is the antimicrobial reduction of the number of viable microorganisms on a product or surface to a level previously specified as appropriate for its intended further handling or use. This chapter considers the most widely used methods of physical disinfection, including heat (moist- and dry-heat methods), cold, radiation, and filtration. Filtration methods are not considered truly biocidal, because the basic principle of action is the physical removal of microbial contamination from liquids and gases (including air) rather than their inactivation; despite this, some consideration is given to filtration as a method of physical disinfection or sterilization. Physical biocidal methods include high and low temperatures; heat-based processes are among the most efficient and convenient techniques of disinfection including specific and widely utilized processes such as pasteurization for the treatment of solid and liquid food. Nonionizing radiation methods, including low-energy UV light, are also considered to be disinfectants, with ionizing radiation technologies further considered in chapter 5, since they are primarily used as sterilization methods.

2.2 HEAT

2.2.1 Types

Physical methods using heat are some of the most widely used and reliable techniques of disinfection. Heat is a form of energy that can be transferred from one system to another due to the difference in their temperatures. Heat can be transferred by conduction (energy transfer from a surface), by convection (transfer by liquid or gas), or by radiation (energy transfer in the form of electromagnetic waves or particles). Here, we are primarily concerned with heat convection and conduction, with further consideration of radiation (for disinfection) in section 2.4.

Heat-based methods can be separated into two basic types:

1. Wet (moist) heat

a. Heating of liquids, including pasteurization and boiling (disinfection)

b. Steam under atmospheric pressure (disinfection)

c. Steam under subatmospheric pressure or low temperature (disinfection)

d. Steam (or water) under pressure (disinfection or sterilization)

2. Dry heat
a. Incineration (sterilization)
b. Hot air (disinfection or sterilization)

Wet heat is an efficient method, because it contains water in a liquid or gaseous (steam) form, which has a higher capacity to carry and transfer heat to a surface than dry air. Dry heat is rarely used as a disinfection process but has been useful for some applications at <140°C, with higher temperature defined as sterilization processes (see chapter 5, section 5.3). Moist heat disinfection methods include immersion in hot water, the direct use of steam, and heating of a liquid or suspension (e.g., pasteurization).

Heat is essentially lethal to all microorganisms, but each type has its own intrinsic tolerance. For example, many common bacterial pathogens (including *Staphylococcus* and *Streptococcus*) are inactivated at moist heat temperatures of ~55 to 60°C, while some spore-producing bacteria are unaffected even at 100°C. The mechanisms behind these resistance profiles are discussed in more detail in chapter 8, section 8.1. Furthermore, lethality is affected by the initial microbial population, temperature distribution, contact time, and materials surrounding the microorganisms (including organic [e.g., protein] and inorganic [e.g., salt] soils).

At the minimum temperature that a microorganism is sensitive to heat thermal inactivation, the rate of microbial lethality is generally considered to be logarithmic and can be plotted as a time/log reduction relationship (Fig. 2.1).

From this plot the decimal reduction time, or *D* value, can be calculated, defined as the time (in minutes or seconds) required at a given temperature to kill 1 log (or 90%) of a given microbial population under stated test conditions. From this graph, the average *D* value can also be determined as the negative reciprocal of the slope of the plotted relationship (−1/slope). With knowledge of the initial population of the target organism, the thermal death time can be determined as the time to achieve a population of 0 (no remaining viable organisms) at the test temperature for a given application. It is expected that as the temperature increases, so does the lethal effect on the test microorganism, thereby reducing the *D* value and the thermal death time. Therefore, a further relationship which can be determined is the effect of various temperatures on the *D* value (Fig. 2.2). This relationship is also considered logarithmic, and from it can be calculated the *Z* value, which is defined as the temperature change required to produce a change in the *D* value by a factor of 10. Therefore, the *D* value is expressed as a time and the *Z* value as a temperature.

The *D* values and *Z* values are the basis for determining the heat-sensitivity of microorganisms. For heat-based disinfection processes, it is typical to choose a test organism with the highest resistance to heat and determine the *D* and *Z* values. For example, *Mycobacterium tuberculosis* or *Coxiella burnetii* may be used in determining the values for pasteurization processes, *Enterococcus* or *Legionella* species for device disinfection, and *Geobacillus stearothermophilus* spores for sterilization processes. From these values, the disinfection time can be determined, depending on the desired (or tolerated) temperature and required level of microbial log reduction. Because the chosen test organism demonstrates greater resistance than other organisms that could be typically present, it is expected that the disinfection process will be efficient for the intended application.

As water is heated to 100°C at atmospheric pressure, steam is formed. Steam is used as a direct disinfecting agent or as a source of heat for other methods. The temperature at which steam is formed is dependent on the pressure. For example, when the pressure is reduced (by pulling a vacuum or under subatmospheric conditions), the temperature at which steam is formed is lowered; equally, as the pressure is increased, the temperature of steam rises. These processes require special chambers to achieve the necessary pressure levels, with the latter (steam-under-pressure) description as the basis of steam sterilization, which is discussed in more detail in chapter 5, section 5.2.

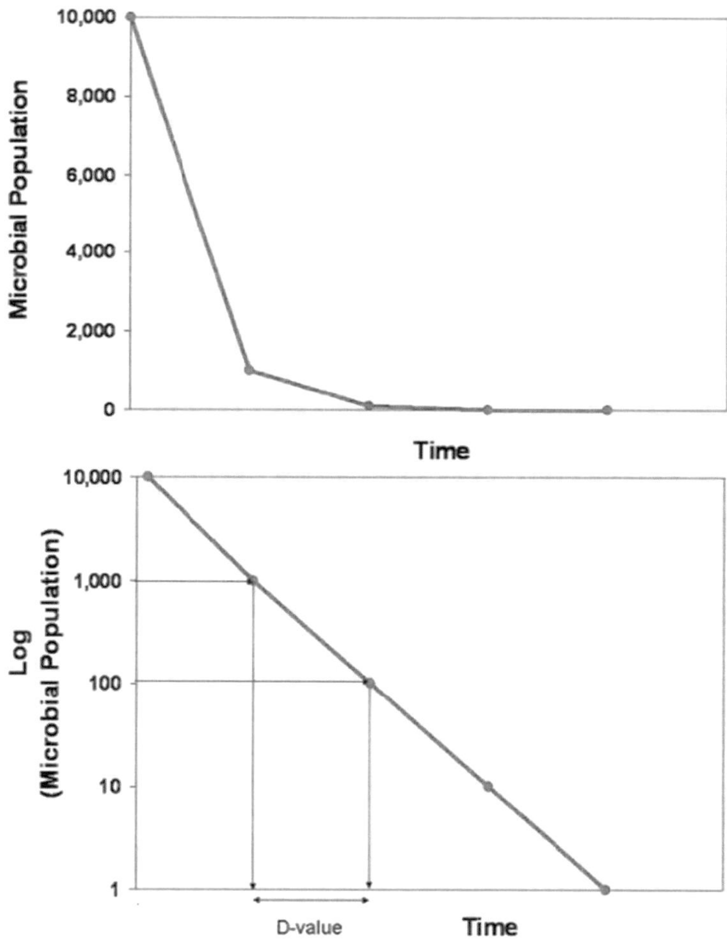

FIGURE 2.1 Typical microbial sensitivity to moist heat disinfection.

2.2.2 Applications

Moist heat-based disinfection can be routinely obtained by heating to temperatures greater than 60 to 65°C, at which most bacteria, viruses, fungi, and other pathogens or unwanted microbial contaminants are inactivated (Fig. 2.4, in section 2.2.3), with the exception of some bacterial spores. Simple applications include the boiling of drinking water or immersion of surgical instruments or other materials into heated water for the required disinfection time. The boiling of instruments in water for ≥5 minutes is a useful process for rapid disinfection, in particular, in emergency situations. Hot water is the method of choice for routine disinfection of temperature-resistant materials. Applications include automated washer-disinfector machines (for reusable surgical devices, bed-pans, and other materials) (see chapter 1, section 1.4.8) and laundry disinfection. In general, the disinfection time depends on the temperature. Recommended examples of overkill moist-heat disinfection times for medical or veterinary surgical devices include:

- 100 minutes at 70°C
- 10 minutes at 80°C
- 1 minute at 90°C
- 0.1 minute at 100°C

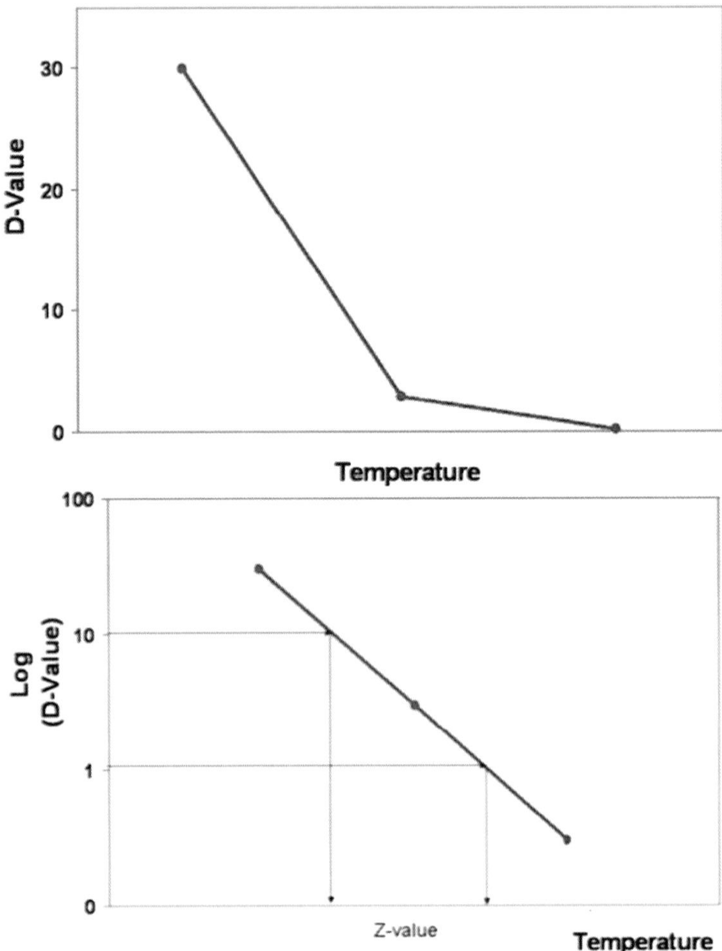

FIGURE 2.2 Effect of temperature on microbial lethality and *Z*-value determination.

Pasteurization is considered a mild disinfection process generally applied to foods or other liquids to reduce the risk of the presence of pathogens and to improve the shelf life of the product by reducing the presence of food spoilage organisms. It is widely used for the treatment of milk and milk products, beer, juices, and vaccines (Fig. 2.3) and as an alternative to boiling for device disinfection in water.

Typical pasteurization processes are developed at a temperature and time that do not destroy the product but provide a level of disinfection acceptable for the subsequent use of the product (e.g., human consumption). Examples include traditional processes at 63 to 66°C for ≥30 minutes and "flash" pasteurization processes at 71 to 72°C for ≥15 to 16 seconds. Pasteurization can be performed as a batch or as a continuous-duty process. Following heat treatment, the product shelf life can be further extended by storing the product at a low temperature (<10°C), which inhibits the growth of spoilage organisms. An alternative process to pasteurization for food products is ultra-high-temperature processing. The product is treated at temperatures ≥100°C (e.g., 140°C for 4 seconds) and then aseptically placed into presterilized storage containers. Ultra-high-temperature

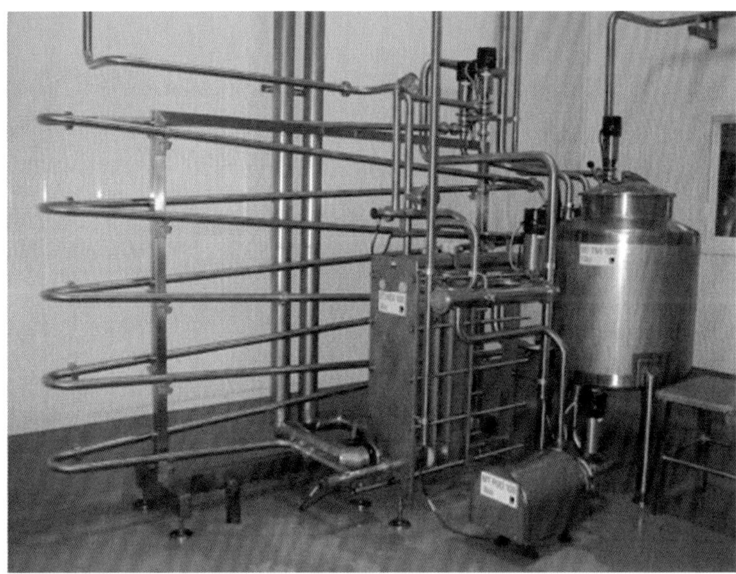

FIGURE 2.3 A pasteurizer for heat treatment of liquids. Image courtesy of System Projects, Ltd.

(UHT) processes are generally performed as continuous-duty processes by the direct injection of steam under pressure (convection) or other indirect heated surfaces (conduction).

Steam may be used directly for rapid disinfection of general surfaces (e.g., steam cleaning). Low-temperature steam (or steam under vacuum) can be used for the disinfection of fabrics and temperature-sensitive instruments, generally at 70 to 95°C. It is also used as a rapid humidification process prior to exposure to chemical sterilants and fumigants, including ethylene oxide, formaldehyde, chlorine dioxide, and ozone (chapters 3 and 6). A method known as tyndallization is used for the disinfection of liquids, in particular, temperature-sensitive liquids that contain proteins or carbohydrates. This process involves repeated cycles of heating (by conduction or direct injection of steam) and cooling over 3 days to allow initial disinfection of vegetative organisms, germination of any spore-forming bacteria or fungi, and subsequent redisinfection.

Dry heat is rarely used as a true disinfection process, but it can be useful for the treatment of resistant materials including glassware and metal at temperatures <140°C. While dry heat has some direct antimicrobial effect, it also causes drying of (or the removal of moisture from) microorganisms, which is biostatic and even biocidal to many bacteria and viruses. Drying is a useful method of preserving the sterility or disinfected state of surfaces and reducing the risk of subsequent microbial growth.

Finally, heat plays an essential role in the overall efficacy of cleaning and biocidal disinfection processes. Most cleaning processes are more effective at temperatures >30 but <60°C, at which point proteins can coagulate and become difficult to remove from contaminated surfaces. An example is enzymatic-based cleaners, which are typically more active in the 40 to 60°C range (chapter 1, section 1.4.8). The role of humidification has already been described as being required for the antimicrobial activity of many chemical biocides. It is also used in combination with other biocides to enhance their activities; in general, as the temperature increases, the antimicrobial effect also increases, although in some cases higher temperature may also cause greater biocide degradation. Examples of various standards and guidelines for heat disinfection are given in Table 2.1.

TABLE 2.1 Examples of standards and guidelines on heat disinfection

Reference[a]	Title	Summary
FDA/CFSAN	Grade A pasteurized milk ordinance	Regulations on the safety and sanitation of milk
FDA/CDRH	Class II special controls guidance document: medical washers and medical washer-disinfectors	Guidance on the content and format for registration of washer-disinfectors, including disinfection testing
ISO 15883-1	Washer-disinfectors - part 1: general requirements, definitions and tests	Requirements for washer-disinfectors, including heat disinfection testing and requirements
AS 4187	Cleaning, disinfecting and sterilizing reusable medical and surgical instruments and equipment, and maintenance of associated environments in health care facilities	Guideline on disinfection and sterilization practices in health care facilities
CFIS (2001)	Recommendations for the production and distribution of juice in Canada	Recommendations on the heat treatment and pasteurization of juices

[a]FDA/CFSAN, U.S. Food and Drug Administration, Center for Food Safety and Applied Nutrition; FDA/CDRH: U.S. FDA, Center for Devices and Radiological Health; ISO, International Standards Organization; AS, Australian standard; CFIS, Canadian Food Inspection Agency

2.2.3 Spectrum of Activity

In general, as temperature increases, so does the activity against microorganisms with variable intrinsic and acquired resistance mechanisms to heat (Fig. 2.4).

Most pathogenic and spoilage microorganisms are readily inactivated at temperatures greater than 65°C. Some vegetative bacteria and viruses demonstrate unusual tolerance to heat; these microorganisms are known as thermophiles and may be defined as microorganisms that can live or survive temperatures above 45 to 50°C (see chapter 8, sections 8.3.9 and 8.3.10). Some examples include *Legionella*, *Enterococcus*, *Coxiella*, and *Mycobacterium* spp., as well as viruses such as parvoviruses and noroviruses. In general, the thermophiles are readily inactivated at 70 to 90°C, although the overall tolerance to heat is affected by the suspension media and growth conditions, as well as specific developmental responses in bacteria and fungi to heat treatment (e.g., the heat shock response [see section 8.3.3]). A dramatic developmental response is the production of spores, which

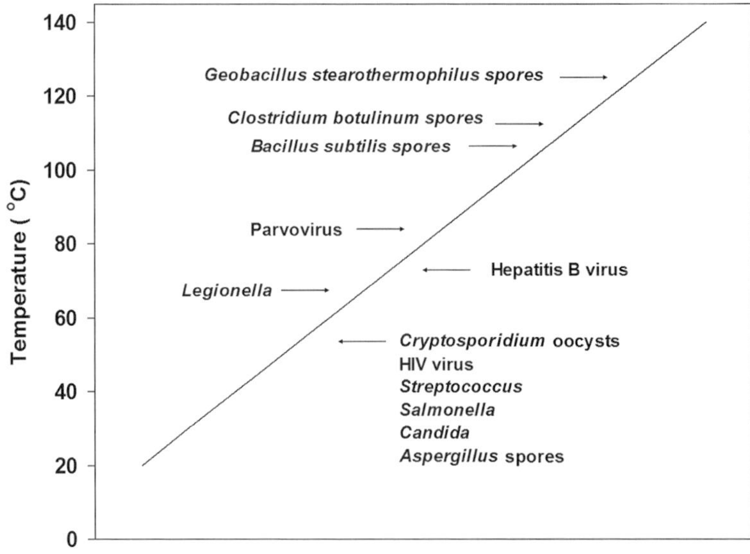

FIGURE 2.4 Moist heat resistance of microorganisms.

consist of a central dormant and modified cell surrounded by multiple protective layers that present a significant barrier to the effects of chemical and physical agents (the development, structure, and resistance of spores are discussed in greater detail in section 8.3.11). Fungi and some bacteria produce spores, but the bacterial spores, including *Bacillus*, *Geobacillus*, and *Clostridium* spores, are considered the most resistant to heat, with heat treatments requiring temperatures in excess of 100°C to be effective. Another group of thermophiles (known as extreme or "hyperthermophiles"), which are capable of growing and surviving at temperatures >80 to 90°C, have also been described (see section 8.3.10). These include archaea species such as *Thermocrinis ruber*, *Thermotoga maritime*, and *Thermus aquaticus*, which have been isolated from hot springs and deep sea vents. Some species have been described as growing at up to 160°C and owe their resistance to unique protective mechanisms including protein design, DNA repair and protection functions, and unique cell wall/cell membrane structures. These organisms are not considered to be feasible pathogens or contaminants and are not considered a concern for routine disinfection or sterilization processes.

Although many bacterial and fungal toxins are readily inactivated by heat, bacterial endotoxins are resistant to moist and dry heat, with high dry sterilization temperatures required for effective destruction. Prions have also shown dramatic resistance to heat-based disinfection processes, although these results may be at least partially due to protective effects (such as fixed protein and lipids) preventing heat penetration. In particular, prions are highly resistant to dry heat but have been shown to be partially reduced by boiling in water for extended times. Hydration appears to play an important role in the activity of heat-based processes against prions.

2.2.4 Advantages

Heat disinfection methods (in particular, moist heat) are easy to use, flexible for various applications, readily available, and cost-effective. They are the most widely accepted methods for being reliable, broad spectrum, and well-described. With *D*- and *Z*-value determinations, heat-based methods can be predictive and allow for simple verification of efficiency by temperature monitoring. Pasteurization methods reduce the risk of pathogen contamination in foodstuffs and extend the shelf life of products. Moist heat is an effective method for the humidification and heating of materials for subsequent sterilization by heat and/or chemicals, while dry heat is effective for drying surfaces post-disinfection/-sterilization. Finally, heat is a synergistic agent for many chemical biocidal processes.

2.2.5 Disadvantages

Care should be taken in the handling of heating methods or treated materials/surfaces due to the risk of burning. Surfaces and liquids should be allowed to cool down before use. In the case of boiling surgical devices, they should be used immediately following cool down and should not be stored prior to use. Heating can damage liquids (in particular, if they contain biological materials such as proteins that need to be preserved) and surfaces, such as many temperature-sensitive polymers. Damage can also occur on temperature-resistant materials from stress-cracking, warping, and corrosion. Pasteurization can change the taste of foodstuffs, but this can generally be controlled by process optimization. Dry-heat disinfection typically can be used for inanimate surfaces such as metals and glass.

It is necessary to ensure that all surfaces are exposed to the minimum disinfection temperature for the required disinfection time. Similarly, the temperature distribution in a liquid needs to be uniform, because cold spots can occur that may not be adequately disinfected. The quality of the water may affect the efficacy and safety of moist heating processes (chapter 1, section 1.4.9). Heat disinfection can cause the release of endotoxin from some Gram-negative bacteria, which is resistant to disinfection temperatures; endotoxins can cause pyrogenic reactions (i.e., fever) if introduced directly into the bloodstream (section 1.3.7). The efficacy of heat can be reduced in the presence of organic and inorganic soils, in particular, dried salts, due to lack of heat penetration to the target microbial population.

2.2.6 Mode of Action

Heat clearly has multiple effects on the viability of microorganisms. High temperatures can initially cause the denaturation of structural and functional proteins, unwinding of nucleic acids, and destabilization of surface structures, including cell walls, cell membranes, and viral envelopes. These effects alone cause the release of cytoplasmic materials and can accumulate to lead to cell death or loss of viral infectivity. As the temperature increases further, proteins and other biomolecules precipitate, leading to further loss of structure, function, and cell lysis. Higher temperatures are required to penetrate the multiple protective layers of bacterial spores and have an effect on the more sensitive inner core. Heat treatment leads to the release of dipicolinic acid and calcium from spores; dipicolinic acid and calcium are considered to play a role in protecting proteins in the inner core from heat damage and are examples of the multiple resistance mechanisms that protect spores from the effects of heat (these are further discussed in chapter 8, section 8.3.11).

2.3 COLD TEMPERATURES

Cold temperatures—cooling to temperatures of $<10°C$ and freezing at $<0°C$—have biostatic and some biocidal effects. At a minimum, cold conditions can prevent or reduce the growth of microorganisms due to the need for specific temperatures for the activity of cellular enzymes. These are generally considered effective and widely used preservative methods (e.g., refrigeration and freezing for the storage of microbial cultures). However, some bacteria, including *Listeria*, and fungi can multiply at refrigeration temperatures (4 to 10°C); these microorganisms are known as psychrophiles. In most cases, microorganisms remain viable under these conditions and grow when the necessary temperatures and growth conditions are restored.

Freezing as a microbial preservation method can include storage at −10 to −80°C, usually in the presence of a stabilizer such as glycerol and dimethyl sulfoxide, or by freeze-drying, a method of removing water from a frozen product directly into a gas by a process known as sublimation. Immersion in liquid nitrogen (at −196°C) is also used as a rapid freezing process. Freeze-thawing cycles can cause inactivation of proteins and cell wall/membrane structure damage/lysis (due to ice crystal formation), leading to the death of vegetative microorganisms.

2.4 RADIATION

Radiation is energy in motion and refers to a natural process in which unstable atoms of an element emit (or radiate) excess energy in the form of particles or electromagnetic waves. For the purpose of this discussion, radiation sources will be considered as isotopes (naturally occurring or manufactured unstable atoms) or other sources of electromagnetic radiation. Electromagnetic radiation is energy transmitted in the form of waves or rays including X rays, UV, and infrared, which are considered to be within the electromagnetic spectrum.

2.4.1 Isotopes

In its simplest form, an atom is a unit of matter which is indivisible by chemical means. It consists of a nucleus, consisting of positively charged protons and neutral neutrons, surrounded by negatively charged electrons contained within defined orbits, or energy levels, around the central nucleus (Fig. 2.5).

There are at least 118 known natural and synthetic elements (as listed in the periodic table of elements), including the building blocks of biological materials such as carbon, hydrogen, and oxygen, which have an overall neutral charge; i.e., in each atom the number of protons equals the number of electrons. Where there is an overall positive or negative charge, the atom is known as an isotope (e.g., ^{35}sulfur, ^{32}phosphorus, ^{60}cobalt). Isotopes are unstable and spontaneously decay, causing the release of radiation (Fig. 2.5) from an atom in the form of streaming particulates (α or β

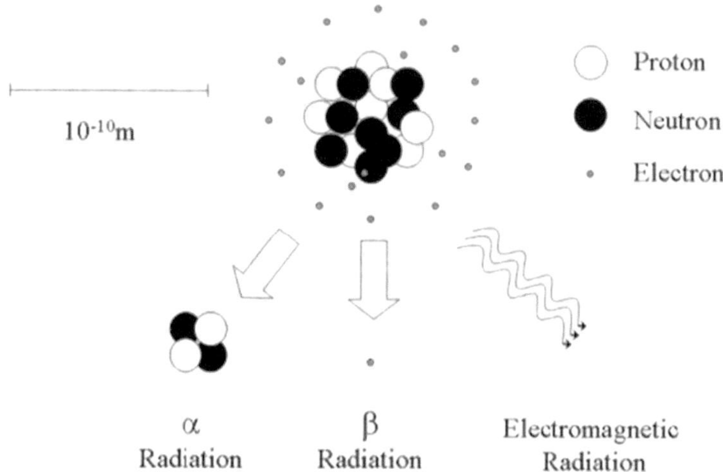

FIGURE 2.5 Atomic structure and the source of radiation.

radiation) or electromagnetic waves (for example, γ radiation). These energy particles or waves have a lethal effect on microorganisms, but their energies or penetration capabilities vary. α particles consist of 2 protons and 2 neutrons (essentially the helium nucleus, ^{4}He) and have a +2 charge. α radiation, although reactive, is not considered further as a disinfection method because it is not highly penetrating; for example, α radiation does not pass through paper or skin. β particles, when accelerated, and γ radiation are widely used for industrial processes, including sterilization, deinfestation, food preservation, and decontamination of devices, materials (e.g., bandages), cosmetics, and foodstuffs. β particles are electrons (with a −1 charge), which demonstrate greater penetration than α particles but can still be shielded by soft metals such as aluminum. β radiation-emitting isotopes (e.g., ^{32}P) are not generally used as direct sources for disinfection, but β particles can be more readily produced from an electron gun (e.g., a heated filament) and are then accelerated by passage through an electrical field to enhance their penetration capabilities. γ radiation is directly sourced from radioisotopes, including ^{60}Co and ^{137}Cs, which release γ radiation at specific energies and are direct sources. γ radiation is a high-energy form of electromagnetic radiation and is used for disinfection, sterilization, and deinfestation. Both β (accelerated) and γ radiation methods are considered in more detail as sterilization processes in chapter 5, section 5.4, with consideration of other sources of electromagnetic radiation in this section.

2.4.2 Electromagnetic Radiation

Electromagnetic radiation is by definition light waves or, more specifically, fluctuations of electric and magnetic fields in space. The basic unit or particle of electromagnetic radiation is the photon, which (unlike particle radiation) has no mass or electric charge and travels at the speed of light in a wave-like pattern. There are many types of electromagnetic radiation, ranging from radio waves to γ waves, which differ and are classified by their respective energies and wavelengths (Fig. 2.6). A wavelength can be defined as the length in meters of a single wave of photon energy or the distance between the two adjacent wave peaks. As the wavelength (given as λ) becomes shorter, the frequency (number of waves that pass a given point at a given time, recorded in hertz) increases. For example, radio waves have very long wavelengths, low frequency, and low energy, in contrast to γ rays, which have very short wavelengths, high frequency, and high energy (Table 2.2).

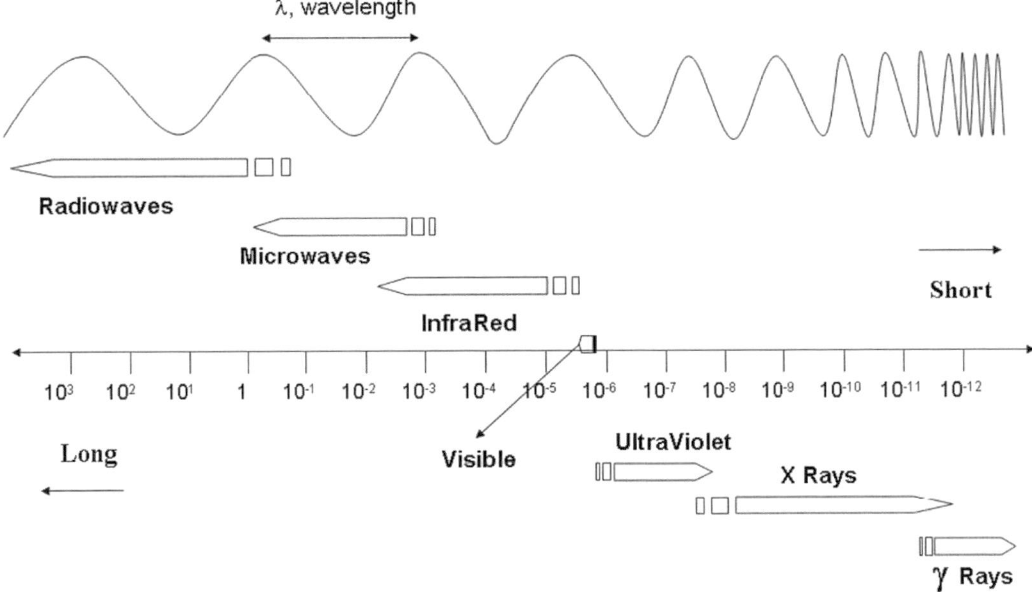

FIGURE 2.6 The electromagnetic spectrum. The range of wavelengths is shown on the axis in meters, with the longest wavelengths on the left (radio waves) and shortest on the right (γ rays).

As disinfection agents, higher-energy types of radiation are clearly more effective and penetrating. For disinfection purposes, the electromagnetic spectrum can be divided into ionizing or nonionizing radiation. Ionizing radiation has enough energy to cause the release of electrons from the target atom, which therefore becomes charged. Both γ and X rays are ionizing radiation; they are often differentiated by their source: γ radiation is released from the decay of the nuclei, and X rays, from the orbiting electrons of atoms. Nonionizing radiation causes the excitation of electrons and in some cases electron transitions from one orbit to another, which can lead to an increase in temperature depending on the exposure time and energy; nonionizing radiation used for disinfection includes UV, infrared, and microwaves. Visible light itself can be antimicrobial under excessive exposure but is generally not used as a disinfection method (with the exception of pulsed light technology discussed in chapter 5, section 5.6.2).

TABLE 2.2 The wavelengths and energies of electromagnetic radiation

Radiation	Wavelength (λ) (meters)	Energy (joules)
Nonionizing		
Radio waves	$>1 \times 10^{-1}$	$<2 \times 10^{-24}$
Microwaves	$1 \times 10^{-1} - 1 \times 10^{-3}$	$2 \times 10^{-24} - 2 \times 10^{-22}$
Infrared	$1 \times 10^{-3} - 7 \times 10^{-7}$	$2 \times 10^{-22} - 3 \times 10^{-19}$
Visual	$7 \times 10^{7} - 4 \times 10^{-7}$ (violet........blue)	$3 \times 10^{19} - 5 \times 10^{-19}$
UV	$4 \times 10^{-7} - 1 \times 10^{-8}$	$5 \times 10^{-19} - 2 \times 10^{-17}$
Ionizing		
X rays	$1 \times 10^{-8} - 1 \times 10^{-11}$	$2 \times 10^{-17} - 2 \times 10^{-14}$
γ rays	$<1 \times 10^{-11}$	$> 2 \times 10^{-14}$

2.4.3 Types

Ionizing radiation (γ and X rays) is used for disinfection and deinfestation but is further considered as a physical sterilization method (chapter 5, section 5.4). Nonionizing radiation methods used for disinfection include UV, infrared, and microwaves. Nonionizing radiation is emitted from atoms when electrons in an excited stage transition from a higher to a lower energy state to give photons in their respective wavelength/energy range (Table 2.2).

2.4.3.1 Ultraviolet. The main source of UV radiation is simple UV lights, including mercury vapor lamps, fluorescent lights, pulsed UV lamps, and "black-light" lamps. A typical representation of a mercury vapor lamp is shown in Fig. 2.7. Lamps can range in diameter and length, for example, 15 to 25 mm and 100 to 1,200 mm, respectively. A typical lamp consists of a sealed tube of UV-transmitting material (e.g., quartz) with an electrode on both ends and containing a small amount of mercury and an inert gas (typically argon) under pressure. UV light is produced by applying electricity (voltage) to the lamp to cause an electric arc and the subsequent excitation of the electrons in the available mercury vapor. When these excited atoms return to their ground state, they release photons within the UV wavelength range (~350 to 100 nm). The inert (argon) gas has only an extraneous function, including extending the lamp life and reducing thermal loss (noting that heat is another form of energy and will reduce light output).

A variety of UV lamps is available, including the following:

- Low-pressure mercury lamps (see, for example, Fig. 2.7). A low amount of mercury vapor is maintained at very low internal lamp pressures (typically <0.001 kilopascal). Some designs include small amounts of other metals (including gallium and indium), which can increase the UV output. These are probably the most widely used UV sources and have a standard output of UV at 254 nm (primarily) and 185 nm. The energy output is considered low, but they are efficient and have a long effective life. Typical operating temperatures are 40 to 100°C.
- Medium-pressure mercury lamps. These lamps have fundamentally the same design as low-pressure lamps but contain a higher amount of mercury, maintained at or near atmospheric pressure, and emit a wider range of wavelengths (200

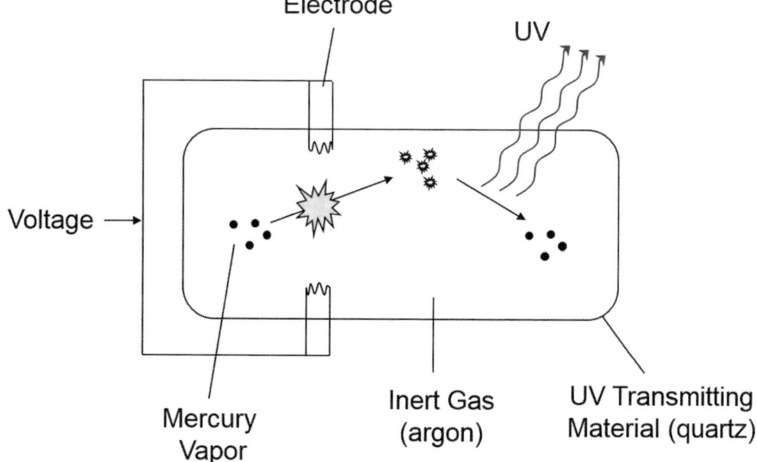

FIGURE 2.7 A representation of a typical UV (low-pressure UV mercury) lamp and the generation of UV radiation.

TABLE 2.3 Types of UV radiation

UV type	Common name	Wavelength range (nm)	Comments
UV-A	Long wave	315–400	"Fluorescent" light, black light
UV-B	Medium wave	280–315	Responsible for sunburn
UV-C	Short wave	200–280	Germicidal range

to 400 nm). These lamps have a characteristic higher UV output but shorter usable life.

- "Flash" lamps are usually operated above atmospheric pressure and also emit a wide wavelength range (170 to 400 nm). These include pulsed-light and eximer lamps. Pulsed-light lamps typically contain xenon gas and require a high voltage supply pulse (up to 30 times a second) to provide a high output of UV light. Eximer lamps use rare gas-halogen mixtures, including KrCl (which emits at 222 nm) and XeBr (emits at 281 nm). Flash lamps have a shorter life, require more power, and are less used than low- and medium-pressure lamps.

Not all UV wavelengths are effective against microorganisms (Table 2.3). The most effective range is the UV-C, or "short" UV wavelengths, in the 200- to 280-nm range. The most effective wavelength has been found to be ~265 nm.

2.4.3.2 Infrared. The infrared radiation range spans the ~0.7- to 1,000-μm wavelength range and can be further subdivided into near, middle, and far infrared (Table 2.4). The near (or short to medium) infrared range is the most widely used for heating/disinfection purposes. Even within this range, infrared does not tend to cause electron transitions and is only adsorbed by atoms with small energy differences in their orbiting electrons. Therefore, infrared is used for surface treatments only and provides a source of heat directly on those surfaces, which can range from 50 to 1,000°C, depending on the wattage of the source lamp. Therefore, infrared can be considered a method of dry heat disinfection or sterilization (chapter 5, section 5.3). Infrared (or "heat") lamps consist of single or multiple heated filaments, which use low energy and heat quickly to release within the desired wavelength in the infrared range. The lamp itself can be made of red or clear glass, but the infrared light emitted is not visible to the human eye (because it is below the red wavelength range of the visible spectrum). In more complicated lamp sources, the released light can be reflected (for example, by aluminum and ceramics) to focus the light from the source, and due to the high heat outputs, lamps may be cooled by air or water.

TABLE 2.4 The infrared wavelength range

Infrared	Wavelength range (μm)
Near	0.7–2.5
Middle	2.5–50
Far[a]	50–1,000

[a]Far infrared is often further subdivided into far and far-far ranges.

2.4.3.3 Microwaves. Microwaves are electromagnetic radiation within the wavelength range ~1 mm to 1 m. Although microwaves may have negligible direct antimicrobial activity, the primary mechanism of action is due to the rapid generation of heat from water and should therefore be considered a heat disinfection method (section 2.2). Microwaves can be conveniently produced in widely available ovens, at a typical frequency of ~2,500 MHz. In these ovens, a standard electricity supply (or voltage) is transformed to a higher voltage (~3,000 V) and supplied to a magnetron tube, which generates microwaves that are released into the oven interior. The magnetron tube is a simple device consisting of a central cathode, surrounded by anodes and contained within an electrical field (Fig. 2.8). When voltage is applied to the cathode, it heats

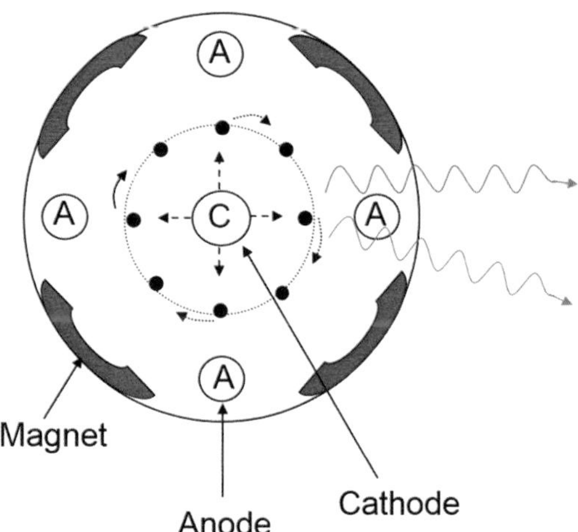

FIGURE 2.8 Simple structure of a magnetron used for the production of microwaves. Voltage applied to a central cathode causes the release of electrons (shown as black circles), which are forced to circulate by the attraction to the anode and the effect of the surrounding magnetic field. Microwaves are released as the circulating electrons lose their energy.

up to release electrons, which, being negatively charged, attempt to travel to surrounding anodes but are prevented by an applied magnetic source. The electrons therefore travel in a circular path around the central cathode and release electromagnetic energy within the microwave wavelength range. Dry items can be placed in the oven for treatment, but the antimicrobial process is more effective in the presence of water. Within the oven, it is optimal for items to be circulated, usually on a rotating table, and for the microwave energy to be pulsed to ensure even heat distribution.

2.4.4 Applications

2.4.4.1 UV. UV light is used for a variety of germicidal applications including liquid, air, and surface disinfection. Typical continuous or batch liquid applications involve the close passage of the liquid past a UV-emitting source for a controlled exposure time, determined by flow and output of the UV source. These simple systems are normally encased in a protective metal to prevent direct human exposure (Fig. 2.9).

Liquids that can be routinely disinfected with UV light include water (drinking and wastewater), emulsions, and liquid foods. UV treatment of water is particularly used in the treatment of drinking water in certain parts of Europe, at typical dosages ranging between 16 and 40 mJ/cm^2. The type of UV lamp used depends on the quality of the water and the flow rate required; higher-capacity lamps are required for higher flow rates and low qualities of water. Multiple low-pressure lamps may also be used, depending on the application. In addition to antimicrobial effects, UV radiation can also be used for deodorization, dechlorination, deozonation, and organic pollutant control. UV radiation is also used for area and equipment decontamination, including the periodic treatment of isolators, laminar flow cabinets, drying cabinets, chambers, rooms (including surgical suites, general hospital wards, and food processing areas), and air conditioning/air handling systems. These systems are easy to apply and cost-effective. They can be as simple as UV lamps installed at various positions within a room, cabinet, or ductwork. Transportable UV systems are also available that typically contain multiple UV lights and can be temporarily placed in an area for disinfection; such systems have been widely used for periodic disinfection of health care facility and manufacturing areas. It is particularly important to ensure that all areas are visible to the UV light in large-area applications, to ensure that the right UV dose is applied to all surfaces. This can be effectively monitored using a series of UV intensity sensors, which can monitor the exposure dose

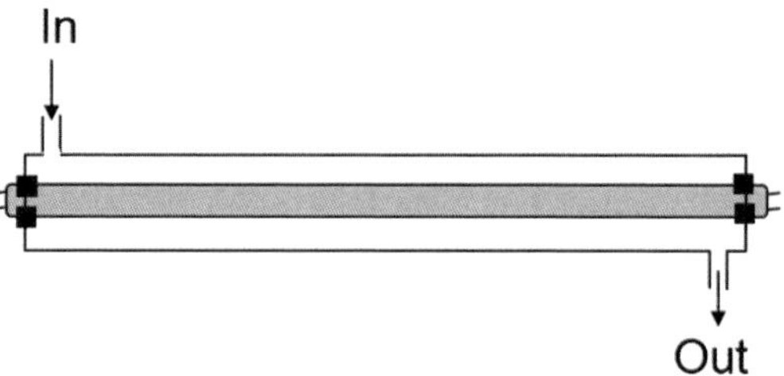

FIGURE 2.9 A simple continuous-duty UV disinfection system for liquids. The UV light is encased centrally in a chamber through which the liquid flows.

applied to a given surface or liquid or to ensure that the UV intensity is sufficient at the source.

Other applications include the direct treatment of food and packaging materials and in combination with other decontamination methods. Examples include air handling control in combination with air filtration and hydrogen peroxide gas (chapter 3, section 3.13) and as an activator for surfaces coated with titanium dioxide (TiO_2) or zinc oxide (ZnO). When TiO_2 is activated with UV light, it produces active oxygen species, including hydroxyl radicals and super oxide ions, which are effective against microorganisms (in particular, bacteria and viruses) and in the reduction of organic pollutants, such as ethylene vapors (section 3.17.2). Flash lamps have also been successfully employed for some unique sterilization applications, including aseptic filling lines (blow-fill-seal aseptic manufacturing of liquids) and simple medical devices. The use of pulsed light is further considered as a sterilization method in chapter 5, section 5.6.2.

2.4.4.2 Infrared. Infrared is used for a variety of applications, including detection, monitoring, and therapeutic applications and data transmission. Infrared lamps can also be used in smaller (e.g., ovens) or larger areas for dry heat disinfection. The heat absorption on surfaces can then be transferred by convection or conduction. The efficacy of a given process depends on the temperature provided to a given surface and can range from disinfection at temperatures <100°C and sterilization at temperatures in the typical 120 to 200°C range, although higher-wattage lamps can provide the much higher temperatures required for some industrial applications. Typical uses have included the treatment of glass, ceramics, and other temperature-resistant materials. Sterilization processes for glass syringes have been described in which the product was passed through an infrared oven on conveyor belts for the required exposure time, although such processes are not widely used. Disinfection processes can include a variety of surfaces including inanimate object and food surfaces. Infrared ovens are used as alternatives for dry-heat ovens, as described in section 2.2 and chapter 5, section 5.3. Due to the transfer of heat, infrared radiation can be an efficient method of drying or heating surfaces and areas.

2.4.4.3 Microwaves. Microwave radiation is routinely used as a household method of rapid and controlled heating of foods and liquids. The rapid application of heat is itself antimicrobial, to the same levels as discussed for moist heat disinfection (see section 2.2). Microwave ovens can be used as a flash disinfection method for wet devices and laboratory utensils, although these methods are not widely used or investigated. Systems are available for the treatment (disinfection) of medical wastes, as an alternative to incineration. With these methods, the waste is initially shredded, sprayed with water or steam to moisten, and heated to ~95°C using microwaves. Other applications that have been described include the low-level disinfection of contact lenses in water, antifungal treatment of paper, and as an alternative energy source for other antimicrobial processes (e.g., electrode-free UV lights can use microwaves for activation with applications in water, air, and surface decontamination).

2.4.5 Spectrum of Activity

2.4.5.1 UV. UV radiation (at the optimal germicidal wavelengths within the UV-C range) is an effective broad-spectrum antimicrobial, with the level of activity dependent on the exposure time and output of the UV source (see Table 2.3). In both room and liquid applications, UV radiation is an effective bactericide against Gram-positive and Gram-negative bacteria at typical doses >5 mJ/cm^2 (as a measure of UV intensity, as the energy per unit surface area). Higher than minimal doses are recommended because many bacteria can reverse the damage caused by UV radiation on nucleic acids at bacteriostatic exposure conditions and be subsequently reactivated to become viable; this intrinsic mode of resistance is further discussed in chapter 8, section 8.3.12.

Important bactericidal applications of UV radiation include the control of *Legionella*, which can be transmitted in water and in aerosols, and *M. tuberculosis*, which can be transmitted by aerosols. Some bacteria, for example, *Deinococcus radiodurans*, have notable resistance to radiation, presumably due to multiple protective mechanisms, including efficient repair processes (chapter 8, section 8.3.9); similar resistance mechanisms can decrease the sensitivity of other bacteria to UV radiation, including *Escherichia coli*. Efficacy has also been reported against *Cryptosporidium* oocysts, *Giardia* cysts, and some viruses at 5 to 10 mJ/cm^2, which has led to the greater acceptance of UV radiation as a method of potable water disinfection. Fungi and viruses, in particular, nonenveloped viruses, often demonstrate greater resistance, with higher dosage levels required for effectiveness (>20 mJ/cm^2). Bacterial spores are also quite resistant to UV-C, but sporicidal effects are observed at longer exposure times and at greater energy outputs similar to fungi. *Bacillus pumulis* spores have been described for use in monitoring the effectiveness of UV radiation treatments. There may be differences in the intrinsic resistance of microorganisms in water and when dried on surfaces; this may be related to the protection of target organisms in organic and/or inorganic soils, which can prevent penetration of UV waves. These protective effects can be reduced by using medium-pressure and flash lamps, which have greater germicidal activity and demonstrate greater efficacy for higher flow rates in liquid applications.

2.4.5.2 Infrared. Infrared radiation is a source of heat for dry-heat disinfection and therefore shows a typical profile for antimicrobial efficacy dependent on the temperature and time (as discussed in section 2.2). Under these conditions, dry heat is an effective bactericide, fungicide, and virucide, with higher temperatures and contact times needed for the required sporicidal activity for sterilization processes.

2.4.5.3 Microwaves. Because the mode of action of microwaves is considered to occur primarily through the action of water heating, the spectrum of activity is dependent on the temperature achieved over time (as discussed in section 2.2). Therefore, efficacy has been described against bacteria, fungi, and viruses, with little to no activity against bacterial spores that demonstrate extreme heat resistance (e.g., *G. stearothermophilus* spores). Sporicidal activity can be achieved, such as that described for microwave-based waste-disposal systems monitored by *Bacillus atrophaeus* (previously known as *Bacillus subtilis* var. *niger*) spores, due to greater heat sensitivity. Efficacy is significantly more efficient in the presence of water, in contrast to dried surfaces.

2.4.6 Advantages

2.4.6.1 UV. UV radiation is a broad-spectrum antimicrobial. Its use for the treatment of water, air, and surfaces is preferred over chemical methods due to the lack of chemical residuals or by-products, in particular, as an alternative to chlorine (for water disinfection) and formaldehyde (for area fumigation). UV radiation is easy to handle, and applications are usually compact and can be monitored to ensure that an effective dose is applied over time and over the life of the UV lamp source. Safety switches that reduce the risk of exposure to UV radiation can be employed. In addition to antimicrobial activity, UV radiation can also be used for reducing chlorine, ozone, and organic pollutants, in particular, with medium-pressure and flash lamps.

2.4.6.2 Infrared. Infrared lamps are convenient, cheap, and economical sources of heat. As heat sources, the antimicrobial effects have been well described. The efficacy of processes can be easily monitored by temperature profiling. In general, applications can be easy to control and risks of exposure are easily minimized.

2.4.6.3 Microwaves. Microwaves are cheap and easy to produce in conveniently available ovens. As a method of heat transfer, microwaves are rapid, with significantly less heating-up time than conventional dry ovens. They can also be used to enhance drying and, due to the specific reaction with water and other biological molecules, microwaves may cause less damage to metals, plastics, and other materials due to nonabsorption or reflection. Microwaves are a useful source of energy for other processes (including UV light production) and may be used synergistically with other chemical antimicrobials.

2.4.7 Disadvantages

2.4.7.1 UV. UV radiation can damage the skin and eyes on direct exposure over time, dependent on the wavelength, dosage time, and output. In general, these effects are delayed and not permanent, but UV light can cause skin burns and irreversible damage to eye tissue. Some damage to surfaces can be observed (including color bleaching and effects on plastics), which is primarily thought to be due to the localized production on surfaces of ozone or reactive radicals, in particular, at maximum germicidal wavelengths. These effects appear to be more pronounced with long exposure times and lower-energy lamps. Efficacy is dramatically reduced in the presence of organic or inorganic soils, due to the lack of contact with the target microorganisms. This is particularly important in the treatment of water due to the presence of iron, hardness, and total dissolved solids or in the case of high contamination levels, where dead microorganisms can shield viable organisms from receiving an effective dose. Overall, UV radiation has low penetration and is also absorbed by glass, plastics, and metals, which limits applications to direct exposure to a given surface or liquid. Effective dose outputs can also be reduced at higher temperatures (in particular, low-pressure lamp applications due to loss of heat energy instead of release of radiation energy) and, in the case of air or surface applications, higher relative humidity. UV radiation does not leave any residual activity, which increases the risk of downstream contamination following UV disinfection of water or air, as in the case of air-handling duct work. Resistance mechanisms (in bacteria and fungi) can allow the reactivation of microorganisms following UV treatment to repair damage and allow for multiplication.

2.4.7.2 Infrared. Infrared radiation has limited penetration; only exposed surfaces can be adequately treated, although heat can be subsequently transferred by convection or conduction. Care should be taken to ensure that all surfaces are exposed and not shielded from the light. Uneven heat distribution can cause damage to surfaces, where only temperature-sensitive materials can be adequately disinfected. Further, cold spots in a given load may prevent the required disinfection times and temperatures. High-temperature sources should be adequately controlled to limit any potential exposure, which can cause severe burns.

2.4.7.3 Microwaves. Microwaves can produce uneven temperature distribution, depending on the density and type of load or material treated. Hot spots can be damaging to the treated material, while cold spots are not adequately disinfected. The presence of moisture or other absorbing materials is essential to ensure adequate heat distribution; therefore, dry materials may not be adequately disinfected. The rapid transfer of heat can also be difficult to control and can cause heat conduction to temperature-sensitive plastics and other materials, leading to damage. With the exception of some waste-disposal processes, microwave applications have not been widely tested or validated. Care should be taken to minimize any exposure to microwave energy, due to the risk of internal organ damage from localized heating.

2.4.8 Mode of Action

2.4.8.1 UV. The main targets for UV radiation, like other sources of electromagnetic radiation, are nucleic acids, such as DNA and RNA, in particular, at 280 nm. UV radiation is specifically known to cause photochemical reactions, particularly with pyrimidine bases, to form covalent linkages between adjacent bases (cytosine and thymine dimers) in the DNA helical structure, and to cause other structural damage affecting adsorption of energy and excitation of atom structures (see chapter 7, section 7.3 for a discussion of the structure of DNA). This prevents the normal functions of DNA—transcription and replication—which prevents cell multiplication and viral infection. Higher doses of photons also cause protein damage (in particular, at 260 nm), leading to loss of structure, function, and cell lysis.

2.4.8.2 Infrared. The mode of action of infrared radiation is predominantly if not totally due to the transfer of heat to a surface or microorganism (see section 2.2 for a discussion of the effects of heat), which culminates in cell death and loss of infectivity.

2.4.8.3 Microwaves. Little is known about the direct antimicrobial effects of microwaves, because application to surfaces causes heat transfer, which is thought to be primarily responsible for their biocidal activity. Microwaves are an efficient method of heating in the presence of water. At widely used frequency ranges, microwaves are rapidly absorbed by water and other molecules including fats and sugars to cause heating and disruption of structure and function. In contrast, many materials such as plastics, glass, and ceramics do not absorb the energy, and with some metals microwaves cause deflection. For further discussion refer to the mode of action of heat (section 2.2).

2.5 FILTRATION

2.5.1 Types and Applications

Filtration is one of the oldest and most widely used physical methods for the removal of contaminants from liquids and gases (Fig. 2.10). Filtration methods are not true biocidal processes because they are based on the physical removal of microorganisms rather than their inactivation; however, in some cases biocides or biocidal processes have been integrated into filter designs. Filtration is used for air quality control, disinfection, and sterilization applications.

The liquid or gas can be passed through a variety of filter (or membrane) types, which retard the passage of contaminants based on their sizes (Fig. 2.11).

A wide variety of filters are available, consisting of flat sheets (often pleated), hollow fibers, or coated tubes of a range of media types. These include inorganic (e.g., glass, ceramics, and metals) and organic materials. Organic materials further encompass natural polymers (e.g., polysaccharides and polypeptides) and synthetic polymers, including plastics. Filter types can also be classified as being screen or depth filters (Fig. 2.10). Simple screen filters prevent the passage of particles due to a given dead-end pore size, while depth filters prevent passage through a given matrix. Because these filters can become quickly blocked by retained particles, filter life can be extended by periodically flushing (e.g., backflowing, or reversing the flow across the filter) or constantly (cross-flow filtration) removing contaminants from the filter surface (as shown in Fig. 2.10C).

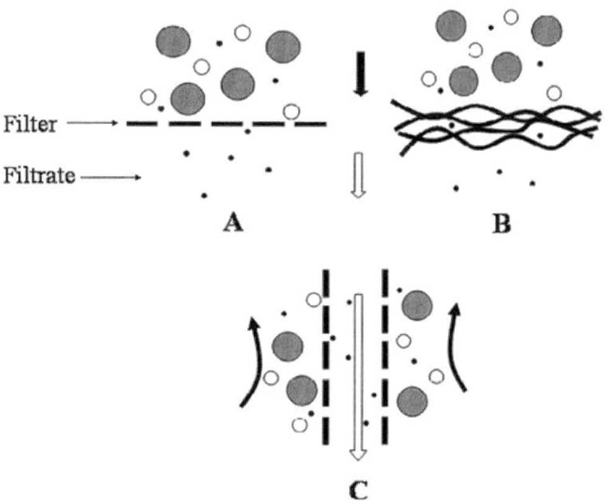

FIGURE 2.10 The theory of filtration. Various types of filtration processes are shown, with larger particles being retained by the filter and smaller particles allowed through the filter. Dead end (A and B) and cross-flow filters (C) are shown. **(A)** Simple screen filter. **(B)** Depth screen filter. **(C)** Cross-flow filter.

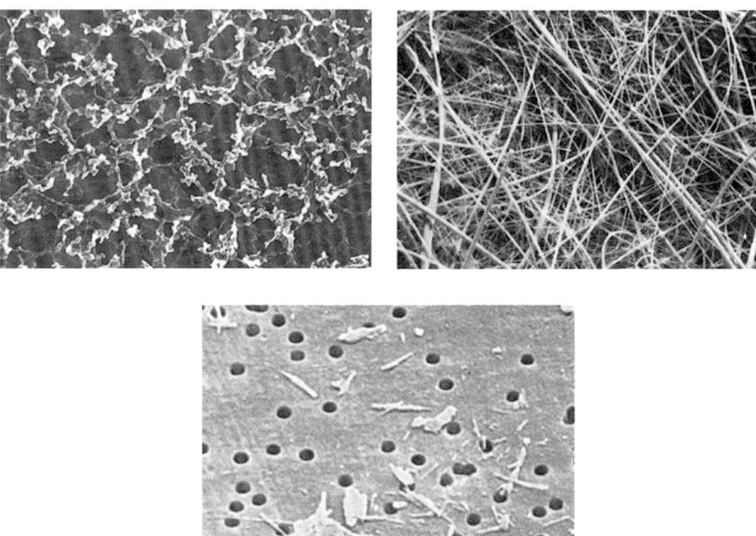

FIGURE 2.11 The microscopic structure of the surface of three filter materials. Image courtesy of GE Healthcare Lifesciences, with permission.

Due to their flexibility and ease of use, filters are widely used for the decontamination of liquids, including water, and gases, including air (Table 2.5 and Fig. 2.12).

Liquid filtration is widely used for the pretreatment, disinfection, or sterilization of water. Pretreatment applications include reduction of microbial load and generation of water for steam production. Critical applications include the production of water for injection, water for dialysis, and sterile water for rinsing manufacturing vessels or medical devices (e.g., following chemical disinfection). Similarly, many temperature-sensitive liquids can be filtered to reduce the risk of contamination; examples include the sterile production of antibiotics, vaccines, and other pharmaceuticals and the concentration of (or removal of water from) a product. Filters are widely used to test liquids and air for the presence of contaminants for the purpose of quality control. Filtration is extensively used for the removal of contaminants in gases, especially air. Air contamination control is employed to reduce the presence of pathogens or other airborne contaminants in critical areas. Many microorganisms can be spread in aerosols (e.g., *M. tuberculosis*) and/or in a dry state (e.g., bacterial or fungal spores). The control of these contaminants is particularly important to prevent cross-infection, product contamination, or spoilage. Typical examples include the use of clean rooms or separative enclosures (e.g., isolators or restricted-access barrier systems) by pharmaceutical, hospital-

TABLE 2.5 Typical uses of filtration for liquid and gas applications

Liquid applications	Gas applications
Water or other liquid sanitization or disinfection	Air used in clean rooms, isolators, and work cabinets
Sterile water production	Air used in ventilators, operating theaters
Sterilization of temperature-sensitive products, e.g., antibiotics, tissue culture media, vaccines	Odor control
Determination of contamination	Air sampling
Sample concentration	Medicinal-gas delivery

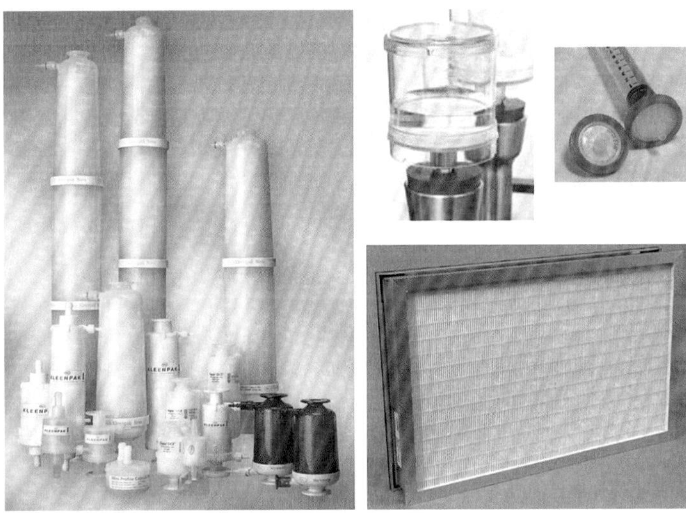

FIGURE 2.12 Examples of various types of filters used for liquids (left), in laboratories (upper right), and for air filtration (HEPA filter; lower right). Images courtesy of Pall Corporation. © PallCorporation, 2017.

dispensing, semiconductor, and other facilities for contamination control. Clean rooms are defined as rooms in which the concentration of airborne particles is controlled and maintained. Separative enclosures can provide the same control within a defined, enclosed area and include different types of isolators as barrier systems, which separate a process or activity from the operator and/or external environment (Fig. 2.13).

Other applications of air filtration include vacuuming to reduce surface contamination and filtering for medicinal gas (e.g., oxygen) delivery and for venting air from or into various processes (e.g., washer-disinfectors and sterilizers).

Filters are also used to reduce the potential for infection in critical hospital environments (operating rooms, ventilators) or research laboratories (containment rooms, laminar flow

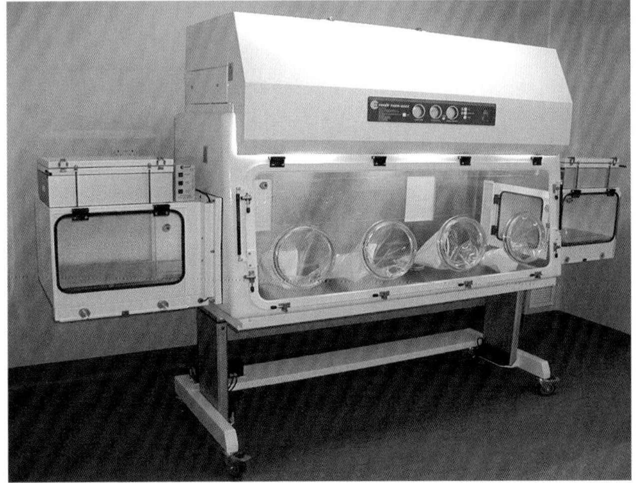

FIGURE 2.13 A rigid-wall isolator system, with glove access ports on the front and transfer hatches on either side.

cabinets), both for the protection of a patient or sample and for those working in these environments. Similar to liquid filters, this can be achieved by both physical retention and/or electrostatic interactions of the filter. The most widely used air filters are high-efficiency particulate air (HEPA) filters, which are fiberglass depth filters of various efficiencies. These are generally rated as microfilters (see below) to remove contaminants of ≥0.3 µm; some have also been described to remove smaller virus particles (0.1 µm) due to adsorption.

In addition to the use of filters, the design of the air handling system in a given room or enclosed area (e.g., a cabinet or isolator) is important for microbial control. The first consideration is air pressure (Fig. 2.14).

When an area is placed under negative pressure, contamination may be kept within the area (as air is drawn into the area), which is an important consideration when handling high concentrations of pathogenic microorganisms. The opposite is true for areas under positive air pressure, which keeps contamination out of the area and is important in the design of areas such as clean rooms and operating rooms.

The next consideration is the uniform control of air flow in the area, which can be used to maintain the air in a room at a given microbial level. This is the concept behind the laminar-flow principle, which controls the flow of air at a standard velocity and direction within an enclosed area while minimizing air turbulence.

Enclosed areas under positive pressure, including clean rooms and isolators, can be maintained at various levels of cleanliness, depending on the risks associated with potential contamination in the area. This can be achieved by the area design, air velocity, and efficiency of the filters. The quality of air in a given environment can be classified based on the maximum number of particles (e.g., of ≥0.5 µm) for a given volume of air. Various classification systems for clean rooms are described and compared in Table 2.6.

Biological control or safety cabinets use the same principles to reduce the levels of contaminants in a smaller enclosed environment. These can be simple designs that flow HEPA-filtered air over a work area, either away from or toward a user, depending on the use of the cabinet. More complicated designs are used for critical applications. For example, various classes of biological safety cabinets can be designated based on their design and intended use (Fig. 2.15).

Biological safety cabinet classes I, II, and III are all run under negative pressure and are designed to protect the user of the cabinet from the microorganism under investigation. In class

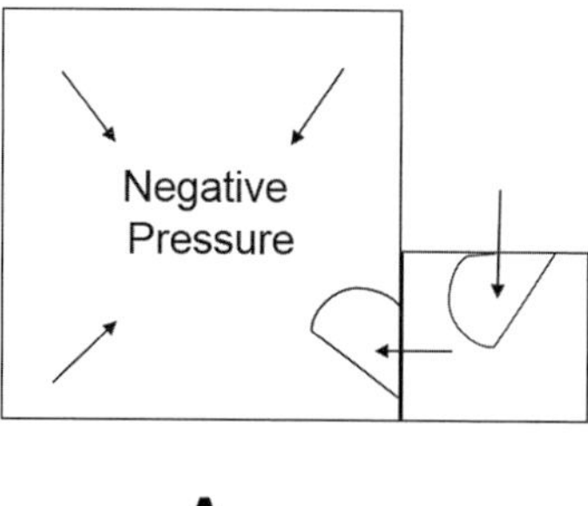

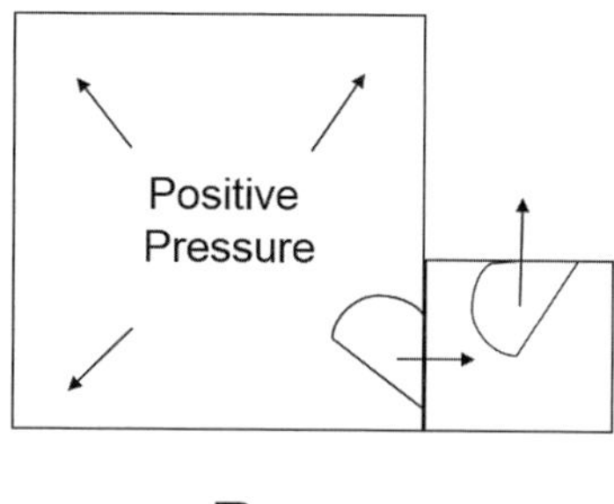

FIGURE 2.14 Air pressure in environmental controlled enclosed areas. **(A)** Rooms under negative pressure draw air into the room, maintaining microorganisms within the room. Negative pressure is typically used in rooms or cabinets where pathogenic microorganisms are manipulated. **(B)** Rooms under positive pressure force air out of the room to reduce the risk of contaminants entering the room. Uses of positive pressure include clean rooms and sterility test isolators.

TABLE 2.6 The classification of clean rooms, based on number of particles of ≥0.5 μm detected within a given volume of air

Maximum number of detected particles (meter^3)[a]	Maximum number of detected particles (feet^3)[a]	FDA FS 209[b]	ISO 14644-1[c]	EU GGMP[d]
35	1	1	3	
352	10	10	4	
3,520	100	100	5	A, B[e]
35,200	1,000	1,000	6	
352,000	10,000	10,000	7	C
3,520,000	100,000	100,000	8	D

[a]One cubic meter is approximately equal to 35 cubic feet.

[b]Federal Standard 209, "Cleanroom and workstation requirements, controlled environments," U.S. Food and Drug Administration, 1992. Withdrawn in 2001 but still widely cited.

[c]ISO 14644-1, "Cleanrooms and associated controlled environments - Part 1: classification of controlled environments by particle concentration."

[d]"EU Guidelines to Good Manufacturing Practice Medicinal Products for Human and Veterinary Use" (European Commission, 2008).

[e]Classes A and B differ in the permissible particle counts when the room is "in operation" or "at rest."

I cabinets the air is drawn into the cabinet and exhausted away from the user and through a microbiological-grade filter. In class II cabinets, the user and the specimen under investigation are protected, because the incoming air is filtered and a laminar flow of air is passed over the working area; the air is then directed out of the cabinet through an additional filter. Finally, class III cabinets are totally enclosed and designed to be airtight. They are used for

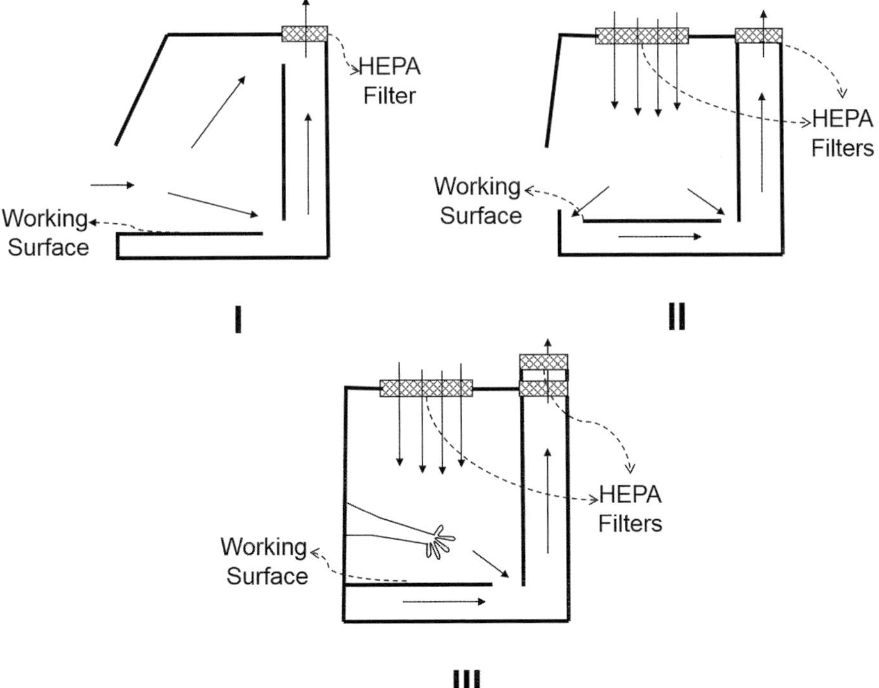

FIGURE 2.15 Biological safety classes I, II, and III. Class I cabinets provide the lowest level of biological control, with all air leaving the cabinet passing through a HEPA filter. In contrast, class III cabinets provide the highest level of control; they are totally enclosed, with access using a glove-port, as shown.

handling higher-risk pathogens. The agent is handled through gloves or a half-suit, and the air leaving the cabinet is typically passed through two filters. These designs may also include special handling pass-through ports or even be directly connected to a steam sterilizer to allow for the safe handling of materials in and out of the cabinet. Examples of standards and guidelines on the use of filtration for disinfection and sterilization are given in Table 2.7.

2.5.2 Spectrum of Activity

Filters can be used to remove a variety of particulates and contaminants including microorganisms, biological molecules (e.g., proteins, endotoxins, etc.), and chemicals such as metals and salts. Filtration methods can be defined based on the size range of contaminants they can remove (Fig. 2.16).

Coarse filters are generally used as prefilters to remove gross contaminants, including large-molecular-weight substances. Typical materials used include sand, activated-carbon (charcoal activated with oxygen), cotton, polypropylene, and cellulose. In addition to gross physical removal, other contaminants can be reduced in the filtrate due to chemical interactions; for example, activated-carbon filters can also remove low-molecular-weight microorganisms and halogens (including chlorine) due to affinity adsorption to the filter surface.

Microfiltration can remove particles as small as 0.05 µm, depending on the filter type, and therefore is widely used to remove a broad range of pathogenic organisms including parasitic cysts, bacteria, fungi, and many viruses. Typical filters used for bacteria-free water filtration include 0.2- and 0.1-µm filters. Surface and depth filters can be used; they are manufactured with a

TABLE 2.7 Examples of standards and guidelines on disinfection and sterilization filtration applications

Reference[a]	Title	Summary
ISO 13408-2	Aseptic processing of health care products - part 2: filtration	Requirements for sterilizing filtration as part of aseptic processing of health care products, including requirements for set-up, validation, and routine operation of a sterilizing filtration process
ISO 13408-6	Aseptic processing of healthcare products - part 6: isolator systems	Requirements for isolator systems used for aseptic processing, including guidance on qualification, biodecontamination, validation, operation, and control
ISO 14644-1	Cleanrooms and associated controlled environments - part 1: classification of air cleanliness	Guideline on the classification of air quality used in clean rooms and other environments
ISO 14698-1	Cleanrooms and associated controlled environments - biocontamination control - part 1: general principles and methods	Principles and basic methodology for assessing and controlling biological contamination when clean room technology is applied for that purpose
EN 12901	Products used for treatment of water intended for human consumption. Inorganic supporting and filtering materials. Definitions	Definitions on the use of filtration and the treatment of drinking water
PDA technical report 26	Sterilizing filtration of liquids	Guidelines on the use of filtration for liquid (e.g., parenteral drug) sterilization, including validation and filter integrity testing
ASTM F2101-14	Standard test method for evaluating the bacterial filtration efficiency (BFE) of medical face mask materials, using a biological aerosol of *Staphylococcus aureus*	Test method used to measure the bacterial filtration efficiency of medical face mask materials

[a]ISO, International Standards Organization; EN, European Standard; PDA, Parenteral Drug Association; ASTM, American Society for Testing and Materials.

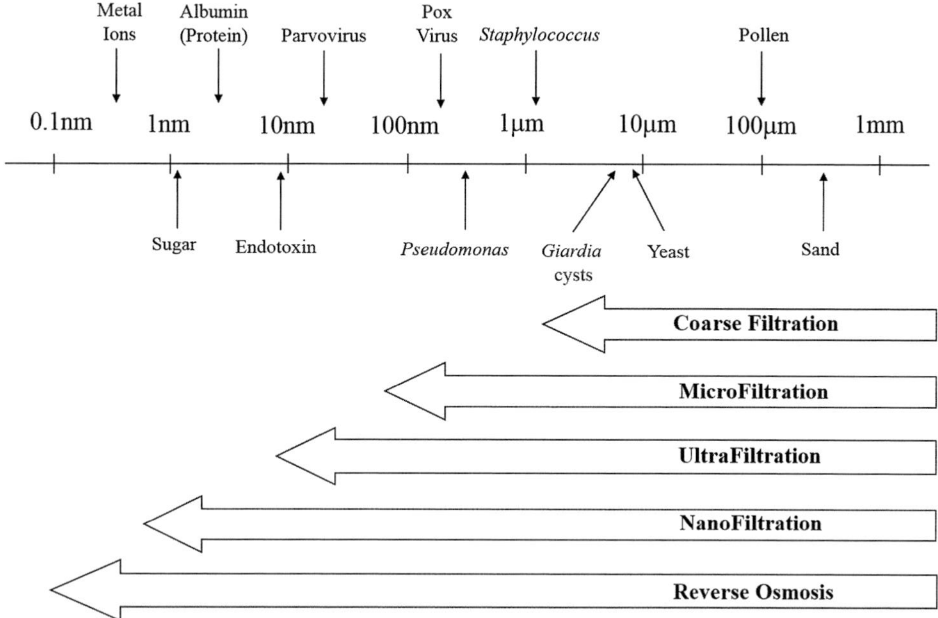

FIGURE 2.16 Range of filtration methods and reference size exclusion capabilities. Note that the size ranges are shown on a log scale.

variety of materials including polymers (polycarbonate, polypropylene, polyethylene, and polytetrafluoroethylene), as well as ceramics and metals (e.g., silver). To increase the effectiveness of surface filters, the surface area for liquid-gas contact can be increased by preparing the filter material in folds or pleats. Similarly, depth filters can be optimized by having a gradient of pore (from larger to smaller) sizes through the filter, to prevent premature clogging of the smaller pore sizes and thereby increasing the life of the filter. Microfilters are generally rated as being "absolute" or "nominal," depending on their retentive capabilities. Absolute filters should not allow the passage of any particle greater than the rated pore size, while nominal filters allow for some passage over time; for example, a nominal depth filter could allow passage of an organism by working through the torturous path of the filter matrix over time.

Contaminants of less than 0.1 to 0.05 μm can be removed by ultrafiltration, nanofiltration, and reverse osmosis (RO). These are all cross-flow filtration methods (Fig. 2.10). The filters are composed of semipermeable membranes in a variety of configurations; the liquid is passed over the filter surface under pressure to allow filtration, and unfiltered molecules are subsequently swept away to prevent fouling of the filter surface. The filter pore size dictates the filtration method. Ultrafiltration methods remove most organic molecules but do not remove salts or other inorganic contaminants. Nanofiltration, in addition, removes endotoxins and other pyrogens, as well as some salts (e.g., it reduces water hardness). Finally, RO is considered an ultimate filtration method, to potentially include nearly all organic molecules and high-efficiency inorganic salts. RO is a combination of filtration and electrochemical interaction; the filter membranes have extremely small pore sizes but are highly adsorptive. Typical membranes used for RO include cellulose acetate and polyamide polymers. RO methods are used as alternatives to physical or chemical purification. Physical methods include water distillation (or the condensation of steam), and chemical methods include deionization (which uses a bed of synthetic resins that can adsorb cations or anions).

2.5.3 Advantages

Filtration can be a simple and cost-effective method to reduce contamination loads in heat-sensitive materials (e.g., pharmaceutical preparations) and to reduce or maintain the contamination levels in enclosed environments such as clean rooms and laminar-flow cabinets. Filtration methods can also be used for efficient sterilization, and many may include the removal of other chemical contaminants (e.g., RO systems can remove chemical and microbiological contamination as a method of water purification). Some filters may contain impregnated biocides that combine physical removal with biocidal activity (see chapter 3, section 3.17.3).

2.5.4 Disadvantages

In general, filtration methods can only remove and not necessarily inactivate microorganisms. Some filter technologies are available that incorporate the presence of biocides to reduce the microbial or can be routinely sterilized, using chemicals or heat. Although coarse and microfiltration methods are cost-effective, as the filter pore size is decreased, the cost of filtration increases. Certain types of smaller bacteria and viruses may pass through these filters due to their sizes. Nominal filters or filtration systems may allow the passage of contaminants over time; in addition, absolute filters have been described to allow the "grow-through" of microorganisms over extended use or if the filter surface is damaged. To reduce this possibility, it is recommended that the filters are routinely changed and/or periodically treated by heat or chemicals. Finally, the efficiency of filtration can be affected by chemicals present in the gas or liquid due to damage of the filter. Filters should be routinely checked for integrity; widely used integrity test methods include microbiological sampling or retention tests (e.g., retention of 10^7 CFU/cm^2 *Brevundimomas diminuta*), the bubble point test, and smoke tests.

2.5.5 Mode of Action

Filters allow for the physical removal of contaminants from gases, fluids, and solids, based on their rated pore sizes. Some filtration materials and processes may also allow for the removal of chemical and/or smaller-than-expected microbial contaminants due to adsorption and other chemical interactions.

CHEMICAL DISINFECTION

3

3.1 INTRODUCTION

Chemical biocides are used for various applications due to their ability to inhibit or inactivate microorganisms. In this chapter, these biocides are classified according to their general chemical types, including alcohols, aldehydes, antimicrobial metals, and halogens. For each major chemical group, the major types of biocides used are described, with consideration of their applications, spectra of activity, advantages, disadvantages, and what is known about their modes of action. The mechanisms of action of biocides are further considered in chapter 7, and the specific uses of some chemical biocides in sterilization processes are discussed in chapter 6. Examples of various guidelines and standards that describe the use and testing of chemical disinfectants are given in Table 3.1.

3.2 ACIDS AND ACID DERIVATIVES

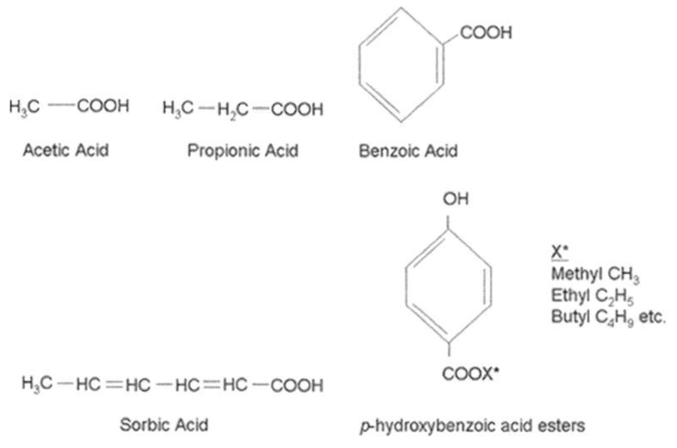

$H_3C-COOH$ Acetic Acid

$H_3C-H_2C-COOH$ Propionic Acid

Benzoic Acid (COOH)

$H_3C-HC=HC-HC=HC-COOH$ Sorbic Acid

p-hydroxybenzoic acid esters (OH; COOX*)

X*: Methyl CH_3, Ethyl C_2H_5, Butyl C_4H_9 etc.

3.2.1 Types

Acids are defined as substances that dissociate in water to provide hydrogen ions (H^+) and are measured under the pH scale as <7. Acids form salts when they are mixed with an alkali (section 3.3). A variety of acids or acid salts are used as preservatives and, to a lesser extent, as disinfectants. These include short-chain-length acids (acetic and propionic acid), longer-chained acids (sorbic and citric acid), and other acid derivatives, including phenolic derivatives (benzoic acid and salicylic acid) and esters. An ester is an organic compound that is formed on the reaction of an acid and an alcohol; the most widely used esters are the *p*-hydroxybenzoic esters. These include methyl-, ethyl-, propyl-, butyl-, and benzyl derivatives.

Strong acids such as hydrochloric acid (HCl) and sulfuric acid (H_2SO_4) readily dissociate in solution to give hydrogen ions, for example:

$$HCl \rightarrow H^+ + Cl^-$$

At lower concentrations (in the pH 3 to 6 range) these acids have been described as being bacteriostatic, while at higher concentrations (pH < 3) they are known to be bactericidal and virucidal and to be effective against other microorganisms. 2.5% HCl has been shown to be effective against *Bacillus anthracis* spores. Despite this, strong acids are limited in use due to concerns about safety and material compatibility.

TABLE 3.1 Examples of guidelines and standards on the use and application of chemical disinfectants

Reference[a]	Title	Summary
ANSI/AAMI ST58:2013	Chemical sterilization and high-level disinfection in health care facilities	Guidelines on the types and uses of chemical disinfectants and sterilization processes for reusable devices in health care settings
CDC HICPAC (2008)	Guideline for disinfection and sterilization in healthcare facilities	Recommendations on cleaning, disinfection, and sterilization of patient-care medical devices and disinfecting the health care environment
FDA (2000)	Content and format of premarket notification [510(k)] submissions for liquid chemical sterilants/high level disinfectants	Guidance on the content and format for registration of liquid chemical sterilants/high-level disinfectants intended for the sterilization and/or high-level disinfection of reusable heat-sensitive critical and semicritical medical devices
EPA (1982) DIS/TSS-1	Efficacy data requirements. Disinfectants for use on hard surfaces	Testing and labeling requirements for disinfectants
Health Canada guidance document (2014)	Safety and efficacy requirements for hard surface disinfectant drugs	General guidelines on safety and efficacy requirements for disinfectants used on environmental surfaces in health care facilities and food contact surfaces
USP ⟨1072⟩	Disinfectants and antiseptics	Guidance on the selection, demonstration of activity, and application of disinfectant in pharmaceutical manufacturing areas
TGA, TGO ⟨54⟩	Therapeutic goods order no. 54 - standard for disinfectants and sterilants	Guidelines for the registration or listing of disinfectants and sterilants in Australia
AS/NZ 4187	Reprocessing of reusable medical devices in health service organizations	Recommendations on cleaning, disinfection, and sterilization practices in health care facilities (Australia and New Zealand)
ASTM E1837-14	Standard test method to determine efficacy of disinfection processes for reusable medical devices (simulated use test)	Method for testing the effectiveness of a disinfection process for reprocessing reusable medical devices when challenged with vegetative cells including mycobacteria
EN 14885	Chemical disinfectants and antiseptics. Application of European standards for chemical disinfectants and antiseptics	Requirements on the testing of chemical disinfectants and antiseptics in the European Union
DPC guideline 9	Fundamentals of cleaning and sanitizing farm milk handling equipment	Guideline on the cleaning and disinfection/sanitization of milk handling equipment
Ministry of Health, China (2006)	Guidance on application of administrative approval license of disinfectants and disinfecting apparatuses	Registration requirements for disinfectants in China

[a]AAMI, Association for the Advancement of Medical Instrumentation; CDC HICPAC, U.S. Centers for Disease Control and Prevention, Healthcare Infection Control Practices Advisory Committee; FDA, Food and Drug Administration (U.S.); EPA, Environmental Protection Agency (U.S.); USP: United States Pharmacopeia; TGA,Therapeutic Goods Administration, Australia; AS/NZ, Australia-New Zealand standard; ASTM, American Society for Testing and Materials; EN, European Standard; DPC, Dairy Practices Council.

In contrast, the weaker acids do not readily dissociate in water and depend on the pH of the formulated solution, e.g., with benzoic acid (Fig. 3.1).

Benzoic acid is usually applied in the salt (sodium benzoate) form. In solution, as the pH increases, the acid demonstrates greater dissociation, while at lower pH values a greater concentration of the undissociated form is observed; in parallel, the antimicrobial efficacy of the acid increases at lower test pH values.

The more widely used antimicrobial acids include acetic acid, propionic acid, benzoic acid, citric acid, and sorbic acid. While acetic acid is used directly, propionic acid, due to its corrosive nature, is generally used as a sodium or calcium salt form. Salicylic acid is considered in more detail as a phenolic compound (section

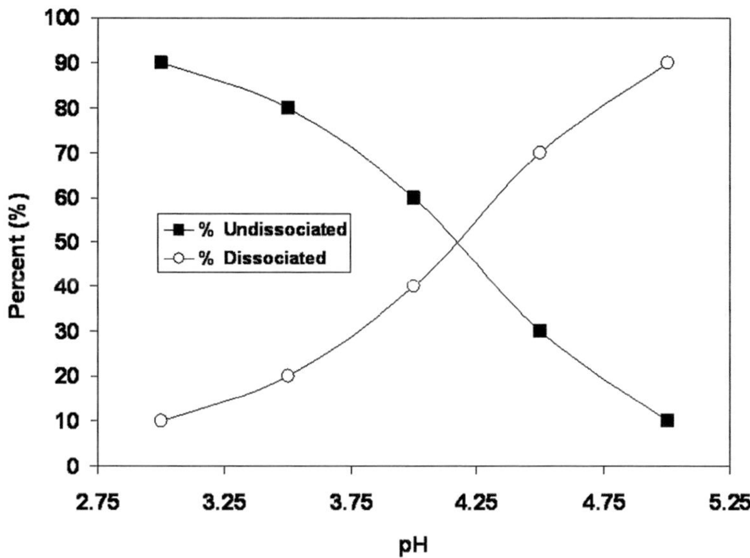

FIGURE 3.1 The dissociation of benzoic acid. As the pH increases, the dissociation of the acid also increases.

3.14), as is peracetic acid (PAA) as a peroxygen (section 3.13). The *p*-hydroxybenzoic esters consist of various chain lengths to give methyl-, ethyl-, and other derivatives, which are commonly known as the parabens. They are colorless, odorless, stable, low-cost, and relatively safe, factors contributing to their widespread use as preservatives.

3.2.2 Applications

The primary uses of acids and acid derivatives are as preservatives for foods, pharmaceuticals, cosmetics, soaps, and other products. The parabens are among the most widely used preservatives in cosmetics at typical use concentrations of ≤0.4% and often in various combinations. They are commonly added to cosmetics, eye drops, lotions, powders, pastes, drugs, and foodstuffs. Many other types of acids are also used a preservative. Acetic acid is used as a food preservative, for example, at 1 to 8% in pickled vegetables and at lower concentrations in products such as salad dressings; vinegar, which can contain 4 to 20% acetic acid in water, is widely used in the food industry (e.g., as a pickling solution). Propionic acid is more often used in baked goods and other foods at concentrations ranging from 0.1 to 0.5%. Benzoic acid is used as a preservative in pharmaceutical, food, and other industries and also as an antiseptic in combination with other biocides; it shows greater efficacy in low pH (2.5 to 4.0) foods such as fruit juices.

Maleic, sorbic, citric, and hydrochloric acids are among the other acids used in combinations for antiseptic, disinfectant, and/or preservative applications. A combination of citric acid and hydrochloric acid has been described as a hard-surface disinfectant against some enveloped viruses (e.g., the foot-and-mouth disease virus). Formulations of citric acid with concentrations ranging from 2.5 to 8% are used as broad-spectrum disinfectants, with efficacy claimed against viruses, fungi, bacteria, and mycobacteria; citric acid is also used as a preservative in beverages (e.g., fruit juices and wines) and as an effective cleaning agent. The acid works in combination with certain biocides, presumably because of its ability to increase the permeability of Gram-negative bacteria cell walls (probably due to chelation and disruption of the cell wall structure [chapter 8, section 8.6]).

The stronger acids, such as HCl and H_2SO_4, have had little cited use as disinfectants or liquid sterilants, but some limited veterinary applications have included the inactivation of the spores of *B. anthracis* on surfaces such as animal hides.

Other acid biocides used as preservatives include dehydroacetic acid, undecenoic acid, and vanillic acid esters. Acidic cleaners, based on formulations containing phosphoric, acetic, citric, lactic, and other acids, are used for removing acid-soluble residues and mineral deposits, including those due to water hardness (calcium carbonate or "scale").

3.2.3 Spectrum of Activity

The acids and acid derivatives demonstrate a range of antimicrobial activities, which also depend on their solubility in water or oil/lipid. These effects are important in the use of acids in various emulsions and other formulations. The parabens are bacteriostatic against Gram-positive bacteria and fungistatic against yeasts and molds, including *Candida*, *Saccharomyces*, *Trichophyton*, *Penicillium*, and *Aspergillus*, at ~100 to 200 μg/ml. Higher concentrations are often described for Gram-negative bacteria, in particular, *Pseudomonas* spp., whose tolerances vary (up to ~1,000 μg/ml), although greater efficacy is observed against *Pseudomonas* with the methyl and ethyl esters. The parabens can also be sporistatic by inhibiting the germination of bacterial spores. In general, the shorter-chained parabens (methyl and ethyl derivatives) are less effective than the longer-chained parabens; however, the solubility of the biocide in water decreases as the chain length increases. Parabens remain effective within a wide pH range (between pH 4 and 8), which makes them attractive as preservatives; the antimicrobial efficacy decreases at pH higher than 8 due to increased ionization of the biocide.

The acids also show variable activity. For example, acetic acid is more effective against bacteria and yeasts than against molds, in contrast to propionic acid which is fungistatic, with little to no activity against yeasts and bacteria. Some yeasts, molds, and bacteria can even use acids, such as lactic and citric acids, as carbon sources for growth. Benzoic acid is particularly active against yeasts at very low concentrations (0.01 to 0.02%), while sorbic acid inhibits the growth of yeasts, molds, and bacteria to a lesser extent. Overall, the antimicrobial activity tends to be microbistatic, with greater activity observed with longer chain lengths, but similar to the parabens, as the chain length increases, the solubility in water decreases. The decrease in pH alone is inhibitory to most bacteria and fungi at pH <4.5, with the exception of acidophilic microorganisms (such as *Acetobacter*). Viruses are particularly sensitive to extremes of pH, as is evident by the use of citric and hydrochloric acids against enveloped viruses; the viral spectrum of activity with acids and parabens has not been well investigated, although some citric acid formulations have been shown to be effective against some viruses (e.g., rhinoviruses).

3.2.4 Advantages

The acids and esters are considerably flexible as preservatives, depending on the required application. The parabens vary in water solubility, while the acids are mostly highly soluble in water. Various ester-acid mixtures can be broad-spectrum preservatives for many products. In addition, most of these biocides are nontoxic, nonirritating, and not known to be carcinogenic. For example, most of the acids, including acetic acid, propionic acid, benzoic acid, and sorbic acid, are naturally broken down in the body or the environment and are therefore often designated as safe for use directly on foodstuffs intended for consumption. Some longer-chained acids, e.g., sorbic acid, can irritate mucous membranes at concentrations of 0.2% or higher. These acids are also widely available and inexpensive. The parabens are colorless, odorless, and stable. Overall, the acids and parabens are useful microbistatic agents.

3.2.5 Disadvantages

At the concentrations most often used, acids are considered to be only bacteriostatic or fungistatic; the exceptions are at higher concentrations in some antiseptic and disinfection applications (for example, citric acid at 2 to 8%). Some bacteria and fungi can use the acids or parabens as carbon sources and can therefore degrade the biocide or preservative over time and overgrow within products; this can be prevented with the use of more than one active agent or, in some cases, by adding a higher concentration of the active agent, depending on the desired shelf life. The parabens have lower water solubility than the acids and are inactivated by nonionic surfactants. At higher concentrations, some of these biocides can be irritating and cause allergic or sensitization reactions. Acetic acid at higher concentrations has a strong pungent odor, which can be undesirable.

3.2.6 Modes of Action

In the use of acids or acidic conditions, the reduction in pH alone can have a dramatic effect on microbial surfaces. With strong acids, in particular, H^+ ions are attracted to such surfaces; the effect on bacterial and fungal cell structures initially is to disrupt the proton motive force (see chapter 8, section 8.3.4), thereby restricting the uptake of essential cell nutrients, oxidative phosphorylation, ATP synthesis, and other essential cell wall and membrane functions. It is also clear that changing the environmental pH disrupts the structure of essential surface and intracellular macromolecules (including in viruses, protozoa, and other microorganisms); the effects on the secondary and tertiary structures of proteins, lipids, carbohydrates, and nucleic acids lead to a cumulative loss of structure and function. However, the mode of action is clearly not that simple with the weaker acids. As shown in Fig. 3.1, the increased accumulation of the undissociated acid with decreased pH correlates with the antimicrobial activity; as the concentration of the undissociated form increases, so does the antimicrobial activity. This may be due to the pH effect alone or more likely acts in combination with direct effects on the structure and function of the microbial cell surface with the undissociated acid. The main effects in these cases have been studied in bacteria and shown to prevent the uptake of essential nutrients due to disruption of the proton motive force, which provides the energy for active uptake (see section 8.3.4). The parabens have demonstrated a similar mode of action, with further inhibition of the electron transport and other proton motive force-related functions. Specific inhibition of various surface and internal enzymes has been reported for acids and ester derivatives; sorbic acid has been reported to covalently bind to sulfhydryl groups (-SH) in proteins, which causes inactivation. Further, disruption of cell permeability (in particular for the longer-chained acids) and inhibition of respiration, nucleic acid, and protein synthesis have also been reported. This may be due to direct interaction with lipid membranes, cell walls, and associated proteins leading to disruption of these structures and functions.

3.3 ALKALIS (BASES)

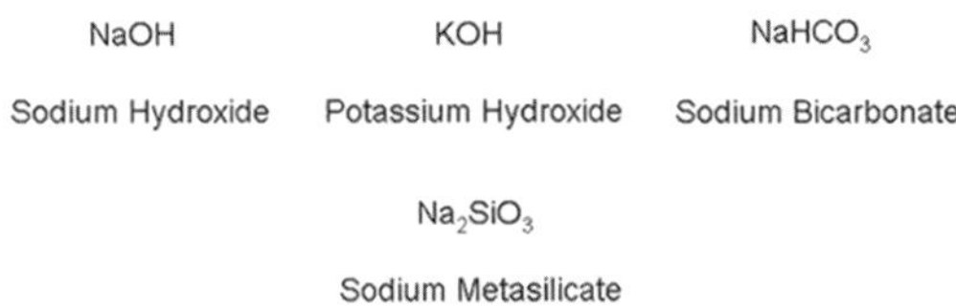

3.3.1 Types

Alkalis (or bases) are defined as substances capable of forming hydroxide (OH^-) ions when dissolved in water and are measured under the pH scale as >7. They are therefore the opposite of acids (section 3.2). Some limited disinfection methods use a high concentration of strong alkali such as NaOH (commonly known as caustic soda or soda lye) and KOH (also known as lye), while lower concentrations of these and weaker alkalis such as sodium bicarbonate (baking soda) and sodium metasilicate are used in various cleaning applications. Other biocides such as the acridines are considered weak bases (see section 3.7).

3.3.2 Applications

High concentrations (0.5 to 2.0 N) of NaOH and KOH are used for the routine cleaning and disinfection of various manufacturing surfaces, including purification and separation equipment such as chromatography columns and fractionation vessels, e.g., those used in the fractionation of blood. These are considered aggressive processes to clean surfaces and inactivate/remove various microorganisms, in particular, bacteria, viruses, and prion contamination. Prions are considered to have the greatest known resistance to disinfection and sterilization methods (chapter 1, section 1.3.6, and chapter 8, section 8.9); contaminated tissues and surfaces are recommended to be decontaminated with 1 to 2 N NaOH for typically 1 hour to ensure priocidal activity, although lower concentrations and contact times have also been shown to be effective for some purposes. Applications include the decontamination of manufacturing equipment (especially those that contact human or animal-derived materials) and reusable medical equipment. Some investigators have recommended boiling in 1 N NaOH as the most effective process against prions, including high-temperature/pressure systems for the destruction of contaminated whole animal carcasses. Alkaline cleaning formulations can include a variety of bases at much lower concentrations, including NaOH, KOH, sodium bicarbonate, and sodium metasilicate, which are effective cleaners due to their ability to emulsify and saponify lipid and fats. In addition, they are effective for protein removal from surfaces and can break down proteins into peptides; some of these formulations have also been shown to be effective against prions and some nonenveloped viruses, presumably due to synergism between the lower concentration of alkali present and other formulation effects (including surfactants, chelating agents, and phosphates). Increased temperatures (e.g., 40 to 60°C) have also been shown to be effective at lower concentrations of specific alkaline formulations against nonenveloped viruses and prion contamination. Sodium metasilicate is widely used as a source of alkalinity in mild alkaline cleaners, because it protects various surfaces from damage by the corrosion often associated with other alkali. Sodium bicarbonate is also used as a deodorizer. Alkalis are used in the manufacture of various soaps and detergents; soaps, for example, are made by reacting alkali (particularly NaOH) with the fatty acids from various fats and oils. Alkaline conditions have been shown to increase the activity of various biocides including phenols and glutaraldehyde and the sporicidal activity of hypochlorites; bacterial spores are more sensitive to heat inactivation under alkaline conditions, presumably due to the destabilization of spore coat structures (section 8.3.11).

3.3.3 Spectrum of Activity

Extremes of alkalinity are inhibitory to microorganisms, with the exception of certain extremophiles (alkaliphiles; chapter 8, section 8.3.10). In general, pH values ≥9 are restrictive for growth of most vegetative microorganisms, including bacteria and fungi. Low concentrations are generally inhibitory, with higher concentrations being bactericidal, fungicidal, and virucidal. Antimicrobial activity has been particularly studied with NaOH and KOH against viruses, due to their use in viral clearance studies. Typical virucidal concentrations are 1 to 2% NaOH and at least 4% sodium carbonate; enveloped viruses (due to envelope disruption) are more sensitive than nonenveloped viruses. Lower concentrations may be enhanced under increased temperature conditions. High concentrations of NaOH (1 to 2 N) are recommended for the inactivation of prions. Alkalis demonstrate activity against bacterial spores over time, such as at 0.5 M for 24 hours. Bacterial endotoxins (see chapter 1, section 1.3.7) are also known to be inactivated by strong alkali in a concentration-time-dependent manner (e.g., 0.1 M NaOH for 24 hours and 1 M NaOH for 4 hours).

3.3.4 Advantages

Alkalis are widely available and inexpensive but are typically used as biocides only under specific, industrial applications. They can be used at lower concentrations as preservatives and at higher concentrations show some microbicidal activity. They are widely used as formulation ingredients and demonstrate enhanced antimicrobial activity in combination with other biocides. Alkalis are the active ingredients in many cleaning formulations, providing excellent cleaning efficacy, in particular against stubborn protein-based (by solubilization and peptidization) and lipid-based (by emulsification and solubilization) soils.

3.3.5 Disadvantages

Alkalis are damaging to various surfaces, depending on the concentration of alkali used and the formulation pH. Concentrated solutions should be handled carefully; for example, NaOH and KOH are extremely damaging to the skin and mucous membranes and can cause severe burns; they are also corrosive to hard surfaces including metals (stainless steel, copper, brass, and aluminum) and various plastics. Reactions with various metals can, under certain circumstances, lead to the release of flammable (hydrogen) gases and when mixed with certain other organic or inorganic chemistries can cause violent reactions. These effects can be minimized by using lower concentrations of alkalis or using them in combination with other formulation effects.

3.3.6 Modes of Action

Alkaline conditions inhibit the growth of microorganisms by restricting various metabolic processes; the structure and function of various macromolecules, including enzymes, are particularly affected. At higher concentrations, alkalis cause the solubilization of bacterial cell walls and membranes, as well as viral envelopes. Studies with enveloped paramyxoviruses have shown disruption of the viral envelope at pH 9 to 11. Reactions with the various types of lipids (including phospholipids) in these membranes can be compared to their reaction with fatty acids in lipids or oils to cause salt (soap) formation. Membrane disruption leads to cell wall destabilization (in the case of Gram-negative bacteria) and loss of membrane structure and function, including disruption of the proton motive force (chapter 8, section 8.3.4) and leakage of cytoplasmic materials. Effects on nonenveloped viruses are presumably due to disruption of the structure of surface proteins, as well as internal nucleic acids. Alkali also causes breakage of peptide bonds and breakdown of proteins, which is presumed to be the major mechanism of action against prions (section 8.9).

3.4 ALDEHYDES

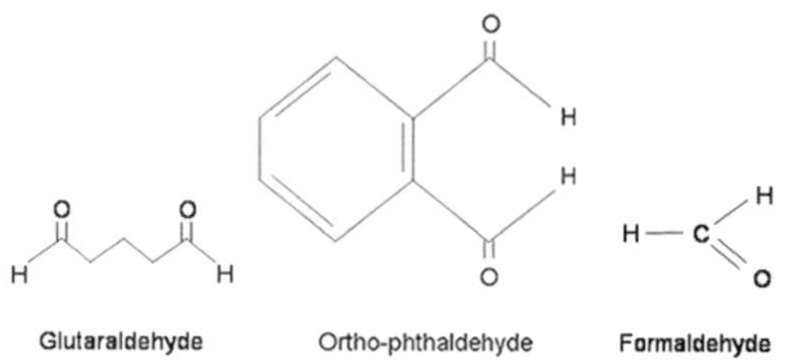

Glutaraldehyde Ortho-phthaldehyde Formaldehyde

3.4.1 Types

Three aldehydes are widely used as potent disinfectants: glutaraldehyde, ortho-phthaldehyde (OPA), and formaldehyde.

3.4.2 Applications

3.4.2.1 Glutaraldehyde and OPA. Glutaraldehyde (1,5-pentanedial) and OPA formulations are widely used as low-temperature, liquid disinfectants for temperature-sensitive medical devices (e.g., flexible endoscopes) and, in the case of glutaraldehyde, as a general surface disinfectant. Examples of glutaraldehyde and OPA solutions are shown in Fig. 3.2.

In addition to its antimicrobial applications, glutaraldehyde is used for many industrial applications and as a fixative for electron microscopy. OPA is used as a detection agent for protein, which turns a gray or black color on contact with OPA, and to provide fluorescence when used in conjunction with a sulfhydryl compound. Glutaraldehyde is a simple molecule with two aldehyde groups that are

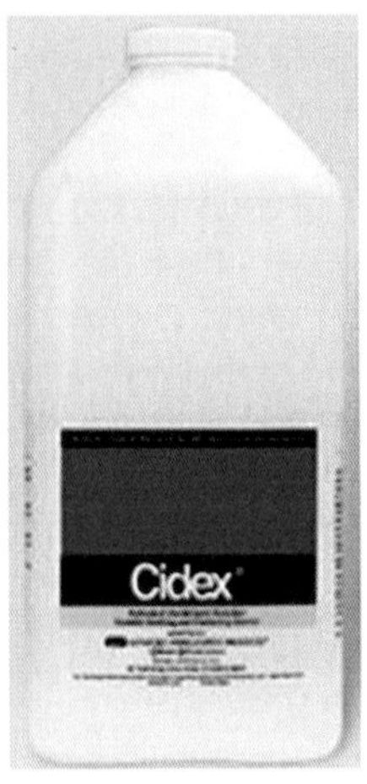

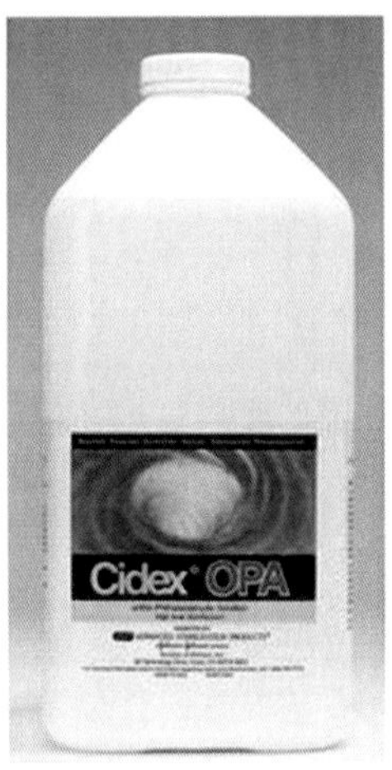

FIGURE 3.2 High-level disinfectants for medical device disinfection based on 2.4% alkaline glutaraldehyde and 0.55% OPA. Images courtesy of Advanced Sterilization Products, with permission. ASP and the ASP logo are trademarks of Advanced Sterilization Products Division of Ethicon, Inc.

keys to its mode of action. Formulations are usually provided at 1.5 to 3.5% (but generally at ~2%) under acidic conditions, which are subsequently activated (or made alkaline to ~pH 8) prior to use. Formulations have also been commercialized in combination with isopropanol (20 to 30%) and ~2% phenol phenate. Glutaraldehyde is a reactive, cross-linking biocide that can be dramatically affected in efficacy and stability based on formulation effects, particularly product pH. As the pH increases from 4 to 9, an increase in antimicrobial activity is observed, but with a concomitant reduction in shelf life; however, glutaraldehyde solutions also have much shorter useful lives at alkaline pHs, due primarily to increased condensation, because the biocide cross-links (or polymerizes) with itself. Stabilized acidic formulations, which do not require activation and have increased sporicidal activity, are also available. Glutaraldehyde solutions are colorless, although many contain a dye to give an amber color, and have a characteristic strong "rotten-apple" odor.

Commercial ready-to-use OPA formulations are also available such as 0.55% at pH 7.5 for temperature-sensitive device disinfection at 20°C, with improved efficacy observed at 35°C. Similarly, a concentrated solution of OPA is also used specifically for dilution in automated washer-disinfectors to provide a final concentration of at least 0.055% OPA for disinfection at 50 to 55°C. In contrast to glutaraldehyde, OPA is stable over a wide pH range (pH 3 to 9) and does not autopolymerize under alkaline conditions. Further, due to a lower vapor pressure, OPA is essentially odorless and less irritating to users. Its antimicrobial activity has been tested over 0.05 to 1% (wt/wt), but solutions at 1% (pH 6 to 8) are required for activity against some bacterial spores over 10 hours of exposure.

3.4.2.2 Formaldehyde. Formaldehyde (methanol, CH_2O) is used for a variety of applications in aqueous or gaseous form. Formaldehyde is a monoaldehyde that exists as a freely water-soluble, colorless gas with a pungent odor. Formaldehyde aqueous solutions (formalin) contain ~34 to 40% (wt/wt) CH_2O in water with methanol (8 to 15%) to delay polymerization. Formaldehyde is also available in polymeric form, as paraformaldehyde, which is available as a white, crystalline powder. Solutions of 4 to 8% formaldehyde in water or alcohol (e.g., 70% ethanol) are used as hard-surface disinfectants, primarily in laboratory applications. Formaldehyde solutions in alcohol were used in the past for device disinfection but are now generally contraindicated due to toxicity and corrosion concerns. Formalin is widely used as a fixative for histological preparations and as a preservative (e.g., in embalming solutions). Formaldehyde is also used in many manufactured products such as resins, adhesives, and vaccines (of poliovirus).

Formaldehyde gas is produced by heating paraformaldehyde, heating formalin solutions, or mixing formalin with potassium permanganate crystals. Formaldehyde is used in gaseous form as an area fumigant (in laboratories, rooms, incubators, etc.) and, in combination with low-temperature steam, as a device sterilization process (see chapter 6, section 6.3). A typical fumigation process uses 6 g of formalin in

40 ml of water for every cubic meter of room area; formaldehyde is vaporized by being heated, held in the room for ~7 hours and then subsequently aerated for up to 2 days, depending on the application. The antimicrobial effects of the gas are dependent on the presence of humidity (>70%), but condensation should be avoided, because formaldehyde rapidly dissolves and becomes significantly less effective, which restricts antimicrobial efficacy in the area.

Novel processes have also utilized formaldehyde-releasing agents for antisepsis, preservation, and other applications (Fig. 3.3).

These applications include the use of a large number of cyclic and acyclic compounds including noxythiolin (oxymethylenethiourea), taurolin (a condensate of two molecules of the aminosulfonic acid taurine with three molecules of formaldehyde), and hexamine (hexamethylenetetramine, methenamine). Hexamine, for example, is a widely used chemical in adhesives and for other industrial purposes. Its primary antimicrobial use is as a preservative or as a urinary tract antiseptic. Other hexamine derivatives are also used as preservatives and antiseptics. All of these agents are claimed to be microbicidal on account of the release of formaldehyde. However, many of them demonstrate greater antimicrobial effects than formaldehyde alone, which may be due to direct or indirect (e.g., synergistic) effects. Low- and high-temperature formaldehyde processes have also been developed for medical, dental, and industrial sterilization applications (chapter 6, sections 6.3 and 6.4).

3.4.3 Spectrum of Activity

3.4.3.1 Glutaraldehyde and OPA. Glutaraldehyde has a broad spectrum of antimicrobial activity, being fungicidal, virucidal, and bactericidal in <10 minutes at 2%, with longer contact times required for sporicidal activity. Acidic formulations demonstrate greater activity at higher temperatures (35°C). Initial reports of protozoal cyst activity *in vitro* could not be verified *in vivo*. Other reports of unexpected resistance to 2% glutaraldehyde include strains of *Mycobacterium chelonae*, *Mycobacterium avium-intracellulare*, and some fungi. Recent reports of the lack of activity of both glutaraldehyde and OPA disinfectants against certain strains of human papillomavirus have been a cause of some concern but do not seem to reflect the demonstrated activity against a wide range of other nonenveloped viruses; these

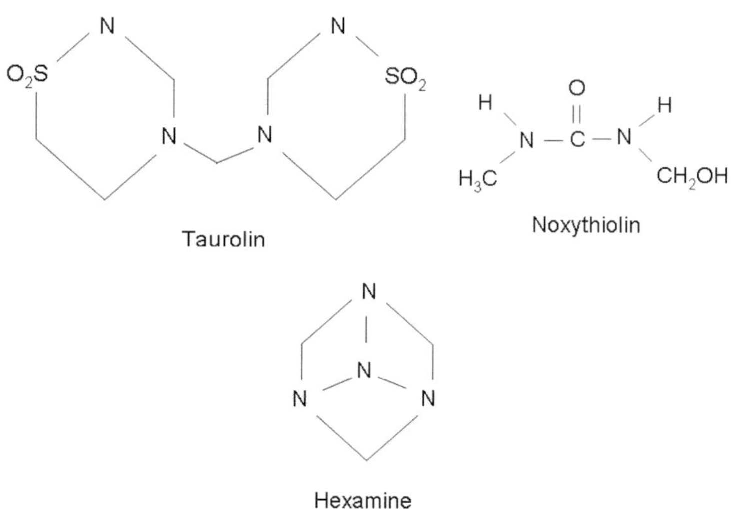

FIGURE 3.3 Examples of formaldehyde-releasing agents.

inconsistent reports deserve further investigation. Glutaraldehyde-based disinfectants are also known to be effective against fungal and bacterial spores, although the latter is reported to require longer exposure times against the spores of certain bacterial strains, depending on their specific formulation (e.g., ranging from 6 to 10 hours).

OPA has a similar efficacy profile, with the notable exceptions of little to no sporicidal activity against certain types of bacterial spores (such as *Bacillus*, but more rapid activity reported against *Clostridium* spores); improved mycobactericidal efficacy has been observed in comparison to glutaraldehyde, including some efficacy against certain strains of glutaraldehyde-resistant mycobacteria, which may be linked to its less cross-reactive nature and (due to its lipophilic nature) greater penetration into bacterial cell walls. Some mycobacteria strains have demonstrated greater resistance to OPA, but this may be formulation-dependent. OPA has also been shown to be rapidly bactericidal, virucidal, and fungicidal.

3.4.3.2 Formaldehyde. Formaldehyde is virucidal, bactericidal, mycobactericidal, fungicidal, and also sporicidal with longer contact times. Typical concentrations used range from 5 to 50 mg/liter. There has been some debate on the extent of sporicidal activity and if the effects are primarily sporistatic; however, this could be due to variations in experimental test methods, in particular, relative humidity levels used during exposure. It is known that the activity of formaldehyde is significantly less effective in the presence of contaminating soil or microorganism clumping. This has been shown in preparations of viral vaccines (polio virus), where particulate clumping protected infectious viruses from inactivation by formaldehyde; such preparations subsequently caused disease (polio) in immunized subjects. Similarly, considering the mode of action, formaldehyde has been shown to be ineffective against prions. In a notable clinical case of medical device (neurological electrodes) transmission of Creutzfeldt-Jakob disease, the material was fixed onto the device surface and remained infectious over time, transmitting disease to multiple patients and experimental animals. Some bacterial species have demonstrated increased tolerance of formaldehyde, due to alterations in outer cell surface structure (*Pseudomonas*) and plasmid-mediated expression of formaldehyde dehydrogenase (*Escherichia*), which degrades the biocide. Formaldehyde gas has been shown to be ineffective against some protozoal cysts and helminth eggs, although these studies require further investigation.

3.4.4 Advantages

3.4.4.1 Glutaraldehyde and OPA. Glutaraldehyde formulations provide rapid low-temperature (generally room temperature at ~20 to 25°C) disinfection of heat-sensitive medical devices and other surfaces. Particularly notable is its noncorrosive nature and lack of deleterious effects on sensitive materials, including plastics, lenses, and rubbers. Many formulations are available and are low cost. These range in antimicrobial and material compatibility claims. OPA-based products are generally more expensive but provide equally good compatibility with materials. They typically demonstrate more rapid activity against mycobacteria, including against several glutaraldehyde-resistant strains. No activation of OPA-based disinfectants is required prior to use, and formulations are considered more stable, increasing the number of times the product can be reused. OPA is a weaker fixative than glutaraldehyde and, due to its lower vapor pressure, is less noxious than glutaraldehyde solutions.

3.4.4.2 Formaldehyde. Fumigation with formaldehyde gas is cost-effective and easy, with no specific apparatus required. It has been traditionally used for control of microorganisms in enclosed areas. Formaldehyde, via conversion to formic acid, breaks down in the environment into carbon dioxide and water, with a typical half-life of within a few hours. Liquid and vapor applications demonstrate broad-spectrum activity, including that against spores over time.

The biocide is compatible with a wide range of metals, plastics, and other materials.

3.4.5 Disadvantages

3.4.5.1 Glutaraldehyde and OPA. Glutaraldehyde fumes are notably irritating and toxic to skin, mucous membranes, and in particular, the respiratory tract. Respiratory tract irritation is observed at concentrations as low as 0.3 ppm. Therefore, good ventilation, preferably in a vented fume cabinet, is strongly recommended when glutaraldehyde is being use. There is conflicting evidence on the mutagenicity associated with the use of this biocide. A further consideration is the absorption of glutaraldehyde into plastics and rubbers, which can cause localized toxicity due to inadequate removal following its use (e.g., colitis in the use of flexible endoscopes). This can be avoided by adequate rinsing in water (over time and over multiple rinsing cycles) in accordance with manufacturers' instructions. Surfaces should be meticulously cleaned prior to treatment, due to the potential of glutaraldehyde fixing material onto surfaces. OPA has not been as well studied but is considered less cross-linking and less toxic than glutaraldehyde; however, due to the mode to fix of action, similar precautions in its use should be taken. The identification of waterborne mycobacteria and certain nonenveloped viruses (e.g., human papillomavirus strains) with higher levels of resistance to both biocides is of some concern and is in need of further investigations. OPA has little to no demonstrated activity against some bacterial spores and protozoan cysts. The biocide stains surfaces (in particular, protein-containing surfaces, including clothing, hard surfaces, and skin) gray or black, which can be undesirable; this should be considered a benefit in the detection of residual soils on cleaned surfaces, which can limit the efficacy of the biocide.

As for many biocides, the activity of aldehydes is dramatically reduced in the presence of contaminating or residual soil (in particular, the presence of amines), presumably due to reactions with the soil and shielding of microorganisms from biocidal activity. Some countries (or areas thereof) have restricted the use and/or disposal of aldehyde wastes in sewer systems or waterways due to toxicity concerns.

3.4.5.2 Formaldehyde. The biggest disadvantage of formaldehyde is the safety concerns: formaldehyde is considered a strong irritant that is toxic, mutagenic, and carcinogenic. The carcinogenic data are conflicting and, with current data, associated with the gaseous form. Permanent damage to olfactory (smelling) tissues and other mucous membranes can occur at toxic levels. Allergic or sensitization reactions to lower concentrations are not uncommon. Formaldehyde can cause eye and mucous membrane irritation at 0.05 ppm, with a proposed safety limit of 0.75 ppm over a typical working day; control and monitoring of these levels can be difficult. Further, chemicals used to generate the biocide or deposited on surfaces following fumigation can be equally hazardous to the user. For example, formalin is an irritant—toxic and caustic—and formalin-permanganate reactions are violently exothermic (heat-producing). Close attention should be paid to ensure that high humidity levels are maintained during biocidal applications, because these are required for antimicrobial efficacy, and, where surfaces can absorb formaldehyde, that sufficient time is allowed for an area to aerate prior to re-entry. Corrosion to some materials may occur. Some countries restrict the venting of formaldehyde into the environment without prior neutralization (e.g., by ammonia or ammonium hydroxide). Removal of gross soil prior to fumigation ensures greater efficacy.

3.4.6 Mode of Action

3.4.6.1 Glutaraldehyde and OPA. The major mode of action of glutaraldehyde is considered to be cross-linking with proteins and inhibition of the synthesis of DNA, RNA, and other macromolecules. Glutaraldehyde is predominantly a surface-reactive biocide. The specific mode of action is due to alkylation reactions with amino groups (primary amines) and sulfhydryls, which form bridges or cross-links in protein structures. Some amino acids (as the primary building blocks in proteins) have free, exposed amino groups (e.g., lysine and arginine), which are the direct targets of coupling reactions with aldehydes such as glutaraldehyde. It is believed that cross-linking of these groups on cell surface proteins leads to rapid inhibition of essential cell functions.

Glutaraldehyde is more active at alkaline than at acidic pH. As the external pH is altered from acid to alkaline, amino groups at the cell surface are converted to the free amine forms and readily react with glutaraldehyde, leading to a more rapid bactericidal effect. The resulting cross-linking prevents the cell from undertaking most, if not all, of its essential, in particular, cell wall- and membrane-related, functions. Novel acidic glutaraldehyde formulations (as alternatives to alkaline glutaraldehyde formulations) have been commercialized that benefit from the greater inherent stability of the aldehyde at lower pH levels. The improved sporicidal activity claimed for these products may be obtained by agents that potentiate the dialdehyde. Glutaraldehyde is also mycobactericidal. Unfortunately, no critical studies have yet been undertaken to evaluate the nature of this action, but some evidence suggests a strong interaction with surface protein structures. Several recent reports have described the identification of *M. chelonae* and other strains with dramatically increased resistance to glutaraldehyde; although the specific resistance factors remain to be identified, differences in the structure of the cell wall in these isolates, in particular, in the wall-associated protein, carbohydrates, and lipids, have been speculated. Investigations have highlighted the lack of surface-associated proteins (in particular, a group of proteins known as porins) in these strains that may render them less sensitive to the effects of the biocide.

Although most studies of glutaraldehyde have involved bacteria, similar modes of action are expected for fungi (interaction with chitin), viruses, and spores. Spore-forming bacteria become more resistant to glutaraldehyde as spore development proceeds. Mature spores bind the biocide to their surface, but uptake has been debated and may be pH-dependent, with alkaline formulation thought to have greater penetration. It has been suggested that changes in pH may also affect the cell or spore surface itself, freeing more amino groups to cross-linking at alkaline pH. The presence of glutaraldehyde can cause spore swelling and inhibits subsequent spore germination, suggesting a direct interaction. Viruses are sensitive to relatively low concentrations of glutaraldehyde; however, it has been noted that free nucleic acid (for example, poliovirus RNA) is more resistant, suggesting a predominant capsid (surface) interaction. Nonenveloped viruses (such as parvoviruses) have higher resistance profiles in comparison to enveloped viruses, with the most resistant types being particularly associated with less reactive surface protein structures. Inhibition of protozoa has also been shown, although the mode of action is currently unknown. Protozoal dormant forms (cysts and oocysts) are notably more resistant to glutaraldehyde than their vegetative forms.

OPA has a similar mode of action to glutaraldehyde but is considered a less aggressive cross-linking agent. OPA covalently binds with proteins via Schiff's base formation with side terminal amino groups and side chain amino groups from lysine and arginine residues, while glutaraldehyde can react with other amino groups in biomolecules. Further, the benzene-ring structure of OPA may limit its ability to interact between adjacent reactive groups due to stearic hindrance. OPA demonstrates more rapid mycobactericidal activity in comparison to glutaraldehyde, presumably due to greater penetration of the lipophilic cell wall structure (see Fig. 1.7). OPA has been shown to be more penetrating than glutaraldehyde and to be effective on proteins within bacterial and fungal cell walls and membranes. This may be due to differences in the structure of OPA under hydrophilic conditions observed at the external surface of the cell, adopting a "locked" structure with unexposed aldehyde groups and allowing penetration of the biocide into the cell. Once within a hydrophobic environment, typical of the cell wall/membrane, it is proposed to assume a more open, exposed form with reactive aldehyde groups (chapter 7, section 7.4.3). Despite this proposed mechanism, some strains of mycobacteria are more resistant to OPA, but this does not always correlate with intrinsic resistance to glutaraldehyde.

3.4.6.2 Formaldehyde. Formaldehyde is an extremely reactive chemical that interacts with protein, DNA, and RNA *in vitro*. It is considered sporicidal by virtue of its ability to penetrate into the interior of bacterial spores. The interaction with protein results from a combination with the primary amide as well as with the amino groups. Formaldehyde is considered mutagenic, presumably by reaction with carboxyl, sulfhydryl, and hydroxyl groups. Formaldehyde reacts extensively with nucleic acids, which form cross-links that inhibit DNA and RNA activity. Lower concentrations of formaldehyde are sporistatic and inhibit germination. A similar mode of action is expected for other microorganisms. Overall, it is difficult to pinpoint accurately the mechanisms responsible for formaldehyde-induced microbial inactivation, because it is more of a ubiquitous toxic substance to a variety of macromolecules. Clearly, its interactive and cross-linking properties play a considerable role in this activity. Further, hydration plays a key role in the antimicrobial activity of formaldehyde, because it is dependent on the presence of water or humidity (at least >60%) for optimal activity.

3.5 ALCOHOLS

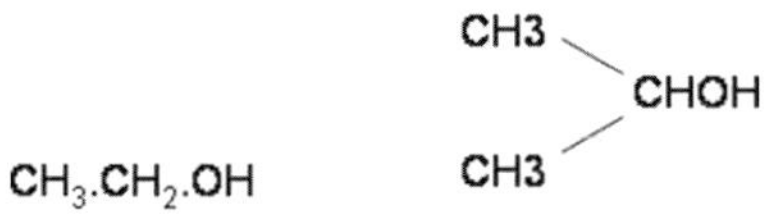

$CH_3.CH_2.OH$

Ethanol

CH3 \ CHOH / CH3

Isopropanol (Propan-2-ol)

3.5.1 Types

Alcohols are compounds with one or more hydroxyl groups (-OH) attached to a carbon atom. A variety of alcohols are used for many chemical and industrial purposes. As antiseptics and disinfectants, the most widely used alcohols are isopropanol (isopropyl alcohol, propan-2-ol, "rubbing alcohol"), ethanol ("alcohol"), and *n*-propanol (propan-1-ol). Many products list "methylated spirits" or IMS as the biocide, which is simply a mixture of 95% ethanol and 5% methanol. Chemically, these are shorter-chained alcohols, which are both water- and lipid-soluble. Alcohols are actually less effective in the absence of water, with typical in-use concentrations ranging from 50 to 90%, the optimum being 60 to 80% (depending on the formulation or mixture with other chemicals). Some alcohols are also used as preservatives at low concentrations, in particular, phenoxyethanol, which is a glycol ether and is commercially available as an oily, viscous liquid.

3.5.2 Applications

Alcohols are used for cleaning, as a drying aid, disinfection, and antisepsis. They can be a good choice for cleaning (in particular, for lipids or lipid-soluble soils), because they rapidly dry following treatment of a surface; however, protein- and carbohydrate-based soils can coagulate on treatment with alcohols. They are often used in formulation with other chemicals as cleaners and disinfectants (Fig. 3.4).

Alcohols are probably the oldest known antiseptics, being used on both intact or broken (wounded) skin. They are commonly used for routine skin disinfection in hospitals and other facilities, both by direct application and in alcohol-impregnated wipes (Fig. 3.4). Recommended concentrations of 70 to 80% alcohols are often cited for routine application on the hands to reduce the risk of pathogen transmission, but products with lower concentrations can be as effective, depending on their formulation. Examples include retarding the evaporation rate of the alcohol (e.g., in antiseptic gels or hand-rubs) and thereby increasing contact time on the skin and achieving greater antimicrobial activity. Alcohols have also been combined with other biocides, such as in cleaning-disinfection formulations with

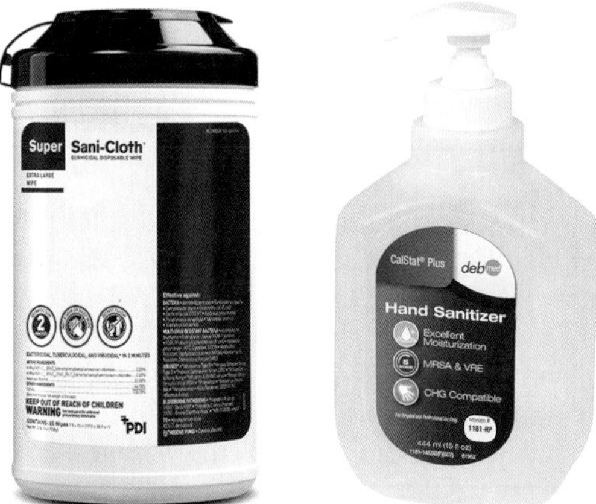

FIGURE 3.4 Alcohol-based antiseptics and disinfectants. An environmental surface disinfectant (left, impregnated wipes), and an antiseptic hand-rub (right). Product images courtesy of Professional Disposables International, Inc., and DebMed USA, with permission.

quaternary ammonium compounds (QACs), chlorhexidine, hydroxides, and hydrogen peroxide. Alcohols are also used at lower concentrations as preservatives and solvents in various antimicrobial formulations.

Phenoxyethanol is particularly used as a preservative in a variety of products including cosmetics, ophthalmological solutions, and pharmaceuticals (including vaccines) at between 0.1 and 2% and usually in combination with other preservatives, such as the parabens (section 3.2). They have also been used in antiseptic hand-washes as alternatives to traditional alcohols such as ethanol and isopropanol (see chapter 4, section 4.5).

3.5.3 Spectrum of Activity

Alcohols have rapid bactericidal and mycobactericidal activity (e.g., 70% ethanol within 30 seconds). Efficacy against fungi and viruses is variable and often slower (>2 minutes with 70% ethanol), with greater activity against enveloped viruses. Alcohols have been reported to have variable activity against nonenveloped viruses, depending on the target virus and type of alcohol or alcohol-containing formulation. Alcohols, in their own right, demonstrate little to no activity against bacterial spores but are sporistatic. Sporicidal activity can be demonstrated over time in combination with other biocides (e.g., surfactants and hydrogen peroxide). There is minimal information on the activity against protozoa, but vegetative forms are rapidly inactivated due the direct effects of the alcohol, and these microorganisms do not survive drying; protozoal cysts and oocysts have demonstrated greater resistance and vary depending on the protozoa strain but have been shown to be inactivated by alcohols over time (e.g., 70% ethanol for 10 minutes). In general, the propanols are often considered to have greater antimicrobial activity than ethanol, but this varies depending on the concentration of alcohol, the formulation of the product, and the microorganism being studied. Phenoxyethanol is primarily a bacteriostatic and fungistatic biocide with a limited spectrum of activity; its antimicrobial activity is particularly marked against Gram-negative bacteria, including *Pseudomonas*, and yeasts but is less effective against Gram-positive bacteria.

3.5.4 Advantages

Alcohols are broad-spectrum, rapid antimicrobials with little to no residues or environmental concerns following application. Cleaning and disinfection can be combined, leaving a dry surface. They are relatively stable, with little odor, inexpensive, nontoxic, and have good compatibility with surfaces (including the skin and inanimate surfaces). They are excellent solvents and are used as preservatives at low concentrations. Phenoxyethanol is stable over a wide pH range (pH 3 to 8.5) and at elevated temperatures. It is not considered toxic at the preservative concentrations typically used; at these concentrations, phenoxyethanol is nonirritating to the eyes, skin, and mucous membranes, is not considered a sensitizer, and is compatible with other types of preservatives (e.g., the parabens).

3.5.5 Disadvantages

Alcohols demonstrate little to no sporicidal activity, and bacterial spores can even survive in alcohol preparations over time. For some high-risk applications (e.g., in pharmaceutical production), sterile alcohol preparations are recommended for use to prevent spore contamination (being sterilized by radiation or filtration). At high concentrations, flammability risks should be controlled. Repeated use on the skin and certain inanimate surfaces can cause drying, irritation, and surface damage over time; alcohols can be irritating to broken skin (short-term stinging sensation). Phenoxyethanol is primarily microbistatic and is thus used mainly as a preservative. Despite a good toxicity record, irritation and allergic reactions have been reported, often related to higher concentrations than those typically used for preservation.

3.5.6 Modes of Action

Little is known about the specific mode of action of alcohols on microorganisms, but multiple toxic effects on structure and metabolism are expected, primarily due to protein denaturation and coagulation. The reactive hydroxyl (-OH) group readily forms hydrogen bonds with proteins, which leads to a loss of structure and function, causing protein and other macromolecules to precipitate. Specific inhibition of enzymes *in vitro* and in whole cells has been described. The hydrogen bonds in the tertiary structure of proteins are particularly sensitive: the alcohol disrupts the amino acid-amino bond to form an amino acid-alcohol hydrogen bond. It is believed that in the use of more concentrated alcohol solutions (>80%) the alcohol rapidly coagulates the protein on the outside of the cell wall and prevents further penetration into the cell, thereby limiting its antimicrobial activity; at 60 to 80% alcohol, greater penetration of the bacterial or fungal cell wall is expected, with further effects on the cell membrane and cytoplasmic proteins. Alcohols also disrupt the structure of any surface lipid-based cell membranes, cell walls, and viral envelopes to cause loss of integrity and function. Alcohols overall lead to cell lysis but have been shown to directly interfere with metabolite production (and therefore cell division). Although not effective against bacterial spores, alcohols do inhibit spore germination and are therefore sporistatic.

Phenoxyethanol appears primarily to target cell membranes. Low concentrations specifically interrupt the membrane proton motive force and cause leakage of cytoplasmic constituents, although these effects have been shown to be reversible in *Escherichia coli*; higher concentrations cause more gross effects on the membrane structure and penetrate into the cytoplasm, with observed inhibition of enzymes and other functions including DNA replication.

3.6 ANILIDES

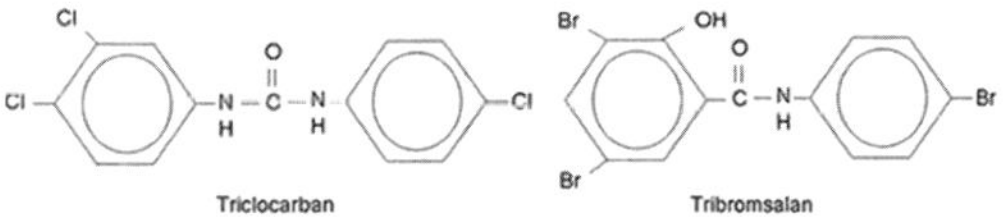

Triclocarban

Tribromsalan

3.6.1 Types

The anilides are derivatives of salicylanides and carbanilides. The most successful antimicrobial derivatives are halogenated, including the carbanilide-based triclocarban (3,4,4′-trichlorocarbanilide) and the salicylanilide-based tribromsalan (3,4′,5-tribromosalicylanide). The anilides are similar in structure to the bisphenols (see sections 3.14 and 3.15).

3.6.2 Applications

The salicylanilides, in particular tribromsalan, are used as preservatives in paper, plastics, and paints. They are also used to a lesser extent in antiseptic soaps and cosmetics. Triclocarban has been used as a cosmetic preservative and is still used in consumer antimicrobial soaps and deodorants. Overall, their use has been limited due to a restrictive spectrum of activity compared to other antiseptic biocides. In addition, tribromsalan has been restricted for use on the skin due to reports of photosensitive eruptions and skin disorders. The anilides have also had limited use as agricultural preservatives and pesticides.

3.6.3 Spectrum of Activity

Anilides, particularly halogenated derivatives, are especially effective bacteriostatic and fungistatic agents. Their specific microbicidal activity varies depending on the specific biocide and its use in formulation, but in general, they have limited fungicidal activity and some bactericidal activity. Triclocarban is particularly active against Gram-positive bacteria, many of which are important pathogenic or odor-causing bacteria on the skin. Bacteriostatic activities are observed at ~1 μg/ml, but higher concentrations are required for fungistatic activity. Triclocarban has little efficacy against Gram-negative bacteria and fungi; the exceptions are some of the fungal skin pathogens (such as *Trichophyton*, *Epidermophyton*, and *Microsporum*), which are inhibited at concentrations below 10 μg/ml. It also lacks appreciable substantivity (persistency) on the skin. The substantivity of an antiseptic may be defined as its property of adsorbing to the skin during washing and subsequently remaining available for antimicrobial activity (see chapter 4). In contrast, tribromsalan demonstrates persistency on the skin, inhibiting the growth of bacteria and fungi, but has seen limited use in antiseptics due to causing irritation and photosensitivity. Little or no activity has been reported against viruses or other microorganisms.

3.6.4 Advantages

Some anilides, in particular, triclocarban, have reasonable safety profiles; others, such as tribromsalan, are restricted in use due to toxicity concerns. Triclocarban and tribromsalan are useful preservatives at relatively low concentrations against a variety of bacterial and fungal species. They are also particularly effective against Gram-positive bacteria, in particular, for odor control. Tribromsalan is persistent on the skin and can provide residual bacteriostatic and fungistatic activity following antiseptic washing.

3.6.5 Disadvantages

Triclocarban is not persistent on the skin, which is a desired attribute present in many other biocides used in antiseptics. In contrast, tribromsalan is persistent but is sensitizing and irritating. Anilides have a limited spectrum of activity, which has restricted their use as preservatives and antiseptics for odor control; they are generally only considered reasonable bacteriostatic and fungistatic biocides. Recent evidence has suggested that triclocarban absorbs into the body and may have long-term toxic effects, including sensitization, disruption of endocrine function, and reproductive effects. It has also been found to be bioaccumulative and therefore may cause environmental concerns such as microbiome disruption and resistance development. The similarities in structure between triclocarban and the bisphenol triclosan (see section 3.15) have caused some concerns in the development of similar tolerance mechanisms and cross-resistance to antibiotics (see section 8.7.2).

3.6.6 Mode of Action

The anilides are thought to act by adsorbing to and destroying the semipermeable character of the cytoplasmic membrane, leading to cell death. The disruption of bacterial surface activities, in particular, has been investigated. Anilides have been shown to cause disruption of the proton motive force across the bacterial surface and interruption of key membrane functions including active transport and energy metabolism. These effects may be due to interference with proteins or the phospholipid bilayer of the membrane to disrupt its structure and function. Of note, the anilides did not specifically cause the leakage of cytoplasmic components in their interaction with bacterial cell membranes, suggesting subtle membrane-associated bacteriostatic effects. Greater antimicrobial activity is observed with increased halogenation of the anilides; the reactions of these groups with various macromolecules (particularly proteins and lipids) appear to contribute to their mode of action. Due to the similarities in their structures, it has been suggested that triclocarban may have similar, specific mechanisms of action to triclosan (see section 3.15), but this has not been specifically investigated to date. In fact, some studies reported that *E. coli* triclosan mutants were not cross-resistant to triclocarban, suggesting different mechanisms of action.

3.7 ANTIMICROBIAL DYES

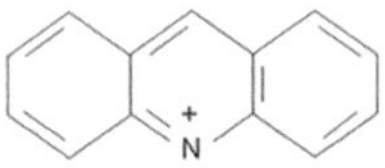

$(CH_3)_2N$ / C= / $N^+(CH_3)_2Cl^-$ / $(CH_3)_2N$ / N / O / O

Acridine 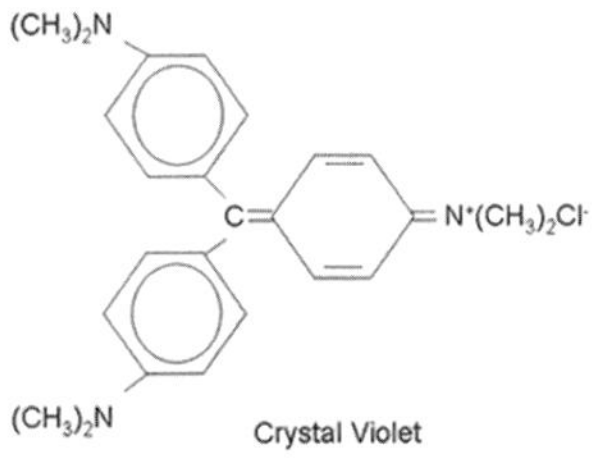 Crystal Violet

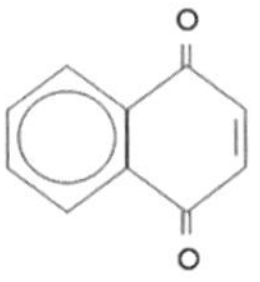

1,4-Naphthaquinone

3.7.1 Types

A variety of antimicrobial dyes have been used as traditional antiseptics and in some cases for water disinfection. These include the acridines and a variety of other dyes. The acridines were first introduced as systemic and topical antimicrobials in the early 1900s, but their use decreased following the introduction of antibiotics. The basic acridine structure is shown above, with a variety of derivatives described with varying antimicrobial or toxic properties. They are essentially hetero-aromatic dyes which have been investigated by a variety of modifications, including the addition of amino groups (known as aminoacridines), halogenation, and nitrification. Various early investigations into specific acridine modifications led to the identification of many therapeutic antiprotozoal drugs including quinoline and quinacrine (chapter 7, section 7.2.4). Further, naturally occurring acridines have been identified, e.g., the acridine alkaloids extracted from plants. The acridines most widely used as antiseptics are the aminoacridines, which include proflavine, euflavine (or acriflavine), and aminacrine (Fig. 3.5). Acriflavine exists in two forms: an acid form (euflavine, shown in Fig. 3.5) and a neutral form; the latter is more widely used due to less irritancy.

Other dyes are the triphenylmethane dyes (in particular, crystal violet and malachite green), the quinones (1,4-naphthaquinone and chloranil), and methylene blue (a phenothiazinium dye).

3.7.2 Applications

Acridine derivatives have been and are currently used in therapeutic and topical applications. Proflavine and euflavine were two of the first used as wound antiseptics, in particular proflavine, which was considered less irritating to the skin. They can be applied in powders or ointments or in soaked gauze. Proflavine, in particular, has been used in wound dressings. Older studies showed that proflavine (and other acridine derivatives) are photosensitive dyes that demonstrated increased activity against bacterial and fungal skin infections when wounds were treated first with the dye and then with various wavelengths of light. Reinvestigation of these applications as logical treatments for antibiotic-resistant bacterial wound infections has been suggested. Various acridines are also added to water for the surface treatment of fish or fish-egg infections, including surface fungal, bacterial, and protozoal infections. An example is the use of acriflavine at 5 to 10 ppm in water for the treatment of open wounds and surface protozoal infections in fish. Aminacrine is still used for the prevention and treatment of mucous membrane infections, including as vaginal suppositories in the treatment of *Trichomonas* infections,

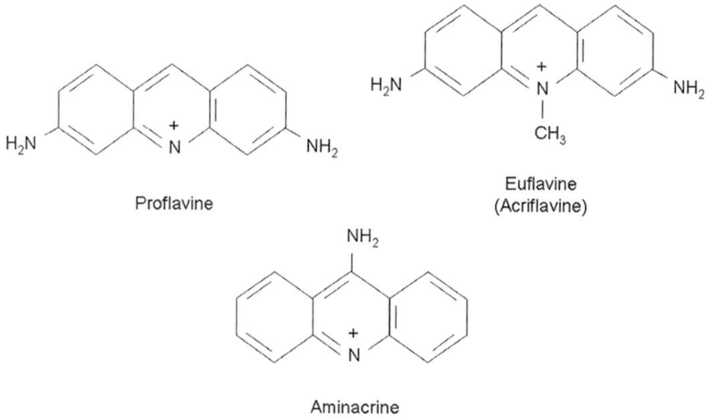

FIGURE 3.5 Aminoacridines commonly used as antiseptics.

and as a topical antiseptic. In recent years, research has focused on the development of new acridine derivatives due to their use as anticancer agents. Many of these developed acridines may also show variable activity against bacterial, fungal, and protozoan pathogens and have future applications as therapeutic antiseptics.

Other dyes such as malachite green and crystal violet have similar antiseptic applications; these dyes have also been used as localized topical antiseptics, in particular in wound applications in animals, but are not widely used on humans. Triphenylmethane dye preparations have been used for the topical treatment of persistent tinea skin infections such as ringworm and athlete's foot. Typical applications include localized treatment with a dye tincture or addition of a few drops of a dye preparation into a water sample, which is used for skin or mucous membrane washings. In addition to specific treatment of infections, a variety of these dyes are also used as general preservatives in aquaculture applications (including fish tanks and ponds) to prevent the overgrowth of bacteria, algae, and other microorganisms. Others such as the quinones are used as agricultural bactericides and fungicides, including the naphthaquinones and chloranil.

Many of these dyes are also routinely used for cytological and microbiological staining; examples include the use of crystal violet to differentiate bacterial types by Gram staining, and fluorescent acridine dyes are used for the staining of chromosomes and other nucleic acid structures.

3.7.3 Spectrum of Activity

The spectrum of activity of the acridines varies depending on their chemical structures and preparation. The dyes that form cations in solutions demonstrate the greatest antimicrobial activity. Cationic acridines are particularly broad-spectrum and retain activity in the presence of organic soils. In general, they are effective against Gram-positive and Gram-negative bacteria to varying degrees and over time. The triphenylmethane dyes are more effective against Gram-positive than Gram-negative bacteria; this is proposed to be due to the increased peptidoglycan layer in Gram-positive bacteria (chapter 8, section 8.5). Increased resistance in some bacteria has been shown to be due to reduced uptake and efflux mechanisms (section 8.3.4). Most are fungistatic but may also be fungicidal against yeasts and molds under some conditions. The acridine dyes have been used for the specific treatment of fungal infections including *Trichophyton*, *Microsporum*, and tinea, for example, in the topical treatment of athlete's foot. Their effects against viruses have not been well studied, with some reports showing activity against enveloped viruses. The mode of action of the acridines against double-stranded nucleic acids suggests activity against a wider range of viruses or inhibition of virus replication;

recent evidence of broad-spectrum activity of certain types of acridine compounds against viruses supports this claim. Acridines and other dyes have varying activity against protozoans, including *Amoeba*, *Leishmania*, and other surface-related parasites. They are often used as preservatives at low concentrations to prevent fungal and algal growth in water tanks and in ponds. Little to no sporicidal activity has been described, presumably due to a lack of penetration, although some dyes have been shown to be sporistatic.

3.7.4 Advantages

Many of the antimicrobial dyes are effective against a wide range of microorganisms at relatively low concentrations, even in the presence of serum or other organic soils, making them useful as antiseptics. Many are odorless and readily soluble in water. Their range of toxicity varies; for example, proflavine is less toxic or irritating to the skin than acriflavine. They are generally stable in preparations and formulations, with characteristically long shelf lives. In aquaculture, they can be used for the treatment of fish pathogens or surface infectious diseases, as well as for preventing the growth of microorganisms, without significant harm to fish or other aquatic life. Nonstaining acridine dyes have also been developed (e.g., aminacrine).

3.7.5 Disadvantages

One of the biggest disadvantages of dyes is aesthetic: the dye colors the skin and mucous membranes, which is often undesirable. This is not a concern with newer acridines, including aminacrine and salacrine. Like other biocides, their antimicrobial activity varies; for example, acriflavine is less effective against fungi and lacks sufficient biocidal activity under acidic (pH <7) conditions. Many of the dyes are toxic at higher concentrations, particularly as the concentration of the dye is increased from preservative to microbicidal levels. Malachite green is toxic to fish but not fish eggs. There have been concerns over the use of some acridines due to evidence of mutagenicity in bacteria and in cell culture experiments. Aminacrine is actually used under laboratory conditions as an experimental mutagen. The potential for mutagenicity may not be surprising considering the mode of action (intercalation of nucleic acid), but these dyes are also photosensitive, which can lead to further irritation (dermatitis) of the skin and other toxic effects. Photosensitization is a process by which a photosensitive molecule (in this case the acridine) adsorbs light radiation to cause a photochemical alteration. In some applications, further investigation into the carcinogenic nature of some dyes is required. Another cited disadvantage of some acridines is the ability of certain bacteria such *Staphylococcus* to acquire increased tolerance to the biocide due to energy-dependent efflux mechanisms; however, it is interesting to note that this has been reported for some acridines (including proflavine) but not for others, such as the aminacrine derivatives.

3.7.6 Mode of Action

The mode of action of the acridines has been well studied, particularly that of the aminoacridines. The primary site of acridine activity is double-stranded nucleic acids. The polycyclic, flat structure of the acridine molecule appears to be well suited to intercalate between adjacent nucleotide base pairs of DNA and other double-stranded nucleic acid structures. This alone disrupts the structure and functions of DNA, but further interactions with the phosphate backbone and the nucleotides also limit the ability of DNA to unravel, which is required for its replication and transcription. The position of the amino group in the aminoacridines appears to be important in these interactions and in the overall activity of the molecule. It is for this reason that the acridines have been investigated as potential anticancer drugs; however, during these investigations different modes of action were described.

Interactions with specific DNA-related (including topoisomerases) and other (cytoplasmic kinases) enzymes have also been described. Multiple effects have been observed in bacterial studies, including inhibition of separation during cell division and strong binding to the bacterial cell envelope. It is clear that other surface effects may contribute to the mode of action. This may be important to consider concerning the mode of action of other dyes, which have been less studied. Many antimicrobial dyes are also believed to result in catalytic production of reactive radicals during intracellular reactions. Intercalation into the bacterial peptidoglycan or interaction with other microbial surfaces appears to play an important role in the overall mechanisms of action. For example, the triphenylmethane dyes (including crystal violet) are more active against Gram-positive bacteria, which may be linked to the greater proportion of peptidoglycan in their cell wall structures (chapter 8, section 8.5). These dyes are difficult to remove from the cell wall surface following application of the dye (as demonstrated in the Gram stain), leading to disruption of associated structures and functions. Further penetration of the cell membrane and into the cytoplasm is also expected, with effects similar to those of general, cellular toxic substances. Although not described, these effects clearly affect the survival of fungi, some viruses, and other microorganisms.

3.8 BIGUANIDES

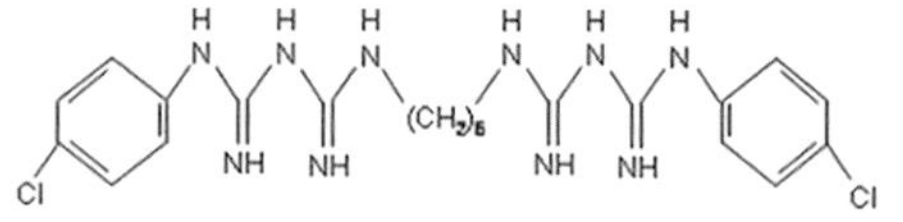

Chlorhexidine

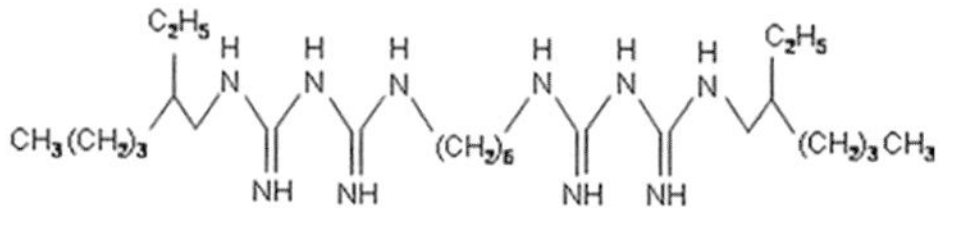

Alexidine

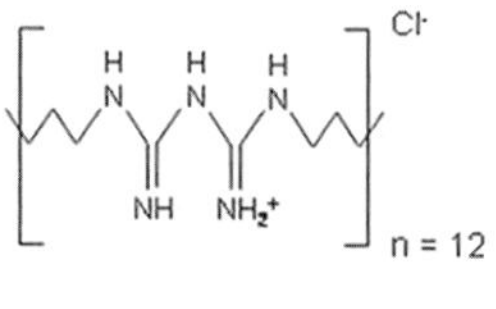

PHMB

3.8.1 Types

Biguanides are compounds that contain the $C_2H_7N_5$ ligand. Chlorhexidine (a bis-biguanide) is insoluble in water and is therefore supplied in salt forms, consisting of the chlorhexidine base reacted with an acid. The chlorhexidine molecule itself consists of a central lipophilic hexamethylene chain with a basic chlorophenyl guanide group on either end, reacted with an acid. Chlorhexidine gluconate, known as CHG, is widely used, but other salts include chlorhexidine diacetate and dihydrobromide. Alexidine differs chemically from chlorhexidine in possessing ethylexyl end-groups. Other similar chemicals, including octenidine, have been described but are less used. A newer class is the polymeric biguanides, which are a heterodisperse mixture of polyhexamethylbiguanides (PHMBs); for example, the general structure of PHMB chlorides is shown to the left. Vantocil™ is a heterodisperse mixture of PHMBs with a molecular weight of approximately 3,000.

3.8.2 Applications

Chlorhexidine is probably the most widely used biguanide, with a range of applications including its use as the biocide in antimicrobial soaps (antiseptics including the widely used Hibiclens and Hibiscrub formulations), biocidal wound dressings, skin decolonization, mouth washes, hair care, and surface disinfectants and as a preservative (e.g., contact lens storage solution). Chlorhexidine (at 0.5 to 4%) is primarily used as an antiseptic for high-risk applications, including in formulation as hospital surgical scrubs, health care personnel hand-washes, and decolonization bathing products (Fig. 3.6). Chlorhexidine is also integrated into various types of skin dressings such as for catheter insertion sites, wound infection (or prevention) treatments, and postoperative treatments.

The widespread use of chlorhexidine is due to its minimal skin irritation (which can be formulation-dependent), broad bactericidal activity, and substantivity to the skin and mucous membranes. Irritation is markedly higher with

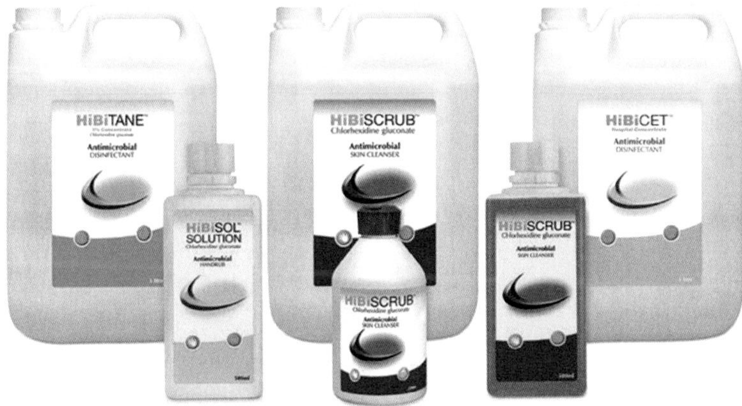

FIGURE 3.6 Examples of chlorhexidine-based antiseptics and disinfectants. ©Molnlycke Health Care AB. Used with permission. The American Society for Microbiology is not employed by, or affiliated with, Molnlycke.

alternative biguanides such as alexidine and octenidine. The broad-spectrum activity of the biguanides can be enhanced in combination with other biocides, in particular with alcohols and QACs (also known as "quats"; see section 3.16), and can be dramatically affected by pH (being more active at pH 5 to 7). PHMBs are widely used for surface disinfection in industrial and medical applications and for water sanitization, particularly as an alternative to chlorine and bromine in swimming pools and water spas. Some biguanides have also been used therapeutically; for example, dimethylbiguanide ("metformin") has been used since medieval times for the control of non-insulin-dependent diabetes and as a malarial prophylactic (e.g., proguanil).

3.8.3 Spectrum of Action

Biguanides are broad-spectrum bactericidal biocides that show rapid action against Gram-positive and Gram-negative bacteria. The PHMBs are also active against Gram-positive and Gram-negative bacteria, although *Pseudomonas aeruginosa* and *Salmonella* spp. have been reported to be less sensitive depending on the specific products being used. In general, biguanides are more active against Gram-positive bacteria, even in the presence of interfering soils such as blood or serum. They are less active against fungi, including yeasts and molds, but their effectiveness can be enhanced in combination with other active agents or by formulation effects. Although chlorhexidine and alexidine have a similar spectrum of activity, alexidine is more rapid in its action. Overall, the formulation of these active agents is important to optimizing their antimicrobial activity and effectiveness on the skin (or other environmental applications). They are not sporicidal but do inhibit the outgrowth (but not the germination) of spores, although some sporicidal activity has been demonstrated in combination with other biocides (alkali, alcohol) or at higher temperatures (>70°C) over time. Biguanides have limited activity against viruses, with some activity against the lipid-enveloped viruses (including significant nosocomial pathogens such as HIV and influenza), due to disruption of the viral envelope, and little to no activity against nonenveloped viruses. As with other biocides, mycobacteria are more resistant than other bacteria, presumably due to a lack of penetration through their unique cell wall structures, but can be growth-inhibited at low concentrations, similar to other bacteria. Some biguanides (e.g., chlorhexidine and the PHMBs) have also been shown to cause damage to active protozoal life stages (including trophozoites and ameobae) but have little to no effect on the viability of cysts or eggs; they have been reported as being algistatic.

3.8.4 Advantages

Biguanides, chlorhexidine in particular, have been widely used for antisepsis due to low irritation of the skin, wounds, and mucous membranes. Skin absorption has been reported as being minimal. Biguanides have similar advantages, as an alternative to chlorine and bromine, in swimming pool maintenance. They are particularly effective in the control of hand transmission of pathogens in hospitals, including antibiotic-resistant bacteria such as methicillin-resistant *Staphylococcus aureus* (MRSA), and in the treatment of wounds with little irritation. In recent years, the use of chlorhexidine for universal patient decolonization (e.g., as a preparation for surgery and in intensive-care units) has been widely cited as being effective in preventing hospital-acquired infections such as those caused by MRSA and vancomycin-resistant *Enterococcus*. Because chlorhexidine and alexidine can remain at bacteriostatic concentrations on the skin following washing, they can control the subsequent regrowth or contamination of the skin over time; this may be particularly important in the prevention of bacterial overgrowth on the skin when under occlusion (for example, when using gloves) during surgical procedures. Similarly, biguanide-impregnated skin or wound dressings have been shown to reduce the rates of catheter- or wound-associated infections by producing a local application of the biocide over time at these higher-risk areas.

3.8.5 Disadvantages

Some bacterial strains have developed increased tolerance to biguanides and have been linked to plasmid-mediated cross-tolerance to antibiotics. Although these changes may not be significant enough to allow growth at the bacteriostatic concentrations of biguanides, or to affect their bactericidal activities, they have been speculated to promote antibiotic resistance (chapter 8, section 8.7.3). Although limited, some cases of sensitivity (including anaphylactic shock) to biguanides have been reported, and contact with the eyes should be avoided. Chlorhexidine and other biguanides can be inactivated by nonionic surfactants, which can be present in some soaps and hand creams, natural soaps, and inorganic water contaminants (such as phosphates and chlorine). Depending on the concentrations, chlorhexidine and the PHMBs may have limited activity against the growth of algae, water-based molds, or bacterial biofilms, which can allow for their selective development over time in treated water.

3.8.6 Modes of Action

The mechanism of action of chlorhexidine against bacteria and yeast has been well studied. Chlorhexidine and generally all biguanides primarily act on cell membranes, causing loss of structure and function. Their biguanide chemical structure allows for rapid absorption through bacterial and fungal cell walls and damage to the inner cell membranes (at higher concentrations), causing cytoplasm leakage and precipitation of proteins and nucleic acids. Direct insertion and interaction with the lipids in the cell membrane are the proposed primary mechanism. The proposed sequence of events during biguanide interaction with the Gram-negative cell envelope is as follows. (i) There is rapid attraction toward the negatively charged bacterial cell surface, with strong and specific adsorption to phosphate-containing compounds. (ii) The integrity of the outer membrane is impaired, allowing further penetration toward the inner membrane. (iii) Direct insertion into the cell membrane or binding to the phospholipids occurs, with an increase in inner membrane permeability (K^+ loss), accompanied by bacteriostasis. In the case of alexidine and the polymeric biguanides, the attraction and interaction with the membrane lipids lead to the formation of lipid domains with dramatic effects on the membrane permeability due to loss of structure. (iv) Complete loss of membrane function occurs, with precipitation of intracellular constituents and bactericidal effect.

Mycobacteria are unique in their cell wall structure (chapter 1, section 1.3.4.1, and chapter 8, section 8.4) and demonstrate varied resistance to chlorhexidine. *M. avium-intracellulare* is considerably more resistant, while other species are inhibited at relatively lower concentrations. This may be due to differences in the various cell wall structures that limit penetration of the biocide to the primary cell membrane target. The trophozoites, or "vegetative" forms of protozoa such as *Acanthamoeba castellanii*, are sensitive to chlorhexidine due to membrane damage; however, the dormant cysts are much less sensitive, presumably due to limited penetration of the biocide. Similarly, chlorhexidine is effective against vegetative forms of bacteria but not bacterial spores. Even with high concentrations of the biguanide, no effects were observed on the viability of *Bacillus* spores at ambient temperatures, although at elevated temperatures a marked sporicidal effect was achieved. Presumably, sufficient changes occur in the spore structure to permit an increased uptake of the biguanide and interaction with internal constituents. Chlorhexidine does not inhibit germination but does inhibit the outgrowth of bacterial spores, supporting a lack of penetration of the intact spore structure and rapid action against the internal cell membrane following germination.

The antiviral activity of chlorhexidine is variable. Studies with different types of bacteriophages have shown that chlorhexidine has no effect on MS2 or K coliphages. High concentrations also failed to inactivate *P. aeruginosa* phage F116 and had no effect on phage DNA within the capsid or on phage proteins; the phage transduction process was more sensitive to chlorhexidine and other biocides than was the phage itself. Chlorhexidine is not considered a particularly effective antiviral agent, and its activity is restricted to the lipid-enveloped viruses. This appears to be due to disruption of the lipid viral envelopes, which can render the virus noninfectious. Chlorhexidine does not significantly inactivate nonenveloped viruses such as rotaviruses, hepatitis A virus, or polioviruses. Any activity appears to be restricted to the nucleic acid core or the outer coat, although it is likely that the latter would be a more important target site.

3.9 DIAMIDINES

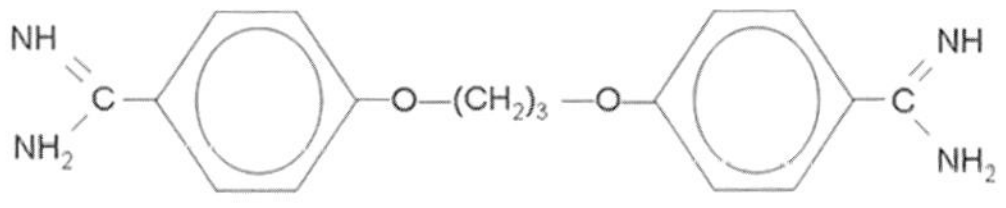

Propamidine

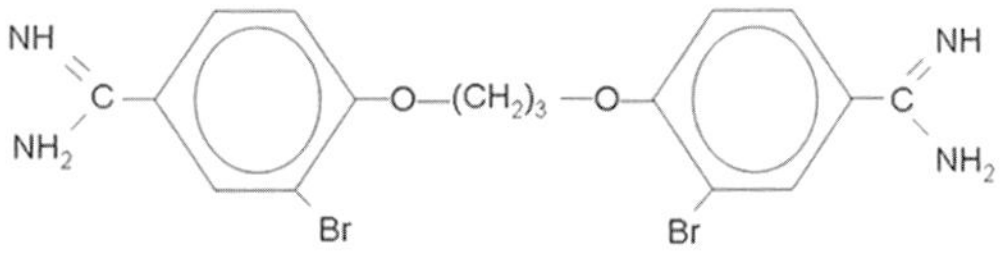

Dibromopropamidine

3.9.1 Types

The diamidines are a group of antimicrobial agents with similar structures that are used as antiseptics. The most widely used are proamidine and the halogened dibromopropamidine. They are both available in the isethionate salt form in drop, ointment, or cream formulations.

3.9.2 Applications

The diamidines are primarily used therapeutically in the treatment of skin, wound, and eye infections. Examples include creams and ointments containing up to 0.15% propamidine or dibromopropamidine which are used for the prevention or topical treatment of wound infections. Further uses are in eye drops and ointments in the treatment of conjunctivitis (bacterial, fungal, and viral) and keratitis due to the amoeba *Acanthamoeba*, which is frequently implicated in contact lens contamination. They have also been used in combination with other antimicrobials such as the biguanides and antibiotics. Therapeutically, the diamidines are used for systemic infections with trypanosomes, such as in *Leishmania* and *Pneumocystis* infections. Diamidine derivatives are the focus of research for further antiparasitic chemotherapy.

3.9.3 Spectrum of Activity

Propamidine and dibromopropamidine have a similar spectrum of activity. They are effective against bacteria, fungi, and some parasites. Antibacterial activity is particularly marked against Gram-positive bacteria, with a typical MIC range of 0.2 to 25 μg/ml, with higher concentrations required to inhibit the growth of some Gram-negative bacteria (25 to 500 μg/ml) and fungi (100 to 1,000 μg/ml). Many antibiotic-resistant strains of *Staphylococcus* (e.g., MRSA strains) and *Pseudomonas* spp. demonstrate higher tolerance to diamidines, but overall, these effects are biocide- and formulation-specific. Activity has also been investigated against *Leishmania*, *Trypanosoma*, and *Pneumocystis*. The diamidines are effective against amoeba, including *Acanthamoeba*, but are poorly cysticidal (but this may be overcome in formulation with other biocides and excipients, such as when combined with 30% dimethyl sulfoxide).

3.9.4 Advantages

The diamidines are not considered toxic in antiseptic applications and are safe for direct use in the eye (dependent on the concentration used). They demonstrate broad-spectrum activity against bacteria, fungi, and protozoa and maintain activity in the presence of organic soils.

3.9.5 Disadvantages

Bacteria, fungi, and parasites resistant to diamidines have been described, including some MRSA strains and *Pseudomonas* spp. (such as common water contaminants). Their activities are dramatically affected under acidic (low-pH) conditions. In some cases, diamidines have caused skin irritation; side effects of renal and hepatic toxicity have also been reported, but primarily in chemotherapeutic applications.

3.9.6 Mode of Action

The mechanisms of action of the diamidines are considered similar to those of cationic surfactants (section 3.16) due to their bipolar structure with interference of cell membrane structure and function. Their exact mechanism of action is unknown, but diamidines have been shown to inhibit membrane uptake, modify cell permeability, and induce leakage of amino acids in bacteria. Their respective charge and hydrophobicity allow for interaction with microbial cell surfaces and affinity with the negatively charged phospholipids of the cell membrane and other intracellular components (e.g., nucleic acids). Specific disruption and damage to the cell surface of *P. aeruginosa*, *Enterobacter cloacae*, and the plasma membrane of amoebae have been described. It is clear that the diamidines (similar to cationic surfactants) can further penetrate into the cytoplasm to cause denaturation and coagulation of proteins and enzymes; specific inhibition of various enzymes has been reported including membrane-associated (e.g., ATPase) and intracellular proteins (e.g., topoisomerases and decarboxylases). The mode of action of the diamidines has been shown to include interaction with DNA, RNA, and nucleoside-containing compounds leading to their precipitation. Interactions with DNA appear to be preferably at adenine-thymine tracts (referred to as the minor grooves in the structure of DNA). In addition to primary effects on microbial membranes, the diamidines clearly inhibit DNA and RNA functions, as well as various proteins and enzymes in the cytoplasm.

3.10 ESSENTIAL OILS AND PLANT EXTRACTS

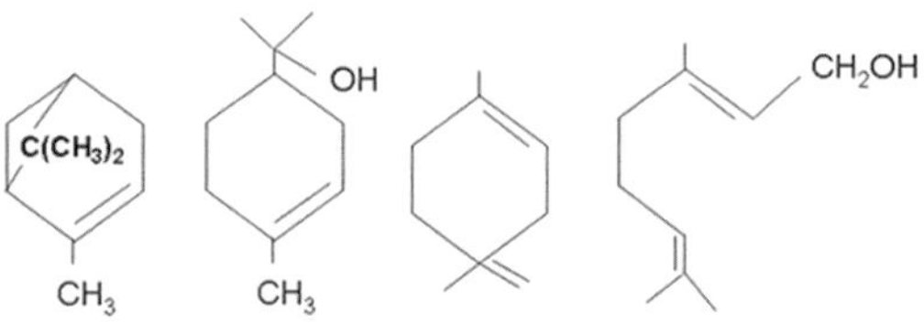

Pinene Terpineol Limonene Geraniol

3.10.1 Types

The essential oils are a complex mixture of chemicals that are extracted from various plants by concentration or distillation. They are widely distributed and isolated from various plant parts including flowers, leaves (or needles), wood, and roots (Table 3.2).

As secondary metabolites from plants, they have been ascribed various functions including as natural biocides for the protection of plant cells from various pathogens. Chemical analysis of these oils has shown that they consist of a range of terpenes, terpenoids, and oxides. Terpenes are hydrocarbons with the molecular formula $(C_5H_8)_n$ and are classified based on the number of repeating isoprene units (five carbon units) that they contain, such as monoterpenes (two isoprene units, e.g., pinene and camphor) and sesquiterpenes (three units, e.g., nerolidal). The terpenoids (or isoprenoids) are chemically modified terpenes (e.g., by oxidation) such as alcohols (geraniol, citronellol), phenols (thymol), aldehydes (neural, citronellal), and ketones (camphor). The oxides include various acids and sulfur compounds (e.g., eucalyptol). Tea tree oil, for example, contains over 100 compounds including monoterpenes, sesquiterpenes, and various alcohols; the major biocide has been found to be the alcohol terpinen-4-ol (generally present at ≥30% in the oil). Pine oil is isolated by steam distillation from wood chips and/or pine needles from various species of *Pinus*, and the major biocides identified are terpineol and pinene.

3.10.2 Applications

Essential oils have characteristic strong yet pleasant odors and have been used in various cleaners and as deodorizers (Fig. 3.7). They are widely used as fragrances and traditionally used as food preservatives (e.g., herbs and species). Some have been used in antiseptics, including in hand-washes, as mouthwashes, and for acne treatment; these include tea tree oil, which has been particularly well studied and used for various antiseptic applications. Pine oil has been widely used in cleaning and disinfection formulations. Its "fresh" smell is often associated with cleanliness; however, in its own right it has little antimicrobial activity and is usually formulated with other biocides (in particular, phenolics, including chlorophenols, and acids) for disinfectant applications. Similarly, lemon oil (containing ~90% limonene) and other citrus oils are used in cleaning and disinfection formulations. Essential oils have also been used for their preservative activities, often in combination with other preservatives. In addition to their biocidal properties, a variety of other chemotherapeutic and medicinal applications have been proposed for essential oils and their components.

3.10.3 Spectrum of Activity

Given the range of essential oils, their spectrum of activity can vary considerably, from potent bactericidal and fungicidal activity to only narrow bacteriostatic and fungistatic activity and, in some cases, no appreciable biocidal activity. In general, essential oils demonstrate greater activity against Gram-positive bacteria than against Gram-negative bacteria, with *Pseudomonas* and *Listeria* strains demonstrating the greatest resistance; exceptions include the activity of pine oils against *Pseudomonas* (although activity is generally less in some Gram-positive bacteria) and the broader bactericidal activity of tea tree oil. The biocidal activity of tea tree oil has been particularly well studied; bactericidal activity has been described within the 0.25 to 0.5% range, with *Pseudomonas* being the most resistant. Tea tree oil is also effective against various fungi, in

TABLE 3.2 Types and sources of essential oils and their use in biocides

Oil	Source	Major biocides
Tea tree	*Melaleuca alternifolia*	Terpinen-4-ol (>30%), cineole (3%)
Pine	*Pinus* spp.	Terpineol, pinene
Lemon	*Citrus limon*	Limonene (90%)
Thyme	*Thymus vulgaris*	Thymol (20–30%)
Geranium	*Cymbopogan* spp.	Geraniol (85–90%)
Eucalyptus	*Eucalyptus globulus*	Cineol (>70%), various terpenes

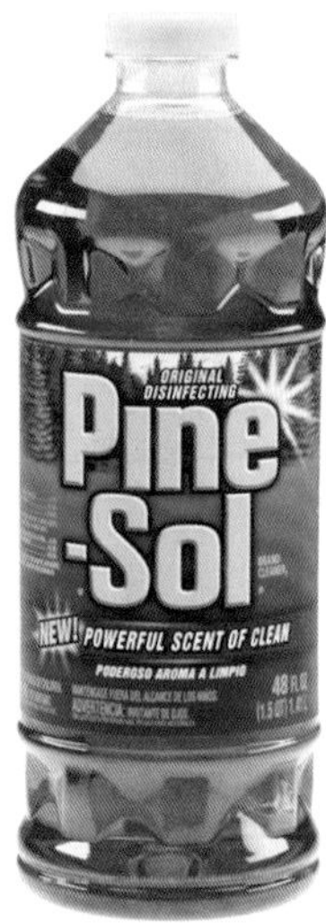

FIGURE 3.7 Example of an essential oil disinfectant. ©2017 The Clorox Company. Reprinted with permission. CLOROX® and PINE-SOL® are registered trademarks of The Clorox Company and are used with permission.

particular yeasts and the dermatophytes (including *Candida* and *Trichophyton*, which can be commonly isolated from skin or mucous membranes), with fungistatic activity at 0.03 to 0.5% and fungicidal activity at 0.06 to 1%. The main compounds with biocidal activity in tea tree oil appear to be terpin-4-ol, linalool, and α-terpineol. Some oils have been shown to inhibit the production of fungal alfatoxins (e.g., geranium oils). The virucidal potential of various oils has not been investigated in any detail, although reports on tea tree oil have suggested activity against some enveloped viruses (such as herpes simplex viruses associated with cold sores and other mucous membrane infections) but not the more resistant nonenveloped viruses. Some essential oils have been found to be mycobacteriostatic and sporistatic.

3.10.4 Advantages

Most essential oils demonstrate bacteriostatic and fungistatic activities at relatively low concentrations. Some oils also have broad bactericidal and fungicidal activities, with little associated irritancy at typically used concentrations. They have pleasant odors and are considered biodegradable. Many have good compatibility with various treated surfaces including skin and hard surfaces. Tea tree and other oils used on the skin have been shown to have some persistency, remaining active on the skin over time.

3.10.5 Disadvantages

The antimicrobial activity of essential oils is dependent on correct formulation, and product efficacy can range considerably. At high concentrations they can be flammable and combustible. In some cases, skin irritancy has been described, and allergic reactions are common; there have been some concerns over skin and mucous membrane toxicity with excessive use leading to poisoning. In some disinfectant applications, incompatibility with various elastomers (such as silicon rubber and PVC) has been described.

3.10.6 Modes of Action

The mechanisms of action of essential oils can be complex, depending on the hydrophobicity or hydrophilicity of the oils and the various biocidal components that can be present, including the potential of synergistic activities between the various biocides present. Overall, they appear to cause effects similar to those described for phenolics (section 3.14), in particular for the predominantly hydrophobic oils (including terpenes). The major site of action is the cell membrane (including the outer membrane in Gram-negative bacteria). Electron microscopy has shown the cell membrane structure to be disrupted, with parallel interference with various membrane functions including disruption of the proton motive force (chapter 7, section 7.4.5, and chapter 8, section 8.3.4) and leakage of cytoplasmic materials. Thymol and tea tree oil have been specifically shown to disrupt the outer and inner membranes of *E. coli*, leading to cytoplasmic leakage and eventual cell lysis; similar effects have been observed in Gram-positive bacteria. As general cell poisons, other effects have been observed including protein coagulation, cell wall disintegration, and inhibition of RNA, DNA, protein, and carbohydrate synthesis in bacteria and fungi. Studies of the fungi *Cladosporium herbarum* with eugenol and carvacrol have shown similar morphological changes, with lower concentrations affecting the activity of various cell wall-associated enzymes, reduced growth rate, and inhibition of stationary phase phenomena such as sporulation and secondary metabolite production.

3.11 HALOGENS AND HALOGEN-RELEASING AGENTS

I - I
Iodine

Br - Br
Bromine

Cl - Cl
Chlorine

3.11.1 Types

Halogens are a group of elements that are physically distinct but show similarities in their chemical reactivity. They include fluorine (F_2), chlorine (Cl_2), bromine (Br_2), and iodine (I_2). Chemically, they have high electronegativity and are highly reactive as oxidizing agents, in the order of $F_2 > Cl_2 > Br_2 > I_2$. Physically, at room temperature and atmospheric pressure, iodine is a solid, bromine is a liquid, and fluorine and chlorine are both gases. Chlorine, iodine, and bromine are widely used as disinfectants and antiseptics. Despite its high reactivity and some studies demonstrating antimicrobial effects of fluorine in the oral cavity, fluorine is not widely used as a biocide.

Iodine (I, atomic weight = 126.9) in its purified form is a bluish-black, shiny solid which is readily soluble in organic solvents (such as alcohol or chloroform) but only slightly soluble in water. It can also sublime into a purple-blue gas with an irritating odor. It is found naturally in seawater and subterranean brines and can be synthesized by reaction of potassium iodide with copper sulfate. The chemistry of iodine in water is complicated by the formation of various iodine-containing species (Fig. 3.8), but only two have been reported to significantly contribute to the overall antimicrobial activity: free, or molecular, iodine (I_2) and hypoiodous acid.

Simple iodine solutions are prepared by dissolving iodine, potassium iodide, or sodium iodide in water or alcohol. Examples include tinctures of iodine (e.g., 2% iodine and 2.4% potassium iodide in ethanol) and Lugol's solution (5% iodine and 10% potassium iodide in water). Alternatively, elemental iodine can be complexed or bound with high-molecular-weight neutral polymers, including alcohol, amide, and sugar polymers. These complexes are known as iodophors and have the benefits of increasing the solubility and stability of iodine by allowing the active iodine species to be slowly released over time. The most widely used iodophor is poly(*N*-vinyl-2-pyrrolidone), which is complexed with iodine in the triiodide form (povidone-iodine [PVPI]) (Fig. 3.9). PVPI solutions or formulations can be prepared in an aqueous (water) or organic (e.g., alcohol) base; for example, a 10% PVPI solution in water gives an active iodine (I_2) concentration of 0.03 to 0.04% (see Fig. 3.10). Another example of an iodophor is poloxamer-iodine.

Chlorine (Cl, atomic weight = 35.45 g) is a yellow-green gas with a strong, irritating odor. It is found in reduced forms in nature as sodium (NaCl, or common salt), calcium, and potassium salts. For antiseptic and disinfection purposes, "chlorine" refers to the presence of active, or oxidized, chlorine compounds which are formed in water (Fig. 3.11). These include Cl_2 (elemental chlorine), OCl^- (the hypochlorite ion), and HOCl (hypochlorous acid).

The antimicrobial activity of chlorine in water (or free available chlorine) is a combination of Cl_2, HOCl, and OCl^-, but is predominantly due to HOCl. Chloride ions (Cl^-) are inactive. Inorganic chloramines or other nitro-chloro compounds may also be formed by the reaction of chlorine with ammonia and other nitrogen-containing compounds. These include monochloramine (NH_2Cl) and dichloramine ($NHCl_2$), which can act as chlorine-releasing agents but are considered weak disinfectants. The antimicrobial activity of available

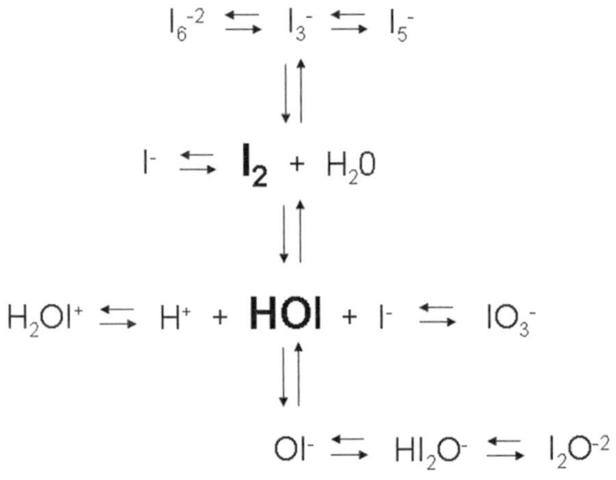

$$I_6^{-2} \rightleftarrows I_3^- \rightleftarrows I_5^-$$

$$\downarrow\uparrow$$

$$I^- \rightleftarrows \mathbf{I_2} + H_2O$$

$$\downarrow\uparrow$$

$$H_2OI^+ \rightleftarrows H^+ + \mathbf{HOI} + I^- \rightleftarrows IO_3^-$$

$$\downarrow\uparrow$$

$$OI^- \rightleftarrows HI_2O^- \rightleftarrows I_2O^{-2}$$

FIGURE 3.8 A simplified chemistry of iodine in water, demonstrating species important for biocidal activity.

chlorine varies depending on its concentration, temperature, and pH. Like other biocides, its efficacy increases with temperature and concentration. The dissociation of HOCl increases at higher pH, with greater production of OCl^- and subsequently less antimicrobial efficacy; the optimal pH for activity is 4 to 7, under which conditions HOCl is the most dominant species. Further, the presence of reducing agents such as iron and copper ions catalyzes dissociation and reduces available chlorine. Similar decreases in activity can be observed in the presence of protein, other organic material, and UV light.

The most important sources of chlorine are chlorine gas, hypochlorites, and the chloramines. Chlorine gas is provided as a compressed, amber-colored liquid, which rapidly forms a gas on release at atmospheric pressure and room temperature. It is extremely irritating and corrosive, with a detectable odor at as low as 3.5 ppm, and is considered fatal at 1,000 ppm. It can be added directly to water to form HOCl but is rarely used as a fumigant gas due to safety risks. Hypochlorites are the most widely used sources of chlorine and include powders and liquid preparations. Powders or tablets include sodium and potassium hypo-

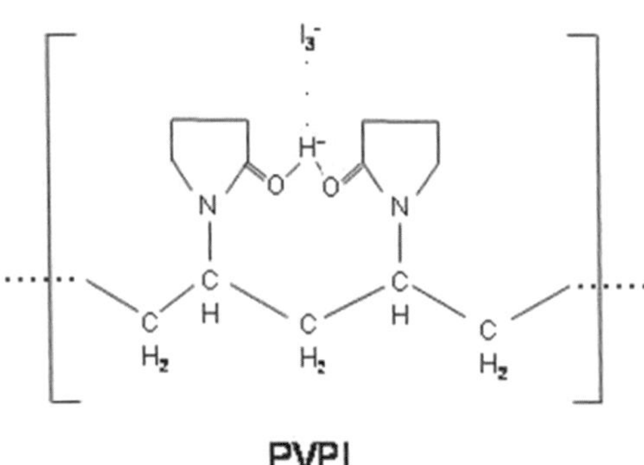

FIGURE 3.9 The structure of PVPI. The polymer consists of repeating units of the base structure shown, with particle sizes of 90 to 140 μm.

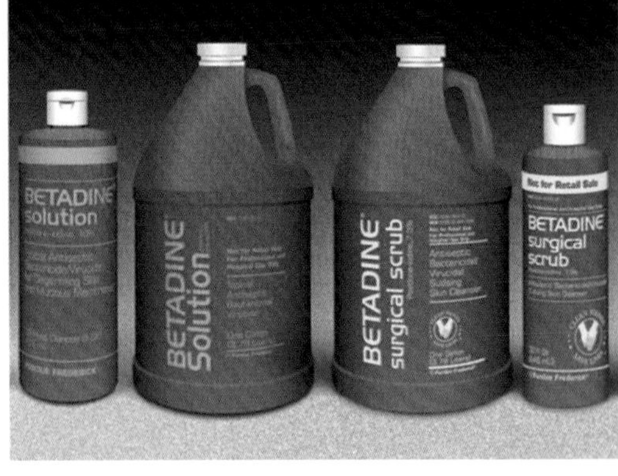

FIGURE 3.10 Various types of PVPI antiseptic products. Image courtesy of Purdue Pharma, LLC, with permission.

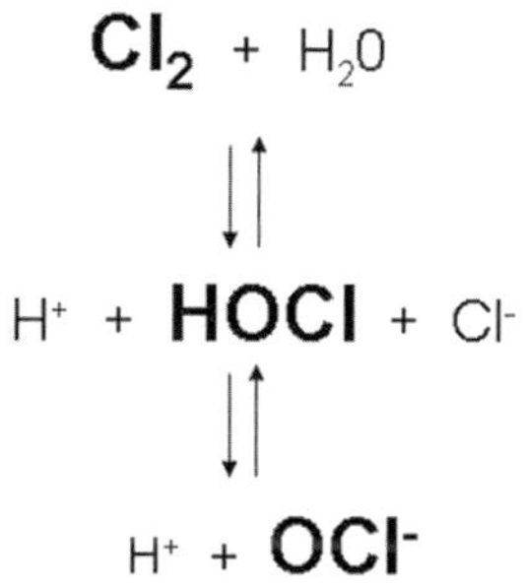

$$Cl_2 + H_2O$$
$$\rightleftarrows$$
$$H^+ + HOCl + Cl^-$$
$$\rightleftarrows$$
$$H^+ + OCl^-$$

FIGURE 3.11 A simplified chemistry of chlorine in water, demonstrating species important for biocidal activity.

chlorites mixed with trisodium phosphate. Calcium hypochlorite ($Ca(OCl)_2$) is a dry, white solid used in powdered or tablet form, which can be added directly to a surface or water. Liquid formulations typically include sodium or potassium hypochlorite solutions and can range from 1 to 15% available chlorine. Commercially available products can include a range of concentrated products (for dilution in water prior to use), ready-to-use formulations, and impregnated wipes. Sodium hypochlorite (NaOCl) solutions have a clear to light yellow color (depending on the concentration and formulation) with a distinctive chlorine odor. These include household bleach solutions, which are generally at ~5% NaOCl and include product stabilizers. Certain household formulations can include essential oils at low concentrations for aesthetic purposes (e.g., masking the strong chlorine smell often associated with these products).

A variety of chloramines (in liquid and powder formulations) also possess antimicrobial activity, although they are often cited to be less effective than the hypochlorites; this depends on their formulation and biocide concentration. They include inorganic chloramines such as monochloramine and dichloramine (discussed above) and organic chloramines, including chloramine T (sodium p-toluene sulfonchloramide), sodium dichloroisocyanurate (NaDCC), and halazone (p-sulfondichloramidobenzoic acid) (Fig. 3.12). NaDCC, for example, is provided in detergent-based effervescent tablets, which when prepared in water can demonstrate broad-spectrum (including sporicidal) activity in the range of 200 to 5,000 ppm hypochlorous acid. Organic

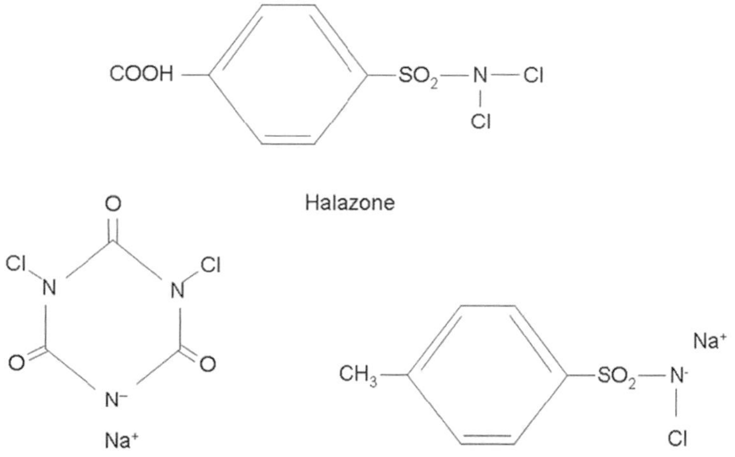

Halazone

Sodium dichloroisocyanurate (NaDCC)

Chloramine T

FIGURE 3.12 Examples of organic chloramines.

chloramines are formed by reaction of HOCl with amine or imine compounds. In general, they are less irritating and more stable but release lower concentrations of active chlorine in solution. Other chlorine-releasing compounds include interhalogens such as bromine chloride (in which bromine is the key antimicrobial when added to water) and the *N*-halamines. The *N*-halamines are nitrogen-containing compounds with anchored chlorine or bromine atoms, which can be released on contact with microorganisms. They can be used integrated into antimicrobial surfaces (as polymers) or as water-soluble monomers, which can subsequently be reactivated by application of a chlorine- or bromine-containing liquid formulation. Chlorine-releasing examples include 1-chloro-2,2,5,5-tetramethyl-1,3-imidazolidin-4-one (water-soluble, monomeric) and poly-1,3-dichloro-5-methyl-5-(4′-vinylphenyl) (water-insoluble, polymeric). Chlorine has also been successfully used in combination with other halogens such as low concentrations of iodine and bromine (e.g., *N*-bromo-*N*-chlorodimethylhydantoin). Newer methods of chlorine production include the use of electrolysis of sodium chloride (or other chloride salts) to form chlorine compounds and other oxidizing agents, which have rapid antimicrobial activity. Another important chlorinated compound is chlorine dioxide, which is considered in section 3.13).

Bromine (Br, atomic weight = 79.9) is a volatile, reddish-brown liquid that can give off a red vapor with an unpleasant and irritating odor. Care should be taken in the handling of liquid bromine because it poses a serious health risk. Bromine occurs naturally and is extracted in the form of bromide from seawater as a sodium salt (NaBr). When bromine is dissolved in water, hypobromous acid (HOBr) and the hypobromite ion (OBr^-) are formed, which are both responsible for the antimicrobial activity observed. Further reaction of bromine with ammonia or nitrogen compounds produces bromamines, which also contribute to the microbicidal activity. The bromide ion (Br^-) itself is inactive but can be reactivated to active bromine species (Br_2, HOBr, and OBr^-) by reaction with a strong oxidizer such as chlorine species and potassium peroxymonosulfate. Typical bromine sources for water or liquid disinfection include liquid bromine, sodium bromide (NaBr together with an activating agent), bromine chloride (BrCl), and bromine-releasing agents (Fig. 3.13) such as BCDMH (1-bromo-3-chloro-5,5-dimethylhydantoin; $BrClC_5H_6O_2N_2$), DBDMH (1,3-dibromo-5,5-dimethylhydantoin; $C_5H_6Br_2N_2O_2$), STABREX (a stabilized liquid of oxidized bromide), and bronopol (2-bromo-2-nitro-1,3-propanediol; $C_3H_6BrNO_4$). Typical bromine-releasing agents including BCDMH are supplied as tablets, which when dissolved in water release HOBr and HOCl, in which the available chlorine can further activate bromide species (Br^-) to give other active HOBr and OBr^- species. Similarly, sodium bromide is usually provided as a two-step method, first with the addition and dissolution of NaBr in water to produce Br^-, which is subsequently activated by a strong oxidizer.

More recent applications have included the impregnation of bromine into resins or polymers, e.g., polyethylenimine, poly(4-vinyl-*N*-alkylpyridinium bromide), and bromine-based *N*-halamines (Fig. 3.13). The *N*-halamines are nitrogen-containing compounds with anchored bromine which are released on contact with microorganisms. An example is poly(1,3-dibromo-5-methyl-5-(4′vinylphenyl) hydantoin) (PSHB), which is a water-insoluble polymeric *N*-halamine (Fig. 3.13). Bromine-based compounds are also used as corrosion inhibitors in biocide formulations, e.g., benzoltriazole. Methyl bromide (CH_3Br) is used for restrictive applications as a stable gas, both on its own or in combination with chloropicrin (a rarely cited chlorinated biocide, initially used as poisonous gas and in certain unique situations used for fumigation, e.g., pest control in soil). At typically used concentrations, methyl bromide is colorless, tasteless, odorless, and nonflammable. It is supplied as a compressed liquid which rapidly vaporizes on release at room temperature. Due to safety and environmental concerns, methyl

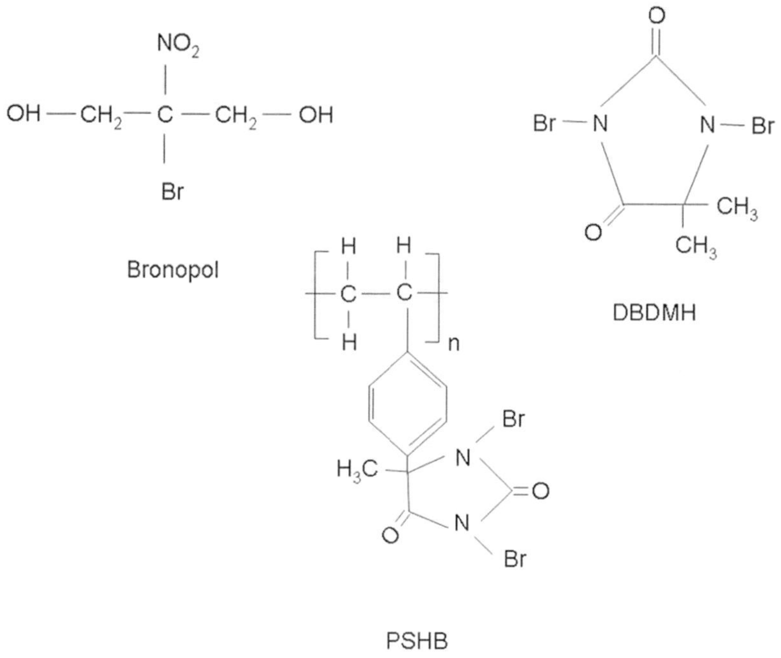

FIGURE 3.13 Typical bromine-releasing agents. PSHB is an example of a water-insoluble polymeric *N*-halamine.

bromide is not widely used and requires special handling for fumigation applications such as insecticide in soil.

Fluorine (F, atomic weight = 18.99) is one of the most reactive chemicals known. It is a pale yellow gas with a pungent odor, detectable at very low concentrations (in the parts per billion range). It is widely used for industrial purposes, including the production of uranium and fluorochemicals, including antibiotics (fluoroquinolones), plastics, and refrigerants. Its presence in water as fluoride (at <1 mg/liter) is claimed to reduce the incidence of dental cavities by direct reaction with tooth enamel hydroxyapatite and some bacteriostatic effects. A variety of fluoride compounds are used for water treatment, laundry detergents, and toothpastes, mouthwashes, and dental varnishes. These include silicofluorides (e.g., sodium fluorosilicates), stannous fluoride, and amine fluorides. Oral antiseptic treatments may play a role in controlling periodontal (below the gum line) infections. Sodium and potassium fluoride have been used as preservatives, but concerns about toxicity have limited their use. These compounds are not considered further.

3.11.2 Applications

3.11.2.1 Iodine. Iodine has been widely used as an antiseptic. Its uses include the reduction of microbial populations on intact skin in preoperative preparations or surgical scrubs and for therapeutic applications on wounds and burns. Traditional solutions in water or alcohol are still used for wound and other topical localized applications. These include tincture of iodine and Lugol's solutions. However, these solutions can be irritating, particularly on repeated applications. Iodophors have allowed for a greater flexibility in the use of iodine in antiseptic and disinfectant liquids, dry powders, and lotions. A variety of formulations are available, including solutions with surfactants and buffers which are used as surgical scrubs, preoperative preparations, shampoos (antidandruff), and wound cleansers (for further discussion see chapter

4, section 4.5 on hand-washing). Iodophor formulations are also used as general surface sanitizers and disinfectants, in particular, in agricultural, food, and veterinary applications, and for equipment, walls, and floors. They are less used for medical device disinfection, and generally only for noncritical applications. "Iodination" is defined as the use of iodine for water disinfection, including drinking water, wastewater, and swimming pool treatment. Low-level iodination (such as at ~1 mg/liter for bactericidal activity) is recommended in urgent cases (or for example, for those traveling in areas with no source of public health treated water), which can include the addition of iodine-releasing tablets or direct addition of a few drops of an iodine solution to drinking water. Some reported synergistic applications are the addition of inactive iodide (I^-), which is activated by reaction with another oxidizing agent, such as hypochloride (HOCl). Air fumigation with iodine vapor has been described, but applications have been limited due to the risks of severe irritation and respiratory damage.

3.11.2.2 Chlorine. Available chlorine has been widely used for water disinfection. In fact, drinking water chlorination has significantly contributed to the control of formerly widespread diseases such as cholera (caused by *Vibrio cholerae*) and typhoid (caused by *Salmonella enterica* serovar Typhi). Typically used concentrations for drinking water range from 0.5 to 1 mg/liter available chlorine, particularly provided by addition of elemental chlorine or calcium hypochlorite. Chloramines such as sodium dichloroisocyanurate have been recommended as alternatives to hypochlorites due to their delayed release of chlorine and potential for greater activity over time in the presence of contaminating soils (e.g., organic materials). Hypochlorites are also used as bleaching agents for laundry and other applications. Other water applications include recreational water (swimming pools and hot tubs) and wastewater, both at typical higher concentrations of 1 to 3 mg/liter of available chlorine. In addition to microbial control, chlorine and chloramines are useful for neutralizing sulfide odors due to oxidation of compounds such as hydrogen sulfide and dimethyltrisulfide and for masking other odors. Chlorine is also widely used for the routine sanitization of water supply systems and pipework (including biofilm control). Hypochlorites, particularly liquid sodium hypochlorite, or "bleach" solutions, are commonly used for a range of surface disinfection applications in households, health care facilities, food-handling establishments, and other industrial settings (Fig. 3.14).

These include direct applications (sprays and wipes) and indirect fogging methods. Direct application to food has also been shown to be effective in reducing the risk of pathogen contamination, including *Salmonella* and *Listeria*. Chlorine has been used in the past for wound and mucous membrane antiseptics, including calcium hypochlorite powders, chloramine T, and Dakin's solution (based on sodium hypochlorite). The *N*-halamines and other chlorine-releasing agents have been incorporated into surface polymers (such as clothing, benchtops, and filters) to provide intrinsic antimicrobial activity; the *N*-halamines have the advantage of being regenerated by application of a hypochlorite solution.

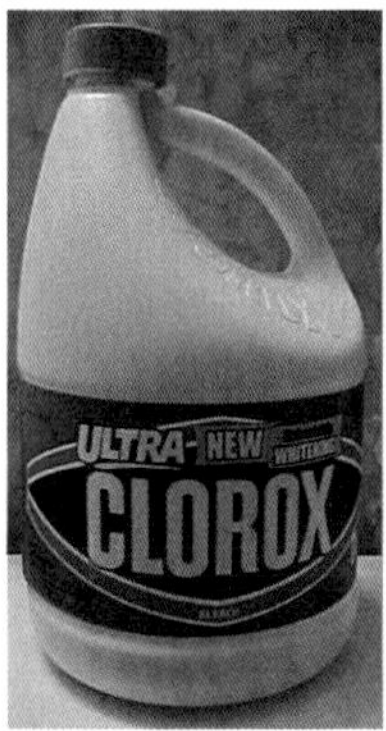

FIGURE 3.14 Sodium hypochlorite (bleach)-based disinfectant. A concentrate which is diluted in water prior to use is shown. ©2017 The Clorox Company. Reprinted with permission. CLOROX® and PINE-SOL® are registered trademarks of The Clorox Company and are used with permission.

In some applications, it is necessary to remove residual chlorine following disinfection and use of the water; an example is the use of water to produce steam, where the presence of chlorine gas causes corrosion to stainless steel and other metals. This can be achieved by reaction with neutralizers including activated carbon, sodium metabisulfite, sodium bisulfite, and sulfur dioxide.

3.11.2.3 Bromine. Applications for bromine and bromine-releasing agents are primarily for recreational and industrial water disinfection, including swimming pools, spas, and cooling systems and towers. They are available in various formulations including as liquids, granules, and tablets. Some bromine (hypobromous acid)-containing products have been approved for surface disinfection on foods. Other applications include wastewater treatment and odor control, but to a much lesser extent for drinking water. Typical applications are at 2 to 4 mg/liter over a wide temperature (5 to 45°C) and pH (6.5 to 9.5) range. Bromine has also been used as a broad-spectrum disinfectant, including fogging applications, and for control of fungal diseases of plants. Methyl bromide has limited applications as a fumigant, in particular as an insecticide, nematocide, herbicide, and fungicide for crops, plants, and soil. The gas can be used on its own or in combination with other biocides as a fumigant. Typical applications use methyl bromide at 16 to 24 g/m^3 at room temperature (15 to 25°C) and for 12 to 24 hours. Primary applications are generally restricted to agricultural uses, including foodstuffs, clothing, soil fumigation, and plants. Similar to chlorine-based *N*-halamines, bromine *N*-halamines have been integrated into various surfaces to provide an antimicrobial barrier.

3.11.3 Spectrum of Activity

The halogens have similar broad-spectrum antimicrobial profiles, dependent on the concentration and control of their applications.

3.11.3.1 Iodine. Molecular iodine (I_2) and, to a lesser extent, hypoiodous acid are broad-spectrum biocides with potent bactericidal, fungicidal, tuberculocidal, and virucidal activity. Activity has also been reported against actinomycetes and rickettsias. Observed antimicrobial activity varies depending on the formulation (particularly availability and concentration of the biocides) and test conditions (pH, temperature, etc.). Aqueous iodine solutions are more active under acidic pH due to the optimal presence of active molecular iodine species, with the prevalence of other ions at alkaline pH. Iodophors can be formulated over a wider pH range due to the slow release of iodine. Although the antimicrobial activity is maintained over time, iodophors are considered less active against certain fungi and spores compared to tinctures. Iodine can be sporicidal, particularly in hard-surface disinfectants, but generally not at the concentrations used for antiseptic applications. For example, vegetative bacteria are rapidly killed at 0.01 to 1 mg available iodine/liter in 1 minute, in contrast to requiring 10 mg/liter for bacterial spore activity for up to 5 hours of contact time. Nonenveloped viruses, like other halogens, demonstrate high resistance to iodine but are generally sensitive at concentrations as low as 15 μg/liter. The microbicidal effects can be improved by various formulation effects, particularly for application on hard surfaces. Activity has been reported against the encysted form of *Giardia*, but less so against *Cryptosporidium* oocysts. Iodine had poor algicidal activity in reported studies but was shown to be an effective insecticide and nematocide.

3.11.3.2 Chlorine. Available chlorine is well established as a broad-spectrum biocide. Vegetative bacteria are readily sensitive to very low concentrations of chlorine (0.1 to 0.3 mg/liter within 30 seconds), but mycobacteria, fungi, protozoan cysts, algae, viruses, and bacterial spores are significantly more resistant. Chlorine has also been used for the removal and disinfection of biofilms common in water systems to control pathogens such as pseudomonads and *Legionella*. Chlorine can be effective against both enveloped and nonenveloped viruses, even in the presence of soil contamination under some concentrations tested. Other forms of life, including fish, frogs, and plants, are also affected at higher concentrations. Special consideration should be given to the control of protozoan cysts, particularly *Cryptosporidium* oocysts, and parasitic worm eggs, which demonstrate greater tolerance to chlorine but are sensitive to higher concentrations in drinking water. Chlorine is slowly effective in the control of algal growth. *N*-chloro compounds, including chloramines, are considered less effective than hypochlorites but have demonstrated greater activity under acidic conditions and in the presence of organic soils. Sodium hypochlorite solutions (at 2.5%, or 25,000 mg, of available chlorine/liter for one hour) have been shown to be effective against prion-contaminated tissue preparations.

3.11.3.3 Bromine. Bromine demonstrates broad-spectrum activity, including bactericidal, mycobactericidal, fungicidal, slimicidal, cysticidal, and virucidal activity. Enveloped viruses and bacteria are sensitive at relatively low concentrations (0.3 mg/liter); in the case of nonenveloped viruses, higher concentrations (10 to 20 mg/liter) are required to achieve total inactivation and degradation of the viral structure and nucleic acid. Bromine has algicidal activity similar to that of chlorine; protozoan (*Entameoba*) cysts were reported to be inactivated at 1.5 mg/liter. Bromine has also been used for biofilm control (removal and disinfection) in water systems.

3.11.4 Advantages

3.11.4.1 Iodine. As topical biocides, iodine solutions are widely available and easy to prepare. They demonstrate broad-spectrum antimicrobial activity at relatively low concentrations on the skin and may have some short-lived persistent activity, remaining on the skin after application to offer residual antimicrobial activity. Iodophors present the greatest advantages, because they are generally nonstaining and water-soluble, have little to no odor, have increased stability of active iodine species released in solution, and minimize the concentration of iodine required for antimicrobial activity. The use of lower concentrations of iodine reduces the risks associated with toxicity, discoloration, and irritation. As disinfectants, iodophors and iodine solutions can better tolerate the presence of contaminating soils in comparison to other halogens such as chlorine. As water disinfectants, they have little to no odor or taste and are not irritating to the eyes at typically used concentrations; iodine is generally used for water treatment only in emergency situations.

3.11.4.2 Chlorine. Chlorine is well accepted as an antimicrobial with reliable broad-spectrum activity. At typical water and surface disinfection concentrations, it is colorless, cost-effective, and easy to handle (but higher concentrations can be noxious). It retains some activity in the presence of some organic materials and at high water hardness levels, depending on the chlorine and soil concentrations. Chlorine-releasing agents are more stable and allow for demand-release over time for preservation efficacy. At typically used concentrations, chlorine is not toxic and can be routinely monitored. In addition to microbicidal activity, chlorine also oxidizes some unwanted and harmful organic and inorganic compounds that may be present, in particular, for sulfide odor control. At lower concentrations, chlorine can be an efficient wound cleanser. Due to its bleaching activity, chlorine solutions are used for removing stains on surfaces and clothing.

3.11.4.3 Bromine. Bromine compounds are well-established, broad-spectrum antimicrobials. Compared to chlorine, bromine is considered less volatile and less toxic to aquatic life over time, but with a similar level of irritation. Bronopol, in particular, is considered to have a lower toxicity profile. It is also claimed to be less corrosive, odorless, relatively safe for use, and easier to handle. Residual bromide ions (Br^-) formed following reaction of active bromine species with microorganisms can be reactivated by use of a strong oxidizer. Bromine is more effective at higher pH than chlorine and demonstrates good algicidal activity at lower concentrations than other halogens. Methyl bromide is a particularly efficacious and low-cost fumigant.

3.11.5 Disadvantages

3.11.5.1 Iodine. Iodine causes brown stains on certain surfaces, including the skin, clothing, and porous materials such as plastics. Iodine solutions are poisonous at high concentrations (>5%) and can be irritating to broken skin and mucous membranes, particularly in combination with alcohol. Surface compatibility can be a concern with some metal (corrosion) and plastic surfaces. It should be noted that many of these disadvantages can be significantly reduced with the use of iodophors such as PVPI. Although it is not fully substantiated, there has been some speculation regarding health complications, e.g., effects on thyroid function and iodine-induced goiter; this is considered unlikely with the concentrations of iodine typically used over time and may be linked to individual sensitivity related to underlying thyroid disease.

3.11.5.2 Chlorine. Chlorine is an aggressive chemical that can promote corrosion of metal surfaces, especially at higher concentrations. This is particularly important when water is heated, which can cause the release of chlorine gas, which is corrosive, as well as being poisonous. Gas can also be released from chlorine solutions on reaction with acids that are commonly used in domestic and industrial cleaners. Studies estimated that the toxic effects of chlorine gas range from ~1 to 3 ppm (with some mucous membrane irritation) to more aggressive effects at higher concentrations (e.g., chest pain and coughing at ~30 ppm and toxic pneumonitis at ~60 ppm). At higher concentrations, chlorine solutions can be irritating to users and can lead to hypersensitivity. This is primarily due to the production of inorganic chloramines on reaction with ammonia and nitrogen-containing compounds, which are also responsible for the strong chlorine odors associated with treated water and surfaces. Further, chlorine and chlorinated by-products can be toxic to fish and other aquatic species over time. Concentrated solutions should be handled with care because they can be toxic to humans. Reaction of chlorine with some organic molecules can lead to the production of disinfection by-products such as trihalomethanes (THMs), including chloroform and bromodichloromethane. THMs are potential carcinogens and are monitored for acceptable levels in drinking water. Typical chlorine odors are detected at ~0.3 mg/liter, with further odorous by-products that can be formed by reactions with phenols (chlorophenols) and amino acids/peptides (aldehydes, including methional and acetaldehyde). Contaminating protein, inorganic ions (including iron), and reducing agents neutralize chlorine but can be compensated for by increasing the biocide dosage. Chlorine antiseptics are not widely used due to concerns over delayed healing and wound irritation.

3.11.5.3 Bromine. The formation of bromate, THMs and haloacetic acids as by-products of water disinfection is a concern, since they have been labeled as potential human carcinogens. Although it is less toxic than chlorine, high concentrations of bromine are considered a hazard to aquatic life. Bromine, similar to other halogens, is degraded by UV light and the presence of reducing agents, which can decrease the overall efficacy of disinfection. In general, bromine is considered more expensive than chlorine for water disinfection. Bromine is also considered less corrosive than chlorine but can still result in significant surface damage over time and at higher concentrations. Methyl bromide has been banned in certain countries due to occupational risks related to respiratory damage and long-term accumulation in body tissues leading to severe damage. It is also known to be a delayed neurotoxin. Its ability to damage the Earth's ozone layer is another cited concern.

3.11.6 Mode of Action

3.11.6.1 Iodine. As with other halogens, the exact modes of action of iodine are unknown. However, active iodine species (as reactive oxidizing agents) have multiple effects on the cell surface (cell wall and membrane) and in the cytoplasm. Iodine has a dramatic effect on microbial surfaces but also rapidly penetrates into microorganisms. Reactive iodine species have been shown to attack amino acids (in particular, lysine, histidine, cysteine, and arginine) to cause protein disruption and loss of structure and function. Iodine reacts with and substitutes with various functional groups on these amino acids. Further, iodine reacts with nucleic acids, lipids, and fatty acids (including those in the cell membrane structures). These various effects culminate in loss of cell function and death. Less is known about iodine's antiviral action, but nonlipid viruses and parvoviruses are less sensitive to it than are lipid enveloped viruses. It is likely that iodine attacks the surface proteins of enveloped viruses, but it may also destabilize membrane fatty acids by reacting with unsaturated carbon bonds. Similar effects are observed against nonenveloped viruses, particularly with any exposure to protein amino acids. The effects of iodine and iodophors against protozoan parasites and prions have not been well investigated.

3.11.6.2 Chlorine. The mode of action of chlorine has been investigated, and it clearly has multiple modes of action by oxidation of proteins, lipids, and carbohydrates. These are expected, because chlorine and chlorine-releasing agents are highly active oxidizing agents. Potentiation of oxidation may occur at low pH (pH 4 to 7), where chlorine activity is maximal, although increased penetration of outer cell layers may be achieved in the neutral state. Hypochlorous acid has long been considered the active moiety responsible for bacterial inactivation, with the OCl^- ion having a minor effect compared to HOCl. This correlates with the observation that chlorine activity is greatest when the percentage of detectable HOCl is highest. This concept also applies to chlorine-releasing agents. The primary mode of action is believed to be against structural and functional proteins, both on the microorganism surface as well as internally. Sulfhydral groups of essential enzymes appear to be particularly targeted, as well as nitrogen interactions on amino acids. Even low concentrations have a dramatic effect on the activity of metabolic enzymes *in vitro*. Direct protein degradation into smaller peptides and precipitation have been shown and are believed to be the main mode of action against prions. Other observed effects include cell wall and membrane disruption from attacks on structural proteins, lipids, and carbohydrates. Hypochlorous acid has also been found to disrupt oxidative phosphorylation and other membrane-associated enzyme activities. Further effects have been reported on nucleic acids, including the formation of chlorinated derivatives of nucleotide bases. Studies on the specific effects on the growth of *E. coli* have shown inhibition of bacterial growth by hypochlorous acid. At relatively low concentrations (~50 μM or ~3 ppm active chlorine), growth inhibition was observed within 5 minutes, with nearly complete inhibition of DNA synthesis but only partial inhibition of protein synthesis and no obvious membrane disruption, suggesting that intercellular DNA synthesis was a particularly sensitive target at an inhibitory concentration of chlorine. Specific effects on viral nucleic acids are expected and have been reported. Direct degradation of poliovirus RNA into fragments has been reported, in addition to severe morphological changes and disintegration of viral capsid structures.

Direct effects on macromolecules are probably responsible for the observed sporicidal activity of chlorine. Direct studies with chlorine on spores have shown that they lose refractivity, followed by separation of the spore coats from the cortex and inner cortex lysis. Other studies have reported an increased permeability of the normally resistant spore coat, which leads to further biocide penetration and spore death.

3.11.6.3 Bromine. Similar to other halogens, bromine oxidizes organic molecules, including proteins, nucleic acids, and lipids. It is generally accepted that the culmination of the resulting structural and functional damage leads to cell death and loss of viral-particle infectivity. Direct reaction with viral coats and nucleic acids has been described. Methyl bromide has been shown to react with the sulfhydryl groups of proteins and enzymes, which leads to the inhibition of cellular biochemical processes.

3.12 METALS

Ag^{+2}	Cu^{+2}
Silver	Copper

3.12.1 Types

Metals are a group of elements that may be chemically defined as having a shiny or lustrous surface and are generally good conductors of electricity and heat. Metals form positive ions (cations) in water, which are the basis for their antimicrobial and toxic effects. It should be noted that many metals (including sodium, potassium, calcium, and iron) are essential for life, but at high concentrations they are toxic by disruption of cellular functions and structure. The metals that are specifically used as antiseptics and disinfectants are often termed "heavy" metals. This is a vague term which does not have a precise chemical definition but generally is used to describe metallic elements with a specific density greater than 4 or 5, with the corresponding "light" metals (such as calcium and sodium) having lower densities. The heavy metals include known toxic elements such as mercury, cadmium, arsenic, and lead, as well as the less toxic and more widely used silver- and copper-containing compounds. Many metals that had traditionally been used as biocides in the past are no longer widely used due to bioaccumulation and toxicity concerns. For example, mercury in its natural form is a unique liquid metal and has been used in various forms (such as elemental mercury and in inorganic and inorganic compounds) in antiseptics, disinfectants, and preservatives. Examples include merbromin, nitromersol, and mercurochrome. Other metals that are less used today are arsenic and tin compounds. Tin compounds, including tributyltin oxide and tributyltin acetate, are considered less toxic than mercury for preservative applications. Similar organic and inorganic arsenic compounds (such as copper arsenate and arsenic trioxide) have been used in the past as pharmaceuticals, soil disinfectants, and wood preservatives, but not significantly since the voluntary banning of many of these compounds in such applications over the past 30 years. Due to their decreased use, mercury, tin, and arsenic compounds are not further considered in detail.

The most widely used biocidal metals are copper and silver compounds. Copper (Cu; atomic weight = 63.55 g) is an essential element in minute quantities for plants, animals, and other forms of life. It is commercially available in a variety of forms with a typical copper (yellow-brown) color. Elemental copper was rarely used in the past, with copper sulfate ($CuSO_4$) and other copper-containing compounds (including cupric chloride, copper-8-quinolinolate, copper naphthenate, and cuprous oxide) being more frequently used. Copper sulfate pentahydrate is a blue crystalline solid that is readily soluble in water. The copper ion (Cu^{+2}) is the actual biocide but may be used in combination with other active agents. Copper alloys (traditional alloys such as bronze [copper with 12% tin and other metals] and brass [copper and zinc combinations], as well as a variety of other alloys ranging from 60 to 99.99% copper, have been successfully used in recent years as antimicrobial surfaces in health care and industrial applications. Copper-containing nanoparticles have also been described for antimicrobial (including antiprotozoal) applications.

Silver (Ag, atomic weight = 107.87) is not an essential element but is a widely known precious metal. Commonly used biocidal silver compounds include silver nitrate ($AgNO_3$), silver iodate ($AgIO_3$), pentasilver hexaoxoiodate (Ag_5IO_4), silver oxide (Ag_2O), and silver sulfadiazine ($C_{10}H_9AgN_4O_2S$, or AgSD), where the silver ion (Ag^{+2}) is the active, ionic species. The nonionized form of silver is considered to be inert and not an effective biocide. Silver nitrate, for example, is a white crystalline powder that readily dissolves in water. Silver sulfadiazine (Fig. 3.15) is generally provided as a cream or in liquid solutions (e.g., as a 1% white, water-dispersible cream). It is essentially a combination of two antibacterial agents: silver ions and sulfadazine, a sulfonamide antibiotic. Silver-containing liquid preparations have also included formulations with other biocides such as chlorhexidine, cerium nitrate, and copper ions. Other silver-releasing agents include silver zeolites (porous mixtures of sodium aluminosilicate that have silver integrated into their structure) and silver nanoparticles (ranging in size from 7 to 100 nm diameter). Silver (as metallic silver, silver iodate, pentasilver hexaoxoiodate, silver nitrate, and silver oxide) has also been deposited or integrated into polymers, filters, and other surfaces to allow for slow release over time. Traditionally, these included the deposition of metallic silver onto surfaces, but these were often claimed to have low release of the active silver ion from such surfaces. Recent medical implants, catheters, and wound dressings have been successfully impregnated with silver iodate compounds (silver iodate itself or in mixtures with other compounds such as pentasilver hexaoxoiodate, silver periodate, and silver orthoperiodate), with effectiveness against Gram-positive and Gram-negative bacteria, as well as yeast, and effectiveness in preventing biofilm formation.

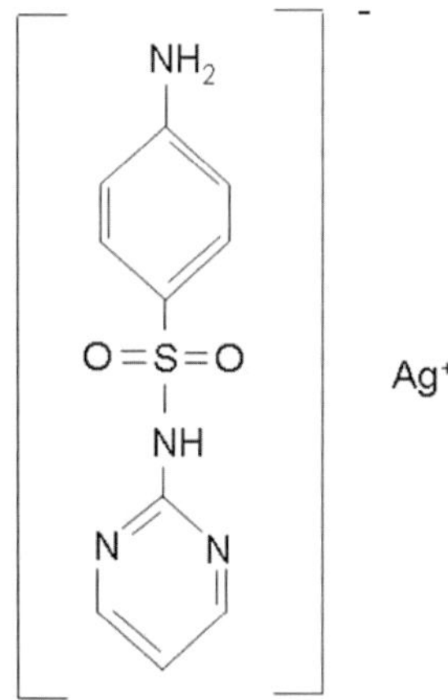

FIGURE 3.15 Silver sulfadiazine.

3.12.2 Applications

3.12.2.1 Copper. Copper has been widely used as a fungicide for agricultural applications, including direct applications to plants. An example is the Bordeaux mixture (first used in France on grape vines), a mixture of copper sulfate and calcium hydroxide, which is used as a crop spray. Other applications include water treatment and preservation. Copper is an effective water disinfectant at low concentrations, including for drinking and recreational water. A typical application for swimming pools is at <3 μg of copper sulfate/ml, particularly for control of algae. Electrolytic generators may also be used, including for *Legionella* control in hospital and industrial hot and cold water supply pipes, as an alternative to chlorine treatment. These consist of an electrode cell with copper-containing anodes to which a current is supplied to cause the release of copper ions into the water flow. Typically, these generators are provided with copper and silver anodes to produce effective ion concentrations at approximately 0.4 and 0.04 mg/liter, respectively. The ion levels can be controlled by varying the applied current to the cell. An example of a copper-silver ionization system is shown in Fig. 3.16.

Copper-containing mixtures and compounds are also used as preservatives in paints, cement, fabrics, and wood; higher concentrations may be used in some paints to provide an antimicrobial barrier to surfaces, in particular for fungal control. Examples of wood preser-

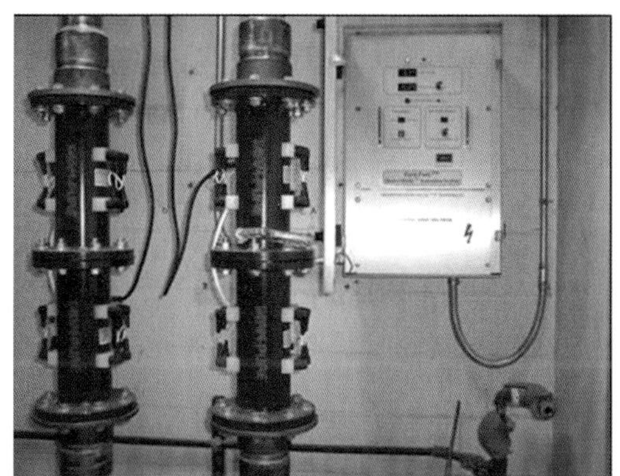

FIGURE 3.16 A typical copper-silver ionization system. An end view of the electrode cell is shown with the copper/silver electrodes and central titanium electrode. Image courtesy of Tarn-Pure, with permission.

vatives include ground copper alone or as a mixture with QACs (e.g., alkaline copper quaternary, which includes copper and dodecyl ammonium chloride) or triazoles (e.g., copper azole, a mixture with triazoles such as tebuconazole as antifungal drugs; see chapter 7, section 7.2.2). Some older copper-containing antiseptics have been used for topical treatments on humans and animals. Metallic copper or copper alloy-containing surfaces can release a low concentration of copper over time, which has been used to prevent the attachment and growth of microorganisms. These have been particularly well studied in recent years and have shown some benefits in critical applications such as "high-touch" surfaces in health care facilities (e.g., door handles, table tops, tap handles, etc.). The antimicrobial effects can vary depending on the copper alloy used (generally >60% copper), but some have shown success as "self-sanitizing" surfaces and in reducing the rates of health care-associated infections from bacteria (e.g., *S. aureus*, *P. aeruginosa*, *Acinetobacter baumanii*) and yeasts (*Candida albicans*) in controlled studies.

3.12.2.2 Silver. Topical (antiseptic) silver applications include 1% silver sulfadiazine cream or solutions for direct application to chemical or heat burns and 1% silver nitrate solutions for instillation into the eye and cleaning/preventing wound or mucous membrane infections. These applications have been used for the prevention of wound infections by *S. aureus* and *Pseudomonas* and mixed-bacteria infections of the eye in newborns. Silver has also been used for drinking water (in particular, in Europe) and recreational water (including swimming pools) disinfection and as a food preservative at a typical concentration range of 0.02 to 10 μg/ml. Examples are the silver-copper ionization systems (which use copper and silver electrodes as sources of ions when an electrical current is applied) for *Legionella* control in water, as described for copper above. Surfaces impregnated with metallic silver or silver compounds (including polymers such as polyethylene and nylon) have been used for wound dressings and on the surfaces of indwelling medical devices such as implants and catheters, which are often prone to bacterial colonization and infection. The slow release of silver (at 1 to 2 μg/ml) from these surfaces can reduce the attachment and proliferation of bacteria (such as *S. aureus*) on these surfaces. Typically, surfaces are impregnated with metallic silver or silver salts such as silver chloride, sodium iodate, pentasilver hexaoxoiodate, and silver calcium phosphate; silver-containing nanoparticles; or silver-containing zeolites (microporous crystals of aluminosilicate that retain and slowly release cations such as Ag^+). Other examples of silver-releasing surface applications have included the use of nanoparticles.

Other heavy metal-based compounds (including mercury- and tin-based compounds) are used as effective preservatives for clothing, paints, pharmaceuticals, and cosmetics at relatively low concentrations.

3.12.3 Spectrum of Activity

3.12.3.1 Copper. Copper, in its active form, is particularly bactericidal at very low concentrations but is also effective against fungi (yeast and molds), being both a fungistatic and fungicidal biocide over time. Copper is also an effective algicide and molluscicide; the control of molluscs (slugs and snails) in the parts-per-million range is important for the indirect control of carriers of parasites (e.g., in the control of schistosomiasis in humans and liver fluke in animals). Copper is an effective virucide against enveloped viruses but to a much lesser extent against nonenveloped viruses (although this may be strain-, concentration-, and formulation-dependent). Copper is not considered sporicidal but is sporistatic at typically used concentrations.

3.12.3.2 Silver. Silver is an effective bacteristatic and bactericidal agent at relatively low concentrations, particularly against Gram-positive bacteria. Depending on the concentration of active ions, silver-impregnated or -coated surfaces have been shown to inhibit the attachment and growth of bacterial biofilms. Less activity has been reported against yeasts and molds. Silver is algistatic and algicidal, although little viricidal activity (except some activity against enveloped viruses such as HIV) has been reported at typical concentrations.

3.12.4 Advantages

3.12.4.1 Copper. Copper is a powerful, stable biocide at relatively low concentrations. Depending on its particular use, it appears to have broader antimicrobial effects than silver. It is cost-effective, easy to use, and colorless/odorless at typically used concentrations. Copper-silver ionization methods are not considered corrosive as alternatives for chlorine water treatment; they are easy to install and cost-effective to maintain. Copper alloy surfaces are also reasonably priced for widespread use, are durable over time, are nonirritating, and are considered safe for use in the environment because copper is slowly released from the alloys over time.

3.12.4.2 Silver. Silver is particularly active against bacteria and is not irritating to the skin or mucous membranes at effective concentrations. Side effects are rarely reported. Silver has affinity for many surfaces, which can provide a residual, sustaining antibacterial and fungistatic barrier. As described for ionization methods that use copper, silver is less aggressive on surfaces as an alternative to chlorine treatment of water.

3.12.5 Disadvantages

3.12.5.1 Copper. Copper is considered toxic at high concentrations, including skin irritancy. When used in liquid formulations or as a preservative, it is stable in the environment and can be bioaccumulated by aquatic life. Some bacteria, fungi, and protozoa, including *E. coli*, *Legionella*, *Candida*, and *Paramaecium*, can develop resistance to copper ions. This can develop due to conversion to nontoxic forms, sequestration, or uptake reduction (e.g., efflux); these are considered in more detail in chapter 8, section 8.3. High concentrations of copper in water supplies can react with other chemicals to form unwanted (e.g., toxic) deposits on surfaces, including medical devices. Levels of contaminants including phosphates, protein, and chlorides can reduce the activity of copper ions by neutralization or sequestration. Copper is less effective in liquid applications at pH >8.

3.12.5.2 Silver. Overuse of silver (at high concentrations) can cause burns to the skin and mucous membrane and may impede wound healing. Silver nitrate causes black discoloration of the skin and other materials, as well as electrolyte loss in patients with extended use, which should be monitored. At high concentrations, silver can cause a blue-gray discoloration of the skin (argyria) and severe toxicity, although these have been rarely reported. The long-term effects of silver are unknown. In addition to limited activity against fungi, which can also cause wound infections or biofouling, resistance development has been described in bacteria, including active efflux (in *E. coli*) and complex formation (in *Pseudomonas stutzeri*); this is discussed in more detail in chapter 8, section 8.3. Levels of phosphates, calcium (e.g., water hardness), protein, and chlorides can reduce the activity of silver in water treatment applications.

3.12.6 Mode of Action

3.12.6.1 Copper. Although a low level of copper is required for the normal activities of many types of cellular enzymes, the toxic effects of copper are typical of other heavy metals, demonstrating multiple effects on cells and viruses at higher concentrations. Positively charged ions have a rapid affinity for negatively charged microbial surfaces. Proteins are a particular target, where ions can disrupt tertiary and secondary structures required for functional (enzymatic) and structural activity. Copper has been shown to interact with amino, carboxylate, and sulfur groups in proteins, with thiol (sulfhydryl, -SH) groups being particularly sensitive. Lower concentrations of copper are growth-inhibitory (and also reversible), but higher concentrations lead to protein denaturation and precipitation, the cumulative effects of which are cell death and loss of infectivity. Cell surface attack (including surface proteins and lipids) has a particular initial impact leading to altered permeability and disruption of cell wall/membrane functions. This includes decreased membrane integrity, inhibition of respiration, and leakage of cytoplasmic components. Copper has also been shown to bind to the phosphate group backbone of DNA, causing unraveling of the helix and subsequent degradation. Further reactions in cells (copper-mediated catalysis) can lead to the production of oxidizing agents (such as hydrogen peroxide and superoxide during oxidative stress), which also damage proteins, lipids, and particularly, nucleic acids. Although the antimicrobial effects of copper have been less studied with viruses, structural (loss of capsid integrity) and viral nucleic acid damage has been observed in some studies with both enveloped and nonenveloped viruses.

3.12.6.2 Silver. Silver ions are also rapidly attracted to the surface of microorganisms, which can lead to disruption of cell wall/membrane functions by affecting the structure and function of proteins. Silver binds to sulfyhdral, amino, and carboxyl groups on amino acids, which leads to protein denaturation. Sulfhydryl (thiol, -SH) groups appear to be particular targets, as demonstrated with amino acids such as cysteine (CySH), and other compounds containing thiol groups such as sodium thioglycolate neutralize the activity of silver ions against bacteria. In contrast, amino acids containing disulfide (SS) bonds, non-sulfur-containing amino acids, sulfur-containing compounds such as cystathione, cysteic acid, L-methionine, taurine, sodium bisulfite, and sodium thiosulfate were all unable to neutralize silver activity. These and other findings imply that the interaction of silver with thiol groups in enzymes and proteins plays an essential role in bacterial inactivation, although other cellular components may be involved. These include other amino acid groups and effects on hydrogen bonding. Specific interference with protein structure is believed to be responsible for increased permeability of the cell membrane, as observed with the release of potassium from target cells. These mechanisms may have some subtle effects on bacteria at low concentrations, such as by inhibiting bacterial adhesion and therefore biofilm formation on device surfaces.

Virucidal and fungicidal properties might also be explained by binding to sulfhydryl groups. Silver has been shown to specifically inhibit cell wall metabolism, respiration (cytochromes b and d), and electron transport (e.g., disruption of the proton motive force). It also has been shown to bind to DNA (specifically, the nucleotide bases) and inhibit replication and transcription. These effects overall are responsible for the various morphological changes in microorganisms that have been observed. These include deposition of silver in vacuoles and as granules in the cell wall of the fungi *Cryptococcus neoformans*, damage to bacterial cell walls and cell division, increase in size, and other structural abnormalities. The mode of action of silver sulfadiazine may be due to a synergistic effect of silver and sulfadiazine.

Differences in the mode of action in comparison to silver nitrate have been observed, particularly on the surface of bacteria, which is indicative of cell wall/membrane damage. Unlike the action of silver ions alone, silver sulfadiazine produces surface and membrane blebs in susceptible bacteria, suggesting greater damage to the cell wall/membrane. Silver sulfadiazine also binds to cell components, including DNA. The polymeric structure of the biocide is proposed to consist of six silver atoms linked to the nitrogen's six sulfadiazine molecules, which bind to sufficient base pairs in the DNA helix to inhibit transcription and replication. A similar effect may contribute to the mode of action against microorganisms, including viruses.

3.13 PEROXYGENS AND OTHER FORMS OF OXYGEN

Hydrogen Peroxide Peracetic Acid Ozone

Chlorine Dioxide Nitrogen Dioxide

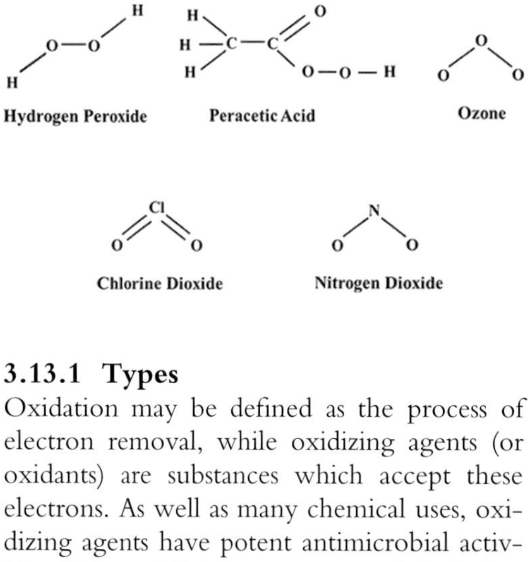

3.13.1 Types

Oxidation may be defined as the process of electron removal, while oxidizing agents (or oxidants) are substances which accept these electrons. As well as many chemical uses, oxidizing agents have potent antimicrobial activities. Many oxidizing agents are used, including halogens (chlorine, bromine, and iodine [see section 3.11]), peroxygens, and other forms of oxygen. Peroxygens are an important group of oxidizing agents that includes hydrogen peroxide, PAA, and chlorine dioxide.

Hydrogen peroxide is a strong oxidizing agent and probably one of the most widely used biocides for medical, industrial, and household applications in liquid and gas form. It is commercially available as a colorless liquid at various dilutions (generally 3 to 90%) in water. Pure hydrogen peroxide is relatively stable, but most dilutions contain a stabilizer (e.g., acetanilide or phenol) to prevent decomposition. Peroxide is considered environmentally friendly, because it decomposes into water and oxygen on exposure to increased temperature and various catalysts, including organic molecules, enzymes (e.g., catalase or peroxidases), and most metals (e.g., iron, copper, and manganese). Some organic peroxides are also used as biocides, with the most prevalent being benzoyl peroxide (Fig. 3.17).

Many other oxygen- and/or hydrogen peroxide-releasing compounds are used for various industrial and biocidal applications, with examples given in Table 3.3.

PAA is commercially available as a colorless liquid, with a strong, pungent (vinegar-like) odor at 5 to 37%. It is significantly less stable than hydrogen peroxide solutions and is therefore provided in equilibrium with water, hydrogen peroxide, and acetic acid. For example, 35% PAA is provided with 7% hydrogen peroxide, 40% acetic acid, and 17% water; in some cases a stabilizer (e.g., sodium pyrophosphate or hydroxyquinolone) may be added. For most medical disinfection and sanitization purposes, PAA is used in formulation with hydrogen peroxide/acetic acid and other components to improve its stability and compatibility with a wider range of material surfaces. Formulations may contain either one or two components (the PAA/hydrogen peroxide component

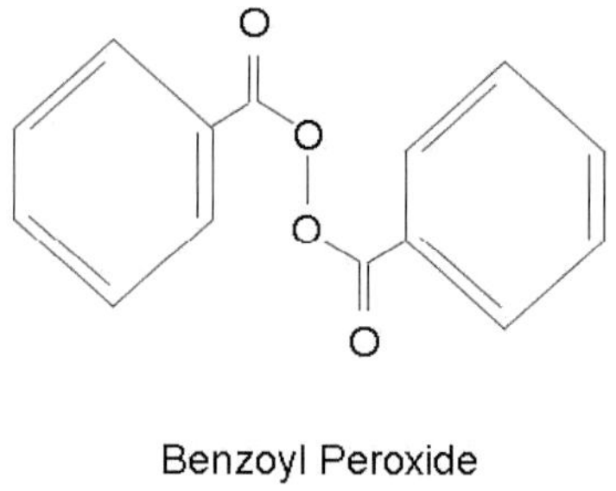

Benzoyl Peroxide

FIGURE 3.17 The structure of benzoyl peroxide.

TABLE 3.3 Oxygen- and hydrogen peroxide-releasing compounds other than benzoyl peroxide

Compound	Formula	Characteristics	Applications
Potassium monopersulfate (potassium peroxymonosulfate)	$KHSO_5$	White powder, readily soluble in water; releases oxygen on contact with moisture	Sanitization and organic waste removal ("shocking") in pools/spas; disinfection formulations; bleaching applications
Ammonium, potassium, and sodium persulfate	$(NH_4)_2S_2O_8$ $K_2S_2O_8$ $Na_2S_2O_8$	Colorless crystals or white powders; liberate oxygen on contact with moisture; react with hydrogen peroxide to boost oxidative process	Skin and hair bleaching, deodorizers
Sodium percarbonate	$2Na_2CO_3.3H_2O_2$	Dry, white powder which contains ~30% (wt/wt) hydrogen peroxide; releases hydrogen peroxide when dissolved in water	Cleaning and disinfection formulations; food and laundry bleaching
Sodium perborate	$NaBO_3.H_2O$ (monohydrate)	White crystalline granules; releases hydrogen peroxide when dissolved in water	Cleaning, disinfection, and antiseptic formulations; dental and industrial bleaching; deodorization
Calcium peroxide	CaO_2	White/yellow solid; slowly decomposes to release oxygen on contact with moisture	Remediation (including of soil and water); disinfection and cleaning formulations (in particular, agricultural applications); bleaching

separated from the base formulation), the latter requiring mixing together prior to use. PAA may also be produced *in situ*, by reaction of sodium perborate or sodium percarbonate with an acetyl donor such as acetylsalicylic acid (aspirin) or tetraacetyl ethylene diamine (Fig. 3.18). Such formulations give longer shelf lives, because they are supplied dry and are activated by dilution in water prior to use; however, they require protection from humidity sources to prevent activation during distribution.

Some other peroxygen compounds have also been used, including performic and perpropionic acid, with efficacy and compatibility profiles similar, if not inferior, to those of PAA.

A consideration of the chemistry of oxygen is also useful, because many active oxygen species are responsible for the antimicrobial activity of mixed-oxidant (or "activated") gases and liquids. Elemental oxygen is found abundantly as a diatomic molecule (dioxygen or O_2). As an allotropic element (i.e., existing in two or more forms), it is also naturally found as atomic oxygen (O) and as ozone (O_3), both of which are highly reactive and unstable oxidizing agents. Ozone is a naturally occurring water-soluble gas. For example, the upper atmospheric ozone layer protects the earth from damaging UV radiation from the sun. At low concentrations (<0.01 mg/liter) it is colorless and odorless, but at higher concentrations it has a slight blue color (>5 mg/liter) and a distinctive, fresh, acrid odor (>0.1 mg/liter). Ozone is relatively stable in clean air over a few hours but rapidly degrades on contact with particles and surfaces, and in water. Other reactive forms of oxygen are formed by electron acceptance of oxygen to give various other reactive, short-lived species, including superoxide (O_2^-) and peroxide (O_2^{2-}) ions. Further, by protonation, other species are generated, including the hydroxyl ($^{\bullet}OH$) and hydroperoxyl (HO_2) radicals. All these species are highly reactive and can damage microorganisms, culminating in cell death.

Other oxidizing agents to be considered in this section are chlorine dioxide and nitrogen dioxide. Chlorine dioxide (ClO_2) is a water-soluble gas, existing as a reactive free radical.

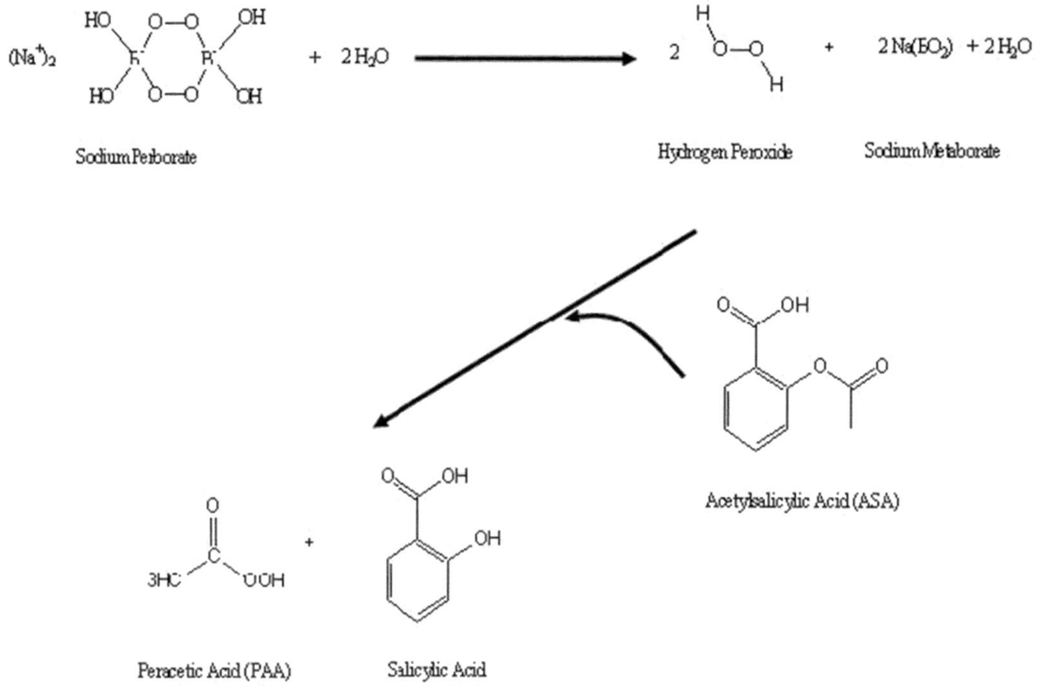

FIGURE 3.18 Example of the generation of PAA from sodium perborate and acetylsalicylic acid.

Due to its unstable and explosive nature (at high concentrations), it is typically manufactured at the site of its use but is also available as a liquid concentrate. A variety of methods are used for generation, particularly from sodium chlorite ($NaClO_2$) and sodium chlorate ($NaClO_3$) by acidification with HCl, H_2SO_4, or organic acids; reactions with chlorine or sodium hypochlorite; and electrolysis. Typical examples are shown in Fig. 3.19.

These methods may be conducted in a gaseous state (e.g., by passing chlorine gas through columns of sodium chlorite) or in liquid (e.g., mixing a solution of sodium chlorite with acids, in some cases including sodium hypochlorite) and subsequently supplied to an air or water application. In addition to direct generation into water or liquid, typically for surface disinfection, applications are provided in two-part systems, which can include formulation excipients such as preservatives, buffers, and corrosion inhibitors to improve efficacy, stability, and surface compatibility. Dry or stabilized mixtures that are activated on mixture with water are also available. In the gaseous phase, chlorine dioxide is reactive and short-lived, breaking down into chlorine gas and

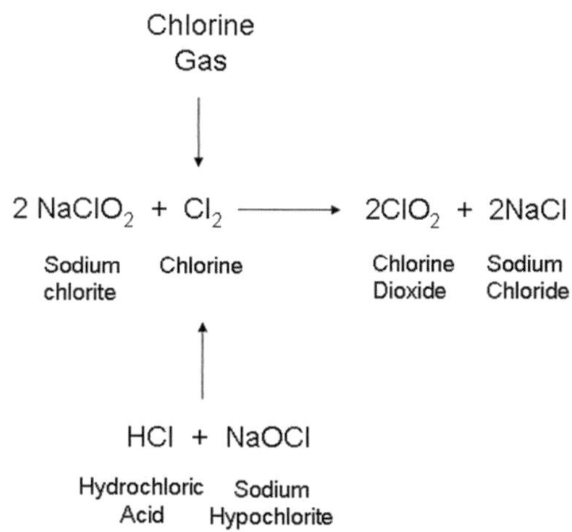

FIGURE 3.19 Examples of the production of chlorine dioxide from chlorine sources.

oxygen. It can be much more stable in water, depending on the presence of light, the concentration, the temperature, the presence of neutralizing agents, and formulation effects.

Chlorine dioxide boils at 11°C and is therefore a gas at room temperature, with a slight yellow-green color (similar to that of chlorine gas) and a pungent, irritating chlorine odor. In solution, a similar color is observed, but it can vary in color (e.g., light red, amber, or blue) depending on the concentration in water and formulation effects. It is soluble in water and can be stored at up to 10 g/liter at 4°C (depending on the partial pressure in air and temperature), although typical disinfection concentrations are <500 mg/liter in liquid and <2 mg/liter in gas.

Nitrogen dioxide (NO_2) is a highly reactive oxidizing agent. At room temperature (>21°C [70°F]) and atmospheric pressure it is a gas, with a distinctive reddish-brown color and a sharp pungent odor. It is commercially available as a yellowish-brown liquid at low temperatures (<21°C [70°F]) or, more commonly, under pressure (as a liquefied gas). Under these conditions nitrogen dioxide is in equilibrium with its dimer, nitrogen tetroxide (N_2O_4). In liquid form a greater proportion is in the dimer form, while under gas conditions the dimer is typically at ~10%. It is a well-known pollutant, being formed as a by-product of combustion (or burning, such as fires, incineration, engines, etc.), but has recently been investigated for disinfection and, predominantly, sterilization applications. It is also a widely used chemical in industrial applications such as in nitric acid production, flour whitening, and rocket fuels. The use of nitrogen dioxide for chemical sterilization is further considered in chapter 6, section 6.6.6.

Other similar chemicals such as nitric oxide (NO [a short-lived gas]) have been investigated for antiseptic and disinfection applications but have not been widely commercialized to date. NO has been particularly investigated as a natural antimicrobial in the immune system (being produced by phagocytic cells in response to inflammation). It is known to react with oxygen to spontaneously produce a variety of reactive nitrogen and oxygen intermediates with antimicrobial potential by reacting with various cellular targets (e.g., nucleic acid, lipids, and proteins). Gaseous disinfection has been described to reduce surface contamination of fruits and vegetables following harvest (e.g., for fungal and bacterial control) at 25°C at 50 to 500 μl/liter gas for 8 days. Overall, to date, such applications have been described as difficult to control and have had limited commercial success. Research has also focused on novel therapeutic and antiseptic applications. Examples include a probiotic patch that locally generates NO from the reaction of a nitrate salt with lactic acid (produced by immobilized lactobacilli from glucose) and acidified nitrate creams. Both applications have described antimicrobial effects on the skin, including against bacteria and fungi. The potential use of NO for such applications is being researched (for efficacy and safety) and is not further considered.

3.13.2 Applications

3.13.2.1 Ozone. Due to its reactive, unstable nature, ozone is produced at the point of use. Ozone generators effectively pass air (which is ~20% oxygen or, in cases where high concentrations are required, pure oxygen) through a high-energy source. The resulting physiochemical reaction leads to the formation of ozone, which can then be used directly for area or surface disinfection or, when bubbled or injected into water or other liquids, for liquid disinfection. Widely used high-energy sources include UV light, electrochemical cells, and more commonly, corona discharge. A corona is formed by an electrical discharge (or spark) around a gas, which causes ionization and ozone production. It should be noted that a corona is therefore a plasma in its formation stage (see chapter 5, section 5.6.1), with ozone being produced as a by-product. Ozone production is most effective in a temperature-controlled environment, since the stability of ozone decreases as the temperature increases. A variety of generators are available for applications as far-ranging as odor control, taste and color remediation, preservation and sanitization of foods, area fumigation, and sterilization (Fig. 3.20).

Ozone disinfection of water and wastewater is widely used worldwide. The typical concentrations used range from 0.2 to 0.4 mg/liter at pH 6 to 7, with up to 5 mg/liter required for wastewater treatment due to increased organic load, which readily reacts with and neutralizes ozone. Currently, due to restrictions in maintaining high concentrations in a given area (0.5 to 3 mg/liter), the use of ozone is primarily for odor control fumigation. Higher-capacity ozone generators have been recently described based on corona plasma technology, to include uses in a variety of industrial, food, and health care applications. A typical fumigation disinfection cycle includes area prehumidification (to 70 to 80%), ozone disinfection (while maintaining required humidity levels), and aeration (to below 0.1 ppm). The recommended safe level of ozone is 0.1 ppm over a typical 8-hour working day, with a minimum short-term exposure level at 0.3 ppm for 15 minutes. Cycle times vary depending on the area size, desired level of disinfection, and area contents. The difficulty of maintaining effective ozone concentrations limited its use, but recent advances in generator technology have seen an increased use of ozone for both water- and air-based systems. A number of medical device sterilization systems have also recently been developed, using ozone either directly for sterilization or in combination with hydrogen peroxide gas (see chapter 6, section 6.6.4).

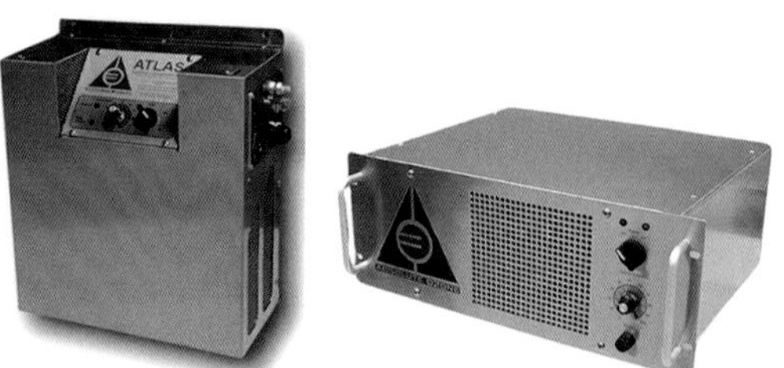

FIGURE 3.20 Examples of ozone generators. Images courtesy of AbsoluteOzone®, with permission.

Although generally not referred to as "ozone-generation," it is clear that ozone plays an important part in the overall efficacy observed in many mixed-oxidant-generation systems. Mixed-oxidant ("oxygenated") species are formed by passing liquids or gases through any high-energy source, including electrochemical cells, ionizing radiation, or corona/plasma-generation systems. In these systems, where oxygen is present, it can be expected that a certain concentration of ozone may be generated, as well as other reactive species. These species not only have direct antimicrobial activity, but also react with other air/water components (including chlorine) to form additional active species; however, many of the generated species may also have undesirable consequences (such as material incompatibility or toxic substances).

3.13.2.2 Hydrogen Peroxide. Hydrogen peroxide is used as a preservative, antiseptic, disinfectant, fumigant, and sterilant. Applications can include the direct use of hydrogen peroxide dilutions in water or in gas form but also in synergistic combinations with other biocides or formulations. Liquid peroxide is generally stored in vented plastic (e.g., polyethylene) containers to allow for the release of oxygen over time as hydrogen peroxide degrades into water and oxygen. It is typically used as an antiseptic at 3 to 3.5% in water or in creams/gels, such as in the cleaning or treatment of wound infections, and treatment of skin or mucous membrane infections (e.g., as an oral mouth rinse). Formulations of 3 to 3.5% are also used for cleaning and disinfecting contact lenses and other hard-surface (noncritical) disinfection applications. Interestingly, it has been proposed for cancer and other therapeutic applications, but little clinical data are available to support these applications.

Inorganic and organic peroxides have been used for various industrial biocidal applications, with benzoyl peroxide being one of the most widely used for the treatment of acne vulgaris. Acne is a common skin condition in young adults and is often associated with *Propionibacterium acnes* and other bacteria on the skin. Benzoyl peroxide is also used as an antifungal antiseptic, with typical concentrations in the 1 to 10% range in many formulations of creams, lotions, gels, and cleansing low-level disinfection solutions. Formulations are often combined with other antimicrobials such as antibiotics (e.g., erythromycin), salicylic acid, retinoids (chemicals similar in structure to vitamin A, such as adapalene), and tertiary amines.

Hydrogen peroxide (5 to 6%) is used as a bleaching agent (e.g., for hair and paper) and as a laboratory surface disinfectant. Higher liquid concentrations are used for a variety of industrial and medical purposes. Typical concentrations include 22%, 35%, and 50%, with higher concentrations generally not used for biocidal applications due to increased safety considerations. General industrial applications include pollution control and chemical manufacturing. Due to rapid degradation into innocuous by-products, hydrogen peroxide is widely used in the food industry for general or critical surface disinfection/sterilization. As a rapidly active biocide, including a sporicidal agent, it is also used as a general surface and water disinfectant. The generally low rate of microbicidal action of hydrogen peroxide-based liquids can be accelerated by various formulation effects including the addition of certain detergents as well as the inclusion of anticorrosive agents to improve material compatibility. Formulations at 2 to 7.5% alone (in particular, under acidic conditions) and in combination with PAA are used for low-temperature medical device and other critical surface (e.g., clean room surfaces) disinfection, to include sporicidal activity with some formulations over time. The impact of formulation in these products is important to optimize antimicrobial activity while minimizing material compatibility concerns; these are good examples of the impact offormulation in comparison to the biocide alone for surface disinfection. High-speed sterilization processes use liquid peroxide at 35 to 50% and up to 70 to 80°C, with the temperature playing an important role in optimizing the antimicrobial effects in these applications. Preservative and immersion disinfection applications include contact lens solutions and bacteria/algae control in water.

The antimicrobial activity of hydrogen peroxide gas is more efficient at lower concentrations than in liquid, and it is used for odor control, fumigation, and sterilization processes (Table 3.4).

Typical concentrations range from 0.1 to 10 mg/liter (0.00001 to 0.001%), depending on the exposure temperature, which can range from 4 to 80°C. For example, a >6 log reduction of bacterial spores is observed within ~10 seconds with hydrogen peroxide gas at 4.5 mg/liter and 45°C at atmospheric pressure. Peroxide gas can be simply produced by heating or pulling a vacuum on a peroxide solution or both. For fumigation applications, peroxide gas is typically flash-vaporized by applying liquid directly to a heated (>100°C) surface, which forms a mixture of hydrogen peroxide and water gases. Gas generator and control systems are used for the fumigation of industrial critical environments (e.g., aseptic production isolators, clean rooms), rooms, buildings, and vehicles (Fig. 3.21). Applications have also included military uses, building remediation (notably, following the *B. anthracis* spore bioterrorism events in 2001 in the United States), and as an infection prevention and control measure in health care facilities (e.g., during outbreaks of norovirus, MRSA, and *Clostridium difficile*). In addition to the antimicrobial

TABLE 3.4 Comparison of the sporicidal efficacy of liquid and gaseous hydrogen peroxide at 20 to 25°C against bacterial spores

Bacterial spores	*D* value[a]	
	Liquid peroxide (250,000 mg/liter; 25%)	Peroxide vapor (1.5 mg/liter; 0.00015%)
Geobacillus stearothermophilus	1.5	1–2
Bacillus atrophaeus	2.0–7.3	0.5–1
Clostridium sporogenes	0.8	0.5–1

[a]Time to kill 1 $\log_{10}$ of the test organism in minutes.

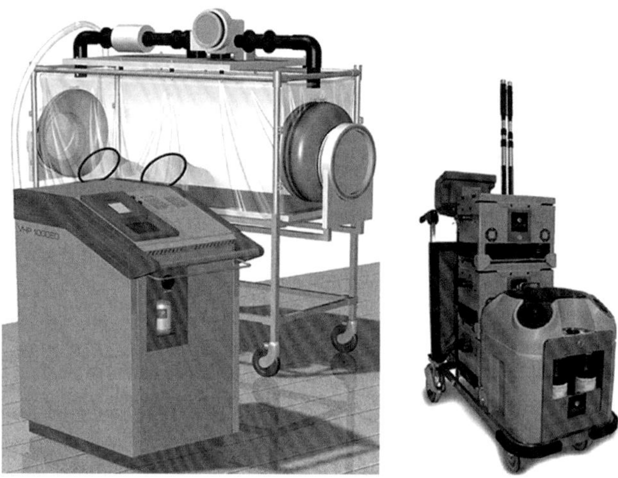

FIGURE 3.21 Examples of hydrogen peroxide gas generators. The example on the left shows a larger, shelf-contained generator system that is connected to a flexible walled isolator for disinfection. On the right is a room disinfection generator system, which consists of multiple modules. Generators can be mobile (as shown) or integrated into an area or facility. Images courtesy of STERIS, with permission.

activity of hydrogen peroxide gas, the biocide has also been shown to neutralize toxins (such as anthrax and botulism toxins) and chemical warfare agents (e.g., blistering agents such as mustard gas [HD] and nerve agents such as VX).

These generator systems are connected to, or are placed directly inside, an enclosed area and typically introduce peroxide gas into the area by controlling the flow of air through the system in a closed loop (Fig. 3.22).

A typical fumigation cycle can consist of up to four phases: dehumidification, conditioning, disinfection, and aeration. During the initial dehumidification phase, the relative humidity in the area can be reduced to below 50% if desired (to subsequently achieve optimal hydrogen peroxide gas concentrations). Hydrogen peroxide gas (and water gas, depending on the concentration of the starting hydrogen peroxide-water solution used to generate the gas mixture) is introduced into the room for conditioning to reach a desired level of hydrogen peroxide in the area for disinfection. As the concentration of peroxide (and water) increases in the area, it reaches a dew point (condensation point or saturation) dependent on the temperature (and, to a lesser extent, relatively humidity), where condensation can occur. Hydrogen peroxide in gas form is a vapor and can therefore readily condense under saturated conditions to return to its preferred liquid state. It is optimal to maintain the concentration of hydrogen peroxide and water gas below the condensation point for efficient antimicrobial activity, safety, and material compatibility. Disinfection can be achieved by simply introducing peroxide gas into an area and holding it for a desired time until it naturally breaks down in the environment to safe entry levels. The natural dissipation of the gas can take an extended amount of time depending on the area design and its contents. More efficient applications that are used continually remove and replenish the gas mixture in the area during the disinfection phase of the cycle to maintain the hydrogen peroxide gas concentration consistently over a programmed exposure time. This may be particularly important because peroxide gas breaks down on contact with surfaces, causing the build up of water vapor and reduced efficacy over time. In other applications, the concentration of peroxide and water is deliberately increased over the condensation point to allow for the deposition of high concentrations of liquid peroxide (condensing out at >70%) on

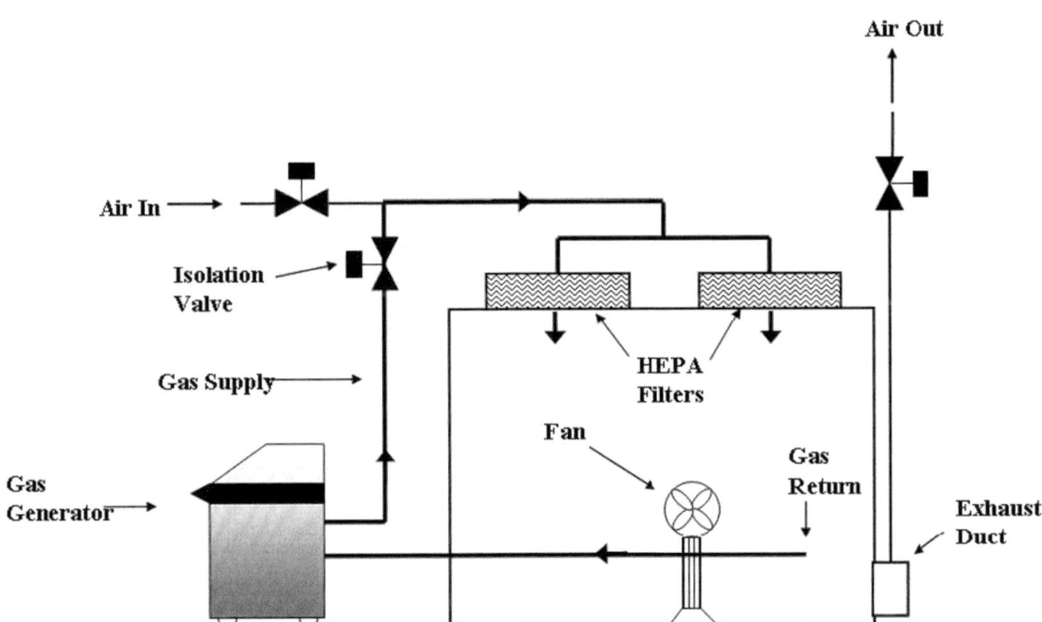

FIGURE 3.22 Typical room fumigation setup with a hydrogen peroxide gas generator. During fumigation, the air-handling system for the room is turned off and the gas is fed into the room. In the case shown below, fumigation includes the room as well as the air-handling ductwork, using the room ventilation system for gas distribution. Alternatively, the generator can be placed directly in the room.

surfaces, which is also an antimicrobial process but may lead to risks of surface damage and safety concerns due to the potential presence of high, and localized, liquid peroxide concentrations. Following disinfection, the area is aerated by passing fresh air into the room and removing peroxide gas residuals by neutralization (e.g., through a catalytic converter) to safe entry levels (generally to <1 to 2 ppm).

Hydrogen peroxide gas diffuses passively when introduced into an area, and therefore constant movement of the gas is often recommended to ensure that all surfaces are contacted over time. This can be aided at atmospheric pressure by using fans or air-handling systems or by introducing a slight positive or negative pressure in the area being fumigated. High-speed container sterilization systems have been described that rapidly introduce a high concentration of peroxide gas to the containers under slight pressure conditions for sterilization in seconds and rapidly remove the gas to prevent residual accumulation. For other sterilization methods, it is often more effective to introduce the gas under vacuum (low pressure) conditions, which ensures greater penetration of the biocide into a complex load. Hydrogen peroxide gas sterilization systems are used for industrial and medical applications. These include simple peroxide gas cycles and combination systems with other agents, particularly plasma and ozone (these systems are described in more detail in chapter 6, section 6.5).

Many novel formulations or processes have been described that use hydrogen peroxide in combination with other biocides or processes. These are often considered synergistic, because the efficacy of a given concentration of hydrogen peroxide has been shown to be greater in the presence of these biocides. It is often difficult to differentiate between true synergistic effects over the individual impacts of each biocide in a given application. Synergism with hydrogen peroxide has been shown in both liquid and gaseous phase. These applications can be by simple combination with heat, as well as in combination with other chemical and physical agents (Table 3.5).

3.13.2.3 PAA. Liquid PAA is used industrially for chemical manufacturing (e.g., for epoxidation), as a catalyst, and for paper bleaching. It is also widely used directly and in formulation for cleaning, sanitization, disinfection, and sterilization. As mentioned above, all solutions and formulations are provided with PAA in equilibrium with hydrogen peroxide, water, and acetic acid. PAA can also be produced *in situ* by dilution of dry formulations in water (Fig. 3.18). Formulation, including mixtures with anticorrosives, surfactants, and chelating agents, is important for the stability, efficacy, and material compatibility of PAA and formulated products can therefore vary considerably. Stability can be improved at lower pH, at higher concentrations of hydrogen peroxide, and by storage at lower temperatures. The overall efficacies of these formulations increase at higher concentrations of PAA and at higher temperatures; however, the degradation rate of PAA also increases at higher temperatures.

Typical concentrations for disinfection and sterilization are <0.35% (or 3,500 mg/liter). Due to its natural breakdown into water and a low concentration of acetic acid, PAA is extensively used in the food industry, directly on food and for sanitization of food contact surfaces; many applications do not require rinsing, which is an advantage due to costs and the potential of cross-contamination. For medical applications, PAA formulations have become popular alternatives to glutaraldehyde, and other aldehyde, liquids for low-temperature disinfection of reusable medical devices, including flexible endoscopes. Formulations include 1 to 7% hydrogen peroxide and 0.1 to 0.25% PAA, as well as *in situ* generation formulations based on acetylsalicylic acid. Liquid PAA-based sterilization processes are discussed further in chapter 6, section 6.6.1. Other medical applications include the treatment of solid and liquid waste, hemodialyzer machine reprocessing, and tissue (e.g., bone) disinfection. PAA is also used

TABLE 3.5 Hydrogen peroxide-based synergistic formulations and processes

Synergistic agent	Application	Description
Copper, iron, manganese	Reaction with liquid or gas	Results in the production of free radicals (including ·OH)
Heat	Heating up to 80°C	As the temperature increases, the activity of peroxide increases, but in parallel to some increase in the degradation rate of peroxide. As a gas, the higher the temperature, the greater the concentration of peroxide (and thus, antimicrobial activity) that can be maintained in air without condensation
UV	Reaction in liquid or gas	Results in the production of free radicals (including ·OH)
Ultrasonics[a]	Applied in liquid	Unknown; proposed to increase the production of free radicals and to increase the penetration of peroxide into target cells. May also cause cells to disassociate to allow direct contact with the biocide
PAA	Combined in formulation or as a gas	Unknown, but both active agents are powerful oxidizing agents and may be effective by different mechanisms; may promote the production of free radicals
Ozone	Combined in liquid or as a gas	Unknown, but both active agents are powerful oxidizing agents; may promote the production of free radicals
Plasma	Combined as a gas and proposed in liquid	Plasma causes the breakdown of peroxide, giving a higher localized concentration of free radicals, in combination with the effects of plasma itself

[a]Ultrasonics: the generation of high-frequency sound waves in liquid.

directly on surfaces for general environmental disinfection, due to its rapid antimicrobial (including sporicidal) activity; this is particularly important for critical environments such as in manufacturing or research clean rooms and aseptic isolators. Other uses have included the use of PAA in ointments and lotions (at 0.05 to 0.1%) as antiseptics, for sewage treatment, for biofilm removal (due to its powerful oxidizing agent activity, which improves cleaning, in particular, for carbohydrate and lipid materials), and for water or water surface (e.g., pipework) disinfection or remediation (e.g., for *Legionella* control). In addition to hydrogen peroxide, formulations with low concentrations of PAA have been described with alcohols to provide sporicidal activity during antisepsis.

Gaseous PAA has been less used than liquid applications for disinfection. This is primarily due to its corrosive nature, which can be better controlled in liquid formulations, and its pungent odor. Similar to hydrogen peroxide, the efficacy of gaseous PAA is greater at lower concentrations than in liquid; overall, efficacy can be considered to be a combination of PAA and hydrogen peroxide gas effects. Applications have included enclosed area fumigation, food sanitization, and medical device sterilization. The use of PAA gas sterilization is considered in chapter 6, section 6.6.3.

3.13.2.4 Chlorine Dioxide. Chlorine dioxide is used primarily in liquid form and, to a lesser extent, in gas applications. Industrial uses include paper bleaching and potable water, wastewater (e.g., slime reduction), and water contact surface disinfection. Examples of chlorine dioxide generator systems are shown in Fig. 3.23.

As an alternative to chlorine, chlorine dioxide is not considered to leave as strong a residual taste or odor in water applications; typical concentrations used range from 0.1 to 5 mg/liter. Due to the degradation of phenols, cyanides, aldehydes, and other undesirable compounds in such applications, it has been used to improve water taste and potable quality. It is used in the food industry (both directly and in formulation) for food-contact surface and food surface sanitization and disinfection. A similar variety of formulations have been used in many countries for low-temperature medical device disinfection, veterinary applications, and general surface disinfection (Fig. 3.24).

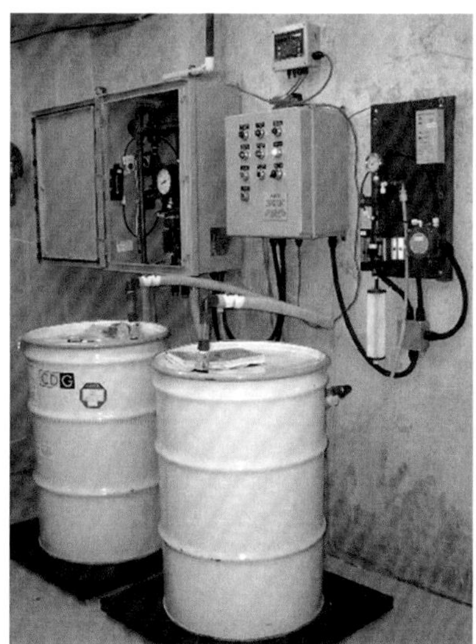

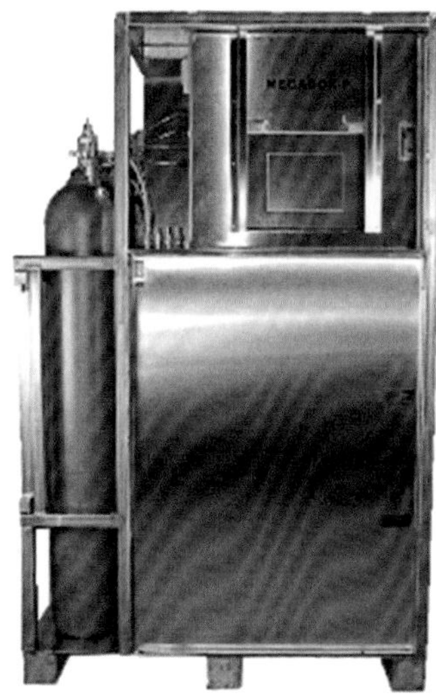

FIGURE 3.23 Chlorine dioxide generator systems for liquid disinfection (left) and gas fumigation (right) applications. Images courtesy of CDG Environmental, LLC and ClorDiSys Solutions Inc., with permission.

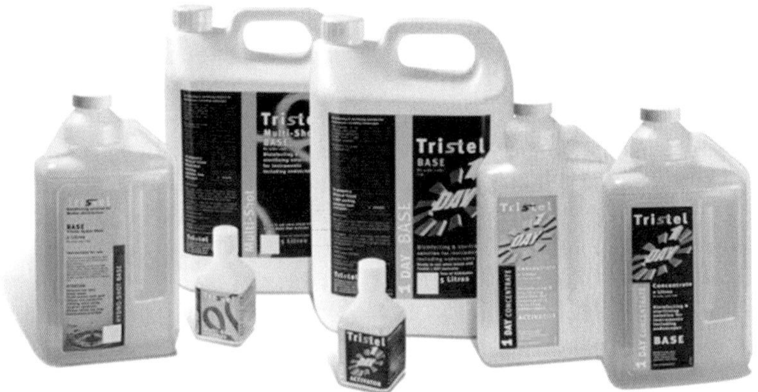

FIGURE 3.24 A range of chlorine dioxide-based liquid formulations for medical device disinfection. Image courtesy of Tristel Solutions Ltd., with permission.

These include a variety of two-component formulations (in dry and liquid forms) and delivery systems, including impregnated wipes. Typical concentrations for critical applications (including sporicidal activity) are 200 to 500 mg/liter for 5 to 30 minutes, but these conditions vary depending on the formulation and its use.

Chlorine dioxide gas is a more effective antimicrobial at lower concentrations (with typical use concentrations varying from 0.5 to 30 mg/liter). As a gas, it is used for odor control, area fumigation, remediation, and sterilization. A brief description of the use of chlorine dioxide under vacuum for biomedical and industrial sterilization processes is given in chapter 6, section 6.6.5. Atmospheric applications include the fumigation of manufacturing and laboratory equipment, isolators, and rooms (including clean rooms) and for large-area remediation. For example, chlorine dioxide gas (at >65% relative humidity) was successfully used for the remediation of contaminated buildings (at ~2 mg/liter or 750 ppm, at >65% humidity for 12 hours). Mobile and fixed gas generator systems that allow automation of fumigation processes are commercially available (Fig. 3.23).

A typical fumigation process includes humidification of the area (generally, 70 to 80% humidity is preferred), exposure to chlorine dioxide, and subsequent aeration to below the safe level of 0.1 ppm (Fig. 3.25). Aeration can be safely achieved by chemical neutralization of the gas, such as by passing it through sodium bisulfite.

Chlorine dioxide has also been used at low concentrations as an antiseptic, including for skin disinfection (e.g., mastitis control), mouthwashes, and toothpastes. An example is the activation of 0.1% sodium chlorite with 0.3% mandelic acid for immediate use as a preoperative preparation.

3.13.3 Spectrum of Activity

3.13.3.1 Ozone. At the concentrations typically used (0.2 to 0.5 mg/liter), ozone is an effective bactericide and virucide, with greater resistance observed with mycobacteria and bacterial spores. For gas-based processes, sporicidal activity requires high levels of relative humidity (75 to 95%) to be effective. Yeasts and molds have been reported to have a wide range of resistance profiles but are generally less resistant than bacterial spores. Similar ranges of activity have been reported for other mixed-oxidant systems. Numerous studies with ozone have focused on protozoal and cysticidal activities, due to a number of notable outbreaks of *Giardia* and *Cryptosporidium* in contaminated water. Ozone was reported as being one of the most effective water disinfectants in comparison to chlorine dioxide,

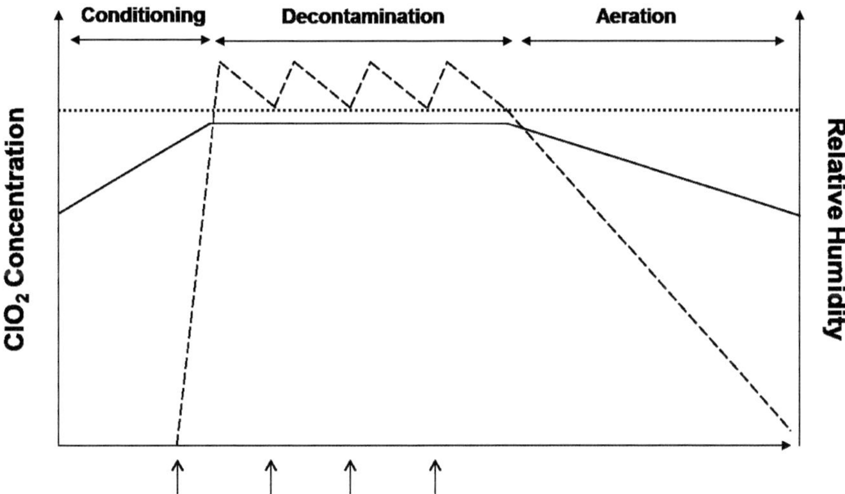

FIGURE 3.25 Typical chlorine dioxide fumigation cycle. The biocide concentration is shown as a dashed line, and humidity as a solid line. The dotted line indicates the minimum concentration required for activity, which depends on the application. As chlorine dioxide breaks down during the disinfection phase, the concentration can be increased by further injection of gas (as shown by arrows).

chlorine, and monochloramine, with *Cryptosporidium* oocysts demonstrating the highest resistance. Ozone has also been used for the treatment of wastewater, which is often heavily contaminated, including for the control of algae. Higher ozone concentrations are generally required in these cases due to the interaction with and neutralization by high organic loads. For fumigation or surface sterilization applications, antimicrobial activity is dependent on the presence and maintenance of 70 to 80% relative humidity, below which little practical activity is observed against bacterial spores. Ozone, under these conditions, has some activity in neutralizing protein toxins, including mycotoxins, and some reports have suggested prion inactivation.

3.13.3.2 Hydrogen Peroxide. Hydrogen peroxide, depending on its concentration and formulation, demonstrates broad-spectrum efficacy against viruses, bacteria, mycobacteria fungi, and bacterial spores. Greater efficacy is seen at much lower concentrations with hydrogen peroxide gas compared to liquid (Table 3.4). Higher concentrations of liquid peroxide (10 to 55%) and longer contact times are required for sporicidal and cysticidal activity, in contrast to gaseous peroxide. Hydrogen peroxide is generally more effective against Gram-positive than Gram-negative bacteria; however, the presence of catalase or other peroxidases (in particular, in Gram-positive bacteria such as *S. aureus* and other staphylococci) can allow for increased tolerance to peroxide due to enzymatic degradation of peroxide. In general, concentrations of peroxide above 3% are bactericidal, and <3% concentrations demonstrate good bacteriostatic, fungistatic, and algistatic activity. Efficacy against *Cryptosporidium* and *Giardia* has been described at 6 to 7% liquid peroxide and in gaseous form at 1 to 6 mg/liter; 3% peroxide formulations, which are used for contact lens disinfection, have been shown to be effective against *Acanthamoeba* cysts over 4 hours. Further studies suggested that different cyst isolates can vary in resistance to peroxide concentrations (in water) from 3 to 8% and over time but that hydrogen peroxide-based formulations at 2% peroxide in acidic conditions were more rapidly and consistently effective. Hydrogen peroxide gas has also been shown to be effective against parasite eggs (including *Caenorhabditis*, *Enterobius*, and *Sphacia*). Although liquid peroxide dilutions have been shown to have little to no effect on prions, hydrogen peroxide gas was shown to be effective in both atmospheric and vacuum applications; further, it was shown that these effects vary from process to process, presumably due to the variations in the potential for condensation to have occurred during exposure conditions. The specific activity of gaseous peroxide to be effective against prions may be linked to its mode of action to include protein fragmentation, unlike what has been seen in studies with liquid peroxide solutions in water (see section 7.4.2). This difference in mechanism of action may be linked to the demonstrated efficacy of hydrogen peroxide gas to neutralize protein toxins and bacterial endotoxins. In addition to biological applications, peroxide is also used for pollution control and chemical neutralization due to its potent oxidizing activity.

Benzoyl peroxide is considered bactericidal and fungicidal at the 2 to 10% range, but its activity is considered slow based on *in vitro* investigations. Interestingly, the activity of benzoyl peroxide is enhanced in the presence of lipids (on the skin) and also breaks down to form benzoic acid, which is itself an antimicrobial agent (section 3.2). The antimicrobial activity of benzoyl peroxide against *P. acnes* has been particularly well studied, and that against the dermatophytes (skin-based fungi such as *Trichophyton*), to a lesser extent.

3.13.3.3 PAA. PAA is generally considered to be a more potent biocide than hydrogen peroxide. It is considered sporicidal, bactericidal, tuberculocidal, virucidal, and fungicidal at low concentrations (<0.35%) at room temperature. Bactericidal and fungicidal activity is rapid, even at concentrations as low as 0.003%. Virucidal activity varies, with the nonenveloped viruses demonstrating the greatest resistance at 0.2% at room temperature; in contrast, enveloped viruses have been shown to be sensitive to PAA at as low as 0.001%. Similar to other biocides, the effect of temperature (Fig. 3.26) and concentration can be significant. For example, for sterilization purposes a sterility assurance level of 10^{-6} has been demonstrated with PAA in formulation at 1,000 mg/liter and 50°C for ~2 minutes.

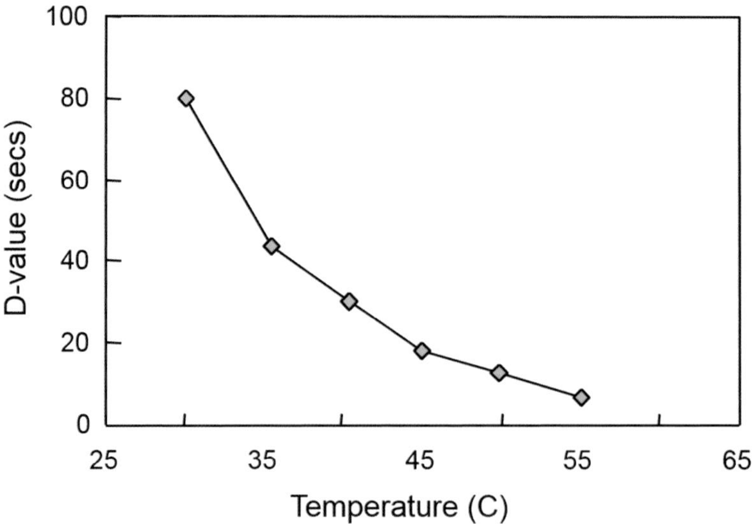

FIGURE 3.26 The effect of temperature on the sporicidal efficacy of PAA. The average *D* value (in seconds) was determined for *Geobacillus stearothermophilus* spores at 1,000 mg/liter PAA in formulation at various test temperatures.

Some liquid PAA-based formulations have been shown to have significant cleaning effects (particularly for lipid and carbohydrate removal from surfaces), which have been useful for biofilm remediation or prevention, although this activity appears to be dependent on the product formulation. Studies that have compared the cleaning effects of PAA-based disinfection formulations have shown that some are effective, while others caused proteins and other materials to be fixed onto test surfaces, thereby posing a risk of further biofilm development. Unlike hydrogen peroxide, PAA is not broken down by the enzymatic activities of catalases and peroxidases, and it demonstrates greater efficacy in the presence of contaminating soils. For example, liquid PAA can dissolve inorganic salts that can be a penetration challenge for other disinfection and sterilization methods such as steam and ethylene oxide gas. Studies have shown some efficacy against *Cryptosporidium* and *Giardia* depending on the PAA formulation being tested, but the activity increased with temperature. Of further note, PAA has been reported to neutralize pyrogens (including endotoxins) and may have some limited effect against prions, dependent on the temperature, concentration, and formulation.

3.13.3.4 Chlorine Dioxide. Chlorine dioxide has a spectrum of activity similar to, if not greater than, that of chlorine or other chlorinated compounds (section 3.11). It is active over a wider pH range (pH 6 to 10, with greater activity at the higher alkaline range) and demonstrated greater activity at increased temperatures. Relatively low concentrations are required for bactericidal and virucidal activities (0.2 to 0.7 mg/liter at room temperature and pH 7). Chlorine dioxide has been used as a cleaner, for biofilm control, and as an algicide. Cysticidal activity has been demonstrated against *Giardia*, *Naegleria*, and *Cryptosporidium* in water at ~1 mg/liter. Higher concentrations (1 to 2 mg/liter) are required to ensure sporicidal activity for some applications. Although reports have suggested activity against prions, this requires further investigation.

3.13.4 Advantages

3.13.4.1 Ozone. Ozone and other oxidants are potent antimicrobials that are effective at relatively low concentrations. They are considered environmentally friendly methods for liquid disinfection, because they rapidly break down into oxygen and water; the lack of significant residual tastes or smells is an aesthetic advantage over alternatives such as chlorine and bromine. In addition, ozone is an efficient agent for taste and odor control (as a chemical neutralizer) in water treatment and can further neutralize algal toxins. Ozone is effective at neutralizing chemical contamination, including cyanides, phenols, some detergents, and metals (e.g., iron). For area decontamination, little to no aeration time is required following exposure, because it breaks down rapidly in the environment, and ozone has a reasonable safety profile (it is considered safe to work in an area at 0.1 ppm ozone over a typical 8-hour day).

3.13.4.2 Hydrogen Peroxide. Hydrogen peroxide is a potent biocide that is effective at low concentrations against vegetative organisms, with higher concentrations required for sporicidal activity. Hydrogen peroxide is considered environmentally friendly and nontoxic, because it can rapidly degrade into water and oxygen. Peroxide solutions are generally safe for use directly on the skin and other surfaces at 3 to 6%; however, at higher concentrations (35 to 50%) burns and material damage can occur. At concentrations greater than 50% the broad use of peroxide is limited due to significant safety concerns. Hydrogen peroxide gas, particularly when maintained below the condensation point at a given temperature, demonstrates a broad material compatibility profile for low-temperature fumigation and sterilization uses; applications have included the safe use of peroxide gas on electronic equipment (including computerized systems) and other sensitive materials that cannot withstand liquid treatments. Fumigation with peroxide is more rapid and safer than traditional formaldehyde methods, and reports have also suggested chemical neutralization activity (e.g., chemical warfare agents, such as VX [$C_{11}H_{26}NO_2PS$] gas, and bacterial toxins). The recommended safety level for a typical 8-hour working day is 1 ppm of peroxide gas, which is readily detected using available detector and alarm systems. With a sufficient concentration of the biocide, peroxide can demonstrate antimicrobial efficacy in the presence of contaminating organic or inorganic soil loads.

Benzoyl peroxide has been successfully used as a treatment for skin-associated infections, in particular, acne vulgaris, due to its keratinolytic (exfoliative) activity, drying of the skin (with reduced production of sebum), and good lipid solubility; *P. acnes* is generally found deep within the outer surface skin layers, and benzoyl peroxide is considered to be more penetrating to these layers than other antiseptic biocides (see chapter 4, section 4.3).

3.13.4.3 PAA. PAA provides broad-spectrum activity at relatively low concentrations. It also decomposes to safe, nontoxic by-products (a low concentration of acetic acid and water) but has the added advantages over hydrogen peroxide of being free from decomposition by peroxidases and having greater activity in the presence of organic/inorganic soils. There have been no reports of resistance development, presumably due to its rapid breakdown in the environment, and it is not considered carcinogenic. PAA is compatible with stainless steel and other surfaces; however, efficacy and material compatibility are dependent on the biocide formulation and application.

3.13.4.4 Chlorine Dioxide. Chlorine dioxide is a potent biocide at relatively low concentrations and, at sufficient concentrations, even in the presence of soils. It is often preferred over chlorine for water disinfection, due to the lack of taste and odor at typical use concentrations. There are no known health effects at the concentrations typically used in water, and it is not currently considered carcinogenic or mutagenic. Chlorine dioxide reacts and neutralizes many harmful or undesired chemicals (including phenols and aldehydes), and unlike chlorine, does not react to form THMs or chloramine derivatives. For applications in the gaseous form, chlorine dioxide can be detected at harmful concentrations (>0.1 ppm) and provides rapid fumigation in comparison to formaldehyde. Unlike hydrogen peroxide gas, for which there are concerns about condensation, chlorine dioxide can tolerate a greater range of temperatures and is less likely to condense under typical use conditions. The biocide degrades into nontoxic residuals, although it is recommended that chlorine dioxide should be neutralized prior to release into the environment.

3.13.5 Disadvantages

3.13.5.1 Ozone. Ozone's restricted material compatibility is probably its greatest disadvantage, because it is a very reactive oxidizing agent and can be corrosive on surfaces. Similar profiles have been described for mixed-oxidant systems. Materials can be manufactured or pretreated to be corrosion-resistant, including high-quality stainless steel, titanium, ceramics, and some polymers; however, even in these cases, damage can occur, such as premature rusting on stainless steel. Rust (FeO_2) forms on exposure of available iron (e.g., on stainless steel surfaces) to ozone. Maintenance of higher concentrations is required for sporicidal activity over longer exposure times (in particular, for sterilization applications), which are also more aggressive on surfaces. For fumigation applications, the requirement for humidification may also be restrictive in some cases and, as for other gaseous peroxygens, applications that contain adsorptive or proteinaceous materials require special consideration due to neutralization of the biocide. Finally, ozone is an irritant to the mucous membranes and can cause significant damage to tissues at typically used concentrations.

3.13.5.2 Hydrogen Peroxide. Hydrogen peroxide in some applications can cause bleaching of surfaces, including some colored anodized aluminum devices. Contact with various surfaces, including organic material, cellulosic materials (such as paper or wood), brass, copper, and iron, can cause the rapid degradation of peroxide. Direct exposure to high liquid concentrations can cause skin burns and, in gaseous form, irritation and damage to mucous membranes even at lower concentrations (e.g., 10 to 20 ppm). For applications in the gaseous phase, liquids (including water) cannot be disinfected or sterilized. High concentrations of liquid peroxide (e.g., on condensation) can pose a risk of fire or explosion on contact with certain surfaces (e.g., certain solvents).

Benzoyl peroxide has low solubility and is considered unstable, which is an important consideration for optimal formulation of the biocide. The major disadvantage in its use as an antiseptic is skin irritancy, including itching and burning in some applications (depending on the concentration and formulation of the biocide). Allergic reactions and some toxicity concerns (due to adsorption into the blood and breakdown to benzoic acid) have been reported, although these effects have been reported to be reduced when benzoyl peroxide is provided as nanoparticles. At typically used concentrations, benzoyl peroxide is an eye and respiratory irritant.

3.13.5.3 PAA. Concentrated PAA has a strong pungent odor, which can be irritating to the eyes, mucous membranes, and respiratory system. Direct exposure at high concentrations, which should be avoided and is not believed to have long-term effects, can also cause nausea and is generally reversed by exposure to fresh air. Adequate ventilation is therefore recommended in areas where high concentrations of PAA are stored or used in open applications. PAA should be stored in vented containers to prevent explosion, due to the buildup of oxygen on degradation over time. Material compatibility can be a concern, in particular, on copper, brass, aluminum, and some plastics; these effects can be minimized by correct formulation of the biocide. PAA also causes burns to the skin at >3% and damage to the eyes at >0.3%. PAA is unstable (e.g., 35% solutions in water will decrease by 0.4% per month at room temperature), and controls should be in place to ensure that adequate use concentrations are present for the required application in accordance with manufacturers' instructions.

3.13.5.4 Chlorine Dioxide. Chlorine dioxide typically needs to be generated on-site and is short-lived, although some stable formulations or two-component generation and delivery systems have been developed. Many of the chemicals used for generation may also pose some safety concerns and should be controlled. For liquid applications, care should be taken to ensure that prepared solutions are at the required concentration for their intended use. There remains some discussion regarding health effects of chlorite and chlorate by-products in the use of chlorine dioxide. It can be explosive at >10% in air; therefore, care should be taken to control its manufacture in large-volume applications. The recommended safety level is 0.1 ppm, above which it is a respiratory, eye, and mucous membrane irritant; at higher concentrations (e.g., 19 ppm) exposure can be lethal. The biocide is light-sensitive, so applications are best conducted in the dark. Chlorine dioxide can be corrosive to certain metals (including copper and brass) and plastics (e.g., polycarbonate and polyurethane), depending on the application. Bleaching of colored surfaces may also be observed, as with other oxidizing agents. Liquid chlorine dioxide is often considered more corrosive, in particular, due to the various acids involved in generation processes, although this can vary depending on the product formulation. Breakdown products (in particular, chlorine gas) can contribute to the observed surface incompatibility profile and can be minimized by reducing the concentration used, by formulation effects (in liquid), and by performing gas fumigation processes in darkness. For fumigation processes, humidity needs to be maintained above 65% for efficacy, and a fine white powder has been reported from some applications on surfaces, but this was not considered toxic. Like other gaseous oxidizing agent-based processes, standing liquids cannot be disinfected, and efficacy can be limited on cellulosics (e.g., paper) or other absorptive materials.

3.13.6 Modes of Action

3.13.6.1 Ozone. Ozone causes oxidation of external and internal cellular and structural components. As a strong oxidizing agent, ozone has been shown to cause enzyme inactivation and cell wall and membrane damage. Direct effects (degradation) on viral and other nucleic acids, as well as lipids, proteins, and polypeptides, have been reported. These effects are thought to be primarily due to direct interaction with ozone itself, particularly in water applications at acidic pH, although the indirect production of other unstable reactive species (including the short-lived hydroxyl and peroxyl free radicals) may play a greater role at alkaline pH. These effects may also explain the requirement for high humidity (or presence of water) during area fumigation applications. Ozone has been shown to break down various types of oxidizable amino acids, including histidine, tyrosine, and lysine over time, but these effects did not necessarily correlate with the loss of protein structure observed with ozone. In addition to effects on proteins and lipids, ozone has been well described as breakages in the backbone of double-stranded DNA, and this is strongly associated with the participation of hydroxyl radicals.

3.13.6.2 Hydrogen Peroxide. Similar to other peroxygens, the antimicrobial effects of hydrogen peroxide and its oxidizing agent effects occur initially on the surfaces of microorganisms, in combination with the presence of short-lived breakdown products such as the superoxide and hydroxyl radicals (as described for ozone) on reaction with these surface components. The increased presence and local production of these radicals are speculated to be responsible for the greater antimicrobial efficacy observed with gaseous peroxide because it demonstrates greater oxidation potential than in liquid studies. These observations are often cited as being due to the Fenton reaction (the reaction of hydrogen peroxide with catalysts such as iron) to give rise to local concentrations of hydroxyl radicals and their impact on key structural and functional macromolecules. Culminative oxidation impacts of key cellular components, including lipids, proteins and nucleic acids, are proposed to cause cell death and viral inactivation. The effects on proteins may be particularly important in some cases, with observed removal of proteins from spore coats with liquid peroxide and direct breakage of peptide bonds (particularly in the mechanism of action of the gas form). It has been proposed that exposed protein sulfhydryl groups and fatty acid double bonds are particularly targeted. Subtle differences in the mechanisms of action of liquid and gas peroxide have been described and can even vary on the formulation of liquid preparations. For example, peroxide gas had direct effects on degrading proteins (presumably by reacting with or causing the breakdown of peptide bonds, depending on the protein structure), while the impact of liquid peroxide (in water) was predominantly due to the oxidation of amino acid side chains. In some cases, the formulation of peroxide solutions was shown to have mechanisms of action similar to those reported for the gas phase; therefore, the true antimicrobial effects can be subtly different based on these formulation effects. This may be important for some applications, as shown in studies where peroxide (and PAA) in some formulations can react with amino acid side chains and lead to the cross-linking of reactive amino acids within and between adjacent proteins; in contrast, other formulations (and exposure conditions) can lead to protein degradation and greater surface cleaning activities. Although the overall antimicrobial activity may be effective, the specific effects can be different. Recent studies on the effects of hydrogen peroxide, particularly in gas form, against bacterial spores have concluded that the primary mechanism of action is due to interaction with and degradation of nucleic acids. Although low-level damage may be repaired by normal cellular functions, the accumulative effects eventually overwhelm the repair mechanism and lead to cell death. Liquid peroxide may have had some impacts at the spore surface layers, but overall it showed slow penetration and reactivity with the inner spore structures (correlating with the differences observed in the slower sporicidal activity for liquid hydrogen peroxide).

The mode of action of benzoyl peroxide, similar to hydrogen peroxide, is linked to its oxidizing activity and the production of hydroxyl and other radicals. In addition, the biocide degrades to give benzoic acid, which is itself an antimicrobial, acid biocide (section 3.2).

3.13.6.3 PAA. The mode of action of PAA is similar to that of hydrogen peroxide and, presumably, is primarily due to direct effects on microbial surfaces and indirectly by the production of short-lived radicals, in particular, the hydroxyl radical. Specific effects on bacterial cell walls and membrane permeability, and viral capsids, have been studied. PAA has been shown to denature and degrade proteins and enzymes, particularly by disrupting sulfhydryl (-SH) and sulfur (S-S) bonds. These effects can be dependent, similar to hydrogen peroxide, on the formulation or state (e.g., liquid as opposed to gas phase) of PAA. Greater protein degradation has been reported in formulations at higher temperatures (e.g., up to 50°C). Effects on nucleic acids, including DNA and RNA strand breakage, have been observed and are particularly important in antiviral efficacy. It is difficult to study the direct role of PAA in formulations because they always contain a certain concentration of hydrogen peroxide and acetic acid in equilibrium. There are clearly synergistic mechanisms of activity with hydrogen peroxide and PAA, although PAA is considered the potent oxidizing agent. The impact of this has been shown in some subtle studies with bacterial spores, which indicate minor effects of hydrogen peroxide on compromising the spore coat structure as a major spore resistance factor and allowing greater penetration of PAA to inactivate the spore by specific effects on the spore inner membranes that are essential to spore germination. It is also clear that both PAA and hydrogen peroxide cause oxidation of nucleic acids, leading to DNA degradation, fragmentation, and inactivity.

3.13.6.4 Chlorine Dioxide. The chlorine dioxide molecule is a reactive radical, reacting with surfaces on contact. Thus, the main mode of action is believed to be disruption of cell walls/membranes and microbial surfaces, which culminates in cell death or loss of infectivity. Specifically, chlorine dioxide was reported to react with specific amino acids (such as tryptophan, cysteine, and tyrosine), but these results could not be repeated by other investigators, who suggested that more subtle effects cumulated to cause loss of protein and enzyme expression, structure, and function. Direct reaction with fatty acids has been reported. Little to no effects were observed on nucleic acids (DNA or RNA) when tested in liquid form, although it is clear that nucleic acid functions (e.g., replication and transcription) are inhibited (presumably due to protein inhibition); these results are in contrast to the specific effects on nucleic acids observed with chlorine and chlorine-releasing agents (section 3.11).

3.14 PHENOLICS

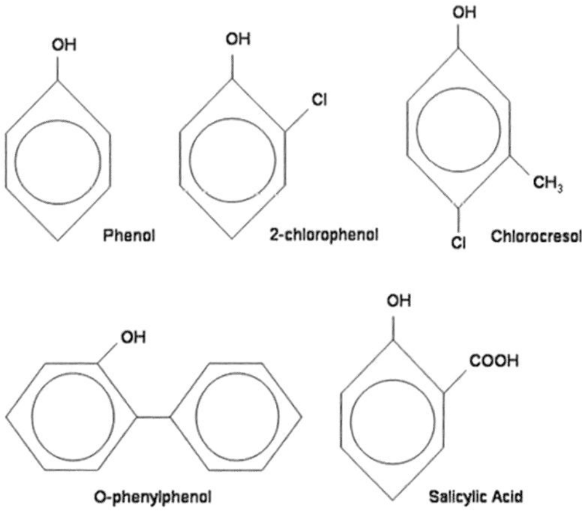

Phenol

2-chlorophenol

Chlorocresol

O-phenylphenol

Salicylic Acid

3.14.1 Types

Phenolics are chemically a class of alcohol compounds with one or more hydroxyl (-OH) groups attached to an aromatic hydrocarbon ring. A wide variety of phenolics are used for disinfection, preservation, and antisepsis (Table 3.6). The traditional range of phenolics, including phenol, cresols, and xylenols, was first identified by fractionation from coal or tar as naturally occurring antimicrobials. Subsequently, many of these and alternative phenolic compounds ("non-coal-tar" phenols) were synthetically produced and investigated, which included modification by halogenation (e.g., chlorination or nitrification) and condensation (e.g., with aldehydes or ketones to produce bisphenols).

3.14.2 Applications

Phenolics and their derivatives are an important class of compounds which are widely used for industrial and medical purposes. In addition to their antimicrobial properties, phenolic compounds are also used as pain killers (e.g., acetylsalicylic acid, or aspirin), as herbicides, and in the manufacture of resins and synthetic fibers. Phenolic compounds have long been used for their antiseptic, disinfectant, and preservative properties. Phenol itself, despite its irritation to the skin, was successfully used during pioneering antiseptic surgical procedures by Joseph Lister (1827-1912). The phenolics most widely used on the skin today are the bisphenols (hexachlorophene and triclosan), chloroxylenol (also commonly known as PCMX [*p*-chloro-*m*-xylenol]), and salicylic acid, which are further discussed for their antiseptic applications (see section 3.15 and chapter 4). Chloroxylenol has also been widely used as a preservative and in some surface disinfectants. Phenol itself is still used in antiseptic ointments and sprays at lower concentrations in combination with other biocides (such as chlorhexidine; section 3.8). Due to their insolubility in water, phenolics are combined (or formulated) with soaps, oils, or synthetic anionic detergents for solubilization and availability. Soaps and surfactants are molecules that change the properties of a liquid at its surface or interface by breaking the surface tension. In both cases, they consist of a water-soluble (ionic, polar, or hydrophilic) part and a longer-chain water-insoluble (nonpolar, or hydrophobic) part. They aid in phenol solubilization by micelle formation, in which the phenolic is solubilized in the central hydrophobic region (see section 1.4.6). Formulation effects, therefore, play a key role in the optimization of phenolic disinfectant activity, so that it is available for optimized antimicrobial activity, as well as remaining soluble (e.g., when diluted in water in concentrated disinfectants). Most phenolic disinfectant formulations contain two or more phenolic types, due to synergistic attributes, including antimicrobial efficacy. Phenolics are widely used as broad-spectrum, intermediate-level disinfectants for general surface disinfection, including walls and floors, such as in health care facilities, veterinary applications, and critical manufacturing areas such as clean rooms (Fig. 3.27).

For some applications (including clean room disinfection), formulations are provided sterilized (by filtration or radiation), to reduce the risk of spore contamination; phenols are sporistatic but not sporicidal and are therefore sterilized to remove any risk of cross-contamination from the product. Phenolics are also used at low concentrations as preservatives, due to broad-spectrum inhibition at relatively low concentrations. Of note, phenol itself has been tradi-

TABLE 3.6 Various types of phenolic compounds

Coal-tar	Non-coal-tar
Phenol	2-Phenylphenol
Cresols	4-Hexylresorcinol
Xylenols	
Naphthols	
Halogenated phenols	**Bisphenols**
4-Chloro-3,5-dimethylphenol (chloroxylenol; PCMX)	Triclosan
4-Nitrophenol	Hexachlorophene
2-Chlorophenol	Fenichlor
Chlorocresol	
Other phenol derivatives	
2,3-Diaminophenol	
Salicylic acid	
8-Hydroxyquinoline	

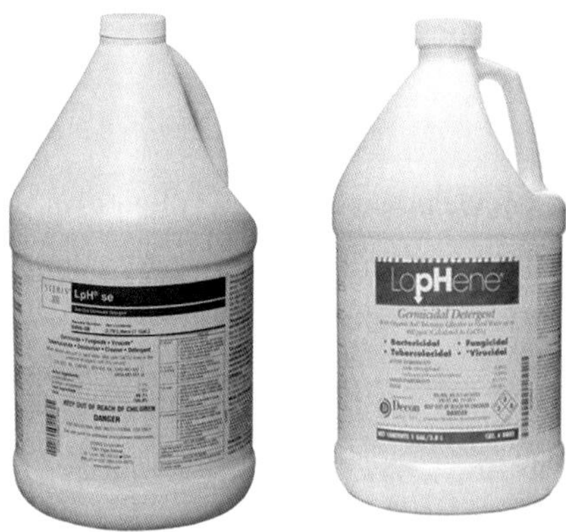

FIGURE 3.27 Phenolic-based disinfectants. Both formulations shown are concentrates that are diluted in water prior to use. Disinfectant formulations are also available as ready-to-use and wipe-based technologies, both in nonsterile and sterilized forms. Image courtesy of STERIS, with permission.

tionally used in a method to standardize the resistance of bacterial and fungal cultures used for disinfection efficacy studies; the Association of Official Analytical Chemists phenol coefficient test exposes a test culture to a known concentration of phenol to determine its intrinsic resistance. Some bisphenols (particularly triclosan) have been successfully integrated into various polymers, including fabrics and miscellaneous surfaces such as cutting boards and toothbrushes, to provide some residual antimicrobial activity.

3.14.3 Spectrum of Activity

Most phenolics demonstrate rapid activity against bacteria (Gram-positive and Gram-negative), fungi, and viruses. In general, phenolics are more effective against Gram-positive than Gram-negative bacteria. Rapid tuberculocidal activity has also been demonstrated, depending on the specific phenolic biocide (or combinations in formulation). The activity varies considerably depending on the phenol types and their formulation; specific attention should be paid to the label claims on products and the test methods used to verify their activity, because they can vary considerably. Most formulations contain two or more phenolic compounds, which generally provide a broader range of activity than the use of a single phenolic. In general, the more lipophilic the phenolic, the greater is the activity observed against lipophilic viruses, and less activity is noted against hydrophilic viruses. Similar conclusions can be drawn for activity against mycobacteria, presumably due to their lipophilic cell wall structure. Many of the bisphenols used as antiseptics have slow activity against Gram-negative bacteria, which can be enhanced in formulation effects, notably by the addition of EDTA or other chelating agents that increase the permeability of the biocides through the cell wall. In contrast, bisphenols are considered to be more rapidly effective against Gram-positive bacteria but also demonstrate little activity against fungi and mycobacteria. Phenolics are sporistatic, with little or no significant sporicidal activity. Although they are not generally considered effective against prions, it is interesting to note that certain types of phenols in formulation have been shown to be effective, although the exact mode of action remains to be determined.

3.14.4 Advantages

Phenolics are widely used as broad-spectrum disinfectants and antiseptics. Most disinfectant formulations have broad-spectrum activities as intermediate-level disinfectants, including tuberculocidal (or mycobactericidal) activity. Phenolics are able to tolerate the presence of interfering substances, including organic and inorganic soil loads, which is of particular importance in the direct clean-up of microbially contaminated soils ("one-step" disinfectants), including blood spills in health care facilities because of blood-borne pathogen transmission risks. In combination with detergents, phenolics can therefore combine cleaning and disinfection advantages. They have an "institutional" odor, which may be useful for odor control. As antiseptics, they demonstrate rapid activity against Gram-positive bacteria on the skin, with some substantive activity (remaining on the skin following washing; see chapter 4). Although irritation varies depending on the specific biocide, triclosan is generally nonirritating and has been described as even inhibiting the inflammation response in some studies. Salicylic acid has good fungicidal and virucidal activity that, combined with its depilatory (or surface skin layer removal) effects, is useful in the treatment of persistent skin infections such as warts. In contrast, phenolic disinfectants are generally labeled as irritants and considered relatively toxic. Residual activity, when the phenolics remain on a surface following application, can be an advantage in certain situations and a disadvantage in others (e.g., on medical devices with skin or mucous membrane contact over time). Most of the widely used phenolics today are considered biodegradable, including *o*-phenyl-phenol and *o*-benzyl-*p*-chloro-phenol.

3.14.5 Disadvantages

Most phenolics are considered irritants to the eyes and skin and can be toxic. They are generally contraindicated for use on food-contact surfaces. The presence of residues may be a concern in other industrial applications due to cross-contamination and necessitate postuse surface rinsing. Restricted use in health care nurseries has been recommended in some countries due to reported adverse reactions in neonates, although this may have been related to improper use of the product. The often strong odors characteristic of phenolic disinfectants may be undesired in certain situations, although newer phenolics often have little odor. Phenolics have little to no activity against bacterial spores, which may limit certain applications, but as disinfectants they are generally considered more efficacious than alternative QAC-based formulations (see section 3.16). Phenolics, dependent on their formulation, can be corrosive to certain plastic and rubber surfaces over extended use. Increased tolerance to some phenolics has been reported in some bacteria, although the significance of this has been debated. It is interesting to note that growing triclosan-tolerant strains of *E. coli* and *Pseudomonas* also demonstrated resistance to isoniazid, which is an antibiotic used to treat mycobacterial infections; this has led to speculation concerning the promotion of antibiotic resistance in the environment due to the use of biocides (see section 3.15 and chapter 8, section 8.7.2). Certain types of phenolics are restricted (or under consideration for restriction) from use because of toxicity concerns such as environmental risks (e.g., in the European Union under the Biocidal Product Regulation) and an ongoing debate over a range of adverse health and environmental effects associated with triclosan in the United States.

3.14.6 Modes of Action

The antibacterial effects of phenols have been well studied. Phenols are general cellular poisons but also have been shown to have cell membrane active properties. The hydroxyl (-OH) group is very reactive and forms hydrogen bonds with macromolecules, but in particular with proteins. Very low concentrations (in the parts per million range) of phenolics result in bacteriostatic activity due to inactivation of essential membrane enzyme functions and increasing cell wall permeability. Phenols induce progressive leakage of intracellular constituents, including the release of potassium ions, the first indication of membrane damage. Specific, rapid cell lysis has been shown for actively growing cultures of Gram-negative (*E. coli*) and Gram-positive (*Staphylococcus* and *Streptococcus*) bacteria which appeared to be independent of internal, cellular autolytic enzymes. Cytoplasmic leakage has also been shown with bisphenols, including fenticlor and triclosan. Fenticlor and triclosan also affected the metabolic activities of *S. aureus* and *E. coli*, including reports of disruption of cell membrane activities leading to an increase in permeability to protons, with a consequent dissipation of the proton motive force and an uncoupling of oxidative phosphorylation. Similar effects have been observed with other phenolics, including chlorocresol. Actively growing bacterial cultures appear to be more sensitive, which may indicate a specific target (or sensitivity) during cell division and separation.

Recent research into the mode of action of triclosan and similar bisphenols such as hexachlorophene at low concentrations has identified specific interaction and disruption of key metabolic processes, including lipid biosynthesis. These studies have shown specific interactions with enzymes involved with lipid biosynthesis; in particular, triclosan forms a complex with the fatty acid synthesis enzyme enoyl reductase and its cofactor NAD+, which causes a conformational change and precipitation of the complex. Triclosan has also been shown to inhibit the activity of other enzymes and to intercalate into the phospholipid membrane, which can lead to disruption of its structure and functions in bacteria and fungi. Further consideration of the mode of action of the bisphenols is given in section 3.15. At higher concentrations, phenols have multiple effects on the cell wall (e.g., lipid disruption), cell membrane, and cytoplasmic components. This includes coagulation of cytoplasmic constituents, which causes irreversible cellular damage.

The mode of action against other microorganisms has been less well studied. Phenolics possess antifungal and antiviral properties. Similar to their bacterial action, their antifungal action probably involves damage to the plasma membrane, resulting in leakage of intracellular constituents and other effects as described for bacteria. Little is known about the specific effects on viruses. Some studies with bacteriophages have shown little to no specific effects on phage DNA but some effects on the capsid proteins. Enveloped viruses are more susceptible, presumably due to coagulating effects on the surface proteins and membrane disruption.

3.15 ANTISEPTIC PHENOLICS

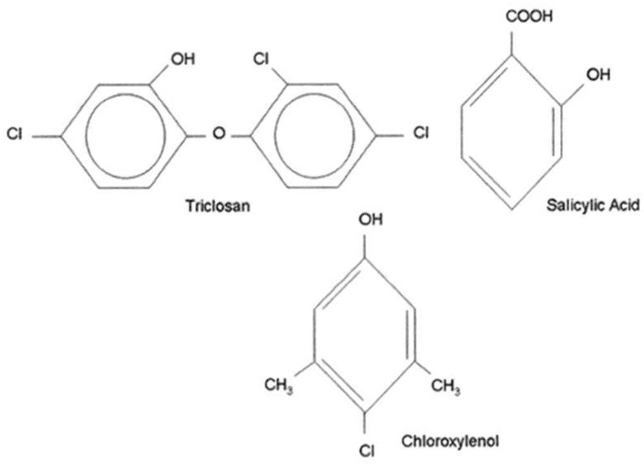

Triclosan

Salicylic Acid

Chloroxylenol

3.15.1 Types

Various phenolics (section 3.14) have been widely used as effective antiseptics and are discussed in this section. These can be subdivided into bisphenols, halophenols, and the organic acid salicylic acid.

The bisphenols are hydroxy-halogenated derivatives of two phenolic groups connected by bridges (Fig. 3.28). They are formed from a condensation of a phenol with an aldehyde or a ketone.

In general, bisphenols exhibit broad-spectrum efficacy against bacteria (particularly Gram-positive vegetative bacteria) and fungi, but have little activity against *P. aeruginosa* and molds, and are sporistatic toward bacterial spores. Activity against Gram-negative bacteria and fungi can be dramatically improved by formulation effects. Triclosan (2,4,4′trichloro-2′hydroxydiphenyl ether; Irgasan DP 300) and hexachlorophene (hexachlorophane; 2-2′-dihydroxy-3,5,6, 3′, 5′,

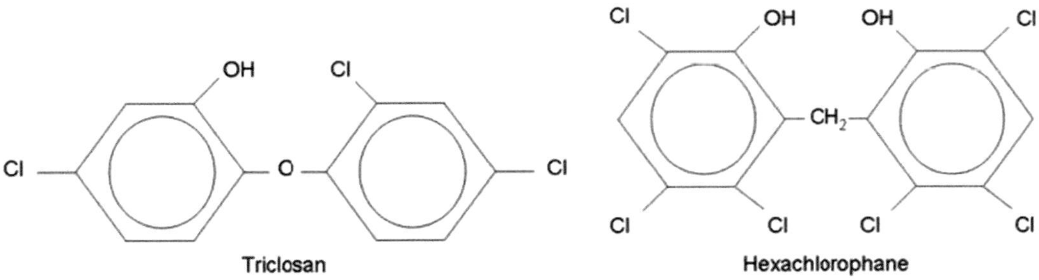

Triclosan

Hexachlorophane

FIGURE 3.28 Typical bisphenolic structures.

6′-hexachloro-diphenylmethane) are the most widely used biocides in this group, especially in antiseptic soaps and many consumer products (such as toothpastes and integrated into various surfaces such as toys). Both compounds have been shown to have some cumulative and persistent effects on the skin. Triclosan is a diphenyl ether and has been one of the most widely used biocides in antiseptics due to its reasonable spectrum of activity against bacteria and mildness to the skin. Hexachlorophene is another chlorinated bisphenol, which was initially widely used as an antiseptic but became less prevalent due to toxicity concerns. Other bisphenols have been described, including fenticlor, but have predominantly been used in veterinary applications.

Halophenols are used as both antiseptics and disinfectants (section 3.14). The most widely used as an antiseptic is chloroxylenol (also known as PCMX, *p*-chloro-*m* xylenol). Chloroxylenol has been particularly used in soap-based hand-washes, both for high-risk and general-use applications. Formulation of the biocide is particularly important to enhance its broad-spectrum activity, especially against Gram-negative bacteria such as *Pseudomonas*.

Salicylic acid (or *o*-hydroxybenzoic acid) is an organic carboxylic acid. In addition to its antiseptic and preservative use, salicylic acid has been used as an anti-inflammatory agent and can be chemically modified to make acetylsalicylic acid (aspirin) and other topical agents used in liniments and tinctures. Salicylic acid is often found in combination with other biocides and formulation agents including isopropanol, sodium thiosulfate, and benzoic acid.

3.15.2 Applications

The bisphenols have been widely used in various antimicrobial soaps. Hexachlorophene was widely used in the 1960s but became restricted in use due to significant toxicity concerns (even linked to deaths in the United States and Europe). Hexachlorophene was typically used in antimicrobial hand- and skin-washes, including specific applications in wound cleaning, surgical scrubs, and antimicrobial powders. Concentrations of the biocide ranged up to 3%, but with the identification of toxicity concerns, its use is now restricted in most countries and usually requires a prescription (typically at concentrations lower than 1%). Hexachlorophene has also been used as an effective preservative in cosmetics (at typical concentrations of ~0.1%) and for agricultural applications (such as soil and plant fungicides).

Triclosan became more widely used as an alternative to hexachlorophene because it was considered a safer alternative, but in recent years its use has been the subject of much debate due to safety concerns, in particular, in the United States and Europe for certain applications (e.g., in general public antiseptic hand-washes). Triclosan has been widely used in antimicrobial soaps, including health care professional (as surgical scrubs and routine hand-washes), industrial, and household uses. There has been a proliferation of antimicrobial soaps, lotions, cleaners, and shampoos over the past 20 years, many of which are based on triclosan as the biocide. These products are known to vary significantly in antimicrobial activity; in most countries the antimicrobial claims on these products are not currently regulated. Applications have included soaps, lotions, deodorants, gels, and antiacne washes. Typical concentrations range from 0.1 to 2%, with higher concentrations used in higher-risk applications (e.g., in health care use). In some cases, triclosan has been combined with other antimicrobials (such as alcohols) to provide persistent activity on the skin over time; there have been some claims of benefits for the use of triclosan as a deodorant and as an odor-control wash. Triclosan is particularly suited as an antiseptic due to its lack of toxicity and irritation to the skin and mucous membranes.

Other applications have included dental mouth rinses and antibacterial toothpastes; these formulations often include other active agents such as zinc citrate and sodium fluoride for the treatment of gingivitis and periodontitis. Triclosan has also been used as a preservative in cosmetics and other products, although usually in combination with other biocides. Due to its thermal and chemical stability, triclosan has been integrated into various plastics and fabrics to provide antibacterial surfaces (e.g., in toys, toothbrushes, and other products). Triclosan has also been recommended therapeutically as an antiparasitic agent, with efficacy reported against *Plasmodium falciparium*, *Toxoplasma gondii*, and *Trypanosoma brucei*. These reports have led to the investigation of alternative drugs in the treatment of diseases such as malaria and toxoplasmosis.

Chloroxylenol has been used in a variety of antimicrobial soaps, including surgical scrubs, preoperative preparations, and hand-washes. Other applications have included shampoos, medicated powders, and impregnated devices. Chloroxylenol may also be used at lower bacteriostatic and fungistatic concentrations as an effective preservative, including in antiseptics and cosmetics, and also in a variety of other products such as paints, textiles, and polishes. Formulations are often in combination with other phenolic compounds including pine oils, terpineols, and alcohols. Typical use concentrations vary from 0.5 to 4%.

Salicylic acid is primarily a skin exfoliant due to its keratinolytic activity. This, combined with antibacterial and antifungal activity, has made it a popular biocide in the treatment of skin disorders such as acne, seborrheic dermatitis (dandruff), and psoriasis. Other formulations are specifically used for the treatment of viral infections such as skin warts caused by papillomaviruses. Although the antimicrobial activity is a benefit in treating diseases like psoriasis, which are prone to bacterial and fungal infections, many of these applications are used particularly for surface skin layer removal rather than for antimicrobial benefits. As an example, psoriasis is a nonspecific, chronic but noncontagious skin disease that benefits from exfoliation of dead skin layers. Similarly, the use of higher concentrations of salicylic acid-based formulations directly on warts allows for the removal of the wart and stimulates the host immune response to target the papillomavirus infection. Also, the presence of the biocide prevents further viral replication and infection. Acne is a complicated disease of the skin, but salicylic acid formulations allow for the combined effects of skin pore cleaning and antibacterial activity against bacteria implicated in acne. A variety of products are available, including general-use shampoos, soaps, and gels and targeted-use paints, drop medicants, and plasters (which release the biocide over time). Other applications include antimicrobial toothpastes and mouthwashes. Concentrations vary depending on the formulation and application. Concentrations from 1 to 6% (generally 1 to 2%) are used for acne and psoriasis applications over wider application areas. An example of a traditional preparation is Whitfield's ointment, containing 6% benzoic acid and 3% salicylic acid. Higher concentrations, ranging from 10 to 17% in antiseptic paints and 20 to 50% in plasters, are also used for limited-area application. Salicylic acid has been used at lower concentrations (0.04 to 0.5%) as a preservative, particularly in acidic foods, because it has an optimum pH range from 4 to 6. Due to toxic restrictions, salicylic acid is not widely used as a preservative and typically at the lower concentration range (<0.1%).

3.15.3 Antimicrobial Activity

The bisphenols are rapidly effective against Gram-positive bacteria and many Gram-negative bacteria. They are much less effective against *Pseudomonas* and other pseudomonads, but activity can be dramatically increased by formulation. An example is synergism with chelating agents (e.g., EDTA), which are known to destabilize the Gram-negative cell wall by chelating associated metal ions, allowing the biocide to penetrate into the cell and contact sensitive cell membrane and intracellular targets. Hexachlorophene is particularly active against Gram-positive bacteria, including pathogenic and antibiotic-resistant *Staphylococcus* strains (such as MRSA). For this reason, hexachlorophene was widely used to prevent and treat wound infections. Some activity is observed against Gram-negative bacteria, but little effect has been reported against mycobacteria, fungi, and (particularly nonenveloped) viruses. Triclosan shows a wider spectrum of activity than hexachlorophene, with particularly rapid activity against Gram-positive bacteria that are prevalent on the skin (e.g., *Staphylococcus* spp.). For example, many staphylococci are sensitive to inhibitory concentrations as low as 0.1 μg/ml, although higher concentrations (>10 μg/ml) are generally required for bactericidal activity. Triclosan is also active against Gram-negative bacteria and yeasts; it has generally poorer activity against some enveloped viruses, some pseudomonads, and fungi. The lack of appreciable activity of triclosan itself against pseudomonads has allowed its use in microbiology laboratory selective media for *Pseudomonas* isolation. The overall antimicrobial activity of triclosan-containing antiseptics can be particularly enhanced by formulation effects, and such formulations can vary widely in antimicrobial activity. Also, applications that use the biocide alone, as when integrated into plastics and other materials, have less broad-spectrum and sustainable antimicrobial activity over time. Recent studies have shown activity against many parasites, including *Plasmodium falciparum*, *T. gondii*, and *T. brucei*; triclosan or similar bisphenols have been recommended as potent inhibitors of blood-borne parasites. Reports have also suggested that in addition to its antibacterial properties, triclosan may have anti-inflammatory activity.

Chloroxylenol demonstrates good bacteriocidal activity against Gram-positive and Gram-negative bacteria. Some Gram-negative bacteria, in particular, *P. aeruginosa* and other pseudomonads, demonstrate higher resistance to the biocide alone, as discussed above for triclosan and hexachlorophene. Chloroxylenol is also effective against a wide range of fungi, particularly yeasts such as *Candida* spp., but some molds (including *Penicillium* and *Mucor*) have demonstrated higher tolerance to its fungistatic effects. Efficacy against pseudomonads and molds can be dramatically increased by various formulation effects; therefore, chloroxylenol-based products vary significantly in antimicrobial activity and claims. For example, similar to other phenolics, the efficacy against *Pseudomonas* can be potentiated by the presence of EDTA or other chelating agents, due to their removal of metal ions from the cell wall and structure destabilization. These formulation effects can also enhance activity of the biocide against mycobacteria and some viruses. Due to disruption of the lipid envelop structure, chloroxylenol formulations are also effective against enveloped viruses, but little activity has been reported against nonenveloped viruses. Chloroxylenol is a stable biocide; it demonstrates good skin penetration and can remain persistent on the skin for several hours following application to provide a further bacteriostatic and fungistatic barrier over time.

Salicylic acid at lower concentrations is an effective bacteriostatic and fungistatic agent. Higher concentrations are also bactericidal and fungicidal. Most studies have focused on bacteria that are associated with skin acne including *Propionibacterium*, *Corynebacteria*, and *Pityrosporum*. Fungicidal activity has been described against yeasts and the dermatophytes, including the fungi that are implicated in various tinea infections (e.g., *Trichophyton* species). Some antiparasitic activity has also been reported. Low concentrations inhibit viral infection and replication, although the antiviral activity of salicylic acid has not been well studied.

3.15.4 Advantages

The bisphenols have potent activity against Gram-positive and, in formulation, Gram-negative bacteria and fungi. They are very stable and persistent biocides on the skin, which can provide bacteriostatic and fungistatic activity following application of the product over an extended period. They can be easily formulated with a variety of soaps and detergents. The bisphenols retain significant activity in the presence of organic soils. These advantages have made them popular in antiseptic applications. Triclosan, in particular, can penetrate into and through the skin and was often cited as having no toxic, allergenic, or mutagenic effects even after extensive investigations and prolonged clinical use. Despite its persistence on the skin, it has not been shown to cause irritation (which, when observed, may be more likely to be due to other constituents of the antiseptic formulation rather that the biocide itself). Its stability and activity are also somewhat preserved in the presence of organic soil and excessive heat, which has allowed the use of triclosan as an integrated antimicrobial barrier in textiles and plastics.

Chloroxylenol is considered a nontoxic biocide at typically used concentrations. It is mild to the skin and, despite its ability to penetrate into the skin, it is rarely shown to be sensitizing or irritating. Chloroxylenol demonstrates good bactericidal and fungicidal activity, in particular, against Gram-positive bacteria. It is a stable biocide and is persistent on the skin, remaining antimicrobial for some time (up to hours) following application.

Salicylic acid is a mild biocide for topical use with little to no side effects reported at the concentrations or in the applications typically used. The biocide is an effective exfoliant, which aids in dead-skin removal but also allows penetration of the active agent into the lower skin layers. It is effective against most common bacterial and fungal skin pathogens.

3.15.5 Disadvantages

The bisphenols demonstrate a restrictive spectrum of activity, are not effective against many pseudomonads (unless enhanced by formulation effects), and are incompatible with nonionic surfactants. Because of their relative stability, they may be biocumulative or ecocumulative in some cases, in particular, with hexachlorophene and in some cases with triclosan. Hexachlorophene has been shown to be particularly toxic to humans and animals at higher concentrations, presumably due to the increased halogenation in comparison to triclosan. Neurologic effects were initially highlighted in the bathing of patients with burns and wounds, and these effects were subsequently verified in animal studies. Hexachlorophene is absorbed through the skin but is particularly contraindicated for those with damaged skin or for the treatment of mucous membranes. The use of hexachlorophene is restricted in most countries, in particular with neonates; for example, in the United States it can only be used with a prescription and under strict regulation.

Triclosan is also stable, is absorbed through the skin, and can be detected in urine. There is much controversy regarding associated toxicity and mutagenicity. Extensive studies and reports of clinical use over many years initially suggested a lack of significant toxic effects. With its increased use over the past 10 to 20 years, it has, however, been found at detectable levels in the environment, including foods, which has raised some concerns over its potential ecological effects. It is estimated that $\sim 3 \times 10^5$ kg per year of triclosan is discharged in the United States alone from wastewater treatment plants. Bioaccumulation has been reported, raising concerns about health and environmental risks. Some evidence has suggested the role of triclosan in disrupting hormonal cycles (particularly thyroid hormones) and even leading to skin cancer following long-term exposure in animals, but the consequences of these effects in humans remain the subject of much debate. The persistence of triclosan in the environment is likely to cause some shifts in the diversity of microbial populations and microbiomes. Another environmental concern is the impact of low levels of triclosan in promoting the development of tolerance (increased MIC) to the biocide, but more significantly, cross-resistance to a wide range of antibiotics in bacteria. These reports have led to recommendations (in the United States and the European Union) for the decreased use of triclosan-containing products, particularly in nonessential applications such as the widespread public use in antiseptics. The use of triclosan (and other antiseptic biocides) in consumer-based antibacterial soaps (hand-washes and body-washes, but not health care formulations and uses) has recently been banned in the United States due to these concerns as well as the considered lack of true antimicrobial benefit over soap-and-water in these cases.

Lower doses of salicylic acid can cause some skin irritation, in particular if combined with other antiseptics such as alcohol, acids, and peroxides. The biocide can cause slight stinging and is not generally recommended for use on broken skin, wounds, or mucous membranes. Specific inactivation of other common topical agents has been reported, including calcipotriene, which is commonly used to treat psoriasis. High concentrations are considered toxic to humans and animals, which can lead to "salicylism," a syndrome that includes gastrointestinal irritation, dizziness, and ringing in the ears. These effects are usually characteristic of overdosing with the biocide.

Chloroxylenol demonstrates a narrower range of antimicrobial activity than other commonly used biocides in antiseptics; although these effects can be enhanced by formulation, products can also vary considerably in antimicrobial activity on the skin or other applications. The activities of chloroxylenol products are highly dependent on formulation attributes. Persistent activity on the skin can be neutralized in the presence of nonionic surfactants, which can be present in some soaps and cleaners.

3.15.6 Mode of Action

3.15.6.1 Triclosan. The mode of action of triclosan has been particularly well studied over the past 20 years, but it is often misrepresented as being similar to many antibiotics with a very specific mechanism of action (see chapter 7). It is clear that triclosan does have some specific effects on certain proteins at low concentrations and additional nonspecific effects, typical of other phenolics, at higher concentrations. Earlier studies identified that the primary effects of triclosan are on the cytoplasmic membrane. In studies with *E. coli*, triclosan at subinhibitory concentrations inhibited the uptake of essential nutrients, while at higher bactericidal concentrations caused the rapid release of cellular components and subsequent cell death. Other investigations have highlighted the importance of fatty acid biosynthesis as a particular target for triclosan. Studies with a divalent ion-dependent *E. coli*-triclosan mutant that exhibited a 10-fold greater triclosan MIC than a wild-type strain showed no significant differences in total envelope protein profiles but did show significant differences in envelope fatty acids. Specifically, a prominent 14:1 fatty acid was absent in the resistant strain, along with minor differences in other fatty acid species. It was proposed that in these mutants the divalent ions and fatty acids may adsorb and limit the permeability of triclosan to its intracellular sites of action.

Minor changes in fatty acid profiles were also found in Gram-positive bacteria (*S. aureus*) isolates that had elevated triclosan MICs but overall had similar minimum bactericidal concentrations. Specific investigations of *E. coli* triclosan-tolerant mutants, which demonstrated increased MICs of triclosan *in vitro*, identified a specific enzyme target for triclosan: enoyl-acyl carrier protein-reductases. Enoyl reductases are involved in type II fatty acid synthesis processes. Type II fatty acid synthase systems in bacteria use a dissociated group of enzymes (in contrast to mammalian type I synthases, which use a multienzymatic polypeptide complex) for the synthesis of fatty acids; this involves the cyclic addition of two carbon units to a growing fatty acid chain. Enoyl reductases catalyze the last stage in this elongation cycle, which is dependent on the presence of the cofactors NADH or NADPH. These cofactors are used as electron carriers during the reaction and vary between bacterial types; for example, NADH (nicotinamide adenine dinucleotide) is specifically used by *E. coli* and *Bacillus subtilis*, while NADPH (NAD phosphate) has been identified in *S. aureus*. The typical reaction is shown in Fig. 3.29.

Triclosan has been shown to specifically interact with the substrate binding site (in particular, tyrosine residues) on the enzyme, simulating the enzyme's natural substrate. It also interacts with the nicotinamide ring of the cofactor, which allows for the tighter, irre-

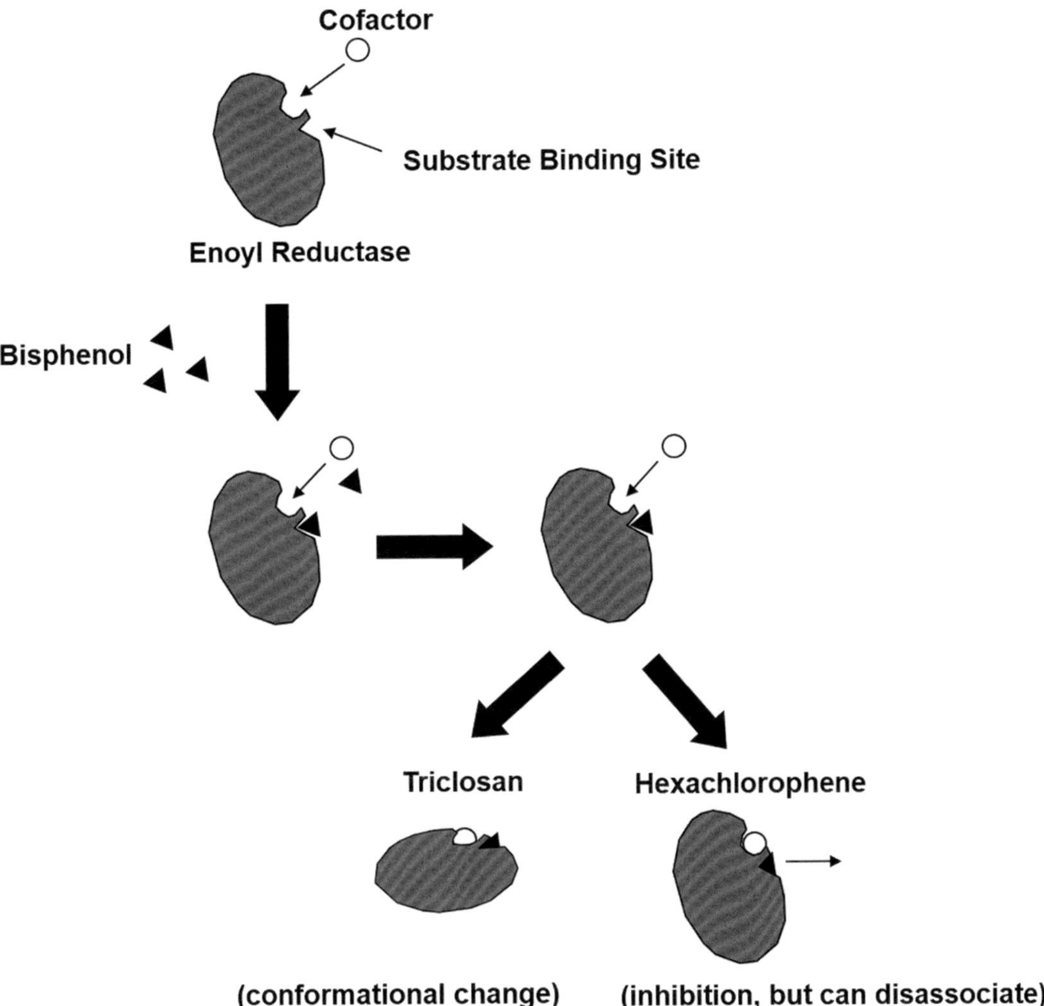

FIGURE 3.29 The mode of action of triclosan and hexachlorophene against enoyl reductases.

versible binding of the biocide. These interactions are noncovalent and are formed by hydrogen bonding, van der Waals forces, and other hydrophobic interactions. Inhibition of enoyl reductases is a key target in bacteria because they play a role in controlling the rate of fatty acid biosynthesis. The effect is referred to as a "slow, tight interaction," whereby the initial, reversible interaction causes a conformation change in the protein/coenzyme structure over time, leading to irreversible complex formation. These effects remove the enzyme from its key role in fatty acid biosynthesis and also cause complex precipitation.

Similar yet distinct effects are observed with the antibiotic isoniazid, the diazoborines, and the bisphenolic biocide hexachlorophene. Isoniazid and the diazoborines form covalent bonds with the cofactors at the enzyme active site, while hexachlorophene forms similar noncovalent interactions to triclosan but does not form the irreversible complex with the enzyme cofactor (Fig. 3.29). Although both biocides bind to the same active site, the effect of hexachlorophene appears to be reversible, does not induce a conformational change, and is not as significant to the overall mode of action. It has been suggested that the ether linkage in the triclosan chemical structure (Fig. 3.28) allows increased flexibility of the biocide to permit greater interaction with the cofactor and the observed conformational changes. Binding of triclosan to enoyl reductases has been observed in Gram-positive (e.g., *S. aureus*) and Gram-negative (e.g., *E. coli*, *P. aeruginosa*, *Haemophilus influenzae*) bacteria, including *Mycobacterium smegmatis* and *M. tuberculosis*. The effect of triclosan at lower concentrations on enoyl reductases clearly plays an important role in its mode of action; however, other specific and nonspecific interactions have been observed. Many examples have been reported in the literature. Overex pression of glucosamine-6-phosphate aminotransferase (which is involved in biosynthesis of various amino sugar-containing macromolecules) also showed increased resistance to triclosan in *E. coli* but not to other biocides, including hexachlorophene or antibiotics. Direct inhibition of other enzymes, including various transferases, has been reported *in vitro*.

Triclosan inhibition of type II fatty acid synthases (in chloroplasts and mitochondria) in plants and parasites has also been observed, although in the case of *Trypanosoma* and *Plasmodium* investigations, fatty acid elongation by enoyl reductases was not specifically inhibited; in these cases the overall activity appeared to be due to nonspecific disruption of the subcellular membrane structure, which disrupted the overall fatty acid biosynthetic pathway. The effect of triclosan on the phospholipid membrane has been specifically investigated in bacteria; studies have shown that the hydrophobic biocide can integrate into the outer region of the membrane via its hydroxyl group, which causes membrane disruption and loss of various functions (including catabolic and anabolic processes) and integrity. These studies confirm that triclosan has multiple effects on key proteins and cell membranes, which have cumulative effects and contribute to bactericidal and fungicidal activity.

Hexachlorophene appears to have similar, multiple mechanisms of action, yet some are distinct from those described for triclosan. Initial studies with *Bacillus megatherium* showed that the primary action of hexachlorophene was inhibition of the membrane-bound part of the electron transport chain, and the other effects noted above are secondary ones that occur only at high concentrations. It also induces cytoplasmic leakage, causes protoplast lysis, and inhibits respiration. Hexachlorophene disrupts the proton motive force on the surface of bacteria, with dramatic effects on structure, motility, and oxidative phosphorylation. These effects are typical for the other phenols, including bisphenols. The threshold concentration for the bactericidal activity of hexachlorophene is 10 μg/ml over a wide range of temperatures, including as low at 0°C. As the concentration was increased, cytological changes were observed at 30 μg/ml and maximal cytoplasmic leakage at 50 μg/ml. Hexachlorophene clearly causes protein structure disruption and enzyme inhibition (both membrane associated and cytoplasmic) at lower concentrations, with macromolecule precipitation and membrane disruption at higher concentrations. It is interesting to note that hexachlorophene, similar to triclosan, has been shown to specifically interact with bacterial enoyl-ACP-reductases, but in a reversible reaction (Fig. 3.29). Specific inhibition of other enzymes has been observed, including esterases and dehydrogenases. These structural interaction and disruption effects have led to some interest in the use of hexachlorophene in cancer therapy and in treating certain neurodegenerative disorders (e.g., Alzheimer's disease).

3.15.6.2 Chloroxylenol. The mode of action of chloroxylenol has not been well studied, despite its widespread use over many years. Because of its phenolic nature, it is thought to have a similar effect on surface proteins and microbial lipid membranes, leading to enzyme inactivation, structure disruption, and loss of viability (section 3.14).

3.15.6.3 Salicylic Acid. Similar to other phenolics, the primary targets of salicylic acid, based on the limited studies performed, are surface and some intracellular proteins. The effects on proteins lead to cell wall and membrane damage, as well as key membrane enzyme inactivation (section 3.14). Specific interference with Gram-negative porin proteins present in the cell wall leading to reduced uptake has been reported; paradoxically, this has also been reported to cause decreased antibiotic uptake and increased tolerance to the antibiotic (chapter 8, section 8.3.4).

3.16 QACs AND OTHER SURFACTANTS

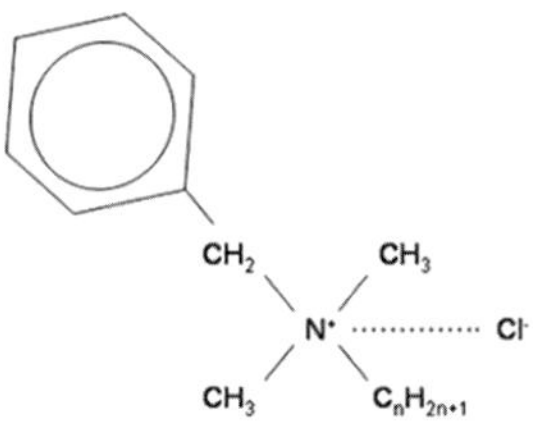

Benzalkonium chloride

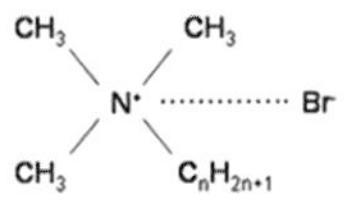

Cetrimide

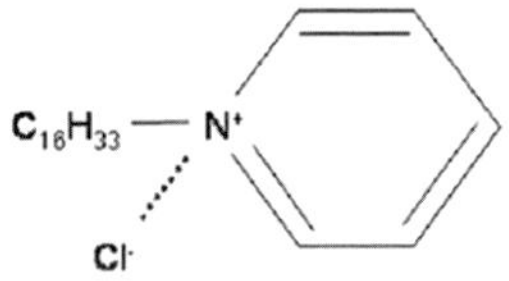

Cetylpyridinium chloride

3.16.1 Types

Surfactants (or "surface-active agents") are a group of compounds with the unique property of having hydrophobic (water-repelling, nonpolar or lipophilic) and hydrophilic (water-attracting, polar or lipophilic) portions (Fig. 3.30). They are referred to as surface-acting because they interact with a liquid (such as water) surface to reduce the surface tension and also form micelles, allowing for dispersion in the liquid. Taking water as an example, the hydrophilic portion of the surfactant molecule is soluble at the water surface, with the hydrophobic end being repelled from the surface. This results in a reduction in surface tension and allows a greater dispersion of water and surfactant mixture across the surface. Dispersion of the surfactant in water also occurs by micelle formation, with the hydrophobic ends interacting to repel the hydrophilic end (Fig. 3.30). Surfactants can therefore be useful as foaming agents (liquid-gas interactions), emulsifiers (liquid-liquid interactions, for example, for mixing oil-like compounds in water), and dispersants (liquid-solid interactions, for example, dispersion of a water-insoluble solid). Surfactants are generally classified based on their overall charge (Table 3.7).

Surfactant classes vary in their observed antimicrobial activities and detergencies. Detergency is their ability to act as a cleaning agent, which is associated with the ability to remove and solubilize soils from contaminated surfaces. For example, anionic and nonionic surfactants often have little to no intrinsic antimicrobial activity but are widely used in cleaners, in formulations, and to enhance the activity of other biocides. Amphoteric surfactants are widely used due to improved antimicrobial activity in combination with good detergency. But from an antimicrobial perspective, cationic surfactants, particularly the QACs, are the most widely used.

The basic QAC structure is shown in Fig. 3.31. The cation (positively charged) portion consists of a central nitrogen with four attached groups, which can contain a variety of structures and is the functional (antimicrobial) part of the molecule. The anion (negatively charged) portion (X^-) is usually chlorine (Cl^-) or bromine (Br^-) and is linked to nitrogen to form the QAC salt. QACs can be subclassified based on their structure (e.g., the anion or nature of the associated [R] groups, which can include several nitrogens, degrees of saturation, branching, and the presence of aromatic groups) or based on their introduction as biocides over time (e.g., first- or second-generation QAC). For example, benzalkonium chloride was a first-generation QAC including an aromatic ring, two methyl (CH_3) groups, and a long chain ethyl (CH_2-CH_3)/ methyl (CH_3) chain structure, which can vary in length from C_{12} to C_{16} (e.g., 40% C_{12},

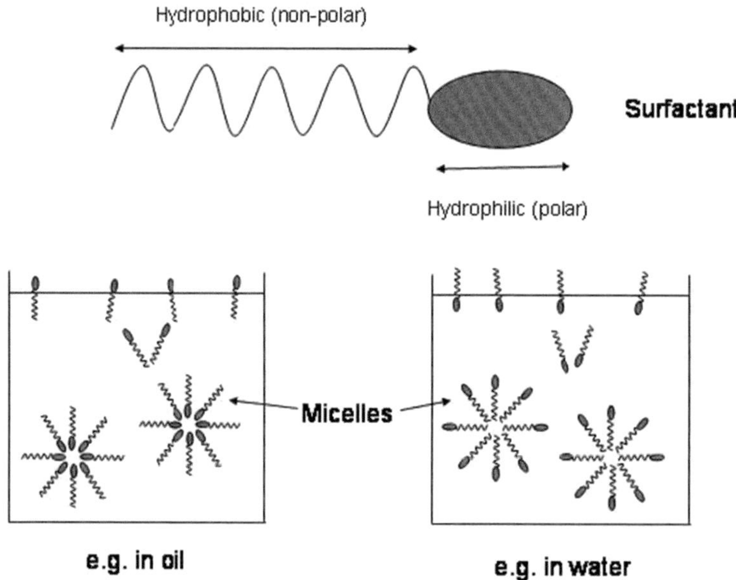

FIGURE 3.30 Basic surfactant and micelle structure.

50% C_{14}, and 10% C_{16}). Further QAC generations were synthesized to improve antimicrobial activity (including observed synergism in various QAC mixtures), detergency, and toxicity. The full chemical names of QACs are often descriptive of their structures. Examples are hexadecyltrimethylammonium bromide (also known as CTAB, or cetrimide), alkylbenzyldimethylammonium chloride (also known as benzalkonium chloride, or BKC), and hexadecylpyridinium chloride (also known as cetylpyridinium chloride, or CPC).

3.16.2 Applications

Nonionic and anionic surfactants are used as preservatives, but their primary applications are in cleaning products, to enhance the efficacy of other active agents (including phenols and QACs) and as excipients or formulants (e.g., as dispersants, emulsifiers, foaming agents, etc.). Anionic and amphoteric surfactants have been used as antimicrobials in food and beverage applications, as surface or direct food sanitizers, and as general surface disinfectants, in particular in combination with cleaning. Amphoteric surfactants have also been used as antiseptics, particularly in combination with other biocides (such as chlorhexidine [discussed in section 3.8]). QACs are extensively used as household, industrial, and general health care surface disinfectants (Fig. 3.32). They are often used for food and other surface disinfection, because

TABLE 3.7 Classification of surfactants

Surfactant type	Antimicrobial efficacy	Detergency	Charge[a] (pH above pKa)	Examples
Cationic	+++	+	+	Benzalkonium chloride, cetrimide
Anionic	+/–	+++	–	Sodium or potassium fatty acid salts (soaps), sodium lauryl sulfate
Nonionic	–	+++	Neutral	Polysorbates (tweens), nonoxynol-9
Amphoteric	+++	++	+/–/neutral[a]	Betaine, alkyldimethyl oxide

[a]Depending on pH.

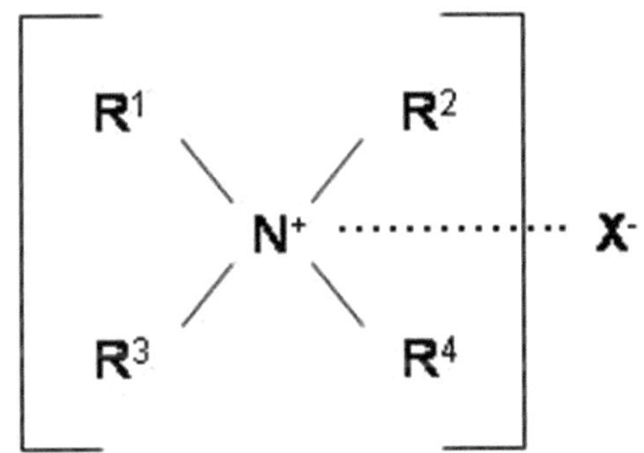

FIGURE 3.31 The basic structure of QACs.

formulations do not generally require post-treatment rinsing with water to remove residuals (unless required for specific uses such as in certain industrial applications).

QACs are formulated for direct spray-and-wipe applications, as QAC-impregnated wipes, and as concentrates that require dilution in accordance with instructions prior to use. These are all widely used directly on tabletops, walls, floors, etc., and can also be provided indirectly by fogging prepared liquid formulations in a room. Due to their lack of sporicidal activity, certain products are provided presterilized (by radiation or filtration) to remove the risk of spore contamination in critical environments such as in manufacturing clean room or isolator applications. QACs are widely used in health care facilities on noncritical devices and surfaces such as bed rails, countertops, etc. As antiseptics, QACs have been used for skin and mucous membrane bioburden reduction, such as in mouthwashes for the control of dental plaque, in wound cleansing, and in antiseptic handwashes and nonalcohol hand rinses (e.g., benzalkonium chloride [see chapter 4, section 4.5]). In addition to disinfection, QAC formulations are widely appreciated for their cleaning and deodorization attributes. Other applications include preservatives (e.g., in paints, contact lens solutions, and cosmetics), fabric and laundry deodorization and softening, hair conditioning, and pool and pond treatment for the control of algae and slime. Biologically active QAC-like chemicals include vitamin B and acetylcholine (a neurotransmitter).

3.16.3 Antimicrobial Efficacy

Nonionic and, in particular, anionic surfactants can demonstrate some bactericidal activity but are generally considered useful inhibitory agents, which can include bacteristatic, fungistatic, and sporistatic activity; these are not considered further as biocidal agents in their own right. Amphoteric surfactants have good bactericidal (including against Gram-positive and Gram-negative bacteria) activity at low concentrations, with greater resistance observed against some pseudomonads, mycobacteria, and fungi (which can be improved by formulation effects). They are generally considered effective against enveloped, but not nonenveloped, viruses. QACs vary in their antimicrobial activity depending on their type and formulation. In general, they are bacteristatic, fungistatic, tuberculostatic, sporistatic, and algistatic at very low concentrations (<500 μg/ml), with Gram-positive bacteria being particularly sensitive (<10 μg/ml). Higher concentrations are generally required for broad-spectrum bactericidal, algicidal, and fungicidal activity (>1 mg/ml). Although generally effective against enveloped viruses (including HIV and hepatitis B virus), QACs are not generally effective against nonenveloped viruses or my-

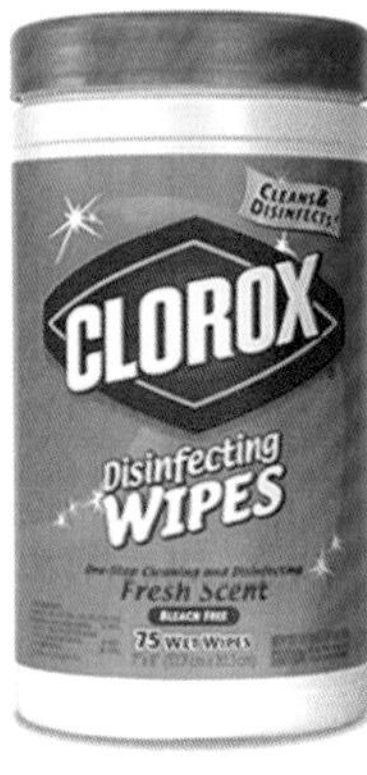

FIGURE 3.32 QAC-based disinfectant. Example shown is a ready-to-use QAC-impregnated wipe. ©2017 The Clorox Company. Reprinted with permission. CLOROX® and PINE-SOL® are registered trademarks of The Clorox Company and are used with permission.

cobacteria; activity can be significantly improved by formulation effects, including the addition of nonionic surfactants and potential synergistic effects between mixtures of QAC types. QACs are not considered sporicidal, although some activity has been observed at higher concentrations and temperatures. They are sporistatic and inhibit the outgrowth of spores but not the actual germination processes (see chapter 8, section 8.3.11).

3.16.4 Advantages

Surfactants provide excellent cleaning ability, which, in the case of QACs and some amphoteric surfactants, can be combined with disinfection activity. This is a useful attribute in a variety of surface disinfection uses such as in health care facilities and food-handling and veterinary applications, where the physical removal of contaminating soils and associated microorganisms can be as important as the antimicrobial effects in certain applications. They are also essential components of formulations such as antimicrobials and cosmetics, including as preservatives and emulsifiers. As sanitizers and disinfectants, they are considered to be gentle (noncorrosive and nonstaining) on surfaces and do not generally require rinsing following application in many cases. They are widely considered to have low toxicity, but this can depend on the specific biocide and/or product formulation. It should be noted that this may be considered an advantage, not only for ease of use, but also because it allows for residual antimicrobial activity on the treated surface; however, it is also a disadvantage due to the difficulty in removing these residues for some applications (e.g., in pharmaceutical or chemical production). QACs, in particular, have the ability to penetrate and solubilize contaminating organic soils that are often associated with microorganisms while retaining antimicrobial efficacy. They have a pleasant, "clean" odor and are regarded as nontoxic under typical conditions of use. They can be used in antiseptics at low concentrations without significant irritation to the skin and mucous membranes.

In addition to the use of surfactants directly as antimicrobials, their ability to form micelles can be a useful delivery system for other molecules and biocides, such as in micro- or nanoemulsions.

3.16.5 Disadvantages

Some formulations (e.g., anionic and amphoteric surfactants formulated at an acid pH) can be aggressive on certain material surfaces such as copper and brass. The antimicrobial efficacy of QACs can be negatively affected in the presence of hard water (if in a diluted product), fatty materials, and anionic surfactants (including soaps); this varies depending on the QAC type and formulation. Surfactants can be difficult to rinse from critical surfaces and can cause excessive foaming, which may not be desired. Most surfactants have poor activity against mycobacteria and nonenveloped viruses, which can limit their use for some applications. Higher concentrations of QACs and other surfactants can cause severe irritation to the skin and mucous membranes. The presence of low-level residues may allow the selective development of bacterial strains with greater tolerance to QACs over time (e.g., *Pseudomonas*); intrinsic and acquired resistance has been described, which has been linked to antibiotic- and other biocide-tolerance profiles (chapter 8). Some surfactants can be detected in wastewater and sediments, creating concerns about their environmental fate, impacts on the environment, and microbial resistance development.

3.16.6 Mode of Action

The primary targets of surfactants, including QACs, are the bacterial and fungal cell walls and membranes. QACs can quickly adsorb to and penetrate bacterial cell walls, which can disrupt their structures and functions. On contact with the cell membrane, they have been shown to react with membrane lipids and proteins (including enzymes), leading to a cascade of effects including loss of structure and function and leakage of cytoplasmic material. Direct insertion into the lipid bilayer has been suggested. Further effects have also been reported on cytoplasmic proteins (including precipitation) and nucleic acids, which culminate in cell death. Direct interaction with viral (enveloped viruses) and spore surface protein may also cause prevention of growth, loss of function, and disintegration. For example, QAC-based products induced disintegration and morphological changes of human hepatitis B virus, which resulted in loss of viral infectivity.

3.17 OTHER MISCELLANEOUS BIOCIDES AND APPLICATIONS

3.17.1 Pyrithiones

Zinc Pyrithione

The most widely used pyrithione is zinc pyrithione (or zinc 2-pyridinethiol *n*-oxide), which is used primarily for its bacteriostatic and fungistatic activity. Chemically, pyrithiones have low solubility in water but are relatively stable and also act as chelating agents. They are used primarily as antiseptics in the topical treatment of psoriasis, dermatitis, and fungal infections (tinea). Examples include the treatment of different forms of seborrhoeic dermatitis, a usually mild, recurring form of dermatitis (e.g., dandruff). Zinc pyrithione is widely used in antidandruff shampoos. Pyrithiones are provided in a variety of product types, including soaps, creams, and sprays. They are known to be deposited and retained on the skin surface to provide some sustained activity over time. An alternative to zinc pyrithione for skin applications is selenium disulfide, an inorganic compound (SeS_2), but this has been less studied as a biocide.

Other applications of the pyrithiones include their use as algicides and as preservatives in adhesive coatings and other surface applications (such as outdoor paints to reduce the growth of mildew and algae). They demonstrate broad-spectrum antimicrobial activity, particularly fungicidal, bactericidal, and algicidal activities. The fungicidal activity of zinc pyrithione has been especially well studied, in particular against *Pityrosporum ovale* (which is often associated with dandruff), but also other fungal skin infections, including the dermatophytes (tinea infections, including various ringworms). They are also effective against bacteria, in particular Gram-positive bacteria, and have been used for the treatment of eczema-related infections. Pyrithiones are unknown to be keratinolytic (i.e., break down keratin, which is associated with the epidermal skin layers [see chapter 4, section 4.3]). They are not considered to be toxic, although some cases of irritation and allergic reactions have been noted. The mode of action of the pyrithiones was initially believed to be specific to DNA interactions and disruption of nucleic acid functions but also due to blocking membrane-bound proton pumps involved in cell surface transport mechanisms. Recent evidence has shown a specific mechanism of action linked to the increased influx and accumulation of cytoplasmic copper (or other metals) in fungal cells and general cell toxicity, particularly targeting cellular iron-sulfur proteins essential for fungal metabolism.

3.17.2 Isothiazolinone Derivatives

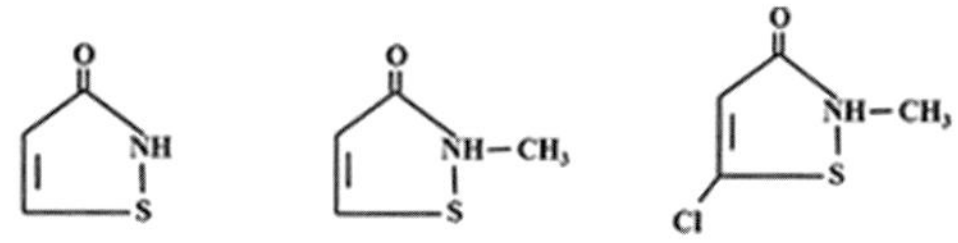

Isothiazolinone Methylisothiazolinone Chloromethylisothiazolinone

The isothiazolinones are a group of sulfur- and nitrogen-containing compounds based on the isothiazolinone structure, such as methylisothiazolinone (MIT) and chloromethylisothiazolinone (CMIT). They have been particularly widely used as preservatives, either alone or in combination (particularly mixtures of MIT and CMIT at different concentrations). Examples are commercialized under the Kathon™ tradename. They are often used in combinations with other preservatives such as the parabens (see section 3.2). Preservative applications include use in water systems (e.g., water tanks, cleaning, and cooling systems), metal-working fluids, wood, paints, and in some cases as preservatives in cosmetic products (such as shampoos, lotions, impregnated wipes, etc.). The individual biocides or combinations of biocides vary in antimicrobial activity but can include broad-spectrum activity against Gram-positive bacteria, Gram-negative bacteria, fungi (yeast and molds), and algae. Some species are more resistant than others at microbiostatic concentrations such as *Streptococcus*, *Flavobacterium*, *Pseudomonas*, and *Aspergillus* spp., depending on the specific biocide, but are inactivated at similar microbicidal concentrations. As an example, a 3:1 mixture of CMIT and MIT is widely used for water treatment, industrial applications, and in various cosmetic products. This combination of isothiazolinones demonstrates broad-spectrum activity against bacteria, fungi, and algae. Reported MICs are very similar to minimal bactericidal concentrations, such as ~0.5 mg/liter against *Aspergillus niger* and *Saccharomyces cerevisiae*. Preservation activity is generally more effective and stable at slightly acidic concentrations. Some activity has also been reported in the presence of biocides and to prevent biofilm development. The biocides are less stable at higher pH (>8) and increased temperatures (>35°C) and in the presence of certain interfering substances such as reducing agents and amines. Toxicity has been reported, including environmental concerns (aquatic toxicity), dermatitis, and hypersensitivity. Concerns about allergic contact dermatitis have led to the reduced use of many isothiazolinones in leave-on cosmetic products, particularly in the European Union.

The mode of action of the isothiazolinones has been studied in some detail. They vary in their rates of cellular uptake but then quickly lead to the shutdown of many normal cellular processes, such as respiration and energy (ATP) synthesis. The specific mechanism of action appeared to be the inhibition of a variety of enzymes, particularly the dehydrogenases, and proteins containing thiol groups. These effects have been shown to initially cause inhibition of cells, but they can be repaired over time. However, the secondary effects of the buildup of free radicals in target cells lead to further damage to biomolecules (including proteins, lipids, and nucleic acids) that culminate in irreversible cell death.

3.17.3 Biocides Integrated into Surfaces

Various types of biocides have been successfully used to create antimicrobial surfaces or surfaces that release the biocide or biocidal activity over time. The most widely used biocides are summarized in Table 3.8. These include metals (e.g., silver- and copper-releasing agents), halogen-releasing agents, biguanides, biophenols, and QACs.

The biocide can be provided by a variety of techniques, including by simple application to the surface (directly or as a coating), impregnation, incorporation into a polymer or during the polymer formation, and fixing onto the surface. Antimicrobial surfaces have found particular applications on the skin and mucous membranes (e.g., antimicrobial dressings and plasters) and devices that are associated with the skin (e.g., catheters). Catheters and other devices that contact and/or penetrate the skin are considered to be high risk for contamination and as a source of infection, in particular when present for extended periods of time and with immunocompromised patients. The slow release of biocides from these surfaces can reduce the risk of bacterial or fungal colonization and prevent wound infections. Other applications include the prevention of biofilms on water-contact surfaces, in textiles, in water or air filters, and on general surfaces such as cutting boards, toys, and food-handling surfaces. It should be noted that their overall benefit to reduce the risk of surface and surface-associated contamination depends on the application, the biocide used, and its practical efficacy over time.

Most of the biocides listed in Table 3.8 are discussed in other sections of this chapter. Further description of titanium dioxide, the

TABLE 3.8 Various biocides used on antimicrobial surfaces

Biocide	Description	Applications
Silver and silver sulfadiazine	Silver-releasing coatings or impregnated surfaces (e.g., silver zeolites, nanoparticles, or silver sulfadiazine) (see section 3.12)	Textiles, wound and skin dressings, devices (e.g., catheters), and packaging materials
Copper	Metallic copper or copper alloys used for surfaces and devices; copper-releasing coatings or impregnated surfaces (see section 3.12)	Various industrial (water pipes, food-handling surfaces, etc.) and medical surfaces
Chlorhexidine	Coatings or impregnated surfaces (see section 3.8)	Wound and skin-care dressings, dental floss, toothpicks, wipes, and some devices (such as catheters)
Triclosan	Coatings or impregnated surfaces (see section 3.15)	Wound and skin-care dressings but also on general surfaces such as toothbrushes, cutting boards, and toys
Benzalkonium chloride and other QACs	Hydrogels and other coatings; impregnated plastics and textiles (see section 3.16)	Reduce biofouling and bacterial adherence; wound and skin dressings, catheters
Titanium dioxide	Photocatalytic, releasing active oxygen species on exposure to UV light	Preservative (e.g., paints) and antimicrobial coating on air filters, food preparation surfaces, medical devices
N-halamines	Halogen (chlorine or bromine)-releasing agents (see section 3.11); includes monomeric or polymeric compounds	General or food-contact surfaces, textiles, water-disinfection, and odor control

N-halamines, and antimicrobial polymers is provided here.

Titanium dioxide (TiO_2 or titania) is the most widely used white pigment in paints, plastics, and paper, as well as used as a food colorant. Cosmetic applications include its use in UV-protective sunblock. It can be applied to surfaces including air filters, metals, and plastics as a thin layer. Some applications have also included the inactivation of Gram-negative bacteria and viruses in wastewater and to prevent biofilm formation on water-contact surfaces. The chemical is photocatalytic, and on exposure to near-UV (<380 nm) light it releases active oxygen species including superoxide ions and hydroxyl radicals (see section 3.13). These active species prevent bacterial and fungal growth and can inactivate microorganisms in contact with the surface over time. The antimicrobial activity is generally slow and sustained and is primarily used to inhibit the growth of bacteria and fungi on surfaces. In addition, due to the reactive nature of released oxygen species, organic pollutants and other chemical contaminants may also be neutralized. Titanium dioxide surfaces are corrosion-resistant and are considered nontoxic.

The *N*-halamines are halogen-releasing agents (section 3.11). They are nitrogen-containing compounds with anchored chlorine or bromine groups, which are released on contact with microorganisms (Fig. 3.33) (other examples are discussed in section 3.11).

N-halamines can be used as water-soluble monomers (e.g., 1-chloro-2,2,5,5-tetramethyl-1,3-imidazolidin-4-one), as preservatives, in disinfectants, and integrated into antimicrobial surfaces [e.g., the chlorinated polystyrene hydantoin, poly-1,3-dichloro-5-methyl-5-(4′-vinylphenyl) hydantoin]. Other bromine-based *N*-halamines include PSHB and DBDMH (section 3.11). Antimicrobial polymers are made by polymerization of the monomers, by attachment to an existing plastic polymer, or by copolymerization. These polymers are stable and odorless. Applications have included their use in various hard surfaces (medical, dental, and industrial), textiles, paper, and antimicrobial paints/coatings and for water disinfection. The choice of *N*-halamine can depend on the application, with slow-releasing compounds used for odor control and biofilm control and as preservatives, while faster-releasing compounds are used for more immediate activity

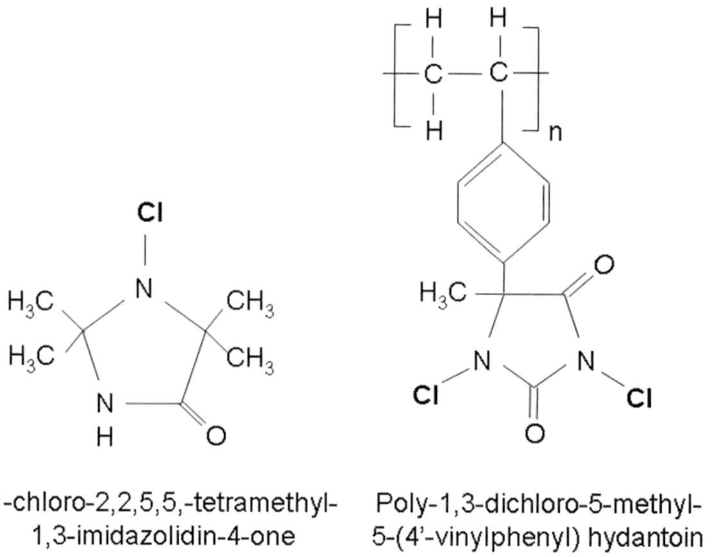

1-chloro-2,2,5,5,-tetramethyl-1,3-imidazolidin-4-one

Poly-1,3-dichloro-5-methyl-5-(4'-vinylphenyl) hydantoin

FIGURE 3.33 Examples of chlorine-based *N*-halamines.

such as on general-use surfaces and for water disinfection. A key advantage of these compounds is that, following exhaustion of the antimicrobial activity, the surface can be reactivated by application of a chlorine- or bromine-containing formulation, which is not the case for other biocidal surfaces. *N*-halamines are broad-spectrum antimicrobials, but their effectiveness varies depending on the type. In general, they are claimed to be stable over a wide pH range (pH 4 to 10) and ambient temperature (4 to 37°C), with efficacy against bacteria, fungi, viruses, and protozoa (such as *Giardia*). Slow cysticidal and sporicidal activity has been reported in some applications. They also have a long functional life and are considered safer to use than higher liquid concentrations of chlorine and bromine (see section 3.11). Their modes of action are considered to be similar to those described for halogens and other halogen-releasing agents (section 3.11).

Other examples of natural and artificial antimicrobial polymers are those based on chitin, chitosan, cellulose, and their derivatives, as well as various types of polyamides, polyesters, and polyurethanes. Their antimicrobial properties can be produced by attaching or inserting various biocides or biocidal groups onto their polymer backbones by alkyl or acetyl linkages. Polymers associated with QACs, phenolics (or phenolic hydroxyl groups), and phosphonium salt (di- and trimethyl-substituted phosphonium salts [PH_4^+] with long alkyl chains) groups have been described for various applications. Phosphonium salts such as tetraphenylphosphonium chloride [$(C_6H_5)_4P^+$ Cl^-] and tetramethylphosphonium iodide [$P(CH_3)_4^+$ I^-] are similar to QAC structures as cationic molecules. Such polymers have been used for garments, vessels, packaging, high-touch surfaces, food-handling areas, wound dressings, and catheters and other medical devices. Investigations to date have focused on health care, the food industry, and water or liquid disinfection applications. Surface applications may have particular benefits in reducing microbial attachment and limiting the impact of biofilm development (see section 8.3.8).

3.17.4 Micro- and Nanoparticles

Microscopic particles can be defined by their diameters: microparticles have diameters of $\sim10^{-6}$ meters and nanoparticles, $\sim10^{-9}$ meters.

These minute particles may also be referred to as nanoclusters, nanocrystals, and ultrafine particles. They can be made of a variety of materials, including liquids (such as water) and solids (including ceramics, polymers, glass, composite materials, and powders). They are generated in a variety of ways, including by wet chemistry, grounding, ultrasonics, radiation exposure, and pyrolysis. The properties of the materials used change when generated into micro- and nanostructures, to include their stability, reactivity, and surface availability. For example, titanium dioxide in its normal form is a white material but in nanoparticle form is more transparent. Nanoparticles have been the subject of various medical and industrial research investigations into applications in optics, electronics, automotive (e.g., on tires), drug delivery, diagnostics, and for liquid-solid dispersion. Their increased stability and reactivity have increased research interest in antimicrobial applications, particularly with metals and metal oxides. The most investigated to date are based on silver, silver oxide, and titanium dioxide. These biocides are already widely used for various antimicrobial applications, such as on surfaces (see section 3.17.2). Other reports have described the antimicrobial activities of nanoparticles based on copper, zinc oxide, gold, selenium, magnesium and calcium oxide, and iron (III) oxide. Titanium dioxide nanoparticles have been described in many applications such as in paints and sunscreens and for water disinfection. Silver nanoparticles have been particularly investigated as antimicrobial coatings, which may release silver slowly over time, and as alternatives to other silver sources (see section 3.12). These include device surfaces and wound dressings. Typical sizes, as determined by microscopy techniques, are in the 1 to 100 nm range. Although their mechanisms of action are similar to those described for silver (see section 3.12), their unique structures appear to prevent particle aggregation, to allow more specific interactions with (or delivery to) bacterial cell wall-membrane structures, and to be associated with lower toxicity profiles due to the more efficient use (or delivery) of silver. However, reports of antimicrobial efficacy of nanosilver particles vary in comparison to other traditional silver solutions, but these may be dependent on the methods used to generate and test the nanoparticles.

A unique application of nanoparticles has been described with water or engineered water nanostructures. These have been investigated for fumigation applications, including air and surface disinfection. In these studies, water vapor was converted into nanostructures in the 20 to 30 nm range at room temperature, and similar to other nanostructures, they have unique properties. First, they appeared to be relatively stable in the environment, being observed after 1 hour postgeneration. They also appeared to be associated with reactive oxygen species (e.g., hydroxyl and superoxide radicals) that provide antimicrobial activity. Studies have shown some efficacy (at 8,000 particles/cm^3 at ~20 nm diameter) against vegetative bacteria over time but little to no activity against bacterial spores. Investigators claimed not to detect any significant concentration of ozone during these studies, which was suspected due to the mechanisms of nanoparticle generation (by adding energy to water vapor in air). Initial inhalation toxicity studies in animals showed minimal toxic effects under these exposure conditions. The broad-spectrum efficacy, process optimization, and any toxicity risks associated with water nanoparticles are of interest for further investigations.

3.17.5 Antimicrobial Enzymes, Proteins, and Peptides

Various types of naturally occurring antimicrobial peptides and proteins have been identified from microorganisms, insects, plants, and animals. Their primary roles are as part of the hosts' intrinsic defenses or immune systems against various types of fungi and bacteria and certain viruses. In general, they have limited applications because they demonstrate restrictive spectra of activity but have been utilized in some instances as biocides. For the purpose of this discussion they are considered antimicrobial enzymes and peptides (Table 3.9).

TABLE 3.9 Various types of proteins, peptides, and enzymes used as biocides

Type	Description	Applications
Antimicrobial enzymes		
Lysozyme	Limited activity against some Gram-positive and Gram-negative bacteria; some investigations have attempted to alter the structure of the enzyme to allow for greater activity against Gram-negative bacteria	Limited to bactericidal and bacteristatic activity; pharmaceutical (eye drops and lozenges) and food (preservative in cheese and wine) applications
Chitinases	Fungistatic and fungicidal activity against chitin-containing fungi	Limited to fungistatic and fungicidal activity; primarily agricultural applications
Proteases	Subtilisins and chitinases; endopeptidases such as keratinases, proteinase K, and other thermostable proteases	Biofilm prevention and control; oral and wound health care; proposed activity against prions
Antimicrobial peptides		
Aprotinin	Polypeptide serine protease inhibitor with some activity against bacteria	Some potential industrial applications as a preservative; used therapeutically to reduce bleeding
Nisin	Isolated from *Lactococcus lactis*; particularly active against Gram-positive bacteria; sporistatic	Food preservative
	Magainins	Isolated from *Xenopus laevis*; bactericidal, fungicidal; some activity against protozoa
	Developing applications, including treatment of impetigo	

Lysozyme is one of the most widely studied enzymes and specifically degrades bacterial peptidoglycan by hydrolysis of the β-1,4 glucosidic linkages between *N*-acetylmuramic acid and *N*-acetylglucosamine (Fig. 3.34).

Due to its specific mode of action, lysozyme is only bacteriostatic or bactericidal against bacteria that contain peptidoglycan, predominantly against Gram-positive bacteria; genetic modification of the enzyme has allowed for the isolation of enzymes with greater penetration and activity against the Gram-negative cell wall. Lysozyme has been used as a preservative in pharmaceutical and food applications such as in eye drops, antibacterial lozenges, wines, and dairy products, the last specifically to limit spoilage by lactic acid bacteria. Many types of enzymes or enzyme mixtures have been specifically investigated to prevent or break down the structures of biofilms (see chapter 8, section 8.3.8). Enzymes include proteases (such as subtilisins, which can hydrolyze adhesion proteins that are associated with biofilm formation in *Pseudomonas* and *Streptococcus*, and lysostaphin, which targets staphylococcal cell wall structures), polysaccharide-hydrolyzing enzymes (e.g., *a*-amylase, with activity against MRSA and *Pseudomonas* biofilms), and oxidative enzymes (e.g., glucose oxidase and superoxide dismutase). Antimicrobial enzymes can have health care, veterinary, and food applications. Examples have included veterinary applications for skin, wound, and ear infections with enzyme mixtures of lactoperoxidase, lactoferrin, and lysozyme, as well as oral care mixtures with mutanase and dextranase.

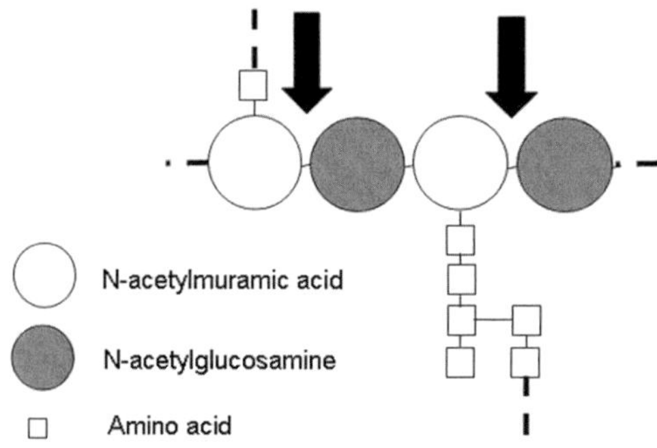

FIGURE 3.34 The enzymatic activity of lysozyme. The structure of peptidoglycan (see chapter 1, section 1.3.4.1) is cleaved at the glycosidic bonds between N-acetylmuramic acid and N-acetylglucosamine in the polymer.

In a similar manner, other enzymes have been used specifically against fungal cell walls. The most widely studied are the chitinases. Chitin is a major polysaccharide component of many fungal cell walls, associated with the inner cell membrane (chapter 1, section 1.3.3.2). Chitin is degraded by various chitinases by hydrolysis of the glycosidic bonds within the polysaccharide. This weakens the cell wall structure and eventually causes cell lysis. Proposed agricultural applications have included the prevention of fungal growth on plants and biopesticidal activity. Other antifungal proteins are glucanases and chitin-binding peptides, which also have fungistatic activity.

Prions are unique infectious agents that are composed exclusively of protein and do not appear to have an associated nucleic acid (chapter 1, section 1.3.6). Although prions have been characterized to have high resistance to proteases, some reports have suggested the use of various endopeptidases to degrade prions over time. These include thermo-resistant proteases such as keratinases, although these reports remain to be verified for practical use as prion inactivation methods.

Various types of antimicrobial peptides have been isolated (with some examples given in Table 3.9). These are characteristically cationic peptides of varying lengths but with a high proportion of basic amino acids (such as lysine and arginine). Their hydrophobic nature appears to be associated with their antimicrobial activity, by affinity to the surface of microorganisms and insertion in cell membranes. In addition to cell membrane structure disruption, other negatively charged macromolecules (such as DNA and some proteins) may also be affected. These peptides have a limited spectrum of activity, and few practical biocidal applications have been described. For example, nisin is particularly active against Gram-positive bacteria and has been shown to be sporistatic (e.g., against *Clostridium botulinum* spores). The primary application for nisin has been as a natural preservative in heat-processed and low-pH foods. Nisin is regarded as safe to use but has little to no effect on Gram-negative bacteria, yeasts, molds, or other microorganisms; however, enhanced activity has been observed with other biocide preservatives, lysozyme, and chelating agents. The magainins are another group of antimicrobial peptides isolated from the frog species *Xenopus laevis* and have been shown to have activity against bacteria, fungi, and protozoa. They range in length from 21 to 27 amino acids and have α-helical, hydrophobic structures. They have also been shown to disrupt lipid bilayers, leading to disruption of cell permeability, and to bind to lipopolysaccharide. Proposed applications have included the treatment of skin infections, including impetigo.

3.17.6 Bacteriophages

Bacteriophages (or "phages") are viruses that specifically infect bacteria and are ubiquitous in nature (see chapter 1, section 1.3.5 and Fig. 1.12). They have been described for many years as potential antibacterial agents, particularly due to their very specific spectra of activity against certain bacteria and therefore lack of particular effect on hosts cells. Overall, phages have seen limited commercial success but have been used as detection systems for bacteria such as *Staphylococcus* (and antibiotic-resistant strains such as MRSA) and as phage cocktails for therapeutic applications (e.g., wound infections) in certain countries. There has been a resurgence of interest in this use of bacteriophages for biocidal, specifically bactericidal, applications, which has included their role in biofilm control, plant and food treatments, and wound infection therapy in humans and animals. In addition, the potency of bacteriophage lysins (as bacterial cell wall peptidoglycan hydrolases) has been of interest as antimicrobial enzymes against Gram-positive bacteria (see section 3.17.4). Recombinant lysins that target a wider range of Gram-positive bacteria have been investigated for mucosal and systemic infection treatments in animals and humans, as well as in plant and food applications.

ANTISEPTICS AND ANTISEPSIS

4

4.1 INTRODUCTION

Antiseptics can be defined as biocidal products that destroy or inhibit the growth of microorganisms in or on living tissue, e.g., on the skin. In theory, any biocide or biocidal process could be used on the skin or mucous membranes, although only a small number are widely used. Living tissues are more sensitive to damage than hard surfaces; therefore, the requirements for safe use restrict the use of antiseptics to those that have limited or no toxicity. Antiseptics can include a variety of formulations and preparations such as antimicrobial hand-washes, hand-rubs ("sanitizers"), surgical scrubs, preoperative preparations, ointments, creams, tinctures, mouthwashes, and toothpastes. Overall, antiseptics should demonstrate the following characteristics:

- A wide spectrum of biocidal activity, in particular, against bacteria, fungi, and viruses
- Rapid biocidal activity
- Little or no damage, irritation, or toxicity to the tissue
- Little or no absorption into the body
- If possible and applicable, some persistent biocidal (or biostatic) activity (Many biocides used in antiseptics can remain on the skin following washing or application, allowing for continuing biocidal or growth-inhibitory action over time.)

4.2 DEFINITIONS SPECIFIC TO ANTISEPTICS

Antimicrobial soap: A soap- or detergent-based formulation that contains one or more antiseptic agents at concentrations necessary to inhibit or kill microorganisms.

Antisepsis: Destruction or inhibition of microorganisms in or on living tissue, e.g., on the skin or mucous membranes. Antiseptics are disinfectant products used for antisepsis. They include washes (which contain soaps or other detergents and are used with water) and rubs (which are applied directly to the skin with no washing, e.g., tinctures and alcohols).

Antiseptic hand-washes or hand-rubs: Antiseptics that are fast-acting, with minimal irritation, and designed for frequent use on the skin, particularly for the reduction of transient microorganisms. These are widely used such as in health care facilities, food-handling areas, agricultural applications, and for general public health. Also known as hygienic hand disinfectants, which may or may not have persistence.

Persistence: The ability of a biocide to demonstrate continued antimicrobial activity on the skin following application of an antiseptic product for a prolonged or extended time to prevent or inhibit the growth of microorganisms. Also known as substantivity or residual activity.

Plain (or bland) soap: A soap- or detergent-based formulation that does not contain specific biocides, except for the purpose of product preservation.

Preoperative preparation: An antiseptic, preferably with persistent activity, to reduce the number of microorganisms on the skin at the site of surgical intervention. Preoperative preparations are used for the localized antisepsis of patient skin prior to surgical incision.

Surgical scrub: An antiseptic, preferably with persistent activity to reduce the number of microorganisms on intact skin prior to surgery. Surgical scrubs are used by surgical staff on hands and forearms prior to a procedure. Sometimes referred to as surgical hand disinfectants.

Wound: Any break in the skin caused by injury or intentional (e.g., surgical) intervention.

4.3 THE STRUCTURE OF SKIN

The skin is the largest human organ, consisting of approximately one-sixth of typical body weight. It has a variety of functions including temperature regulation and energy storage and as a barrier or protection against water loss, various microorganisms, chemicals (including biocides), and radiation (e.g., UV light). Skin has a complex structure consisting of three layers: the outer epidermis, the dermis, and the innermost subcutaneous layer (Fig. 4.1).

The epidermis is the outermost layer and can itself be further defined as various layers

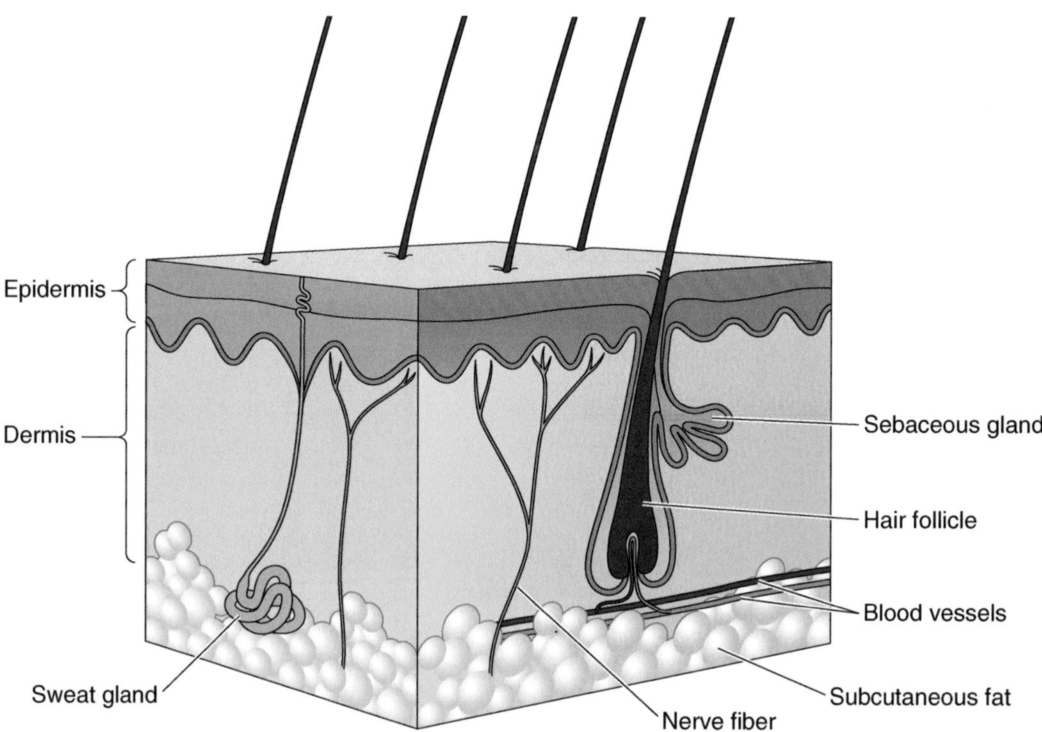

FIGURE 4.1 Cross-section of skin structure. Illustration by Patrick Lane, ScEYEnce Studios.

consisting of an innermost layer (stratum basale) of actively multiplying skin cells (keratinocytes) to the outer layer (stratum corneum) of dead, flattened cells held together by various skin lipids, which are constantly released from the surface and replaced by new cells from the lower epidermal layers. The keratinocytes, which produce keratin as they develop into the skin surface layers, are the most prominent cell types in the epidermis. Another cell type associated with the epidermis, in particular the lower layers, is the melanocytes, which produce the dark pigment (melanin) that gives the skin a tanned color as a protection mechanism on exposure to UV light. The epidermal cells are separated from the lower dermis layer by a basement membrane and are dependent on the dermis for nutrients and oxygen. The dermis largely consists of fibroblast cells, which produce collagen and elastin to give flexibility and strength to the skin. The dermis also contains various glands (such as sebaceous glands), blood and lymph vessels, hair follicles, muscle cells, and nerve endings. Finally, the subcutaneous layer (or subcutis) is composed of larger blood and nerve vessels and sweat glands, with specific fat-storage cells known as adipose cells.

4.4 SKIN MICROBIOLOGY

The overall structure and constituents of the skin, including its thickness, pH, temperature, wetness, density of hair, and distribution of secretory glands, can vary across the body. The microorganisms that can be found on the skin also vary, depending on the above and other environmental factors. Overall, the microbiological ecology of the skin is complicated and varies in type and population from site to site and from individual to individual. For example, the levels of bacteria on the hands, scalp, forearm, and axilla can range from 10^3 to $>10^6$.

Skin floras have traditionally been considered as two types: resident and transient floras. Resident floras are considered to be permanently found and growing on the skin or a given skin area; typical residents include various types of *Corynebacterium*, *Propionibacterium*, *Staphylococcus* (coagulase-negative staphylococci such as *Staphylococcus epidermidis*), and *Micrococcus*. In general, drier areas of the skin (such as the hands) have a larger population of Gram-positive cocci, including *S. epidermidis* and *Micrococcus* spp., while areas associated with higher moisture or the presence of sebum (increased oil content) have more prominent populations of the diphtheroid Gram-positive rods such as *Corynebacterium* and *Propionibacterium* spp. Gram-negative bacteria (including *Klebsiella*, *Escherichia*, and *Enterobacter*), as well as various types of fungi (particularly *Candida* spp.), are found to a lesser extent. Transient residents of the skin are described as being short-lived or simply carried on the skin but are not consistently identified as resident flora in most individuals. Transient populations vary considerably and include bacteria, yeasts, fungi, viruses, and other microorganisms. Many of these can be pathogenic to the skin, particularly within wounds, or can be transmitted from various surfaces and between individuals.

Antiseptics are used to reduce the presence and transfer of resident and transient microbial residents on the skin and mucous membranes; many are also used to reduce the risk or treat the presence of various skin infections, including wound infections. Types of intact skin and wound infections are listed in Table 4.1. Some of the most common wound or surgical site infections are caused by *Staphylococcus aureus* (including methicillin-resistant strains), coagulase-negative staphylococci, *Enterococcus*, *Escherichia coli*, *Enterobacter*, and *Candida albicans*. There is some correlation between the site of the wound and the associated pathogen; for example, Gram-negative bacteria are often associated with intestinal and urologic-related wounds or surgical site infections, because they are often found at high concentrations in these regions of the body.

4.5 ANTISEPTIC APPLICATIONS

Five types of antiseptic applications are considered in this section: routine skin hygiene, skin treatment prior to surgical intervention, treatment of skin or wound infections, treatment of

TABLE 4.1 Common or notable infections of the skin

Microorganism	Comments
Intact skin infections	
Streptococcus pyogenes	Impetigo, an infection of the epidermis, particularly in children (also caused by *S. aureus*); some virulent strains can cause significant damage to the skin, as in the case of necrotizing fasciitis ("flesh-eating bacteria")
S. aureus	Boils and carbuncles such as infections of hair follicles and sebaceous glands
Propionibacterium acnes	Associated with acne
Treponema pallidum	Syphilis, a sexually transmitted disease with lesions in the genital region and other areas of the skin
Herpes simplex virus	Cold sores
Varicella-zoster virus	Chickenpox and shingles
Papillomaviruses	Common and other types of warts that can progress into tumors and malignancies
Dermatophytes (*Trichophyton*, *Microsporum*, and *Epidermophyton*)	Fungal infections of keratinized tissues, including skin, nails, and hair; diseases are referred to as "tinea" or "ringworms," including tinea unguium (nail ringworm), tinea corporis (body ringworm), and tinea pedis (athlete's foot)
Leishmania spp.	Cutaneous leishmaniasis, with skin ulceration on the face and limbs
Onchocera volvulus	Infects the skin subcutaneous layer but can also lead to complications such as "river blindness"
Wound or surgical site infections	
S. aureus	The most prevalent cause of infections in wounds (~15–20%)
Coagulase-negative staphylococci, including *S. epidermidis*	Often associated with bite wounds and catheter-associated infections
Enterococcus spp.	Opportunistic wound infections, including burn contamination with *Enterococcus faecalis*
Clostridium spp.	*Clostridium perfringens* causes gas gangrene, and *Clostridium tetani* causes tetanus, both associated with deep wound infections
E. coli	The most common Gram-negative bacterium associated with wound infections
Acinetobacter baumannii	Opportunistic infections in wounds (including burns); difficult to treat due to intrinsic antibiotic resistance
Pseudomonas aeruginosa	Opportunistic infections in wounds (including burns); difficult to treat due to intrinsic antibiotic resistance
C. albicans	The most common fungi isolated from wounds, in particular, burn infections

mucous membranes, and biocide-impregnated materials used as antiseptics. Some examples of the types of antiseptic products are shown in Fig. 4.2. Examples of guidelines and standards that describe the types, uses, and requirements for antiseptics are given in Table 4.2.

4.5.1 Routine Skin Hygiene

Skin, particularly hand, hygiene is often cited as an important step in reducing the potential of microbial cross-contamination from surfaces to individuals and between individuals. Washing with plain soap can remove a significant level of transient and surface resident flora associated with surface epidermal layers, as well as contaminated soils such as dirt and blood, by mechanical action alone; however, some studies have suggested that washing with plain soap may also increase the shedding of bacteria in some cases. The use of antimicrobial hand-washes and hand-rubs can provide a greater reduction of microorganisms on the skin. This is particularly important in higher-risk situations, for example, for workers in hospitals, surgeries, and other health care facilities, as well as in food-handling and preparation. It should be remembered that the purpose of antiseptics is to reduce the level of contamination; although antiseptics vary considerably in antimicrobial activity on the skin, they do not completely remove all transient and resident microorganisms (section 4.4). There are many reports of the cross-transmission of pathogens from contaminated hands in these situations, and studies have shown that the use of antiseptics can reduce the risks of transmission;

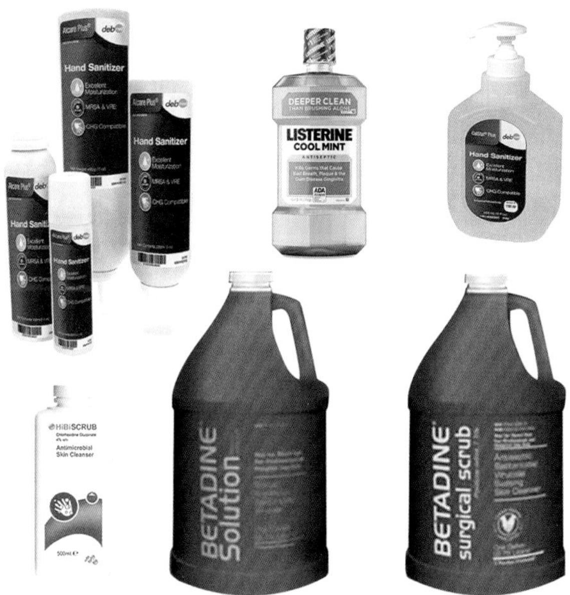

FIGURE 4.2 Examples of types of antiseptic products. HibiScrub bottle: ©Molnlycke Health Care AB. Used with permission. The American Society for Microbiology is not employed by, or affiliated with, Molnlycke. STERIS product: Image courtesy of STERIS, with permission. Betadine Solution: Image courtesy of Purdue Pharma, LLC, with permission. Listerine is a trademark and brand of Johnson & Johnson Consumer, Inc.

their effects vary from formulation to formulation, despite the presence of similar concentrations of different biocides.

Hand-washes are soap- or detergent-based formulations that typically contain biocides such as chlorhexidine, triclosan, chloroxylenol, triclocarban, essential oils (in particular, tea tree oil), benzalkonium chloride, and some iodophors. These products, known as health care personnel hand-washes, are widely used by personnel in health care facilities for routine washing of hands and the body; the most widely used biocides in these products are chlorhexidine, triclosan, and chloroxylenol. These products are required to meet specific antimicrobial claims to meet labeling and registration requirements such as in the United States, Canada, and the European Union, in both *in vitro* and *in vivo* studies (e.g., Table 4.2). In recent years, antibacterial soaps have become popular for general household use (particularly formulations based on triclosan, triclocarban, and essential oils) and are particularly recommended in the handling of food or in food-preparation facilities or for those caring for small children or immunocompromised patients. The efficacy of these products varies significantly depending on the concentration of the biocide and its formulation, as well as on the correct use of the product (washing time, adequate coverage, etc.). Formulation examples include the use of emollients (such as oils and creams), which are used to soften and sooth the skin by reducing water loss and improve the aesthetics.

However, in many countries, including the United States and the European Union, the domestic use of antimicrobial soaps is being discouraged or even restricted due to the risks of using these products compared to any potential antimicrobial benefits. Concerns have included risks due to the persistence of many of these biocides in the environment, particularly triclosan and triclocarban. Some evidence suggests the development of resistance (or increased tolerance) to these biocides, cross-resistance to antibiotics (due to similarities in modes of resistance), changes in microbial

TABLE 4.2 Examples of various guidelines and standards that describe the types, uses, and requirements for antiseptics

Reference[a]	Title	Summary
WHO (2009)	WHO guidelines on hand hygiene in health care: first global patient safety challenge. Clean care is safer care	Hand hygiene guidelines and protocols for caregivers
APIC (2015)	APIC implementation guide: guide to hand hygiene programs for infection prevention	Guidelines for evidence-based strategies in implementing hand hygiene programs in health care settings
CDC, HICPAC (2002)	Guidelines for hand hygiene in healthcare settings	Guidelines on hand-washing and hand antisepsis in health care settings, including recommendations to promote improved hand-hygiene practices and reduce transmission of pathogenic microorganisms
FDA Tentative Final Monograph (2015)	Health care antiseptics	Commercial guidelines on the registration and labeling of health care antiseptics
Health Canada (2009)	Human-use antiseptic drugs	Guidance document for support of the labeled claim of an antiseptic product for human use in Canada
Hand Hygiene Australia (2012)	Hand Hygiene Australia manual	Guidelines for developing and implementing hand hygiene programs
ASTM E-1174	Standard test method for evaluation of the effectiveness of health care personnel hand wash formulations	Test method for demonstrating the *in vivo* efficacy of health care personnel hand-washes by determining the reduction of an indicator microorganism (*Serratia marcescens*)
ASTM E 1173	Standard test method for evaluation of a preoperative, precatheterization, or preinjection skin preparations	Test method for demonstrating the *in vivo* efficacy of a preoperative skin preparation on normal (volunteer) skin flora
EN 1499	Chemical disinfectants and antiseptics. Hygienic hand wash. Test method and requirements (phase 2/step 2)	Test method for demonstrating the *in vivo* efficacy of an antiseptic hand wash
EN 12791	Chemical disinfectants and antiseptics. Surgical hand disinfection. Test method and requirement (phase 2/step 2)	Test method for demonstrating the *in vivo* efficacy of a surgical scrub disinfection method
EN 14885	Chemical disinfectants and antiseptics. Application of European standards for chemical disinfectants and antiseptics	Guideline on the testing of chemical disinfectants and antiseptics

[a]WHO, World Health Organization; APIC, Association for Professionals in Infection Control and Epidemiology; CDC, HICPAC, U.S. Centers for Disease Control and Prevention, Healthcare Infection Control Practices Advisory Committee; ASTM, American Society for Testing and Materials; EN, European Standard (Norm).

populations in wastewater, and the potential of other health effects (from animal studies showing the potential for hormonal cycle disruption and skin cancer on long-term exposure). In addition, strong evidence has not been shown that the antimicrobial effects of many such formulations had significant benefits in comparison to soap-and-water in reducing the population of microorganisms and reducing infection or cross-contamination rates.

Hand-rubs (or hand-rinses) include various types of alcohols (particularly ethanol, isopropanol, and *n*-propanol) at various concentrations, which are applied to the skin without the use of water and rubbed into the skin until they evaporate. Alcohols are the most widely used antiseptic biocides in hand-rubs, but non-alcohol-containing formulations have also been recently commercialized. Unlike some hand-washes (see Table 4.3; section 4.6.2), they are rapidly effective, but once evaporated they do not provide any persistent (or residual) activity (which may be desired in some applications). The efficacy of the alcohols in these

TABLE 4.3 Examples of the most widely used biocides in skin antiseptics and washes[a]

Biocide	Antimicrobial activity	Typical concentrations	Reference	Persistence	Reported toxicity
Alcohols, including ethanol, isopropanol, and *n*-propanol	Bactericidal, fungicidal, virucidal, tuberculocidal	60–92%	Chapter 3, section 3.5	None	Skin drying and some irritancy
Chlorhexidine	Bactericidal, fungistatic, tuberculocidal, some virucidal activity	0.1–4%	Section 3.8	Yes	Keratitis, irritancy, and ototoxicity reported
Iodine and iodophors	Bactericidal, fungicidal, virucidal, tuberculocidal	0.5–10% iodophors 2–5% iodine in tinctures	Section 3.11	Some	Irritation and some toxicity reported
Chloroxylenol (PCMX)	Bactericidal (dependent on formulation), fungistatic, some virucidal	0.5–4%	Section 3.15	Yes	Not reported
Triclosan	Bactericidal (dependent on formulation), fungistatic, tuberculostatic	0.1–2%	Section 3.15	Yes	Preliminary reports of long-term toxicity risks

[a]It should be noted that the characteristics of these biocides vary depending on the antiseptic formulation in which they are used.

formulations can be increased by decreasing the evaporation rate on the skin using various emollients or thickening agents, which can also reduce the drying effects associated with alcohol use by using lower concentrations of the biocide (e.g., 60% compared to 70 to 80% alcohol). Alternatively, lower concentrations of other biocides (e.g., 0.5% chlorhexidine in 70% ethanol or the use of preservatives) can be formulated into the hand-rub to provide residual activity following alcohol evaporation. In these and other cases, the antimicrobial activity can be increased due to combined effects of the biocides in these products. Due to the lack of sporicidal activity of alcohols, certain types of hand-rub products are provided presterilized (by sterile filtration or γ radiation sterilization [see chapter 6]) to reduce the risk of spore contamination in high-risk applications. Alcohol-free hand-rubs have been developed as alternatives to traditional ethanol- or isopropanol-based formulations. In particular, these have included 0.1 to 1% 2-phenoxyethanol or 0.1 to 0.3% benzalkonium chloride in foam or liquid formulations or as single-use wipes. These are claimed to be less irritating to the skin on frequent use (due to less drying of the skin that is often observed with some alcohol-based antiseptics) and have also been reported to have some residual antimicrobial activity on the skin over time.

4.5.2 Pretreatment of Skin Prior to Surgical Intervention

Preoperative preparation of patients' skin is an important application prior to surgical intervention to reduce the introduction of potential pathogens from the skin during surgery and the risk of surgical site infections. Such preparations are also important for any medical intervention through the skin, such as the insertion of a needle (e.g., for injection purposes) or catheter. Surgical site or other wound-associated infections can be caused by microorganisms from endogenous or exogenous sources. Exogenous sources can include medical devices (surgical instruments, needles, catheters, etc.), environmental air and surfaces, and contaminated hands or gloves of health care personnel. Endogenous sources are the patient's own microbial flora, particularly from the skin area at the site of intervention, and are typically found to be the most common sources of infection. Preoperative preparation products are used to clean and disinfect localized skin immediately prior to medical or surgical intervention. The most widely used biocides in these applications are alcohols (e.g., in wipes at 60 to 90%), iodine tinctures or iodophors (e.g., providone-iodine solutions or scrubs at 7.5 to 10%), and chlorhexidine (usually at higher concentration ranges, typically 2 to 4%). For surgical preoperative preparations, products that can have persistent activity on the skin over time are preferred (such as chlorhexidine washes and alcohol-based solutions that contain 0.5 to 1% chlorhexidine). Triclosan and PCMX (chloroxylenol) formulations are often recommended for facial applications due to lower toxicity or to limit the risk of eye contact, but these effects can be formulation-dependent. Chlorhexidine soap formulations are also used for preoperative bathing or showering, which have been shown to have a significant impact in reducing the rates of postoperative infection as part of surgical site infection prevention protocols in health care facilities. Other products that have been used, but less studied for effectiveness, for preoperative bathing are the iodophors and other routine antiseptics (e.g., triclosan hand-washes). In some cases, various impregnated films or barriers are applied to the surgical site (either before or following surgery), which allow for slow release of the biocide over the surgery time; examples are chlorhexidine, iodine or iodophor, triclosan, and silver-impregnated products, which have found particular applications in the prevention of indwelling skin catheter-related infections (for further discussion see section 4.5.5).

In an application similar to preoperative preparations, surgical hand-scrubs and -rubs are used to reduce the transient and resident populations of microorganisms on the hands and forearms of surgery personnel. The rationale behind their use is the frequent occurrence of glove damage or tears during surgery and, in particular, cases where gloves are not used. Typical surgical scrubs are conducted for up to 5 minutes and include washing with chlorhexidine (1 to 4%) or iodophor-containing antiseptics or repeated application and rubbing of alcohol antiseptics for the same duration. Other biocides such as triclosan, hexachlorophene, and chloroxylenol are also labeled for use as surgical scrubs. The residual microstatic activity of biocides such as chlorhexidine and, to a lesser extent, iodophors is considered important to reduce the growth of bacteria under gloves during surgical procedures. But it is also important to confirm that the residual activity does not interfere with the barrier properties of the gloves being used. Specific surgical rub formulations that include alcohols and iodine are also used. Recommended exposure times of surgical scrub or rub application vary depending on the product formulation and country-specific registration efficacy requirements.

4.5.3 Treatment of Skin or Wound Infections

It is common to use a variety of antibiotics and other anti-infectives to treat skin or wound infections, in particular, if the infection is present in the deeper layers of skin (section 4.3). Despite this, various biocides are often used for localized applications to prevent skin infections, to clean and treat wounds (in particular, over larger surfaces such as in the case of burns), or to treat skin surface infections.

In these cases, the objective is similar to that for other antiseptics, i.e., to reduce the microbial population in a wound or skin surface infection without significantly damaging the tissue or interfering with the healing process. A typical application is in cases of eczema, an inflammation of the skin that leads to itching, scaling, and blistering that leaves the patient prone to skin infections; the use of biocides can be helpful to reduce the risk or treat infections that can occur in these and similar conditions. The most common causes of wound infections are Gram-positive bacterial cocci including *Staphylococcus* and *Enterococcus*, although Gram-negative bacteria (particularly *Pseudomonas* and *Acinetobacter* spp.) and some yeasts (e.g., *C. albicans*) are frequently implicated (Table 4.1). Older applications to control these infections included the use of mercuric chloride (and other mercury compounds), diamidines, acridines, and some dyes. Most of these biocides are not widely used today and, in the case of mercury, this is primarily due to risks of toxicity, poisoning, or other adverse effects. Antimicrobial dyes (such as crystal violet) are still used but primarily on animals for wound or mucous membrane treatments (e.g., in cattle). Hydrogen peroxide solutions (ranging from 3 to 6%) or cream formulations (typically in the 1 to 3% range for the treatment of ulcers and pressure sore infections) are widely used for cleaning and disinfection of infected wounds; they are also used to prevent infections following injury to the skin to lower the local bioburden. Low levels of hydrogen peroxide gas and mixed-oxidant liquid solutions have also been described but have not seen widespread use. Of the antimicrobial heavy metals, silver (for example, silver nitrate solutions [see chapter 3, section 3.12]) is also used for topical skin treatments and has also found some applications integrated into wound dressing and catheter materials to prevent or control infections (especially in burn patients and for the treatment of chronic wounds). Some biocides are specifically used to treat infections of intact skin (see Table 4.4).

Various phenolics have been used for wound treatment and are provided in creams, ointments, dusting powders, and liquid formulations. These include hexachlorophene (in particular, 0.33% dusting powder to treat or prevent neonatal staphylococcal infections), triclosan (e.g., washes at 0.5 to 2%), and 2,4,6-trichlorophenol. Some essential oils (and other natural products such as honey that contain intrinsic, particularly bacteriostatic, antimicrobial activity) have been recommended, particularly in the treatment of *S. aureus* infections, although their actual benefits remain inconclusive based on mixed reports in the literature. Iodine tinctures have become less used due to irritation to damaged skin and have been mostly replaced by iodophors. Typically, antiseptics with povidone iodine (PVPI) for wound applications are provided at <5% (e.g., 2.5% powders, sprays, and solutions), in contrast to higher concentrations used for intact skin preoperative preparations of surgical scrubs, due to irritation and wound tissue damage. Iodophor-based dressings are also used for chronic wounds such as ulcers. Other halogen-available solutions, including 1% sodium hypochlorite and 5% chloramines, are used to a much lesser extent, primarily as wound cleaners. Chlorhexidine is also used in various dusting powders, creams, and solutions ranging in concentration from 0.05 to 1%; some formulations are provided as combinations with chlorhexidine, for example, 0.015% with 0.5% cetrimide (a quaternary ammonium compound [QAC]; chapter 3, section 3.16) for wound applications. Other surfactants (including QACs) are frequently used at relatively low concentrations as wound cleaning solutions. Another example of combination formulations includes mixtures of various acids such as salicylic acid, benzoic acid, and maleic acid. Some reports, although limited, have suggested the benefit of using UV (specifically the UV-C wavelength range; chapter 2, section 2.4) for wound treatments at dosage levels in the 100 to 300 $mW/cm^2/second$ range; radiation applications have not found widespread use in antiseptic applications.

The treatment of intact skin infections with biocides is often limited to those that are associated with surface skin layers and that have not spread to deeper layers, which are typically inaccessible to biocidal penetration. Examples are the use of antiseptic skin washes to control bacterial infections such as cellulitis, erythema, impetigo, and acne. These include triclosan, chlorhexidine, iodophors, some essential oils, salicylic acid, benzoyl peroxide, and QACs. In the case of boils and carbuncles, moist or dry heat is often used to help drain the infections and is then followed by an antiseptic ointment to aid in wound healing. Similar biocide-based washes, mouthwashes (in particular, chlorhexidine), lozenges, and suppositories (e.g., boric acid) are recommended in the treatment of candidiasis, which is often associated with various mucous membranes, particularly in immunocompromised patients. Medicated shampoos, skin washes, and local-

TABLE 4.4 Miscellaneous biocides used as antiseptics and their applications

Biocide	Antimicrobial activity	Reference	Applications and comments
Antimicrobial dyes, e.g., acridines and crystal violet	Bactericidal, fungistatic, virucidal (enveloped viruses), algistatic, and some protozoal activity	Chapter 3, section 3.7	Wound and wound dressing (humans, animals, and fish) Mucous membrane infections Various fungal infections, e.g., tinea
Anilides, e.g., triclocarban	Bactericidal, fungistatic	Section 3.6	Preservative, deodorant and antimicrobial soaps
Boric acid	Bactericidal, fungicidal, and virucidal	Section 3.2	Suppositories for the treatment of vaginal yeast and viral infections
Diamidines, e.g., propamidine and dibromopropamidine	Bactericidal, fungicidal, amoebicidal, and some protozoal activity	Section 3.9	Wound or skin infections Eye infections
Metals, e.g., silver, silver sulfadiazine, and mercury	Bactericidal, fungicidal, algicidal, and virucidal (enveloped viruses)	Section 3.12	Burn, wound, and mucous membrane infections Preservative Antimicrobial dressings
QACs, e.g., benzalkonium chloride and cetrimide	Bactericidal, fungicidal, sporostatic, virucidal (enveloped viruses), and algistatic	Section 3.16	Skin and mucous membrane washes Shampoos Treatment of seborrhoea and psoriasis Mouth rinses
Salicylic acid	Bactericidal, fungicidal	Section 3.15	Exfoliant (keratinolytic) Wart removal Acne and other skin infections (e.g., associated with psoriasis and dermatitis), as shampoos, gels, washes, and integrated plasters/swabs
Hydrogen peroxide	Bactericidal, fungicidal, virucidal, mycobactericidal, and some sporicidal activity	Section 3.13	Preservative Wound and wound infection treatment
Benzoyl peroxide	Bactericidal, in particular, studied with *P. acnes*	Section 3.13	Acne control
Chlorine dioxide	Bactericidal, fungicidal, and virucidal	Section 3.13	Mastitis control Preoperative preparations
Essential oils, e.g., tea tree oil and thymol	Bactericidal, fungistatic (some fungicidal), and some virucidal activity (enveloped viruses)	Section 3.10	Mouthwashes Antimicrobial hand and face washes Acne treatment
Pyrithiones, e.g., zinc pyrithione	Bactericidal, fungicidal, and algicidal	Section 3.17.1	Treatment of psoriasis and dermatitis as skin washes, sprays, or creams Antidandruff shampoo

ized skin applications have been useful in controlling the spread of various fungal dermatophytes (tinea) and other fungal infections (Table 4.1). Virus infections causing cold sores, warts, or other skin eruptions are a particular challenge to biocide penetration. Salicylic acid and/or lactic acids (either as liquids or impregnated patch applications) are used to soften the skin to allow the removal of warts over time, although typical application times span a number of weeks; in the case of salicylic acid, this is primarily due to its keratinolytic activity allowing the breakdown of surface skin layers over time. Warts are also conveniently removed by cryotherapy, localized freezing with liquid nitrogen and allowing the wart to flake off following treatment. Most other viral and parasitic skin infections are treated with specific antiviral or antiparasitic drugs. Common biocides used to treat acne, which is associated with *P. acnes* and other bacteria on the skin, are salicylic acid, triclosan, hydrogen peroxide, and particularly, benzoyl peroxide-based antiseptics.

4.5.4 Treatment of Oral and Other Mucous Membranes

A similar range of biocides are used for the treatment of more sensitive oral and other (including urogenital) mucous membranes. These are used to treat specific infections or as a prophylaxis, for example, oral mouth rinses in the treatment of gingivitis, ulcers, and throat infections and prior to oral surgery. Mouth rinses can include various formulations with QACs (such as cetylpyridinium bromide, cetrimide, and dequalinium chloride), chlorhexidine, hydrogen peroxide, essential oils, and PVPI (1% with 8% alcohol). For example, a widely used essential oil-based formulation uses thymol (0.06%), eucalypol (0.09%), and menthol (0.045) in combination with methyl salicylate. In addition to antimicrobial activity, these formulations are often used for odor control (e.g., to treat halitosis).

Some, including lower-hydrogen peroxide solutions and chlorhexidine, have also been used directly on the eye. Antibacterial toothpastes can include triclosan, zinc chlorine, fluoride, and chlorhexidine, although there are mixed reports on the benefit of antibacterial toothpastes to reduce periodontal diseases. Urinary and genital tract infections, including bacterial, fungal, and viral pathogens, can be treated with products including hexamine, silver nitrate, boric acid, chlorhexidine, octenidine, phenols, and QACs; these products include rinses, suppositories, and creams.

4.5.5 Material-Integrated Applications

Polymers, textiles, and other materials have been successfully impregnated with biocides for antiseptic uses (section 3.17.2). These include medical devices such as catheters and needles that can remain in contact with the skin/mucous membranes and bandages, dressings, and patches that are used on the skin or wounds over extended periods of time (Fig. 4.3). Antibacterial wound dressings include various types of hydrocolloids, cellulose, alginates, and polymers (e.g., polyurethane) with biocides such as dyes (methylene blue, gentian violet), iodophors, and silver.

Other applications include surgical drapes and gowns that could contact the skin during surgical procedures. Biocides that have been successfully integrated into these materials and polymers for use on contact with the skin or mucous membranes include triclosan, silver, silver sulfadiazine, and chlorhexidine. These and other biocides have also been used for hard-surface applications (chapter 3). Some applications have shown success in reducing the rate of wound and/or indwelling medical device infections. Antimicrobial surfaces have been developed by incorporation directly into the polymer or by impregnation or coating various materials and surfaces. In some cases they release the biocide over time into the area associated with the device or material, while in others, they remain an intrinsic part of the surface to prevent the attachment and growth of bacteria and fungi (e.g., to prevent biofilm development).

4.6 BIOCIDES USED AS ANTISEPTICS

4.6.1 General Considerations

Antiseptics should provide a spectrum of activity, considering the various transient and resident microbial populations that can be present on the skin and mucous membranes or associated with various skin or wound infections (section 4.4). With the exception of some specific therapeutic applications, emphasis has primarily been on the antibacterial and bacteriostatic properties of these products,

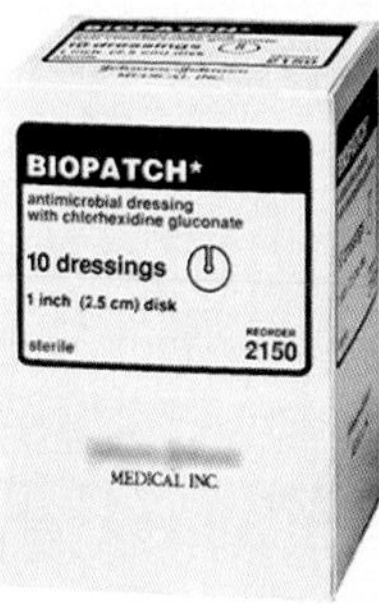

FIGURE 4.3 Example of biocide-impregnated wipes for skin applications. Product Image courtesy of Ethicon, with permission.

with some investigation of their effects on fungi (in particular, *C. albicans*) and viruses. Although the biocide itself has a known spectrum of antimicrobial activity, its formulation into antiseptic products must optimize not only its effectiveness but also its compatibility with the skin or mucous membranes (the effects of formulation are discussed in chapter 1, section 1.4.6). Examples of these effects in antiseptics include the following:

- The use of chelating agents (e.g., EDTA) with triclosan to improve the penetration of the biocide into the cell wall of Gram-negative bacteria.
- The formulation of iodophors as iodine-releasing agents in comparison to the use of high concentrations of iodine in tinctures, which are more irritating.
- The formulation of lower concentrations of alcohols (60 to 70%) in the presence of other excipients that reduce the evaporation rates of alcohols and allow them to remain on the skin longer, to minimize drying and irritation of the skin over multiple uses.
- Inclusion of moisturizing ingredients to counteract the drying of skin from washing or alcohol use (e.g., humectants and emollients such as glycerin and dimethicone).
- Effects of formulation pH and the dissociation constants of biocides in formulations, where un-ionized molecules are considered to penetrate the skin layers better than ionized forms.
- The use of mixtures of biocides for antimicrobial and preservative activity in formulations. In addition to the predominant biocides used in soap or non-alcohol-based hand-washes and hand-rubs, others are used at low concentrations for preservative activity (e.g., the parabens and methylisothiozolinone).

For these and other reasons, the antimicrobial efficacy of antiseptics (similar to disinfectant formulations) can vary significantly even in the presence of similar or varying concentrations of the biocide. Antimicrobial efficacy is also dependent on the use of the product. In some cases, routine hand-washes or -rinses should provide rapid activity within the typical amount of time used to apply the product, which is generally in the range of 5 to 20 seconds. Claims of antimicrobial activity at longer contact times (e.g., 1 to 10 minutes) may be impractical in some situations due to the way the product is routinely used. The correct use of these products is therefore important, not only because of the recommended exposure time, but also to ensure coverage (e.g., over the hands, between the fingers, under the nails, etc.) and adequate rinsing, when required, to remove formulation components that can cause irritation over time. In other cases, as with preoperative preparations and surgical scrubs or rubs, much longer times are generally recommended (~2 to 5 minutes), and given their professional use, it can be easier to ensure compliance with minimum exposure times and application of the product. The condition of the skin can also affect the activity of the product due to variations in soiling (e.g., blood, dirt, or various foods), pH of the skin, microbial load, etc. Finally, when used with hand-washes, the quality of the water (for example, hardness and presence of inactivating substances such as phosphates, chlorine, and other inorganic ions commonly present in water) can also limit the activity of the antiseptic formulation on the skin.

Irritation associated with the use of an antiseptic is also important to consider, because it can limit the product's practical use over time. Similar to the biocidal effects discussed above, the irritation observed with a product can be based on the biocide itself (type, concentration, pH, etc.), various formulations, excipients (such as the choice of surfactants), individual sensitivity, and the way the product is used. Formulation residuals remaining on the skin due to inadequate rinsing are often associated with irritation, which can be exacerbated with extended use of gloves. An increase in sweating under the gloves can lead to a loss of moisture, drying, cracking, and allergic reactions (most often associated with latex gloves; latex itself can be a skin irritant). Most of the commonly used biocides are considered nontoxic, but in some cases, allergic reactions have been reported, and certain restrictions are recommended; for example, chlorhexidine infusion into the ear is often not recommended due to reports of ototoxicity; allergic and toxic effects have been associated with the use of iodine (although these reports are generally associated with tinctures and less so with iodophors), and in a notable extreme case, the use of hexachlorophene is contraindicated for use on broken skin due to neurotoxicity risks. In contrast, some interesting reports have suggested that triclosan (and some other phenolics used on the skin) may inhibit histamine-induced inflammation on the skin and mucous membranes; however, preliminary reports of the role of triclosan in disrupting hormonal cycles and other long-term health effects are the subject of much debate.

Persistence of the biocide on the skin following washing or application is considered an advantage and is associated with a strong affinity for the skin. Persistence has been observed with many biocides including chlorhexidine, triclosan, hexachlorophene, antimicrobial metals and dyes, essential oils, chloroxylenol, and to some extent, the iodophors. The benefit of persistence is the inhibition of the growth of bacteria and fungi on the skin, in particular, for higher-risk applications such as preoperative preparations and surgical scrubs and rubs. The persistence of chlorhexidine, in particular, has been studied in some detail. Chlorhexidine has affinity for the skin and is predominantly found associated with the outermost layers of the epidermis, with little to no significant penetration further into the skin (Fig. 4.4). The stratum corneum is a particular barrier to penetration, although at high concentrations and with damaged skin, the biocide can be found to penetrate deeper into the dermal skin layers.

Persistent activity can be achieved by direct application (e.g., in the case of 0.5% chlorhexidine in alcohol rubs or encapsulated applications) and by single washes of higher concentrations of chlorhexidine-containing products (typically with 2 to 4%) or multiple applications of lower-concentration formulations (0.5 to 2% washes). The persistent concentration is generally sufficient to inhibit the growth of most Gram-positive bacteria, including *S. aureus* (with a typical inhibitory concentration in the 0.2 to 8 mg/liter range), some Gram-negative bacteria, and fungi. However, because chlorhexidine is a cationic surfactant (section 3.8) this activity can be neutralized by various factors including the presence of inorganic anions (such as phosphates and chlorides) in water, organic soils, organic anions (such as soaps), and other detergents and lotions that contain either anionic or certain nonionic surfactants. Similar neutralizing effects have been found with other persistent biocides on the skin.

Some investigations have suggested negative impacts of the presence of low concentrations of biocides on the skin (or indeed in the environment over time). Of particular note is the risk associated with the development of tolerance to inhibitory concentrations of the biocide and cross-resistance to antibiotics in bacteria. Modes of resistance to biocides such as triclosan and chlorhexidine, including cell wall and cell membrane structural alterations, efflux, and even target site modifications, have been shown to increase resistance to certain antibiotics (see chapter 8). Although these mechanisms may have minimal impacts on the antimicrobial effects of the biocides (because they generally have multiple modes of action in bacteria), they can have a more dramatic influence on bacterial resistance to antibiotics that can lead to failure during their use to treat infections.

Overall, there is no perfect antiseptic for all applications, and the choice of the biocide and/or product use varies depending on:

- The application (intact or broken skin, high or low risk of cross-contamination, presence of water, etc.)
- The extent and type of contamination (presence of soils, mechanical removal, microbial load, types of microorganism[s], etc.)

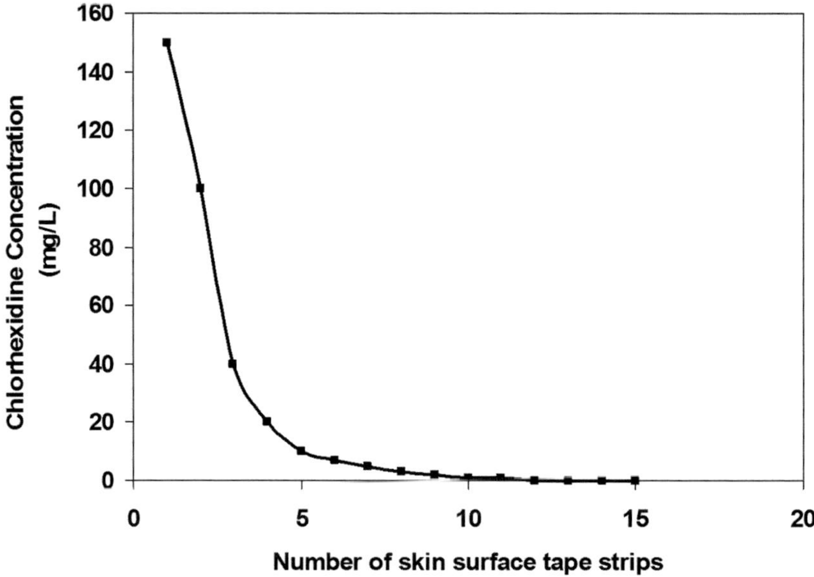

FIGURE 4.4 A representation of the penetration of chlorhexidine into the skin epidermis. The concentration of residual activity varies, depending on the formulation and application of the antiseptic. In this case residual activity was present following washing with a 4% chlorhexidine formulation. The concentration can be determined by removing various layers of the epidermis by tape-stripping (using adhesive tape to remove various layers) or by histologically removing layers by sectioning, followed by chlorhexidine extraction and determination.

- Spectrum of antimicrobial activity (bactericidal, fungicidal, or virucidal)
- Previous reports of irritation, toxicity, and/or allergic reactions (skin condition, personal history, label warnings, and restrictions)
- Labeling and regulatory requirements, which can vary from country to country

4.6.2 Major Types of Biocides in Antiseptic Skin Washes and Rinses

The most-used biocides in antiseptic washes and rinses are summarized in Table 4.3. These biocides are discussed in some detail in chapter 3 and are only briefly discussed in this section with respect to their antiseptic uses.

Alcohols, including ethanol, isopropanol, and *n*-propanol, are widely used as antiseptics, the last primarily in Europe (chapter 3, section 3.5). They are provided as various hand rinse formulations and as impregnated wipes and also in combination with other biocides such as chlorhexidine. They are also used at lower, nonbiocidal concentrations in various other formulations. In general, they have rapid antimicrobial activity over relatively short exposure times at typical antiseptic concentrations ranging from 60 to 92%, with optimal activity reported for the alcohols on their own around the 70% range. Most alcohol antiseptic formulations contain emollients and other excipients to reduce the drying effects often associated with the use of alcohols on the skin and to decrease the evaporation rate, thereby allowing lower concentrations of alcohol (60 to 65%) to be used. Alcohols demonstrate broad-spectrum antimicrobial activity, with the notable exception of having no appreciable effects on bacterial spores (although they are sporostatic). They are rapidly effective against bacteria, including mycobacteria, and fungi, with mixed reports in the literature regarding their efficacy against viruses and fungal spores (which varies depending on the alcohol type and formulation). Enveloped viruses are rapidly sensitive, with varying activity described for nonenveloped viruses. Because they are used as hand-rubs, they have the advantage of not requiring the presence of water for application, but this is also a disadvantage in the presence of soils (such as blood, food, etc.). Although they can be used to treat wounds, in particular, small abrasions, they cause short-lived stinging effects in contact with damaged skin; despite widespread use, alcohols have rarely been associated with any toxic effects, but care should be taken to avoid contact with the eyes at typical concentrations used. Alcohols and their formulations can be flammable and should be stored according to the manufacturer's instructions.

Chlorhexidine is a bisbiguanide used both as a preventative and as a therapeutic antiseptic (chapter 3, section 3.8). It is used in various salt forms, in particular, gluconate, acetate, and hydrochloride salts, but also in combination with other biocides such as QACs (e.g., cetrimide) and alcohols. Chlorhexidine is one of the most widely used and accepted biocides in high-risk hand-washes and rinses, including in higher-risk applications such as health care preoperative preparations and surgical scrubs. Chlorhexidine is also used as a biocide impregnated into various surfaces for release over time into the skin and for treating mucous membrane infections, including in oral mouth rinses for the treatment of minor infections, mouth ulcers, and gingivitis. Chlorhexidine is used for direct application into the eye at concentrations <0.1%; higher concentrations are considered damaging to the eye tissue. Formulations of the biocide vary considerably. An important consideration is pH, with optimal activity at pH 5.5 to 7.0, as well the potential for incompatibility with various anionic and nonionic substances. For example, lotions containing anionic surfactants neutralize residual chlorhexidine concentrations on the skin.

In general, formulations demonstrate broad antibacterial activity, with particularly rapid activity against various Gram-positive bacteria including staphylococci, as well as Gram-negative bacteria. Chlorhexidine is bactericidal at low concentrations, with the highest MICs reported for certain bacterial strains such as *Providencia stuartii*. In general, higher bactericidal concentrations have been reported against Gram-negative bacteria, including pseudomonads. At relatively low concentrations, chlorhexidine is also mycobacteristatic and fungistatic, although its fungicidal effects can be improved in formulation, in particular, against *Candida* spp. that are often associated with skin and membrane infections. Because the primary mode of action of chlorhexidine is considered to be disruption of the lipid membrane (chapter 3, section 3.8), virucidal activity against enveloped viruses has been reported, but little to no effect has been observed against nonenveloped viruses (such as noroviruses). Chlorhexidine also demonstrates residual activity on the skin, providing some protection against microbial growth over time. One of the main reasons for the wide acceptance of chlorhexidine as an antiseptic is the limited reports of adverse effects and toxicity. It is considered nontoxic, with little adsorption into the skin. Many studies have confirmed limited to no toxicity, carcinogenicity, or irritancy, although some cases of irritancy may be related to other formulation effects, and some cases of allergic reactions have been reported; despite this, higher concentrations of chlorhexidine can cause eye damage and ototoxicity. Other biguanides have been used as antiseptics, including alexidine and octenidine (chapter 3, section 3.8).

Iodine is a halogen (chapter 3, section 3.11). Various iodine alcohol and aqueous solutions have been used, although the most effective are the various tinctures of iodine in alcohol, which are predominantly used as preoperative preparations (directly or in swabs or gauzes) and to a lesser extent for wound applications or as general hand-washes. This is primarily due to toxicity, irritation, and staining disadvantages with higher concentrations of iodine in solution. These have been all but replaced by the use of various iodine-releasing agents such as the iodophors, particularly PVPI . They have the advantages of greater solubility for formulation and release-active (or "free") iodine over time and as required and therefore are less irritating and damaging to the skin, depending on the concentrations used. The chemistry of iodine in solution is complicated, with two species primarily associated with antimicrobial activity (free iodine, I_2, and hypoiodous acid, HOI). Therefore, the activity of an iodophor solution is dependent on the concentrations of these species released over time. For example, a freshly prepared 10% PVPI solution contains approximately 1% available iodine (with respect to the total capacity of the iodine reservoir of the iodophor) and releases free iodine in the 0.5 to 5 mg/liter range for antimicrobial activity; however, as the equilibrium between bound and available iodine is disrupted, for example, by dilution or biocidal use, the iodophor can release additional iodine for antimicrobial activity under in-use conditions. Iodophors are provided as various solutions, powders (for wound applications), and lotions.

Depending on the free iodine concentrations, iodophor solutions can be used for routine and high-risk applications, including surgical scrubs and preoperative preparations. Unlike tinctures, they are generally associated with low toxicity, little irritation even in wounds, and are nonstaining, depending on the concentrations used over time; however, allergic and toxic effects, including adsorption into the blood, have been reported. As an oxidizing agent (chapter 3, section 3.11), iodine has been shown to have broad-spectrum antimicrobial activity including bactericidal, fungicidal, virucidal, and mycobactericidal, with some sporicidal and protozoal activity over time. Because it readily reacts with organic soils, the presence of these soils can inhibit penetration to target microorganisms but can be compensated for by the further release of iodine in the case of the iodophors being used during hand-washing. As for other biocides, various formulation effects affect the activity and shelf life of the antiseptic.

Chloroxylenol (or PCMX, for para-chloro-meta-xylenol) is a phenolic biocide used as a skin antiseptic wash and in some cases as a surgical scrub and preoperative preparation (chapter 3, section 3.15). Typical antiseptic concentrations range from 0.5 to 4%. It is also used in medicated shampoos and as a medicated powder for wound applications. Its antimicrobial activity is limited in comparison to other antiseptic biocides, with particular bactericidal activity against Gram-positive and Gram-negative bacteria. Formulation also plays an important role in optimizing the efficacy of chloroxylenol against some Gram-negative bacteria such as *Pseudomonas*, as well as yeasts, molds, and enveloped viruses. Chloroxylenol is mycobacteristatic and sporistatic, but no activity has been reported against nonenveloped viruses. It also has a good safety profile, despite penetration into the epidermis and persistence on the skin, and is considered to have low to no toxicity and little irritancy. In some cases, allergic contact dermatitis has been reported. Similar to chlorhexidine, residual concentrations on the skin can be neutralized by various chemicals including nonionic surfactants.

Triclosan is a diphenyl ether (see discussion of biophenols in chapter 3, section 3.15) and has an antimicrobial profile similar to that of chloroxylenol, with rapid activity against Gram-positive bacteria and yeasts, less against Gram-negative bacteria, and limited to no activity against many fungi and nonenveloped viruses. Formulation plays an important role in optimizing the activity of triclosan on the skin, including the combination with low concentrations of EDTA and other chelating agents to improve the penetration into Gram-negative bacteria, fungi, and some yeasts. Overall, triclosan has limited activity against molds but is fungistatic at relatively low concentrations. Triclosan is used in a variety of antiseptic hand-washes at concentrations ranging from 0.1 to 2%; its primary use is for routine and frequent hand or body washing, although some formulations have been used as health care personnel hand-washes and surgical scrubs. Lower concentrations of triclosan are used for odor control in body washes and deodorants, due to its bacteriostatic activity under these conditions. Other applications include shampoos, lotions, and integration into dressings and bandages for release over time on contact with the skin. Triclosan has demonstrated some residual activity on the skin, although this is due to a different type of binding than a cationic molecule such as chlorhexidine. Triclosan-containing antiseptics have shown particular clinical use for the control of staphylococcal (*S. aureus*, including methicillin-resistant *S. aureus*) carriage on the skin. Although these results may be primarily due to the potent activity against these bacteria, it should also be considered that many triclosan products have good compliance rates due to their associated low irritation. Formulation effects are particularly important to improve efficacy against Gram-negative bacteria, which may be more important in other applications such as in food-handling facilities.

Triclosan is generally nonallergenic and nonmutagenic and was associated with a good safety profile; some long-term toxicity and bacterial resistance concerns may limit the use of this biocide over time. Concerns have been raised about the use of triclosan (and chlorhexidine) due to the development of bacterial resistance (or more correctly, reduced susceptibility or increased tolerance) to low concentrations of the biocide and cross-resistance to some antibiotics (chapter 3, section 3.15, and chapter 8, section 8.7.2). A similar biophenol used as an antiseptic is hexachlorophene (section 3.15), which has a similar range of activity and greater persistence/penetration into the skin; however, confirmed reports of neurotoxicity have led to the limited use of this biocide as an antiseptic, and it is recommended only on intact skin. Other biocides with increased use in antiseptics over the past few years include QACs (particularly benzalkonium chloride [see section 3.16]) and 2-phenoxyethanol [see section 3.5].

4.6.3 Other Antiseptic Biocides

A variety of other biocides are used for other antiseptic applications. A summary of these is given in Table 4.4.

PHYSICAL STERILIZATION

5

5.1 INTRODUCTION

Chapter 2 described the various physical disinfection methods. The basic concepts behind many of these methods also apply to physical sterilization techniques. Sterilization is a process used to render a surface or product free from viable organisms, including bacterial spores. The methods of sterilization discussed in this chapter are the most widely used physical sterilization techniques and include the use of moist heat, dry heat, and radiation. Heat-based methods were previously discussed as physical disinfection methods (chapter 2, section 2.2). Moist heat (steam) processes, based on the application of steam under pressure, are the most widely used methods of heat-based sterilization and are considered the most reliable. High-temperature dry-heat sterilization methods are also used for particular applications, including the incineration of contaminated waste products and materials. Low-temperature alternatives of physical sterilization include the high-energy ionizing radiation methods (including X rays, γ rays, and electron beams [E beams]), although these are used primarily for industrial applications (for an introduction to radiation see section 2.4). This chapter also includes a discussion of some of the developing methods of physical sterilization, including plasma, pulsed light, supercritical fluids, and pulsed electric fields, that have been successfully used in some applications.

5.2 STEAM (OR MOIST-HEAT) STERILIZATION

High-temperature steam (or steam under pressure) is one of the most widely used sterilization methods. Antimicrobial activity is achieved by steam exposure in a time-temperature relationship, similar to that described for moist-heat thermal disinfection (see chapter 2, section 2.2). At higher temperatures the time for disinfection or sterilization decreases, and this can be achieved by increasing the pressure of the process exposure conditions.

Steam is simply a gas that is produced by the heating of water and, therefore, this concept can be explained by the gas laws that consider four variables: volume, temperature, pressure, and the amount of gas.

1. Boyle's law describes the relationship between pressure (P) and volume (V) at a constant temperature and amount of gas. As the pressure rises, the volume of steam decreases, and vice versa:

$$P_1 V_1 = P_2 V_2$$

2. Charles' law describes the relationship between temperature (T) and volume

(V) at a constant pressure and amount of gas. As the temperature increases, the volume increases (the gas expands), and vice versa:

$$\frac{V_1}{T_1} = \frac{V_2}{T_2}$$

3. Combining the equations above, the combined gas law is given as:

$$\frac{P_1 V_1}{T_1} = \frac{P_2 V_2}{T_2}$$

Therefore, if we consider the introduction of a given amount of steam into a fixed volume, the temperature of the steam can be varied by changing the pressure. At atmospheric pressure (101.35 kPa, 14.7 lbp in^{-2} [psi], 1 bar, 760 mmHg [or torr] at sea level), water boils to produce vapor (steam) at 100°C. If the pressure is increased, the boiling temperature of steam also increases, and high sterilization temperatures can be achieved. Equally, as the pressure is decreased (e.g., by pulling a vacuum), the temperature at which steam forms decreases; this is referred to as "low-temperature" steam, which is used in other sterilization and disinfection methods. The relationship between steam temperature and pressure is shown in Fig. 5.1.

At each point along the line, the steam quality is referred to as being "saturated," which is optimal for steam sterilization processes. Under these conditions, steam contains as much water as possible, prior to condensation. At a given point, if the temperature is lowered (for example, where the steam meets a cold surface), water condenses and heats up the surface by the release of thermal energy. Equally, if the temperature is increased, the steam becomes "superheated," or essentially drier (more like dry air), which is less efficient for sterilization.

Steam (as a source of moist heat; see chapter 2, section 2.2) rapidly inactivates most types of microorganisms on contact, but the immediate release of energy on condensation is believed to be particularly effective at inactivating more resistant forms of microorganisms, such as bacterial spores (see chapter 8, section 8.3.11). For example, 1 g of water at 81°C that decreases in temperature to 80°C releases ~1 calorie of

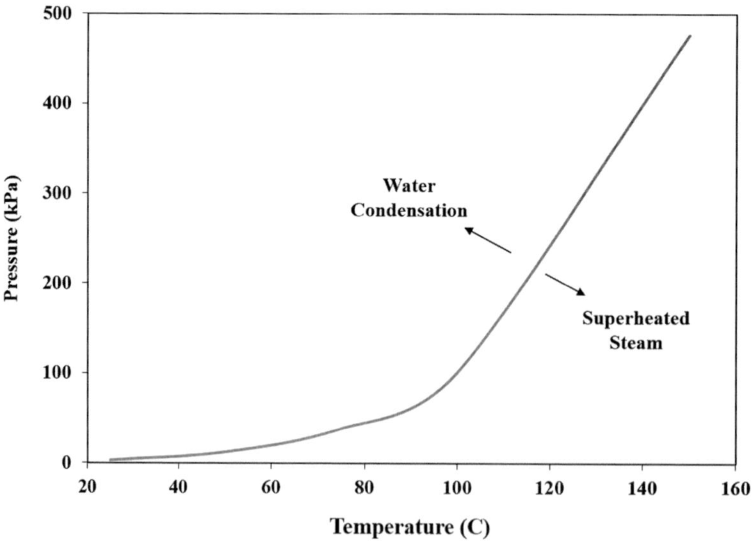

FIGURE 5.1 The relationship between saturated steam temperature and pressure.

energy. In contrast, 1 g of steam at 121°C that condenses into water at 120°C yields ~550 calories of energy. This is known as the latent heat of condensation. In some applications, excessive condensation may need to be avoided, because it restricts the penetration of steam to desired surfaces. In others, the steam is used to heat a surface that then transfers heat (by conduction) to another surface or liquid (such as in the case of the sterilization of liquid in a sealed container) to achieve the desired temperature for sterilization. Therefore, although the use of steam for sterilization may appear straightforward, the control of the sterilization process is important and is dependent on the desired application.

5.2.1 Types

Steam sterilization is performed in controlled vessels (known as autoclaves, steam sterilizers, or pressure vessels) that are capable of safely withstanding the required pressures for sterilization (Fig. 5.2).

Efficient air removal (or mixing in some applications) is essential to ensure steam sterilization, because air will prevent the penetration of steam and leave cold spots within the chamber or load to be sterilized. Most autoclaves are designed for the removal of air from the vessel and its load and can therefore be classified based on the mechanisms of air removal.

Upward-Displacement Autoclaves: Upward-displacement autoclaves are generally small, laboratory-scale autoclaves—a typical example being a pressure cooker (Fig. 5.3). Water is placed at the base of the vessel and heated (e.g., by an electric heater or on a burner) to produce steam. As the steam rises, air and steam are expelled from the vessel under pressure, through a safety valve on the lid, for a given time and then the valve is closed. The vessel is maintained heated during the sterilization time and then allowed to

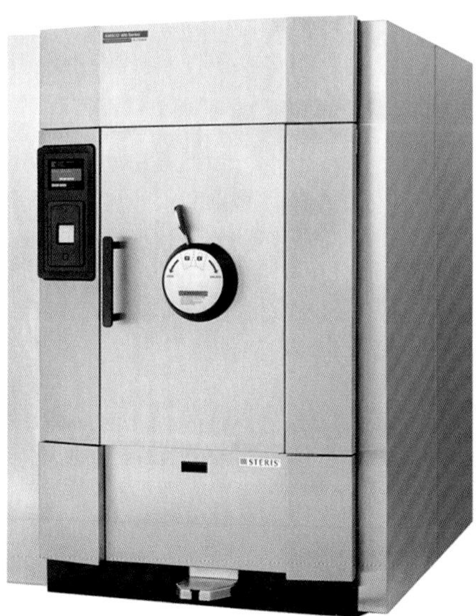

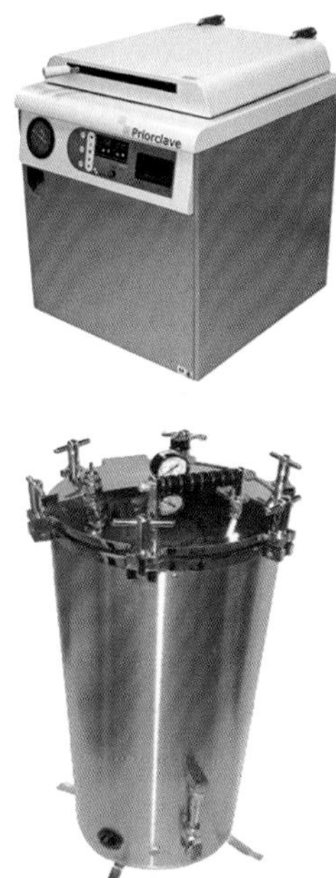

FIGURE 5.2 Steam sterilizers come in a variety of sizes and shapes depending on their application. In addition, the steam sterilization process can be conducted as an intrinsic part of some manufacturing or industrial equipment, which can be routinely sterilized without being disassembled ("steam-in-place").

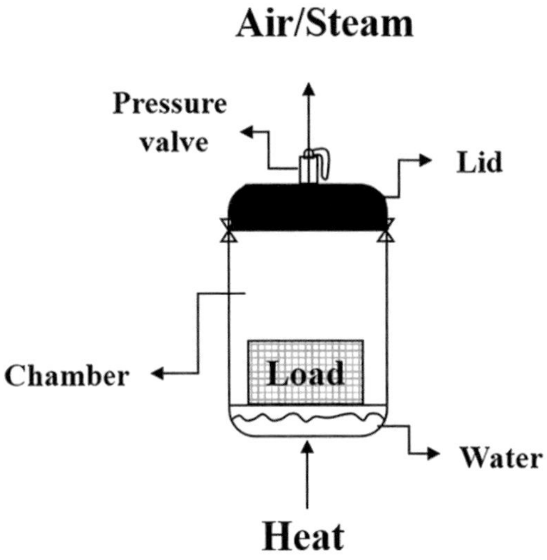

FIGURE 5.3 The basic design of an upward-displacement steam sterilizer.

cool before being opened. These designs can be effective for simple devices but are less reliable for efficient air removal with complex loads.

Downward-Displacement Autoclaves: Downward (or gravity)-displacement steam sterilizers vary in size from small bench-tops to large laboratory, industrial, or hospital autoclaves. They are widely used for liquid and surface (devices, cages, vessels, etc.) sterilization. They are often not recommended as being efficient for the sterilization of porous load materials (such as foodstuffs, towels, etc.), due to limited efficiency of air removal. A simplified design is shown in Fig. 5.4. The pressure vessel is usually jacketed to allow for preheating of the load prior to sterilization (or cooling after sterilization); preheating can be achieved electrically (by dry heat transfer) or by using steam. Steam is then slowly introduced into the top of a pressure vessel and passes though a water separator and baffle. The water separator provides a torturous path for the removal of a significant amount of water that may be carried in the incoming steam from a boiler. Further, the separator or baffle reduces the velocity of steam entering the chamber to reduce mixing with the air, which would result in inefficient air removal. Steam is less dense (lighter) than air and initially fills the chamber from the top; then the mass of steam pushes down through the chamber to force (displace) the air out through a valve at the base of the chamber. Correct control and design of the autoclave optimize the removal of air from the chamber. When the required temperature and pressure are achieved, the incoming steam is shut off and the load is held for the given sterilization time. The temperature is controlled at the coldest point in the chamber, which is at the base of the chamber in the drain line. Following the required sterilization time, air is then introduced into the chamber and the contents are allowed to cool (generally to below 80°C).

Vacuum and Pressure-Pulsing Autoclaves: A variety of designs and sizes of vacuum and pressure-pulsing autoclaves are available for sterilizing porous and non-porous loads. Porous loads include fabrics, towels, and certain wrapped items of plastics, which can trap air, thereby limiting the penetration of steam. The simplest systems use a vacuum pump to draw air out of the chamber ("pulling a vacuum"; Fig. 5.5).

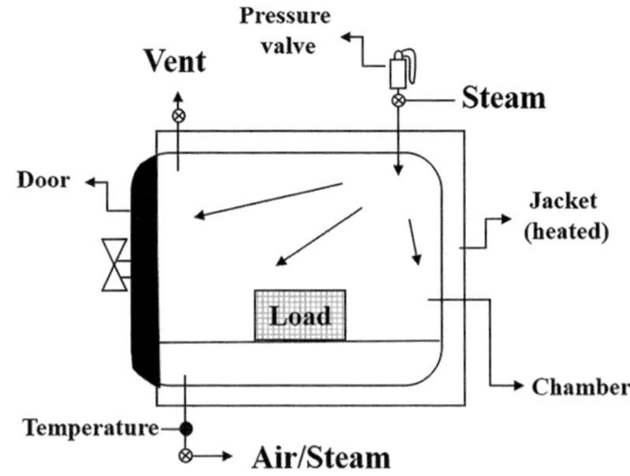

FIGURE 5.4 The basic design of a downward-displacement steam sterilizer.

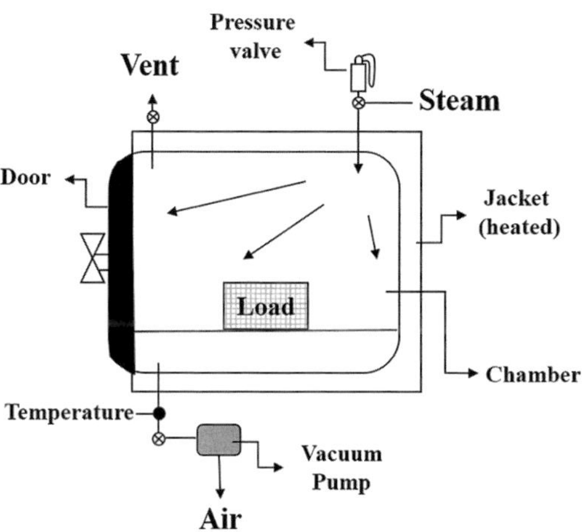

FIGURE 5.5 The basic design of a prevacuum steam sterilizer.

The lower the pressure (or "deeper" the vacuum), the greater the air removal from the chamber and its contents. But it is also important to note that low vacuum levels cause the load to cool during a cycle. Following air evacuation, steam is introduced to heat the load and is placed under positive pressure to reach the desired sterilization temperature for the required time; the chamber is then vented to atmospheric pressure to cool. The load can be more rapidly cooled by pulling a vacuum following sterilization. A typical simple vacuum cycle is shown in Fig. 5.6. There are many alternatives to simple vacuum cycles that can be used. For example, steam can be pulsed into the chamber at various stages to aid in the removal of air and allow even penetration of steam through the load (Fig. 5.6).

These active, pulsing cycles are generally more efficient and can include:

Forced displacement: Steam is introduced into the chamber under pressure and is continually introduced as a vacuum is pulled, followed by an increase in pressure to the desired set point for sterilization. Note that air removal and heating to the sterilization temperature are referred to as conditioning.

Pressure-vacuum pulsing: Steam is introduced into the chamber under pressure, and the air/steam mixture is evacuated by pulling a vacuum. These pulses can be repeated to optimize air removal and load heating.

Pressure pulsing: This is similar to pressure-vacuum pulsing, but the chamber is evacuated to atmospheric (or above atmospheric) pressure only (thereby not requiring a vacuum pump to achieve lower pressures).

Other Types of Autoclaves and Steam Sterilization Cycles: Other types of autoclaves can be designed for specific applications. Examples are those that are used for the sterilization of packaged materials or liquids that may be sensitive to the pressure changes that occur in the previously described autoclave designs (particularly during the heating and cooling phases of sterilization). These are referred to as air pressurization steam cycles and sterilizers. They are designed to retain the pressure balance between the containers or packages and the sterilizer chamber to prevent the rupturing of containers or loss of seal integrity (a concern for the ingress of microorganisms following sterilization). Simple designs can include the use of fans (or other air-movement mechanisms) to allow for the uniform mixing of air and steam at different stages of the sterilization process (e.g., overpressurization of the sterilizer chamber with compressed air to balance with the increased pressure in containers during the process). Other designs include the use of water sprays or even complete water-immersion sterilizers.

When considering steam sterilization, in addition to the temperature and pressure of the process, it is important to understand the factors that can affect the efficiency of steam sterilization:

Air removal: As discussed above, it is important to remove air and other noncondensable gases (gases that do not condense under the conditions of steam sterilization) from the chamber and load. Because

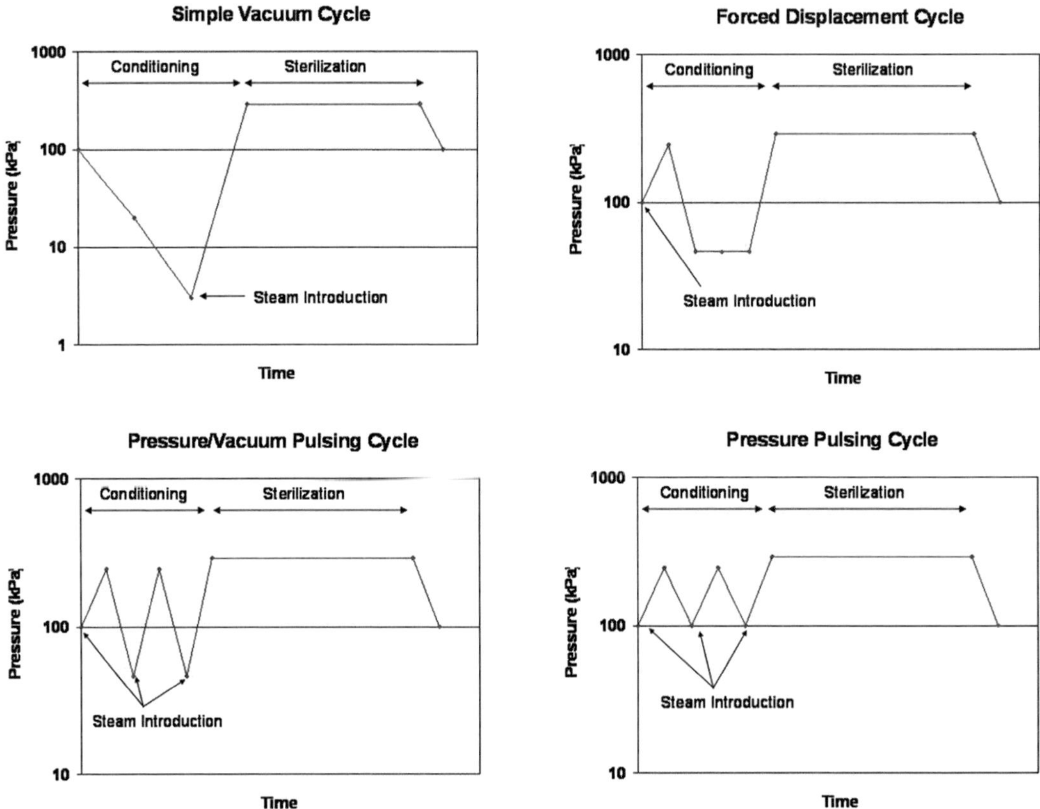

FIGURE 5.6 Typical team sterilization cycles, showing different mechanisms of air removal and load conditioning prior to sterilization.

air cannot condense under conditions of steam sterilization, it impedes the penetration of steam. For prevacuum-based processes, it is particularly important that the chamber is airtight, which can be confirmed by performing a leak test prior to sterilization or conducting other periodic tests to confirm the efficient removal of air. The most common method is called the Bowie-Dick test (Fig. 5.7). This test can be used to measure the efficiency of mechanical air removal and leak detection in a prevacuum sterilizer. As discussed above, specific cycles and sterilizer designs can accommodate or even use the presence of air during the sterilization process, but these cycles need to be developed for specific applications and ensure that a uniform mixture of air and steam is present during sterilization (e.g., by the use of fans).

Water content: Optimal sterilization is achieved using saturated steam, which is dependent on the temperature and pressure (Fig. 5.1). As steam becomes wetter (or supersaturated), condensation forms that can limit steam penetration into a load. Excessive wetness can also leave the load difficult to handle and prone to recontamination (e.g., by bacterial penetration through packaging or sterile barrier systems used over time). In these cases, drying is recommended. Conversely, as steam becomes dryer (defined as superheated, where the water vapor temperature is higher than

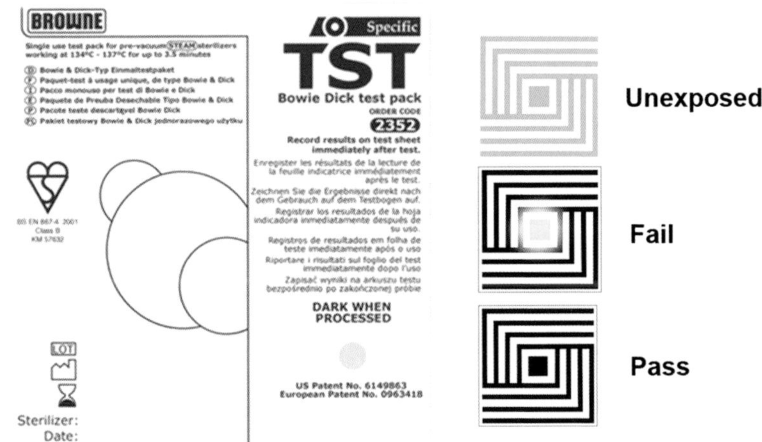

FIGURE 5.7 An example of a Bowie-Dick test pack, a method of testing the steam penetration and air removal capabilities of a vacuum sterilizer. A single-use test pack is shown (left). It consists of a chemical indicator at the center of the test pack, which changes color on exposure to the correct combination of time, temperature, and steam. Examples of unexposed, failed, and pass chemical indicator results are shown (right). Image courtesy of STERIS, with permission.

the boiling point of water at the corresponding pressure), it is less effective for sterilization.

Steam purity: The purity of steam is determined by the quality of water from which it is made and can also be affected during the transfer of the steam from a generator to the steam sterilizer. Many water contaminants can be carried over in steam and deposited onto surfaces, including devices or foods being sterilized, packaging materials, pipework, and the sterilizer itself. These can contaminate surfaces and liquids (e.g., medical device surfaces leading to toxic effects on surgical use) and can cause significant damage to surfaces. The most common contaminants and their effects are shown in Table 5.1.

Because the purity of water can vary significantly, it may be necessary to pretreat the water, control the generation of steam, and protect its quality during distribution to the sterilization vessel. Examples of pretreatment systems are shown in Fig. 5.8.

For certain applications, the steam is required to be "clean," which may be defined as steam whose condensate meets a high requirement for the purity of water, such as water

TABLE 5.1 Common steam contaminants and their effects

Contaminant	Effects
Organic materials	
Pyrogens (e.g., bacterial endotoxins)	Pyrogenic reactions (fever)
Amines	Toxicity
Particulate materials	Discoloration of packaging materials
Inorganic materials	
Toxic metals (e.g., cadmium, lead mercury)	Cumulative poisons
Alkaline earth metals (e.g., calcium, magnesium)	Hardness (calcium carbonate) deposits
Iron	Corrosion (iron oxide)
Chlorides	Corrosion

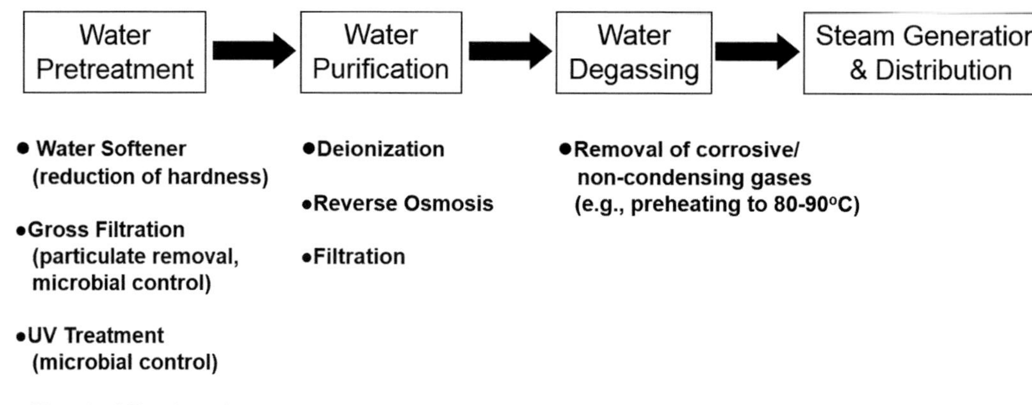

FIGURE 5.8 Typical water pretreatment systems for the production of steam.

for injection. Water for injection has specified limits of organic and inorganic contaminants that have been shown to be safe when injected directly into the bloodstream (e.g., as used for the preparation of dried parenterals or drugs for injection). These requirements are defined in various pharmacopoeias used worldwide (e.g., the U.S. Pharmacopoeia [USP] and the European Pharmacopoeia [EP]; Table 5.2).

5.2.2 Applications

Steam sterilizers can range in size from small benchtop sterilizers to large chamber sterilizers, depending on their use and applications (Fig. 5.2). A variety of steam sterilization cycles may be used depending on the application. Essentially, any combination of temperature-pressure and exposure time that has been demonstrated to provide the necessary microbial reduction and has been validated for the appropriate purpose can be applied. Some of the typical overkill steam sterilization cycles are listed in Table 5.3.

Steam is widely used for reusable device sterilization in medical, dental, and veterinary facilities. Reusable devices are generally cleaned,

TABLE 5.2 Typical quality of water for injection and clean steam[a]

Property	European Pharmacopoeia (EP 4)	U.S. Pharmacopoeia (USP27-NF 22)	EN 285 (2002) steam condensate (clean steam)
Characteristic	Clear, colorless, odorless, and tasteless		Colorless, clear, no sediment
pH	5.0–7.0	5.0–7.0	5.0–7.0
Oxidizable substances	Below detection	Below detection	Below detection
Chlorides	<1 mg/liter		<1 mg/liter
Nitrates	<0.2 mg/liter		<0.2 mg/liter
Sulfates	<1 mg/liter		<1 mg/liter
Ammonium	<0.2 mg/liter		<0.2 mg/liter
Calcium/magnesium	<2 mg/liter/<1 mg/liter		<2 mg/liter/<1 mg/liter
Heavy metals[b]	<0.1 mg/liter		<0.1 mg/liter
TOC[c]		<500 ppb	
Conductivity	<1.1 μS/cm (20°C)	<1.3 μS/cm (25°C)	<3 μS/cm (20°C)
Endotoxin	<0.25 EU/ml	<0.25 EU/ml	<0.25 EU/ml

[a]The permitted levels are based on described methods in the respective guidelines.
[b]Heavy metals include iron, cadmium, and lead.
[c]TOC, total organic carbon.

TABLE 5.3 Typical steam sterilization cycles

Temperature (°C)	Time (mins)
115	≥30
121	≥15
126	≥10
132	≥4
134	≥3

wrapped in steam-penetrable and microbial retentive materials ("sterile barrier systems" that can include paper, plastics, or fabrics), and sterilized. The sterilization cycle includes the removal of air (as described above), a minimum exposure time within a minimum range of temperatures, and then evacuation. Some cycles can be followed by an extended drying cycle. Drying is essential to prevent recontamination of or damage to the material on subsequent storage and depends on the nature and size of the load. In some applications, rapid immediate-use (or "flash") sterilization cycles are used, typically at 132 to 135°C for 3 to 10 minutes in a prevacuum sterilizer (depending on the load). These cycles are primarily designed for emergency situations, e.g., where a specific device is required immediately for a surgical procedure and may have been unavailable or inadvertently contaminated during a procedure. In general, nonporous materials and nonlumened devices required shorter cycle times because air can be efficiently removed from these loads; longer times, or cycles designed with a more efficient conditioning phase for air removal, are often required for porous materials (e.g., textiles such as gowns, towels, and dressings) and lumened devices. So-called porous load cycles are designed to optimize air removal from porous loads or lumened devices. Gravity drain cycles are recommended for use with liquids and generally up to 121°C; as with any steam sterilization process, care should be taken in the design of liquid cycles to ensure even temperature distribution and to prevent boiling over of the product during heating or cooling. Examples include the laboratory or industrial sterilization of microbiology growth media and other liquids. Other loads can be conveniently sterilized by steam so long as they can withstand the required temperature, pressure, and time for sterilization. Examples include single-use devices, water, liquid media, liquid and solid wastes (including infectious materials), foods, containers, utensils, and vials.

Steam sterilization is also used for routine vessel disinfection or sterilization, including manufacturing equipment, freeze-dryers, and aseptic filling lines. It should also be noted that because steam can be generated at higher temperatures and pressures for sterilization, some processes can use the same principle to allow the liquids (including water) to be sterilized. As shown in Fig. 5.1, if the water is heated and maintained at a pressure greater than the saturation line, the water will remain in a liquid stage and be held at that temperature for the required sterilization time. These systems have been described for water and wastewater treatment. Steam production and condensation (by distillation processes) are the preferred method for the manufacture of high-quality, sterile water, including water for cleaning and water for injection, which is used during the manufacturing and use of pharmaceutical products (e.g., dilution and injection of sterile and nonsterile drugs). Steam (in particular, low-temperature steam) is used as an effective humidification and heating method, which is an essential part of other sterilization processes, including those using ethylene oxide, formaldehyde, and some oxidizing agents (such as ozone and chlorine dioxide) (see chapter 6).

Examples of various standards and guidelines for steam sterilization applications are given in Table 5.4.

5.2.3 Spectrum of Activity

The spectrum of activity of heat is discussed in chapter 2, section 2.2. Steam sterilization is widely regarded as having rapid, broad-spectrum activity. The efficacy of steam against bacteria, fungi, viruses, protozoa, and spores has been well described. *Geobacillus stearothermophilus* spores are widely regarded at the most resistant organism to steam sterilization and are therefore used to test, confirm, and validate steam sterilization processes. These processes

TABLE 5.4 Examples of standards and guidelines for steam sterilization applications

Reference[a]	Title	Summary
EN 285	Sterilization. Steam sterilizers. Large sterilizers	Specifies design requirements and the tests for large steam sterilizers primarily used in health care, laboratory, or industrial applications
EN 764-1	Pressure equipment. Vocabulary	Definitions and requirements for pressure equipment used for steam sterilization
ISO 17665-1	Sterilization of health care products. Moist heat. Requirements for the development, validation and routine control of a sterilization process for medical devices	Specifies requirements for the use of moist heat in sterilization processes, including development, validation, and routine control of the sterilization process
AAMI ST8	Hospital steam sterilizers	Construction and performance requirements for larger hospital steam sterilizers
AAMI ST79	Comprehensive guide to steam sterilization and sterility assurance in health care facilities	Guidelines on the processing of reusable devices, including steam sterilization, in health care facilities
HTM 01-01	Management and decontamination of surgical instruments (medical devices) used in acute care. Part C: steam sterilization	Guidance on the design, installation, and operation of clinical steam sterilizers
PDA technical report #1	Validation of moist heat sterilization processes: cycle design, development, qualification and ongoing control	Guidance on the development and validation of steam sterilization cycles in industrial applications

[a]EN, European Norm; ISO, International Standards Organization; AAMI, Association for the Advancement of Medical Instrumentation; HTM, Health Technical Memorandum (United Kingdom); PDA, Parenteral Drug Association.

may include the use of liquid suspensions, standard inoculated materials (such as biological indicators), or direct inoculation onto the surfaces being sterilized. The efficacy of steam against *G. stearothermophilus* spores depends on the intrinsic resistance of the spore crop preparation and the exposed temperature-time. The intrinsic resistance of spores varies depending on a number of factors, including their age and growth conditions, which are discussed in more detail in chapter 8, section 8.3.11. At a given intrinsic resistance (known as the *D* reference), there is a linear relationship between the exposure temperature and average *D* value of a spore preparation, similar to the discussion in section 2.2. The *D* value is defined as the time (in minutes or seconds) required at a given temperature to kill 1 log unit (or 90%) of a given microbial population; a *D* reference is usually given at 121°C (given as D_{121C}). The *Z* value, the temperature change required to change the *D* value by a factor of 10, can also be determined for the spore population. The *D* and *Z* values for a given spore population are determined by exposure to various temperatures and various times. These reference terms are usually provided by the spore or biological indicator manufacturer and are determined in tightly controlled pressure vessels for steam exposure known as BIER vessels. Therefore, for a given spore population with a typical *Z* value of 10°C and a determined *D* reference of 1 minute at 121°C, the predicted log reductions at various exposure temperatures can be calculated and graphed (Fig. 5.9).

Using this graph as a reference, for any given temperature, the minimum sterilization time can be determined based on the required log reduction. For most steam sterilization processes, where overkill is desired with an initial population of 6 $\log_{10}$ spores, a minimum 12 $\log_{10}$ reduction is typically recommended to give a sterility assurance level of 10^{-6} (see chapter 1, section 1.4.3). With the example of Fig. 5.9, a 12 $\log_{10}$ reduction may be achieved at 131°C for 72 seconds (6 seconds × 12 = 72 seconds) or at 141°C for 7.2 seconds (0.6 seconds x 12 = 7.2 seconds). It can therefore be appreciated that for typical steam sterilization processes, contact temperatures and times have an appreciable safety factor built into them. An example is device sterilization cycles at 134°C for >3

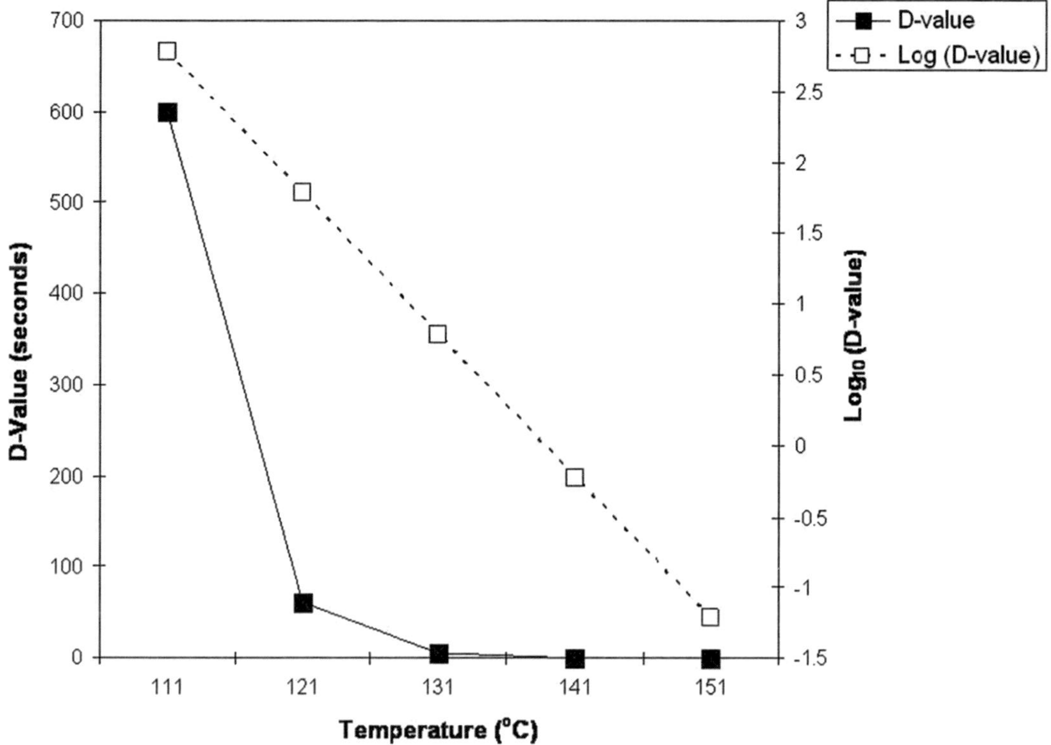

FIGURE 5.9 Effect of temperature on the lethality of a *G. stearothermophilus* spore population with a D_{121C} of 1 minute and a *Z* value of 10°C.

minutes, which can be estimated from Fig. 5.9 to provide a theoretical reduction of ~60 $\log_{10}$ units for the organism most resistant to steam; this is a conservative estimate, because it would not include any additional lethality due to the increase and subsequent decrease in temperature during the conditioning and cool-down phases of the cycle.

Organic and inorganic soils can prevent the penetration of steam. Examples include lipid materials, which can repel water molecules, and to a greater extent, salt crystals, which can form around microorganisms on drying and delay steam access. Practical examples of inorganic salts that can protect microorganisms include calcium carbonate (which can precipitate from hard water, for example, on rinsing following a cleaning process) and iron oxide (which can form as red-brown deposits or rust on a surface). As with any disinfection or sterilization process, it is therefore important that the surface is clean to ensure the optimum efficacy; for wastes or other soiled surfaces, extended sterilization times are usually adopted to ensure adequate penetration and content exposure.

Prion inactivation requires special consideration. Although the exact nature of the infectious agent in transmissible spongiform encephalopathies (chapter 1, section 1.3.6) is unknown, it is widely accepted to be proteinaceous in nature and is termed a "prion," to denote an infectious protein. In experiments, steam sterilization has been shown to significantly reduce the infectivity of prion preparations, but residual infectivity has been identified in many of these investigations. This may be due to the use of grossly soiled preparations (i.e., brain homogenates) in these experiments and incomplete accessibility of steam to the infectious particles. In cases of known or suspected transmissible spongiform encepha-

TABLE 5.5 Typical steam sterilization cycles recommended for prion inactivation on contaminated surfaces.[a] Similar methods are used for liquid or tissue-contaminated materials (see chapter 8, section 8.9)

Sterilizer type	Process	Comments
Gravity displacement	Immersion in 1 N NaOH and autoclave at 121°C for 30 minutes	Can cause damage to the autoclave
	Immersion in 1 N NaOH for 1 hour; remove, place into water, and autoclave at 121°C for 1 hour	NaOH treatment can be substituted with 2–2.5% sodium hypochlorite; devices should be resistant to chemical treatment
	Immersion in 1 N NaOH for 1 hour; remove, rinse in water, remove, and autoclave at 121°C for 1 hour	
	Immersion in water and autoclave at 134°C for 18 minutes	
	121–132°C for ≥1 hour	
Porous load	Immersion in 1 N NaOH for 1 hour; remove, rinse in water, remove, and autoclave at 134°C for 1 hour	NaOH treatment can be substituted with 2–2.5% sodium hypochlorite; devices should be resistant to chemical treatment
	134°C for ≥18 minutes	

[a]Note that in some case the methods given are considered pretreatments, where devices are then further cleaned and sterilized according to normal practices.

lopathy disease, extended steam sterilization cycles are widely recommended (Table 5.5), although in most cases, known contaminated critical devices are generally not reused and are discarded or incinerated.

Prion inactivation by steam sterilization has been shown to be more effective when the contaminated material is kept hydrated by immersion in water or sodium hydroxide (1 to 2 N NaOH). The use of NaOH may cause damage to the sterilizer due to the production of hydroxide aerosols, which can damage the pressure chamber or associated seals/pipework, as well as pose safety risks in the handling of high concentrations of hydroxide. Special applications have been described for the high-temperature/high-pressure liquid sterilization of devices and materials (including whole animals) with 1 to 2 N NaOH in specifically designed pressure vessels.

5.2.4 Advantages

Steam sterilization processes are generally considered reliable and efficient for the sterilization of liquids, foods, and solid materials, including devices. Steam demonstrates broad-spectrum antimicrobial activity, and steam processes often have a significant safety factor built into them to ensure lethality. The processes are flexible and predictable, depending on the required temperature (and pressure), contact time, and minimum log reduction requirements. The apparatuses are economical, widely available, and generally easy to use. Running costs are also considered low. Materials can be sterilized within their packaging for subsequent storage or sterile handling, which is particularly important for provision of sterilized medical devices such as critical surgical implants and instruments.

5.2.5 Disadvantages

Steam sterilization is not suitable for temperature- or pressure-sensitive materials or devices. In some cases, despite the material's resistance to heat, some materials may demonstrate stress cracking or other effects on single or repeated steam sterilization and drying cycles. Care should be taken to ensure that materials have effectively cooled down before handling them; in some cases, the cooling-down time is a disadvantage, for example, in large vessels used in manufacturing facilities. The success of steam penetration is dependent on the optimal removal (or uniform mixing) of trapped air or other noncondensable gases. For this reason, specific steam sterilization cycles are recommended for materials such as porous loads (including fabrics, towels, etc.) and devices that have long internal channels/lumens. Special consideration may also be required for the sterilization of liquids and sealed containers to prevent loss or damage, respectively. Unlike dry heat, steam has not been found to be very effective against endotoxins (although some reduction in endotoxin activity has been reported). Endotoxins are released from the cell wall of Gram-negative bacteria (chapter 1, section 1.3.7) and can be present in water or released at high concentrations from the presence of these organisms following cell death by steam (or during steam generation). In some critical applications, it may be important to control the level of endotoxin on a surface for sterilization (e.g., surgical devices) or in source water (for example, in the production of water for injection). Like all other sterilization methods, the presence of organic and, in particular, inorganic soils can retard the penetration of steam. The purity of the steam should be controlled and is often underestimated; the presence of chlorine (or chlorides, which can promote rusting) and hardness or heavy metals (which can lead to scaling and deposits on surfaces) in steam can lead to surface damage (corrosion) or unwanted deposits. This is a particular concern in the industrial sterilization of critical devices but is a growing concern in hospitals due to device damage.

5.2.6 Mode of Action

Steam, as a source of heat, has multiple effects on the viability of microorganisms, (discussed in chapter 2, section 2.2). An initial increase in temperature causes changes in structure (e.g., unfolding) and then denaturation of proteins, nucleic acids, and lipids. This is rapidly followed by the coagulation of protein and other components to result in cell death. Higher temperatures are required to penetrate the multiple protective layers of bacterial spores, which are primarily responsible for their intrinsic resistance to heat; it should also be noted that the presence of internal spore levels of dipicolinic acid and calcium is considered to play a role in protecting proteins in the inner core against heat damage (further discussed in chapter 8, section 8.3.11).

5.3 DRY HEAT STERILIZATION

5.3.1 Types

Dry heat may be defined as hot air or more specifically as heat at humidity levels of less than 100% (in contrast to saturated steam). Dry heat sterilization methods include the use of ovens and incinerators.

Incineration is essentially burning to ashes, which can be performed by passing material through a naked flame (for example, in microbiological manipulations by flaming) or much larger-scale applications in kilns or furnaces. Larger, modern, industrial-scale furnace designs include processes to move the materials being incinerated during the process (to maximize incineration of the load and have emission control strategies in place to reduce pollution concerns). Examples include moving grate (also referred to as municipal solid waste) incinerators and rotary kiln designs. Typical incineration temperatures are maintained at 800 to 1,300°C (1,472 to 2,372°F), with the required time dependent on the incinerator design, size, and nature of the load.

Dry-heat sterilizers (Fig. 5.10) are simple designs consisting of an oven chamber to hold the load, which is typically fed with electrically heated air at the desired sterilization temperature range. Heat is therefore transmitted to the sterilizer load by air convection. Monitoring of the temperature within the chamber is important to ensure that the correct sterilization temperatures are attained and maintained during the exposure cycle. Dry-heat sterilizer designs include static-heat sterilizers and forced-air sterilizers. In the static-heat designs, air is heated directly from electric coils (usually at the base of the sterilizer chamber) and allowed to permeate through the chamber by gravity (hot air rises). These designs are generally smaller in size and are associated with longer cycle times (due to slower heat-up times to set sterilization temperatures), and it can be difficult to ensure heat uniformity within the load to be sterilized.

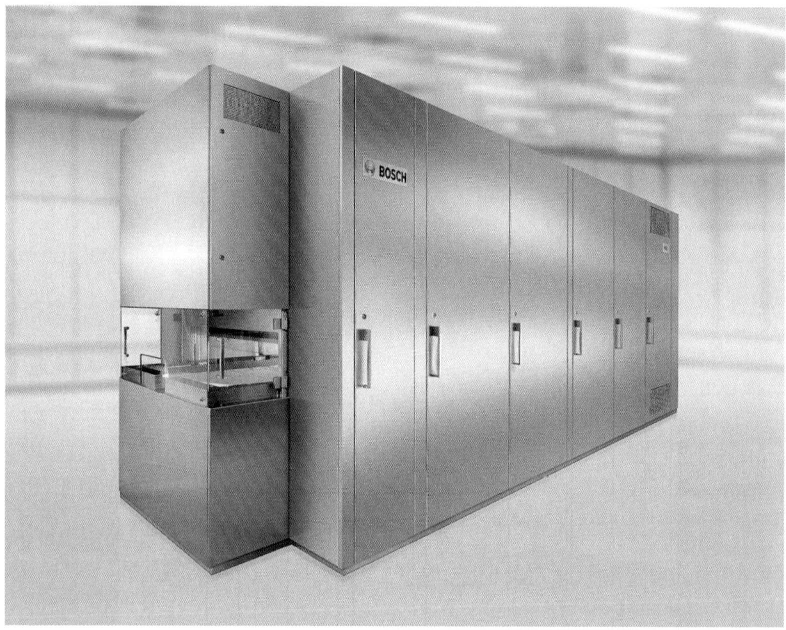

FIGURE 5.10 A series of industrial dry-heat sterilizers used for dry-heat sterilization and depyrogenation. Image courtesy of Bosch.

In contrast, forced-air sterilizers use various blowing mechanisms (e.g., filtered air centrifugal fans) to increase the heat distribution and turbulence within the chamber, thereby improving sterilizer efficiency. Most larger, modern sterilizer ovens contain fans (or other air-movement mechanisms) to ensure equal air temperature distribution and are maintained at a slight positive pressure during sterilization.

Typical dry-air sterilization cycles include conditioning to the specified, uniform temperature, sterilization (under controlled temperature and time), and then cooling to <80°C to allow access to the load. Sterilization temperatures (typically >160°C) are much higher and exposure times longer than moist-heat sterilization, because air is a less efficient conductor of heat than steam (see section 5.2). Typical dry-air sterilization hold conditions include the following:

- 160°C for 120 minutes
- 170°C for 60 minutes
- 180°C for 30 minutes
- 190°C for 6 minutes

Following sterilization, ambient air is introduced through a HEPA filter and circulated through the load for cooling. Additional cooling is often necessary before further handling, but this can be achieved outside the sterilizer chamber under controlled conditions.

5.3.2 Applications

Incineration is used for the disposal of contaminated medical, veterinary, and industrial wastes including needles, sharps, plastics, and other materials. Wastes are usually reduced to <10% of the starting material, so incineration is often a method of choice to significantly reduce the volume of waste in comparison to other methods. Dry-heat sterilizers are rarely used for reusable surgical device sterilization but can be used for sterilization (and disinfection) of temperature-resistant materials including wound dressings, laboratory glassware, materials, some single-use devices, and certain food applications such as oils (Fig. 5.10). Industrial and laboratory applications include the sterilization of powders and water-insoluble materials, including oils, fats, and ointments; essentially, dry heat is used for materials that cannot be sterilized by moist heat due to risks of moisture damage or lack of penetration. Dry heat is also an effective depyrogenation method (e.g., 180°C for 4 hours) for glassware and other laboratory materials, parenteral vials, and other heat-resistant surfaces.

5.3.3 Spectrum of Activity

The antimicrobial activity of dry heat is less understood than that of moist heat, but it is regarded as being rapidly effective against vegetative organisms including bacteria, molds, yeasts, and protozoa. Similar to moist heat, enveloped viruses are sensitive to dry heat at ~60°C, but some nonenveloped viruses (including parvoviruses) have been shown to survive up to 100°C (in some cases with similar resistance for bacterial spores). The activity of dry heat varies depending on the test matrix (for example, dried salts and proteins can protect organisms from heat penetration), the test microbial populations, surface inoculation, the presence of humidity (in the air or load being sterilized), etc. Bacterial spores are recognized as the most resistant organisms to dry heat (Table 5.6), with *Bacillus atrophaeus* (previously known as *Bacillus subtilis* subsp. *niger*) being used as a biological indicator for the purposes of sterilization efficacy validation and routine monitoring. As with moist heat, the exposure time for sterilization is inversely proportional to the temperature, i.e., lower temperatures require longer exposure times, and vice versa.

Dry heat is not considered effective at reducing prion infectivity but is widely used for the reduction of endotoxins and other pyrogens (i.e., depyrogenation). Typical depyrogenation cycles include 250°C for 30 minutes or 200°C for 60 minutes.

TABLE 5.6 Examples of bacterial spore resistance to dry heat at 160°C

Bacteria species	Average *D* value (minutes)[a]
Clostridium sporogenes	1.0
B. atrophaeus	1.8
Bacillus megarterium	0.1
Bacillus cereus	0.05
Bacillus stearothermophilus	1.5

[a]*D* values can vary significantly depending on the spore preparation and test methods.

5.3.4 Advantages

Dry-heat sterilization is less expensive than steam processes, is easy to perform, and demonstrates broad-spectrum antimicrobial efficacy. It is a useful process for the sterilization of moisture-sensitive but heat-resistant surfaces (such as some metals and glass), liquids (oils and ointments), and solids (powders). It may also be a useful alterative to moist-heat sterilization for pressure-sensitive materials and devices. Dry heat is often considered more penetrating than moist heat over time, but this depends on the moist-heat process (e.g., prevacuum or gravity cycles [see section 5.2]). For some materials, dry heat is preferred, due to the lack of corrosion or other effects (e.g., water residuals or damage) that result from moist-heat processes. Incineration is a useful method for the sterilization and management of waste materials, as well as a significant waste-reduction mechanism. Dry heat is a particularly effective depyrogenation method and is widely used for that purpose for laboratories, devices, and pharmaceutical production.

5.3.5 Disadvantages

Dry heat cannot be used for many widely used rubbers, plastics, and other temperature-sensitive materials. It is clear that liquids cannot be effectively sterilized, unless dry heat is used as a heating mechanism alone (and therefore not directly as the sterilant). Higher temperatures and longer cycle times (including attaining, maintaining, and cooling temperatures) are required in comparison to other sterilization processes. This can lead to material damage, in particular on surfaces exposed to multiple cycles over time, despite the general heat resistance of these materials. Examples include stress cracking, warping, and burning.

Hot air rises within the chamber, which may lead to stratification of heat distribution. Therefore, adequate air circulation is required to ensure that the sterilization temperature is attained and is uniform in all areas of the load; it is particularly important that the chamber is not overloaded, because overloading could hinder heat distribution. Care should be taken to ensure that loads have been allowed to cool sufficiently prior to handling them.

Incineration emissions are the subject of increased regulatory controls due to the production of toxic by-products such as dioxins and furans (which are biocumulative and stable in the environment) and chlorine monoxide. Control measures should be considered for reducing these pollution effects.

5.3.6 Mode of Action

The mode of action of dry heat is considered different from moist heat, not only because of the effects of temperature but also due to oxidation (removal of electrons) from cellular and viral particle components. These effects both lead to loss of the structure and function of biomolecules including proteins, lipids, and nucleic acids. It is clear that during conditioning and sterilization exposure dry heat causes any water content in the surrounding environment (e.g., humidity) or intracellular water to heat and eventually boil, which causes effects similar to moist-heat sterilization, including protein degradation and precipitation of cellular components. The water content in the air and in heat-resistant spores plays a role in the observed activity of dry heat, with greater resistance observed at humidity levels between 20 and 40% (Fig. 5.11). Further, the ultimate removal of water causes the loss of biomolecule function and structure. Dry heat causes rapid loss of outer viral envelopes and disintegration of viral particles, although nonenveloped viruses are significantly more resistant to these effects. The mode of action against pyrogens (including lipopolysaccharides) is unknown but is, for example, associated with the loss of endotoxin structure and its effects on the immune system. This may be due to the direct incineration of endotoxin by the dry-heat process, but also due to oxidation effects.

5.4 RADIATION STERILIZATION

5.4.1 Types

As discussed in chapter 2, section 2.4, radiation is energy in the form of particles or electromagnetic waves. For radiation sterilization, only high-energy or ionizing radiation

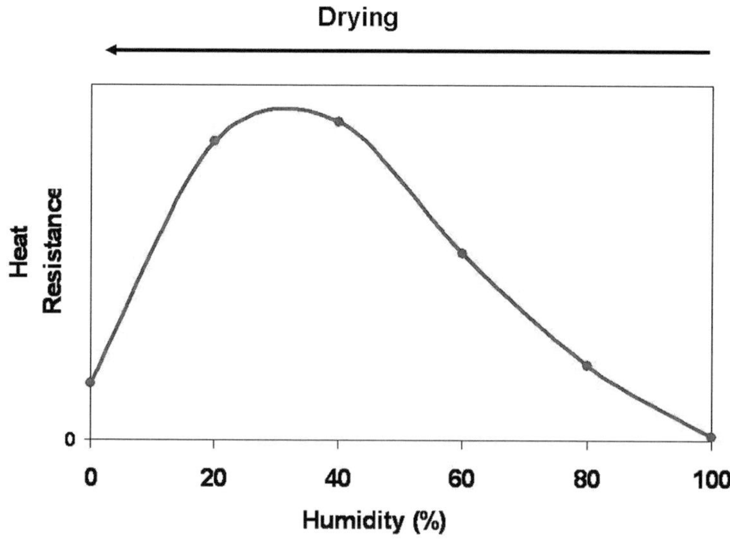

FIGURE 5.11 Representative effect of humidity/water content on the dry-heat resistance of bacterial spores.

sources are utilized due to their greater penetration and antimicrobial efficacy. Ionizing radiation has sufficient energy to cause the release of electrons from target atoms in a given compound, which leads to the loss of essential structure and function and antimicrobial activity. The most widely used ionizing-radiation types are γ radiation, X rays, and electron (or E) beams. γ radiation and X rays are electromagnetic radiation, which is light waves consisting of photons that have no mass or electric charge and travel at the speed of light in a wave-like pattern (see section 2.4). γ radiation is a higher-energy, penetrating source of radiation that is released from radioactive nucleotides, specifically from their unstable nuclei. X rays have less associated energy and penetrating ability that is typically produced from generators, specifically from electrons orbiting their nuclei. Other forms of electromagnetic radiation are mostly used for disinfection purposes, including UV, infrared, and microwaves (section 2.4). An E beam is a source of particle radiation consisting of beams of electrons (or β radiation) that are accelerated to improve their penetration. Like X rays, E-beam particles have sufficient energy to cause the release of electrons from orbiting electrons of target atoms (ionization).

γ radiation is energy in the form of electromagnetic waves (high-energy photons), which are released on the decay of isotopes (or radionucleotides) such as cobalt-60, cesium-137, and iridium-192. Isotopes are unstable atoms that have an overall positive or negative nuclear charge, due to an imbalance in the ratio of neutrons (uncharged) to protons (positively charged) in their nuclei (chapter 2, section 2.4). An example is an isotope of cobalt, ^{60}Co. Elemental cobalt (^{59}Co) is a naturally occurring metal with an atomic number of 27 (i.e., the number of protons or electrons in each atom is 27). ^{60}Co is manufactured by reacting ^{59}Co with neutrons produced from a nuclear reactor, with a subsequent increase in atomic mass (59 to 60). Over time, isotopes spontaneously break down from a higher to lower energy state in a process called radioactive decay (Fig. 5.12).

Radioactive decay proceeds at a predicable rate over time. This rate is specific to the type of isotope and is expressed as its half-life. The half-life is the time required for the radioactive activity to decrease by one-half of its initial value. ^{60}Co, as an example, has a half-life of ~5.3 years and decays to nonradioactive ^{60}Ni (elemental nickel). ^{137}Cs has a much longer half-life at ~30 years and decays in a similar

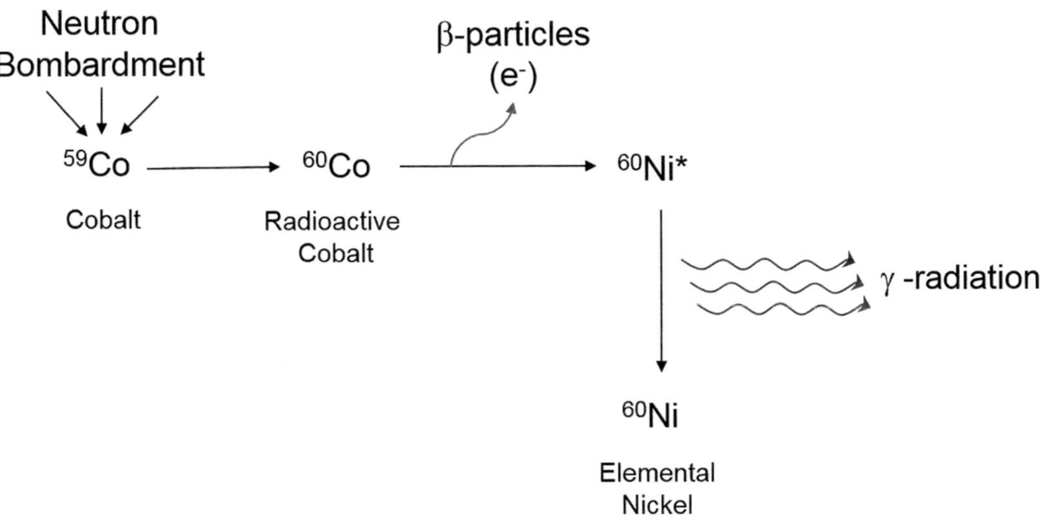

FIGURE 5.12 Generation and decay of ^{60}Co.

fashion to give ^{137}Ba. Radioactive decay causes the release of energy in the form of radiation as streaming particles (α or β radiation) or electromagnetic waves (for example, γ radiation). ^{60}Co, ^{137}Cs, and ^{192}Ir are all γ radiation emitters, but they are not pure γ emitters. As shown in Fig. 5.12, ^{60}Co decays on release of β and γ radiation. During this process, the excess neutrons decay to give a proton and release electrons (β particles). The conversion into an additional proton gives rise to a new element. Due to the lack of significant penetration of β particles, the main source of antimicrobial efficacy during sterilization with ^{60}Co is due to γ radiation alone. γ radiation has extremely short wavelengths ($<1 \times 10^{-11}$), which are high-energy sources (at $>2 \times 10^{-14}$ joules) and are therefore more penetrating and rapidly biocidal. Different isotopes decay to release γ radiation at different wavelength/energy ranges, with ^{60}Co (at 1.17 and 1.3 MeV) being more efficient and penetrating than ^{137}Cs (at 0.67 MeV) for sterilization processes.

X rays are another higher-energy form of electromagnetic radiation in the nanometer wavelength range ($\sim 1 \times 10^{-8}$ to 1×10^{-11} m). X rays have less energy than γ radiation and can be absorbed by many large (or heavier) atoms because they have greater energy differences between the orbiting electrons in their atomic structure; it is this difference between the adsorption of bone, which contains high concentrations of calcium, and smaller atoms present in skin and soft tissues that allows the use of X rays for the visualization of bone structure. Some isotopes (e.g., thalium-170) spontaneously release X rays on decay, but these are generally not used for biocidal processes. X rays are normally artificially generated by the collision of high-speed electrons with a solid metal target (Fig. 5.13).

Typical generators consist of a cathode and anode in a glass vacuum tube. The cathode is a simple filament, which is heated to cause the release of electrons (e^-). These electrons, at high speed and negatively charged, are attracted to the positively charged anode, which is made of a heavy metal such as tungsten or lead. The choice of metal dictates the frequency of X rays produced. X rays can then be generated by two processes as the high-energy electrons approach and collide with the anode metal. The first process is referred to as "brehmsstrahlung," where the electrons are slowed down as they approach the positively charged metal nuclei, causing the release of X rays (Fig. 5.13A). The second process is related to the direct interaction with orbiting electrons in the atom struc-

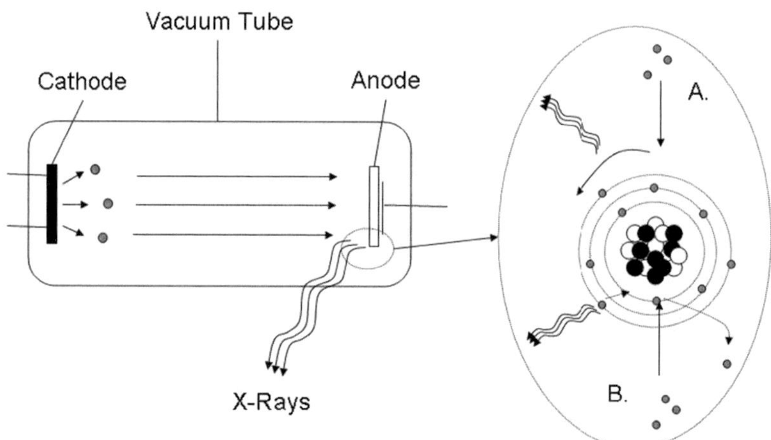

FIGURE 5.13 The generation of X rays. Electrons are produced from the cathode and react with atoms at the anode to produce electrons by two mechanisms discussed in the text.

ture. It should be remembered that electrons are organized around a given nucleus at various energy levels known as orbits. When highly energized electrons from the cathode source collide with the metal atoms, they cause the low-energy electrons orbiting close to the nucleus to be expelled (Fig. 5.13B). This is compensated for by the transition of higher-energy orbiting electrons falling to the lower energy levels with the subsequent release of energy in the form of photons in the X-ray wavelength range. Because these reactions cause the release of heat, X-ray generators are usually cooled (for example, in oil baths) and are contained within a lead shield, which prevents the release of X rays except through a designated window in a controlled manner. X rays are exceptionally biocidal and penetrating, the extent to which depends on the wavelength range produced.

Electrons, or β-particle radiation, are extremely reactive but on their own lack sufficient penetration for most sterilization processes. However, electrons produced from a source can be focused and accelerated in electric or magnetic fields to produce a more effective high-energy beam for sterilization processes, known as electron beam, or E beam. These beams are typically within the 1 to 10 MeV range. E beams are produced and accelerated in a variety of machines known as accelerators (Fig. 5.14). Accelerators can be either linear or circular and vary in design.

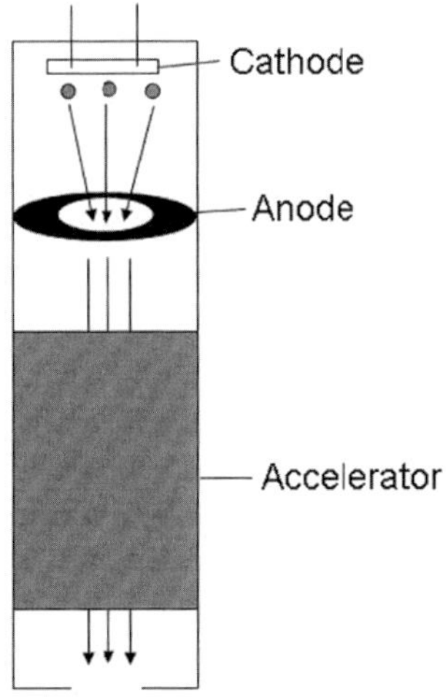

FIGURE 5.14 A simplified linear high-energy E-beam generator.

Electrons are produced in an apparatus known as an electron gun, in a process similar to that described for the generation of X rays. Electrons are generated under vacuum by heating a cathode, for example, by the pulsing or continuous application of an electric current. The cathode is made of a thermionic material, for example, a metal such as tungsten or mixed oxides, which release electrons when heated. The electrons are then attracted to but at the same time deflected from an anode under an electromagnetic field, which focuses the beam into an accelerator. The accelerator uses an electric field to increase the speed of the electrons, depending on the required energy level. Low- and medium-energy accelerators (at <5 MeV) use a high voltage to generate a steady electric field, while high-energy accelerators (at 5 to 10 MeV) use radio frequency or microwave energy. In general, the longer the accelerator, the greater the energy of the E beam. The electron beam can then be controlled under a magnetic field to allow for direct application to a given target product.

5.4.2 Applications

Ionizing radiation sources can be used for a variety of disinfection and sterilization processes, including devices, foods (including pasteurization and insect deinfestation), cosmetics, water, wastewater, and some air/gas applications. Sterilization can be routinely achieved for pharmaceutical products, including ointments, liquids, and dry materials, and prepackaged devices or garments. A typical list of materials that are sterilized or otherwise treated with radiation is given in Table 5.7.

The usual dose applied in each case depends on the load and the required level of biocidal activity. In all radiation processes, the sterilization efficacy can be verified by the amount of adsorbed radiation dose (by dosimetry). Radiation exposure is expressed as the amount of

TABLE 5.7 Example of materials disinfected and/or sterilized by radiation

Liquids	Devices
Alcohol wipes	Pacemakers
Sterile disinfectants	Orthopedic and other implants
Cements	Surgical sutures
Water	Needles and syringes
Serum	
Proteins and enzymes	
Lubrication gels	
Foods	**Other materials**
Fruits and vegetables	Tissues such as excised skin
Meats and poultry	Petri plates and other plasticware
Prepackaged meals	Test tubes
Spices and other dried foods	Cotton balls
	Gloves and gowns
	Bandages
	Bottles and other liquid containers

absorbed dose (or energy) applied to a load and is expressed in grays (Gy or kiloGy [kGy]). Typical dose ranges for radiation processes are given in Table 5.8.

A variety of dosimeters are used to measure the adsorbed dose, including calorimeters and spectrophotometers. Calorimeters monitor the increase in temperature in the load, which is related to the adsorbed dose; for example, a 10-kGy dose will raise the temperature of water by 2.4°C. Spectrophotometric methods are more widely and routinely used to monitor the penetration of radiation into various parts of a sterilization load. These dosimeters can essentially contain any material that has been calibrated to react with radiation over a dose range to change in structure and therefore detect the dose applied. These include various types of radiosensitive dyes or other radiosensitive materials integrated into an indicator (or dosimeter) system. Examples include ferrous ion (Fe^{2+})-containing formulations (which form ferric ions, Fe^{3+}, on exposure), alanine dosimeters (alanine pellets that form stable free radicals on exposure, which is detected by spectroscopy), and a variety of radiochromic dyed plastics, films, and nondyed polymers.

γ and X rays are preferred for the sterilization of denser materials or loads, which can include certain foods and metallic (or mixed-load) medical devices, because they are more penetrating than E beams. These applications include the sterilization of solid and liquid pharmaceutical products, ointments, and raw materials. E-beam applications have traditionally been more limited, depending on the energy level, but have been efficient for surface and small-load sterilization. In time, more advanced E-beam systems and technologies are expected to be able to accommodate a wider range of sterilization loads and materials. The efficiency of E-beam radiation is more dependent on the product load density, size, orientation, and packaging. X-ray and E-beam applications are in general more flexible because they can be conveniently turned off when not in use, unlike the use of isotopes as γ-radiation sources.

Radiation sources may also be used to initiate chemical reactions such as polymerization and physical and chemical material modifications (e.g., cross-linking of polymers to increase rigidity) and to cause the breakdown of unwanted chemicals including organic contaminants such as benzene and toluene. X rays and γ radiation are also used for a variety of medical applications including visualization of internal structures and cancer therapy.

For sterilization, a load is exposed to γ radiation in an irradiator, which can be designed for continuous-duty or batch-type applications (Fig. 5.15). The radiation source is usually stored under water and raised for exposure to the load for the desired exposure time (often

TABLE 5.8 Typical doses of radiation for biocidal and other applications

Typical radiation absorbed doses (kGy)[a]	Applications
<1 kGy	Surface modification, deinfestation, food preservation
1–10 kGy	Disinfection, pasteurization
10–100 kGy	Food, medical device sterilization, polymer and other material modification

[a]1 Gy = 100 rad; 1 kGy = 0.1 Mrad.

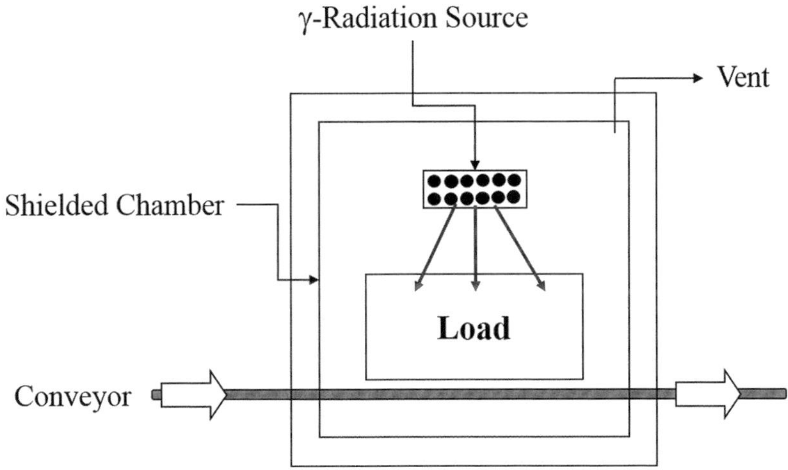

FIGURE 5.15 A typical γ irradiator sterilizer.

over a few minutes) (Fig. 5.16). The exposure chamber, similar to other irradiator chambers, is shielded by concrete (typically up to 10 feet thick) to prevent worker exposure. The conveyor system can be designed to allow rotation of the load around the γ-radiation source to ensure adequate product exposure and penetration. It is important that sterilization cycles are specifically developed for each load type, with consideration of load density, method of conveyance, and minimum exposure time required for the process. Underdosing may not achieve the desired sterilization criteria, while overdosing may lead to load damage. Following cycle development, only the exposure time and age of the radiation source need to be monitored for controlled loads.

A radiation dose of 25 kGy (or 2.5 Mrad) of absorbed energy is generally considered sufficient for γ sterilization in a typical pro-

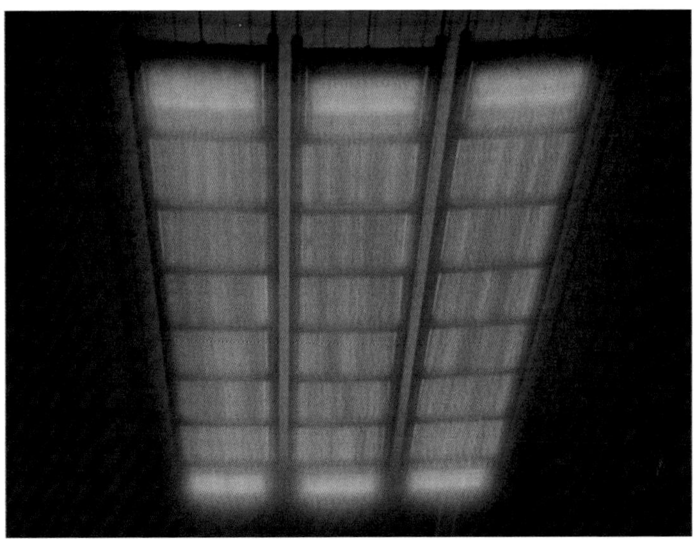

FIGURE 5.16 A typical exposure rack containing ^{60}Co as a γ-radiation source with a γ irradiator sterilizer.

cess, but this can be varied depending on the product bioburden (see chapter 1, section 1.4.2.3), radiation validation method, and load configuration.

X rays or E beams may be applied to a load in a similar fashion. Processes can be as a single batch or, more commonly, as a continuous-duty process, where the product is passed on a conveyor belt through the beam (Fig. 5.17). E beams may be applied in a single direction (as shown in Fig. 5.17) or in multiple directions to increase load penetration. Other applications have included the use of X rays and E beams in pharmaceutical production, e.g., integrated into aseptic filling lines.

In general, radiation sterilization processes are rapid, requiring no preconditioning, exposures times of a few seconds or minutes, and minimal aeration times. During the process, activated species such as ozone and radicals can be formed; they are short-lived and vented from the chamber.

Examples of standards and guidelines for radiation sterilization applications are given in Table 5.9.

5.4.3 Spectrum of Activity

When radiation is applied to a load, antimicrobial effects can be direct and indirect. Directly, radiation can cause a variety of biochemical effects, with the primary target being the nucleic acids, which have been particularly studied for DNA. Indirect effects are caused by the production of free radicals, ozone, and other short-lived and reactive species that have significant antimicrobial effects but can also increase damage to surfaces. For this reason, an increase in oxygen tension in a load can result in a greater production of free radicals and other oxygenated species. The combination of these direct and indirect effects is associated with the broad-spectrum efficacy of radiation methods.

In general, most types of bacteria, viruses, fungi, and protozoa are relatively sensitive to radiation doses of <1 kGy. In addition, ionizing radiation has been shown to neutralize the toxicity of toxins, including endotoxin. Despite this, data in the literature vary due to the different test methods used to determine the antimicrobial effects at various radiation doses. For example, *Escherichia coli* and *Pseudomonas*

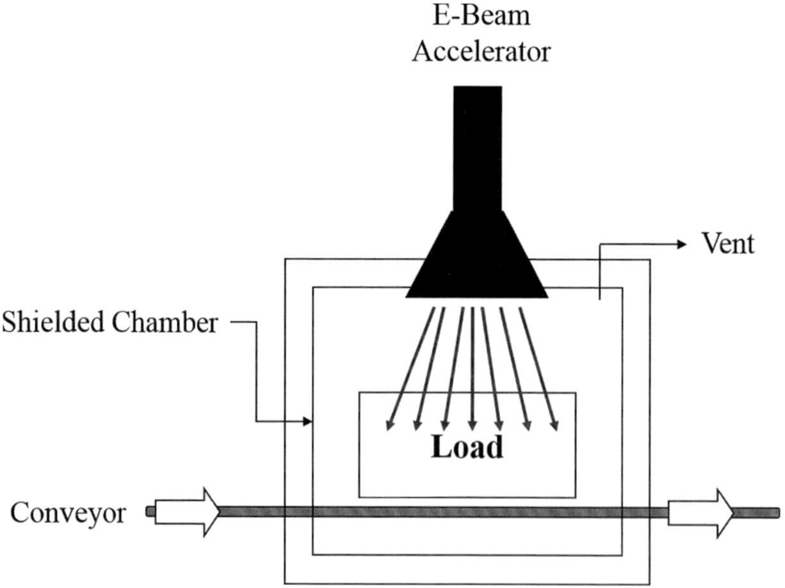

FIGURE 5.17 A typical E-beam sterilizer; an X-ray sterilizer can be in a similar orientation, with an X-ray source as an alternative to the E-beam accelerator.

TABLE 5.9 Examples of standards and guidelines for radiation sterilization applications

Reference[a]	Title	Summary
ISO 11137-1	Sterilization of health care products. Requirements for the development, validation and routine control of a sterilization process for medical devices - radiation - part 1: requirements	Specifies requirements for the development, validation, and routine control of a radiation sterilization process for medical devices, including γ radiation, E beam, and X ray
ISO 11137-2	Sterilization of health care products. Radiation - part 2: establishing the sterilization dose	Guidance on the radiation dose required for sterilization
ISO/ASTM 51702	Standard practice for dosimetry in a gamma facility for radiation processing	General guidelines on the use of γ radiation for sterilization, including installation and dosimetry procedures
PDA technical report 11	Sterilization of parenterals by gamma radiation	Guidance on the development and validation of γ-sterilization processes for drug manufacturing
IAEA radiation technology series 4	Guidelines for the development, validation and routine control of industrial radiation processes	Guidance on meeting the requirements of international standards regarding the development, validation, and routine control of radiation processes

[a]EN, European Norm; AAMI, Association for the Advancement of Medical Instrumentation; ASTM, American Society for Testing and Materials; ISO, International Standards Organization; EAEA, International Atomic Energy Agency; PDA, Parenteral Drug Association.

spp. have been reported to have *D* values (1 $\log_{10}$ reduction of a population) at relatively low doses (~60 Gy), and protozoa (including amoeba) within the 100 to 1,000 Gy range. Vegetative bacteria and fungi were found to range in resistance from 60 to 1,000 Gy. In general, Gram-positive bacteria have been reported to be more sensitive than Gram-negative bacteria, but this varies from strain to strain. Viruses also vary in resistance within this range, with nonenveloped viruses being more resistant than enveloped viruses. Traditionally, as for other sterilization methods, bacterial spores were considered most resistant to radiation, and *Bacillus pumilus* spores were recommended for use in the development and verification of sterilization cycles (although this has been replaced by the use of radiation dose monitoring as described above). The radiation resistance of bacterial spores has been reported in the 0.6 to 4 kGy range. In all these cases, the observed resistance varied depending on the test method and presence of interfering substances. For example, the resistance of *B. pumilus* spores ranged from 1 to 4 kGy depending on whether testing was conducted under dry conditions, liquid conditions, or in the presence of various soils or salts. This is an important consideration for viruses, which are typically associated with extraneous materials; with nonenveloped viruses, suboptimal exposure conditions may elicit capsid and envelope damage but not sufficient nucleic acid damage to render all viruses noninfectious.

However, many types of vegetative bacteria and archaea have been described as ionizing radiation resistance organisms; these may be defined as having unique resistance profiles at radiation doses >1 kGy. Notably, these have included bacterial strains of *Deinococcus radiodurans* and other *Deinococcus* spp. that, in some cases, have been reported to have radiation resistance profiles in the 5- to 30-kGy range. Studies of these strains have shown an accumulation of resistance mechanisms that are responsible for the resistance phenotypes, including active DNA repair mechanisms, and protective and structural effects (see chapter 8, section 8.3.9). Other types of bacteria and archaea with similar resistance profiles include strains of *Geodermatophilus*, *Hymenobacter*, and *Rubrobacter*, as well as certain strains of *Thermococcus* and *Pyrococcus* that have parallel high resistance to thermal disinfection (see chapter 1, section 1.3.4.2, and section 8.3.10). Strains of *Acinetobacter*, *Methylobacterium*, and *Kocuria* have also been isolated with unique resistance profiles to radiation. These strains have been identified as naturally occurring and also can be induced under laboratory conditions by exposure to low doses of radiation over time, such as with strains of *Salmonella enterica* serovar Typhimurium and *E. coli*. In these cases, resistance mechanisms were predominantly due to active or overexpressed repair mechanisms, which can reverse the damage to DNA at suboptimal exposure conditions.

For these reasons, during many applications with radiation and validation procedures, it is important to understand and control the bioburden that is normally present on the material or load to be sterilized (see chapter 1, section 1.4.2.3) to reduce the risks associated with thc presence of these strains. This is an example of a bioburden-based approach to sterilization validation (see section 1.4.3). Periodic dose auditing is recommended to ensure that the bioburden present is adequately inactivated by the radiation sterilization method. This is performed by exposing the material to be sterilized to a lower radiation dose expected to inactivate the bioburden and to confirm sterility, thus confirming the expected sterilization effectiveness of the higher dose used for routine sterilization.

5.4.4 Advantages

The greatest advantages of radiation sterilization methods are reliability and acceptability as a sterilization process. These processes are essentially "cold," although increases in temperatures should be monitored during the various processes due to the heat that can be generated on exposure. Radiation sterilization processes, unlike heat or chemical sterilization, do not require preconditioning for heat or humidity, nor do they require postprocess aeration, because they are essentially chemical- and residue-free. It is important to note that products are exposed to radiation ("irradiated") but are not themselves made "radioactive," which is a common misperception. Products can be packaged in a variety of material types and orientations, including final packaging, and exposure times are rapid (generally from a few seconds to a few minutes). X rays and γ radiation are significantly more penetrating than E beams. E-beam and X-ray machines are generally lower cost (installation and maintenance) than γ-irradiators, with X rays requiring less energy; X rays generally cause a lower increase in temperature and, with γ radiation, provide a more uniform dose to a load.

5.4.5 Disadvantages

Radiation has been limited to industrial applications due to cost and safety considerations. The risks associated with accidental exposure to radiation need to be tightly controlled, which requires significant capital investment. It is for this reason that radiation sterilization is not widely used and is generally restricted to specific facilities that provide contract sterilization services. It is also necessary to ensure that all portions of a load are contacted by the radiation source to ensure adequate contact time and dose; this can be a particular concern with low-dose E-beam exposure. In the case of γ radiation and the use of isotopes, there may be concerns regarding the disposal of radioactive waste, which requires specific handling and control. The bombardment of materials, in particular, certain types of plastic polymers, foods, and biological materials, with radiation may also cause embrittlement or other negative effects. For example, γ radiation is incompatible with polyvinyl chloride, polytetrafluoroethylene, and acetyl, depending on the dose. E beams can also cause damage to plastics (such as polypropylene) and some resins. Overall, materials that require special consideration for radiation sterilization include polyethylene, silicon rubber, polypropylene, and Teflon. These effects can be due to cross-linking and/or chain breakage. It is therefore necessary during cycle development to minimize the radiation dose applied to a load required for sterilization. Alternative approaches include the formulation of polymers with reducing agents, which may limit the negative effects of radiation exposure, while strengthening the material by cross-linking on exposure to high doses of radiation. Because the application of radiation also causes an increase in temperature, further consideration should be given to ensure that the load does not overheat, which could cause damage to temperature-sensitive materials or monitoring processes. Other effects can include discoloration, unpleasant odor generation, changes in taste, and accelerated aging of materials. These effects may restrict applications with certain types of drugs, foodstuffs, or other materials.

5.4.6 Mode of Action

Radiation causes electron disruption (ionization) in the atoms of molecules that can be essential for microbiological structure, metabolism, and survival. This causes direct disruption of structural and functional molecules, including lipids, proteins, and nucleic acids. An example of this is the fact that radiation processes are less effective at lower temperature, presumably due to low metabolic rates. Radiation has been specifically shown to cause mutations in DNA and other nucleic acids, which leads to cell death or lack of viability. Indirectly, the production of free radicals occurs due to the adsorption of energy by water, oxygen, and other molecules within the target organism, leading to the production of free radicals, including OH^- and H^+, and other reactive species. These free radicals also react with various surface and internal structures, leading to a variety of oxidative and reducing effects that can also culminate in microbiological inactivation.

5.5 FILTRATION

Filtration methods can be used for sterilization of gas (such as air) and liquids, including water. These methods and applications are discussed in chapter 2, section 2.5.

5.6 OTHER PHYSICAL STERILIZATION METHODS

5.6.1 Plasma

There are three traditional states of matter: liquid, gas, and solid. Plasma may be considered the fourth state, in which the molecules of a gas are excited (by the addition of energy) to become a plasma when the gas atoms lose their associated electrons and give a highly excited mixture of charged nuclei and free electrons. A true plasma is actually considered to consist of positively and negatively charged particles in approximately equal concentrations. Plasmas can be generated by the application of sufficient energy, in the form of temperature or an electromagnetic field, to a gas. If we take the example of water, when it is at its lowest energy state, it forms a solid, or ice. As energy (in the form of temperature) is applied to ice, it becomes a liquid (water), and with further energy absorption, it boils to produce a gas (steam). A plasma can be subsequently formed by further energy absorption of the gas, which fragments the gas atoms and molecules to give negative ions, positive ions, electrons, and other short-lived reactive species. An example of the reactive species formed in an oxygen plasma is shown in Fig. 5.18.

It should be remembered that an atom of any element consists of a central nucleus (consisting of positively charged protons and neutrons, which have no charge) that is surrounded by negatively charged and paired electrons, which are organized in defined orbits (or orbitals) depending on their energy levels. In this state each atom is balanced with an overall neutral charge with an equal number of electrons and protons. As energy is applied to the atoms/molecules in a gas, the molecules and atoms fragment to give positive ions (because they now have a higher number of protons) and free, negatively charged electrons. In some cases, the electrons react with other atoms, thereby gaining an overall negative charge (negative ions). Further unstable species are also generated, including ozone (in the case of oxygen and air plasmas) and other free radicals. The other free radicals that can be formed include the hydroxyl radical (·OH); these are very reactive in that they have unpaired electrons in their outermost orbitals and therefore bind with electrons from other molecules to produce a chain reaction of electron loss and gain. Therefore, on exposure to microorganisms, a variety of effects occur, which cause structural and functional damage to cell components (including proteins, lipids, and nucleic acids),

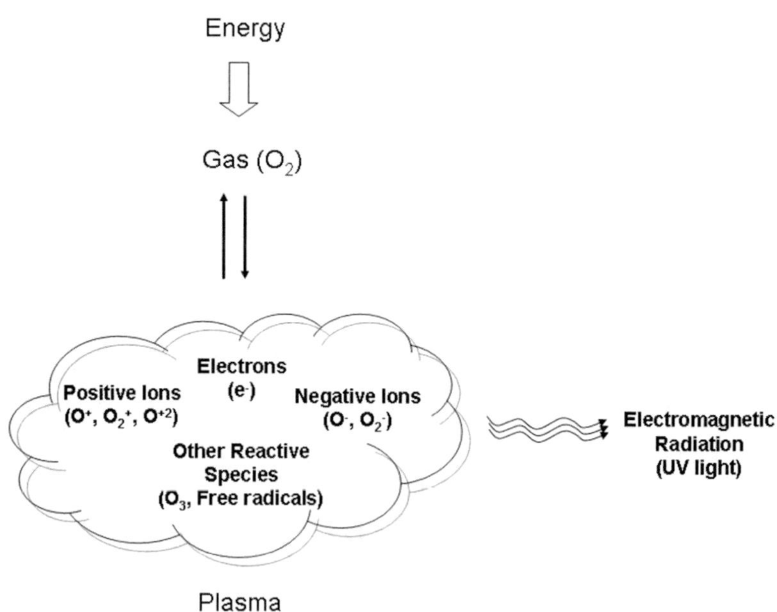

FIGURE 5.18 Example of plasma generation with oxygen gas (O_2).

leading to cell death or loss of viability. Further, with the excitation of electrons between atom orbitals, as they return to their natural states, they give off energy in the form of heat or photons, for example, within the UV wavelength range (see section 2.4). This also contributes to the antimicrobial activity (see chapter 2, section 2.4). When the energy source applied to the gas is turned off, the various species rapidly recombine into lower-energy, stable forms.

A variety of plasmas can be produced, which are usually named after the gas used to create them, e.g., oxygen or neon plasmas. Many gas types have been investigated for plasma generation, including oxygen, neon, argon, nitrogen, hydrogen peroxide, peracetic acid, aldehydes (such as formaldehyde), halogens, and mixtures thereof. As discussed above, plasmas are generated by the application of heat or electromagnetic radiation. Heat is generally not used due to the very high temperatures and pressures required for generation (e.g., up to 3,000°C). Lower-temperature plasmas are usually produced in a gas under vacuum with the application of microwave or high-energy radio frequency energy sources. These plasmas are usually generated under deep vacuums (0.001 to 0.15 kPa) and low temperatures (30 to 50°C).

Applications for plasma have included liquid waste disposal, water disinfection, and surface and air disinfection. Plasmas are used as part of sterilization processes, in particular, in combination with hydrogen peroxide (chapter 6, section 6.5) and peracetic acid (section 6.6.3). In most cases, it is the gaseous chemical (see chapter 6) that is used to provide the desired antimicrobial activity during the process, with the impact of the plasma generation playing a minor role, such as the use of low-energy plasma to generate the gas (from a liquid) for introduction into the sterilization process or the generation of plasma following gas exposure to break down gas residuals during the load aeration (or gas removal phase) of the sterilization cycle. These systems are used for device and material sterilization in health care and industrial applications. An example is the STERRAD series of gas plasma hydrogen peroxide sterilizers (see section 6.5). Plasmas have also been described for the generation of ozone and other reactive species from oxygen, which can then be applied to surfaces. The use of true plasmas of various gases such as nitrogen, argon, hydrogen peroxide, and oxygen and combinations of these and other gases have been investigated but have had few commercial applications to date.

Typical plasma production applications under vacuum can be limited due to the need for treatment within a defined chamber and the difficulty of ensuring the uniformity of the short-lived reactive species in a typical load for sterilization. More recent applications have been the use of plasma production at room temperature and at atmospheric (or slight negative or positive) pressure by dielectric-barrier discharge. This is achieved by the passage of a gas through a pair of electrodes, which are covered by a dielectric material (or simply an insulating or nonconductive material such as quartz glass plates) that prevents arcing when a current is applied. A similar method is used for the production of ozone by corona discharge (chapter 3, section 3.13). In addition to gases, energy or plasmas can be applied to liquids, including water, which can cause similar atom or molecule dissociation; although these may not be considered true plasmas, they are similar to the generation of electrolyzed or activated water (chapter 6, section 6.6.2).

In general, plasmas demonstrate broad-spectrum antimicrobial activity due to the production of many reactive species; not surprisingly, bacterial spores (in particular, aerobic spores including *Bacillus* and *Geobacillus*) demonstrate the greatest resistance, with longer exposure times required for activity. The potency of the plasma depends on the vacuum applied and the gas used to generate the plasma. Many of the efficient antimicrobial plasmas that have been described generally contain a level of air or oxygen during generation, highlighting the importance of oxygen-based reactive species for antimicrobial activity. Plasmas are, however, short-lived, which means they should be generated and applied as close as possible to the surfaces to be treated; for these reasons, they are not considered to be very penetrating into a sterilization load. Antimicrobial processes are generally rapid due to their reactive nature, and little to no associated residuals remain on surfaces following treatment; typically, simple or little aeration is required following exposure. Due to their reactive nature, plasmas can be damaging to various metal and plastic surfaces, which has limited their antimicrobial applications (e.g., plasmas are actually used more widely in industry for surface modification).

Although the exact modes of action of plasmas are unknown, the various reactive species in a typical plasma react with surface and potentially internal proteins, lipids, and other essential molecules. The resulting addition or removal of surface electrons in these molecules leads to the destabilization of these structures, which leads to the loss of structure and function of microbial systems. Certain types of plasma (in particular, those containing oxygen) have been shown to be effective in reducing the infectivity of prions, which was linked to the production of various oxidizing agents that react with and break down the structure and function of these proteinaceous agents.

5.6.2 Pulsed Light

Pulsed-light applications use short, intense pulses of "white" light for the disinfection and/or sterilization of surfaces. The white light includes wavelengths spanning the near-UV to visible-infrared range (~200 to 1,500 nm), although the exact wavelengths used for applications vary depending on the lamp-generating methods used in various systems (chapter 2, section 2.4). Therefore, applications use a range of light-emitting lamps, for example, quartz tubes filled with xenon under vacuum, and some specifically used pulsed light just within the UV range. Although normal white light (sunlight) is generally not effective (apart from as a drying mechanism), the intensity of the light is significantly increased to produce a higher energy range (0.01 to 50 J/cm^2) that can be rapidly microbicidal. This is achieved by short bursts of a high-voltage or high-current electrical field to the lamp. The light is applied to a surface by a short duration of pulses, with each pulse consisting of a number (typically

1 to 20) of short flashes of light, each only a fraction of a second long. The number of pulses varies depending on the application and desired microbial reduction. Multiple lamps can be assembled within a treatment chamber or tunnel to provide simultaneous or sequential pulses (an example of a chamber system is shown in Fig. 5.19). The process can be controlled by monitoring the dosage applied, in particular, the specific UV output of the pulses, and a water-cooling system can be provided to prevent overheating of the lamps.

Pulsed-light technology is not currently widely used. Some applications have included foods and food-packaging material disinfection and sterilization. Food treatments have included fruits, eggs, cheeses, and seafood, primarily to extend their shelf life and to reduce the presence of food-associated pathogens on the surfaces. Other applications are for the treatment of clear liquids (water, vaccines, biopharmaceuticals) and limited sterilization of medical devices and packaging (in particular, transparent) materials. Pharmaceutical investigations have included the use of pulsed light in blow-fill-seal aseptic manufacturing applications.

Pulsed light demonstrates rapid, broad-spectrum activity. Although test results vary depending on the lamps used and doses applied, the technology has been shown to be bactericidal, fungicidal (against yeasts and molds), virucidal, sporicidal, and cysticidal. There are mixed reports regarding the relative resistances of various microorganisms, including high resistance of vegetative fungi and fungal spores (in particular, *Aspergillus niger*) and viruses (for example, poliovirus and other non-enveloped viruses); however, these results may be related to the test method used (presence of soil, distribution of inocula, etc.). Pulsed light is considered sensitive (with reduced antimicrobial activity) to the presence of contaminating soils, is not considered very penetrating (e.g., in the presence of high concentrations of microorganisms or into adsorptive materials), and is only effective in direct contact with surfaces. Despite these concerns about reproducibility and reliability, the technology has many advantages. There are no process residuals (an important consideration in food and pharmaceutical uses); there are minimal utility requirements, rapid cycle times, and good material

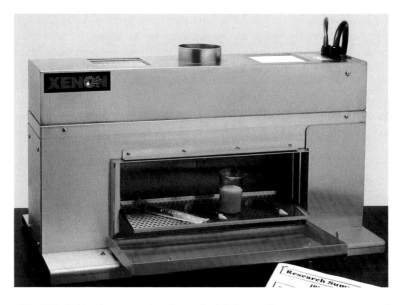

FIGURE 5.19 An example of a pulsed-light sterilizer. Image courtesy of XENON Corporation, with permission.

compatibility (similar to other nonionizing radiation methods; see chapter 2, section 2.4). In food and liquid applications, the technology has been shown to extend the shelf life of products and to cause minimal increases in temperature during treatments; however, some reports have found the technology to induce undesirable products in foods due to various photochemical and photothermal reactions. Applications can require high power consumption, and ozone is likely to be produced during a typical cycle (which should be monitored as a safety risk). Only exposed surfaces can be treated, with further limitations on opaque, colored, or irregular surfaces.

The modes of action of pulsed light are considered similar to those described for nonionizing radiation, with the major target being the nucleic acids, in particular, DNA (chapter 2, section 2.4). Chemical modifications to the DNA (including dimers and other photoproducts) have been described, as well as DNA strand breakage (presumably associated with the higher energy levels applied in comparison to normal UV/infrared applications). Other effects have been reported against proteins, lipid membranes, and other cellular components, which may be due to direct effects of the light energy or due to localized production of ozone and other reactive species.

5.6.3 Supercritical Fluids

Substances can exist in three essential states (solid, liquid, or gas) depending on the temperature and pressure (for example, see the discussion on steam in section 5.2). However, when the substance is above a certain "critical" temperature and pressure it demonstrates the properties of both a liquid and a gas and is referred to as being "supercritical" (Fig. 5.20).

These properties include reduced surface tension of the liquid (similar to the effects of surfactants used in liquids; chapter 3, section 3.16) but with the ability of the liquid to dissolve and maintain a contaminating substance.

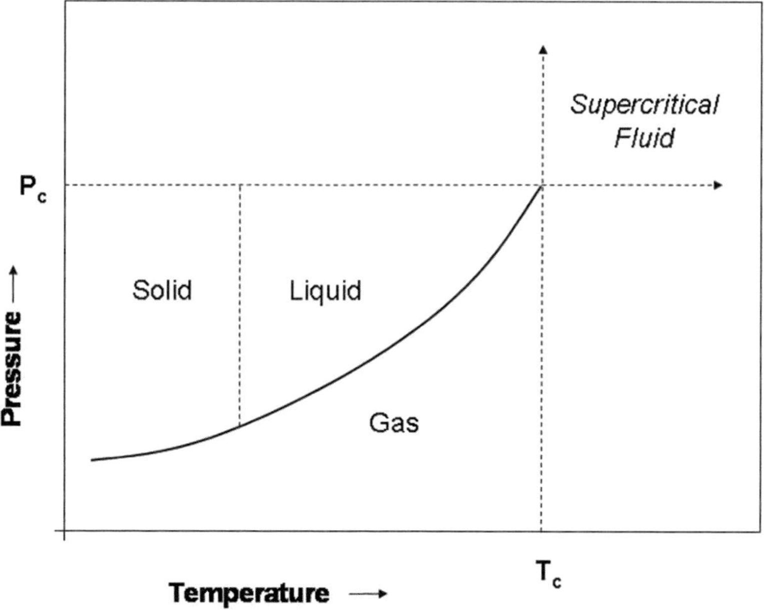

FIGURE 5.20 The relationship between solid, liquid, gas, and supercritical fluid states for a substance. As the temperature and pressure increase, the substance can exist in each state. Above the critical temperature (T_c) and pressure (P_c), the substance demonstrates combined properties of a liquid and a gas and is known as a supercritical fluid.

For example, supercritical carbon dioxide (CO_2), in particular, has been used because it has a relatively low critical temperature (~31°C; 88°F) at a critical pressure of ~7,300 kPa and is considered safe (nontoxic/nonflammable); however, it should be noted that these pressures are relatively high (considering that atmospheric pressure is ~100 kPa and typical steam sterilization cycles are at pressures in the range of 200 to 300 kPa), which has restricted the use of supercritical fluids for general cleaning, disinfection, or sterilization applications.

Supercritical fluids have been particularly used for extraction and purification of various chemicals including oils, fragrances, pigments, and lipids. They have also been used for precision cleaning of intricate or complex materials in industrial applications such as the removal of lubricants, lipids, and adhesives from laser system components, ceramics, and nuclear seals. In a typical application, the component to be cleaned is exposed in an extraction vessel at the given temperature and pressure to supercritical CO_2, which dissolves the soil, and then the CO_2 is passed through a second, "separating" vessel at a reduced pressure to allow for the removal of the soil. In these cases, cleaning is limited to the removal of hydrophobic materials such as oils and other organics, but not particles or salts. Some studies have shown slow bactericidal, fungicidal, and sporicidal activity with supercritical CO_2, as well as physical removal of these contaminants. Associated applications include the pasteurization of thermolabile liquids including foods, blood products, and pharmaceutical preparations. The mode of action appears to be due to diffusion into target cells and direct alteration of intracellular pH, because no direct disruption of the cell wall was observed; however, lipid extraction or disruption may also be expected to occur and to contribute to the antimicrobial activity. Despite these investigations, the spectrum of activity and optimal process requirements have not been investigated in detail.

Advantages of supercritical fluids are that they are dry processes with good cleaning activity, require relatively short exposure times (5 to 15 minutes) for precision applications, and have relatively low operating costs. In contrast, the equipment costs are high, and they have little activity on hydrophilic contaminants, but the primary disadvantage is the requirement for high pressures and the associated safety risks. Supercritical CO_2 is compatible with most metals but can be incompatible with certain plastics and elastomers. Reports of antimicrobial activity are varied and limited.

5.6.4 Pulsed Electric Fields

The pulsing of an electric field through a bacterial or fungal culture demonstrates some antimicrobial activity. These simple processes apply an electric pulse in the 1- to 20-kV/cm range across a liquid, including water, juices, dairy products, and salt solutions. This method is used as a laboratory technique for the introduction of molecules (e.g., plasmid DNA) into a cell in a process known as electroporation, but it can also cause cell death and lysis. Microscopic investigations of this phenomenon have shown that the specific effects of application of the electric field are thinning (compression) of the membrane, leading to pore formation and leaking of the cytoplasm. These effects can be initially reversible but over time cause cell death, depending on the time and strength of the electrical field. Increased antimicrobial activity in the application of the electric field has been noted with an increase in temperature, with supercritical fluids, ozonation, hydrogen peroxide, and other biocides; in many of these cases this is probably due to increased penetration into the already damaged cells. Studies have primarily focused on vegetative bacteria and yeasts. Considering the mode of action, the efficacy against spores and nonenveloped viruses is considered to be limited and may be more applicable for bioburden reduction or disinfection applications. Although there have been reports that pulsed electric fields in combination with other biocides or heat-based processes could be used for disinfection purposes, it seems unlikely that these could be used as true sterilization methods.

CHEMICAL STERILIZATION

6

6.1 INTRODUCTION

Theoretically, any chemical that demonstrates broad-spectrum antimicrobial activity, in particular, those with sporicidal activity, could be developed for use in a sterilization process. Although this may be true depending on the types of microorganisms that are known to be present in certain situations, it is important to remember that because a given process is sporicidal does not necessarily mean that sterilization can be achieved (see discussion in chapter 1, section 1.4.3). Sterilization is a validated process that ensures that a surface or product is free from viable microorganisms, and evidence should be provided to support such a designation of a process. Examples of the requirements for validating such processes are given in the international standard on sterilization of health care products (ISO 14937, "Sterilization of health care products. General requirements for characterization of a sterilizing agent and the development, validation, and routine control of a sterilization process for medical devices"). Although this standard has been designed for use specifically for health care applications, it does specify the minimum requirements for any sterilization process to include the following:

- Characterization of the biocidal agent(s) to include safety, antimicrobial efficacy, and effects of materials
- Characterization of the sterilization process and any delivery equipment
- Definition of the sterilization process for a given application
- Definition of the product to be sterilized within the process
- Validation of the sterilization process for its intended use

Despite the wide variety of chemical biocides (see chapter 3), only a limited number have been developed for use in sterilization processes. These include the epoxides (particularly ethylene oxide [EO]), formaldehyde, hydrogen peroxide-based systems, and other oxidizing agent-based liquid and gaseous processes. These systems are primarily used as alternatives to physical sterilization methods, particularly due to material compatibility concerns, for example, as alternatives to steam for the sterilization of temperature-sensitive materials.

6.2 EPOXIDES

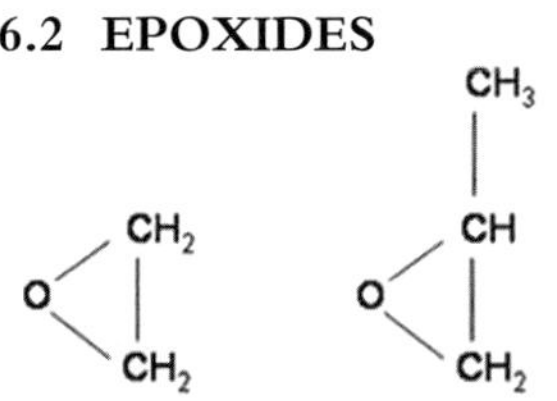

6.2.1 Types

EO (also referred to as ETO or oxirane) is widely used as an intermediate in a variety of chemical-manufacturing processes, including products used in solvents and surfactants. At ambient temperature and atmospheric pressure, it is a colorless gas with a slight sweet, aromatic odor. EO is a flammable, explosive chemical in the presence of ~3% air, which has restricted its use to tightly sealed, enclosed environments where the risk of flammable mixtures has been controlled. EO is industrially produced by oxidation of ethylene with air and oxygen and can then be provided as a 100% liquid in compressed gas cylinders (Fig. 6.1) or as a mixture with inert chemicals such as carbon dioxide or fluoridated hydrocarbons (8 to 10% EO: 90 to 92% carrier; known as EO gas blends).

Propylene oxide has been used for sterilizing foods (e.g., almonds and other nuts), health care materials, and other heat-sensitive products, as well as for fumigation and pasteurization applications but is not as widely used as EO or other gases. Examples include its use for sterilization of some lubricants and as an alternative to methyl bromide (chapter 3, section 3.11) for food applications. Propylene oxide is a colorless, flammable gas and is often considered less toxic than EO (but is reported to be linked to carcinogenicity and genotoxicity). Its antimicrobial effect is lower, requiring higher concentrations for sterilization (800 to 2,000 mg/liter), which can be difficult to achieve in some applications. Propylene oxide breaks down into propylene glycol, which is innocuous and is itself used as a food preservative; toxic residues, including propylene chlorohydrin, can form on reaction with certain salts. The required longer cycle times and safety concerns have restricted the use of propylene oxide, and it is not considered here in further detail.

6.2.2 Applications

As a reactive antimicrobial, EO has been widely used for low-temperature equipment (including device) sterilization, as well as decontamination (including disinfestation) of dried-food and pharmaceutical products. EO is one of the widely used methods for industrial sterilization, in particular for temperature-sensitive medical devices or other materials. It is estimated that greater than 50% of single-use, sterile medical devices in the United States are terminally sterilized using EO processes. Due to its penetration capabilities, EO is successfully used for the fumigation of paper, fabrics, wood, and leather products. Area fumigation applications have been described, but these have been very limited and are not generally used. EO processes have been traditionally used for the low-temperature sterilization of temperature-sensitive medical devices and equipment in health care facilities, but careful monitoring and adequate ventilation are required to reduce

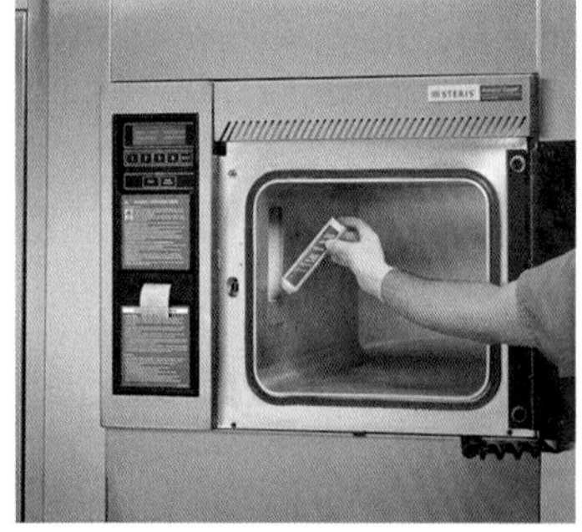

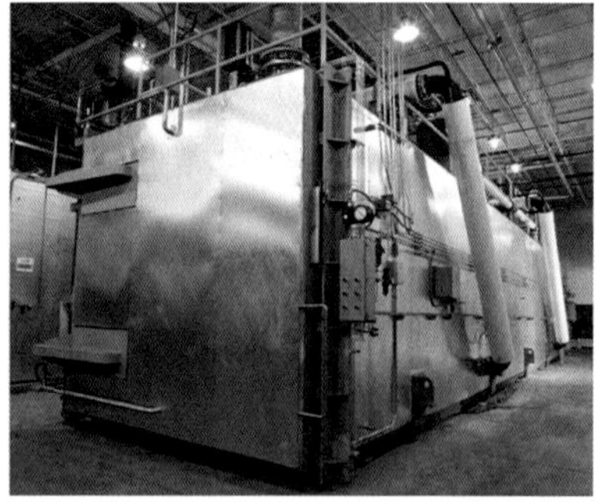

FIGURE 6.1 EO sterilizers. Small, front-loading EO sterilizer chamber (left) into which the load is placed (load not shown) and the insertion of an EO canister which is used to deliver the gas during the sterilization process. Large, industrial-scale EO sterilizer (right). Images courtesy of STERIS, with permission.

the risk of gas exposure even at low concentrations. EO sterilization processes can be particularly effective for porous materials and devices containing permeation challenges (e.g., long lumens or mated surfaces) due to its penetration capabilities. EO is widely used for industrial and contract sterilization of devices and other materials. Examples of EO sterilizer designs are shown in Fig. 6.1 and schematically in Fig. 6.2. Sterilizers can vary in size from small, benchtop units to larger industrial size chambers.

The important variables to ensure efficient sterilization with EO are air removal, temperature, EO concentration, humidity, and time. These are controlled during a typical sterilization process, which includes conditioning, sterilization, and aeration phases (Fig. 6.3).

As with other processes, the sterilization load should be adequately conditioned prior to sterilization. For EO treatment this involves heating the load to the desired sterilization temperature and humidifying the load, usually to >40% relative humidity. Preconditioning may be conducted outside of the actual sterilization chamber, which is common for large-scale applications to maximize the use of the sterilization chamber. It is also essential that air is adequately removed, not only due to the explosion risk (with EO at ≥3% air), but also because air can inhibit the penetration of the biocide and humidity, which are both required for sterilization. The simplest method is by pulling a vacuum and then controlling the introduction of low-temperature steam. Steam is generated at 100°C, but by controlling the pressure within the chamber the steam can be maintained at a lower temperature (for further discussion, see chapter 5, section 5.2); this allows the load to humidify and rapidly heat up to the desired temperature for sterilization. In some cases, where the load to be sterilized is sensitive to the vacuum levels required, air removal can also be achieved using inert gas (e.g., nitrogen) injection to dilute and replace the air. Following conditioning, typical sterilization conditions are maintained at 400 to 1,200 mg/liter EO, 40 to 80% relative humidity, and 30 to 70°C; the higher temperatures and concentrations within these ranges are considered more efficient. Recent efforts have been made to reduce the overall cycle time by reducing the EO concentration to 400 to 450 mg/liter, which can minimize the required aeration time to remove residuals; in general, little efficacy benefit has been reported

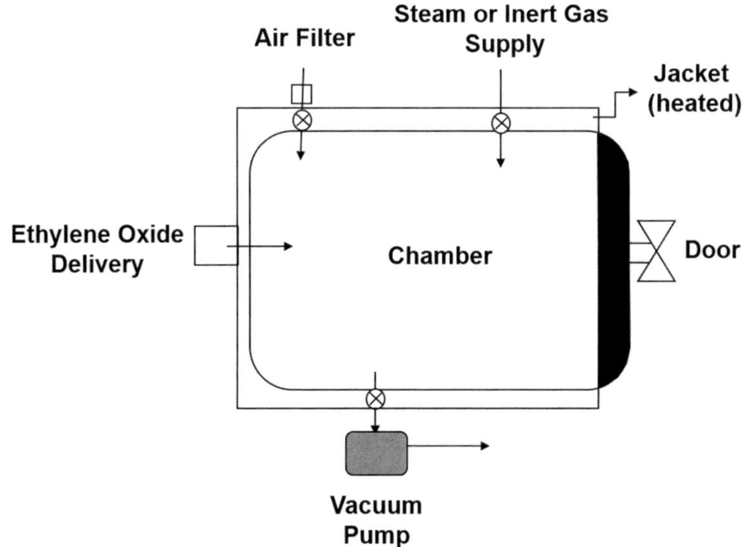

FIGURE 6.2 A typical EO sterilizer.

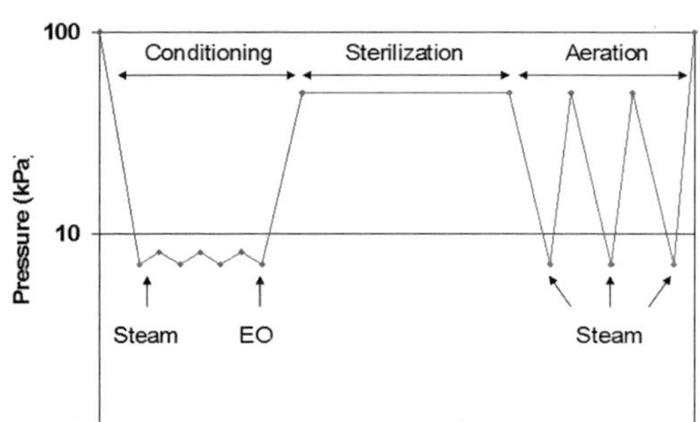

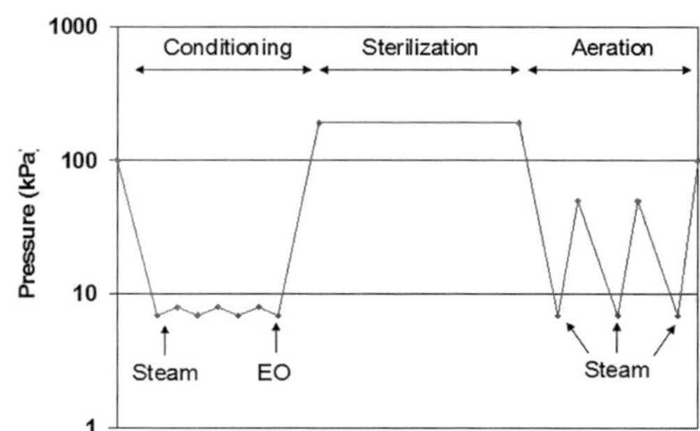

FIGURE 6.3 Typical EO sterilization processes. Vacuum processes (top), in which sterilization is conducted at pressures below atmospheric pressure conditions (i.e., below 101.35 kPa), are generally applied with 100% EO, while pressurized cycles (bottom), in which sterilization is conducted above atmospheric pressure, have traditionally used EO mixtures.

at concentrations >800 mg/liter. Other cycle developments have included the optimization of cycles at lower temperatures. Examples of EO sterilization cycle conditions are given in Table 6.1.

EO has a boiling point at approximately 11°C at atmospheric pressure (101.35 kPa), below which it is a liquid; therefore, pure EO is provided as a liquid within a pressurized canister. The gas can be simply produced by passing the liquid (within the canister) onto a heated surface under vacuum, for example, at 1.3 kPa and 66°C. Under these conditions the load can be held under subatmospheric pressure during sterilization. Alternatively, EO gas blend mixtures (including HCFCs or CO_2 and provided within gas canisters) are required to be put under pressure (28 psi/in^2; 193 kPa) to ensure adequate concentration of EO within the load (Fig. 6.3). Circulation fans or other air movement methods can also be used to increase dispersion of the gas and humidity in the chamber. Following exposure, EO is exhausted from the chamber through a system to remove the gas before venting to the atmosphere. This can be achieved by passing the gas through a catalytic converter, acid scrubber, or other abater system. EO is broken down into carbon dioxide and water. Residual EO within the chamber can be further actively removed by pulsing (washing) with steam or nitrogen gas in a series of vacuum pulses. Despite aeration of the chamber, it is common that extended aeration of the load is required by heating over time (e.g., 8 to 12 hours with dry air at 50 to 60°C, depending

TABLE 6.1 Typical EO sterilization process conditions, based on FDA[a]-approved cycles for health care sterilizer applications[b]

EO source	Concentration (mg/liter)	Relative humidity (%)	Temperature (°C)	Exposure time (hours)
100% EO	700–900	50–80	37–38	4–4.5
100% EO	700–900	50–80	55	1
EO/HCFC[c]	550–650	30–70	38	5–6
EO/HCFC[c]	550–650	30–70	55	2
EO/CO[c]	350–450	30–80	55	7.5

[a]FDA, U.S. Food and Drug Administration.

[b]Note that cycle times do not include extended aeration following the sterilization process, which may be required for some applications.

[c]FHC, fluorinated hydrocarbons, also known as HCFC.

on the load type and volume). This is necessary to remove (also through a catalytic converter) EO residuals, which have been adsorbed into various materials, to a safe level and to reduce the presence of other EO-associated residuals that may have formed on reaction with the biocide (e.g., ethylene chlorohydrin). Extended aeration can be conducted in the sterilizer chamber or, more commonly, in a separate chamber or aerator for up to or greater than 12 hours, depending on the load, with a constant air flow and typically at 50 to 60°C.

Examples of various standards and guidelines for EO sterilization applications are listed in Table 6.2.

6.2.3 Spectrum of Activity

Both EO and propylene oxide are broad-spectrum biocides. Efficacy has been demonstrated against bacteria, viruses, fungi, bacterial spores, and other microorganisms. Antimicrobial activity, in particular against bacterial spores, is dependent on adequate hydration (presence of water), usually between 40 and 80% relative humidity. This may be due to the effect of hydration to lead to germination of the spores and thereby allow easier access to the internal spore structures (see chapter 8, section 8.3.11), or to assist EO in penetrating the outer spore layers. EO sterilization processes can demonstrate log-linear kinetics at constant conditions of humidity, concentration, and temperature. *Bacillus atrophaeus* (previously known as *Bacillus subtilis* subsp. *niger*) spores are considered the organisms most resistant to EO and are widely used to verify the efficacy and validate EO sterilization processes. *B. atrophaeus* spores can show variable resistance to EO sterilization processes and are usually standardized by determining a *D* reference value at a minimum humidity level and temperature (e.g., at 600 mg/liter EO, 60% relative humidity, and 54°C). Microbial resistance is significantly increased in the presence of organic and inorganic soils; the presence of inorganic salts can lead to the protection of microorganisms during drying and salt crystal formation; these effects can be minimized by adequate humidification and EO exposure times.

As along as conditioning has been efficient and uniform prior to the sterilization phase, the efficiency of EO sterilization is dependent on the gas concentration, humidity, temperature, and exposure time. Typical sterilization processes are used within the 400 to 900 mg/liter EO range, with a typical increase in activity observed as the concentration is increased to ~700 mg/liter, with little substantial benefit observed at higher concentrations (Fig. 6.4).

TABLE 6.2 Examples of standards and guidelines for EO sterilization applications

Reference[a]	Title	Summary
ISO 11135	Sterilization of health care products - ethylene oxide - requirements for the development, validation and routine control of a sterilization process for medical devices	Requirements for the development, validation, and routine control of an EO sterilization process for medical devices
ISO 10993-7	Biological evaluation of medical devices. Ethylene oxide sterilization residuals	Specifies allowable limits and methods for detection of residual EO and ethylene chlorohydrin on EO-sterilized medical devices
EN 1422	Sterilizers for medical purposes. Ethylene oxide sterilizers. Requirements and test methods	Guidelines on the design and testing of EO sterilizers
AAMI ST41	Ethylene oxide sterilization in health care facilities: safety and effectiveness	Guidelines on the use of EO in health care settings
AAMI TIR14	Contract sterilization using ethylene oxide	Guidance on the use of EO for sterilization at contract sterilization facilities

[a]ISO, International Standards Organization; EN, European Standard (Norm); AAMI, Association for the Advancement of Medical Instrumentation.

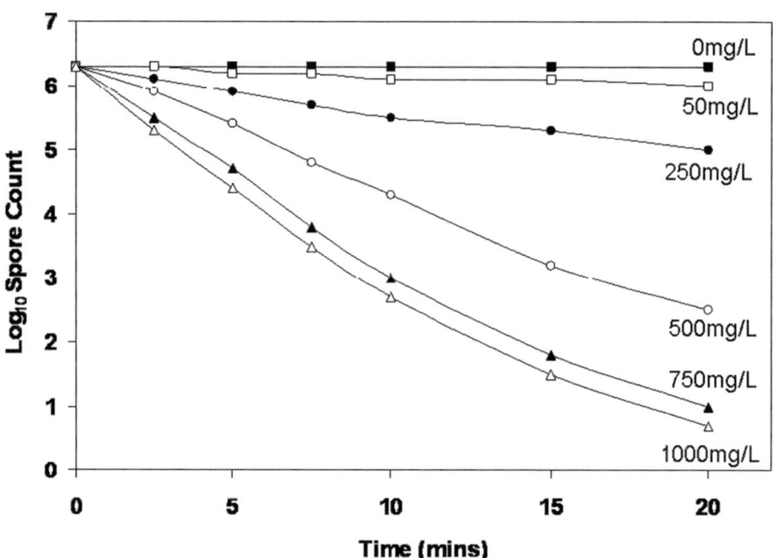

FIGURE 6.4 The sporicidal (*B. atrophaeus*) effect of EO concentration at 60% relative humidity and 54°C.

Greater sporicidal efficacy has also been shown at higher temperatures, typically within the 45 to 65°C range, with restrictions at higher temperatures due to the heat sensitivity of many materials. Lower temperatures are often desired and generally require longer exposure times (see Table 6.2), but these can be optimized for specific applications. Optimal and reproducible sporicidal activity is observed within the 30 to 80% relative humidity range, which is important for the demonstration of linear kinetics and acceptable sterility assurance levels with EO. Lower humidity levels, including essentially dry conditions at 1% relative humidity, demonstrate initial rapid spore log reduction but slow to no further activity. These conditions, which may be due to limited penetration or increased spore resistance in the absence of water, are therefore not generally acceptable for sterilization processes. Other important considerations, which are not unique to EO, are the presence of organic/inorganic soils, which can prevent the penetration of EO and/or water to shielded microorganisms, and variable activity on various material surfaces, due to differences in EO and/or water absorbance. For example, aluminum, nylon, and paper materials have greater resistance to penetration than do some rubbers, polyester, and stainless steel.

In addition to the higher resistance of bacterial spores, fungal strains of *Pyronema domesticum* have demonstrated unusual resistance to EO sterilization (see chapter 8, section 8.10). *P. domesticum* and similar species are fungi in the group Ascomycetes, defined by the production of sexual spores known as ascospores that are produced within an ascus (sac) structure (see chapter 8, Fig. 8.38). Ascospores demonstrate higher resistance profiles to chemical and physical biocidal methods in comparison to other types of fungal spores. In addition, the hyphal growth of *P. domesticum* forms hardened (or desiccated) clumps known as sclerotia, which also demonstrate high resistance to EO sterilization. Sclerotia have been estimated to have resistance to EO gas 10 times greater than *B. atrophaeus* spores (e.g., a *D* value of ~34 minutes at 600 mg/liter EO and 54°C). To address these concerns, in the routine monitoring of EO sterilization processes over time it is common to monitor the natural product bioburden (see chapter 1, section 1.4.2.3) and resistance of the bioburden to EO (via much reduced exposure times compared to those used for sterilization). Ascospores and sclerotia also show higher resistance profiles to γ radiation sterilization (in the *D*-value range of 0.5 to 2 kGy, particularly at the higher end of this range for ascospores; see chapter 5, section 5.4). The risks associated with *P. domesticum* isolates were highlighted in the 1990s with the voluntary recall of contaminated surgical laparotomy sponges (and subsequently other similar cotton-based products) that had used fungi-contaminated raw materials.

6.2.4 Advantages

EO is a broad-spectrum biocide with high penetrability, including efficacy in porous loads and complex equipment. These attributes have seen the use of EO for the reliable (although rare) fumigation and sterilization of temperature-sensitive materials, which cannot be treated by heat or radiation sterilization. Materials for sterilization can be packaged in various plastics or paper wraps, pouches, or containers once they allow adequate penetration of EO and humidity; following sterilization, this allows for sterile storage and maintenance of sterility over time. EO is a very reactive but relatively stable biocide during typical antimicrobial processes. Despite its stability, EO can be rapidly degraded in the environment. In contrast to other chemical biocides, the active agent itself demonstrates broad material compatibility and is not damaging to plastics, metals, and other materials. This is a particular advantage in the treatment of sensitive materials including museum artifacts, paperwork, and medical devices including single-use devices and complex, temperature-sensitive reusable devices (such as flexible endoscopes); however, consideration should also be given to the requirement for adequate humidification and temperature requirements, which may cause some damage in some processes over time and should be controlled to minimize potential damage (e.g., the quality of steam [see chapter 5, section 5.2] and minimum humidity levels). Due to increased safety concerns, it is required that EO is monitored and controlled in a given environment to reduce the risk of accidental exposure; sensitive personnel and area monitoring systems are available for this purpose.

6.2.5 Disadvantages

EO is toxic at relatively low concentrations. The typical recommended daily occupational safety level is given as 1 ppm. Short-term exposure can cause irritation to the eyes, skin, and mucous membranes, which can lead to severe damage over time. Further, EO is sensitizing to the skin and lungs, which can lead to allergic and asthmatic symptoms. The odor detection level is relatively high at >250 ppm, at which level EO can be extremely damaging and dangerous. Nausea and vomiting have been reported in some industrial applications at low concentrations, and concentrations at 800 ppm have been known to be lethal. EO is a listed mutagen, carcinogen, and teratogen (reproductive hazard), which may not be surprising given its reactive nature and mode of action against proteins and nucleic acids. Toxicity concerns have necessitated close monitoring of gas concentrations in the air and, in most cases, the design of dedicated ventilated rooms to house a sterilizer. Other safety risks are related to the flammability and explosive risks of EO due to its reactivity; the flammability risk is reduced with the use of nonflammable blends of EO, but these have become less used in sterilization applications due to environmental concerns. The use of fluorinated hydrocarbons in EO blends has been restricted in favor of 100% EO due to damaging effects to the Earth's protective ozone layer. On the other hand, 100% EO (which is stored as a pressurized liquid) can slowly polymerize over time to form blockages in feed lines and in the sterilization chamber; these effects can be minimized by equipment design and maintenance.

During cycle development for particular applications, care should be taken to ensure that the load is adequately humidified to achieve optimal antimicrobial efficacy; this is particularly important in dried loads or in vacuum cycles (which also cause drying), remembering that greater resistance is observed in spores with a lower water content. Overall cycle times also tend to be extended with EO due to the need for adequate aeration to remove residual EO from the load. This has caused a decrease in the use of EO for sterilization of devices and other materials requiring a rapid turnaround time in health care and other similar applications. Typical aeration times can be up to 10 to 16 hours, particularly in the presence of adsorptive materials such as rubbers and some plastics (e.g., polyvinyl chloride). In addition to toxic concerns with EO, some breakdown or other toxic residual chemical products can be formed during sterilization. These can include EO-based ethers, nonylphenol ethoxylates, and other ethoxylates that are toxic and bio-accumulative. Examples are the reaction of EO with water to form ethylene glycol, which is an eye and skin irritant, and with chlorine (e.g., in polyvinylchloride) to form ethylene chlorohydrin, which is a suspected mutagen. EO cannot be used for the sterilization of liquids.

6.2.6 Modes of Action

EO is a reactive chemical and is effective by alkylation. As an alkylating agent, it acts to replace any available hydrogen atom within a chemical group (including amino, carboxyl, and hydroxyl groups) with a hydroxylethyl radical. This leads to cross-linking within and between proteins and nucleic acids. Therefore, most cellular components including nucleic acids and functional or structural proteins react with EO to inhibit vital functions, which culminates in cell death. Propylene oxide, although less studied, is also an alkylating agent and is believed to have a similar mode of action. In both cases, the presence of water for activity is an important consideration. This may be due to a combination of the activities of water to break the epoxide ring during the sterilization process to allow reaction with sensitive molecules and to allow penetration of external bacterial spore layers. It is also likely that the humidification conditioning requirement for EO processes allows for spore germination and greater access to internal spore structures.

6.3 LOW-TEMPERATURE STEAM-FORMALDEHYDE (LTSF)

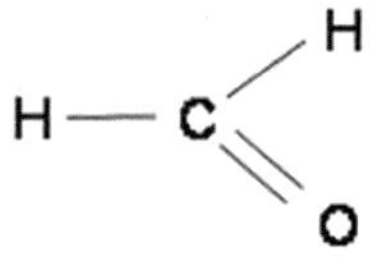

H—C(H)=O

Formaldehyde

6.3.1 Types and Applications

Formaldehyde (methanal) is a monoaldehyde with a characteristic pungent odor. It is widely used as a biocide in liquid or gaseous form for disinfection, preservation, and sterilization (as discussed in chapter 3, section 3.4). Two types of sterilization methods use formaldehyde gas: LTSF, which is discussed in this section, and high-temperature formaldehyde-alcohol sterilization, which is discussed in section 6.4.

Formaldehyde gas requires high humidity for optimal biocidal activity, particularly against bacterial and fungal spores. The concept of low-temperature steam (or steam under vacuum) was introduced in chapter 5, section 5.2, and in LTSF systems it is used to provide both humidity and temperature control during a typical sterilization process. A typical sterilizer design is shown in Fig. 6.5.

In some sterilizer designs, a steam supply is not required, and the chamber temperature is maintained using a heated chamber jacket (by conduction). Most modern LTSF systems are programmed with multiple sterilization cycles which vary in cycle temperature and can range from 50 to 80°C. A typical sterilization process is shown in Fig. 6.6 and can be separated into three phases: conditioning, sterilization, and aeration.

Prior to sterilization, a leak test is often performed to ensure that the sterilizer chamber is airtight and can achieve the desired pressure levels for the process. Some preheating of the chamber and/or load may be required to prevent water condensation and subsequent loss of formaldehyde gas concentration. It should be noted that condensed water on

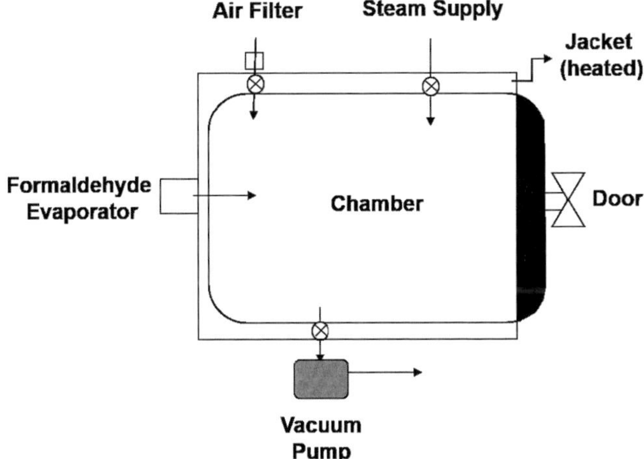

FIGURE 6.5 A typical LTSF sterilization system.

various surfaces can act to readily dissolve formaldehyde, which can reduce the biocidal gas concentration and reduce the efficiency of the process overall. Air and other noncondensable gases are removed by a series of pulses of drawing a vacuum in the chamber and, in parallel, introducing steam, which heats and adds humidity to the load. By controlling the pressure in the chamber, the temperature of steam under vacuum can be closely controlled, generally in the 50 to 80°C range. The extent of humidification should also be controlled to prevent the buildup of excess water on surfaces. Vacuum pulses are then repeated while formaldehyde gas is introduced to equilibrate the load. The gas is generated in a heated evaporator which is supplied with a formalin solution ranging from 2 to 40% formaldehyde in water (which may also contain a low concentration of methanol to prevent formaldehyde

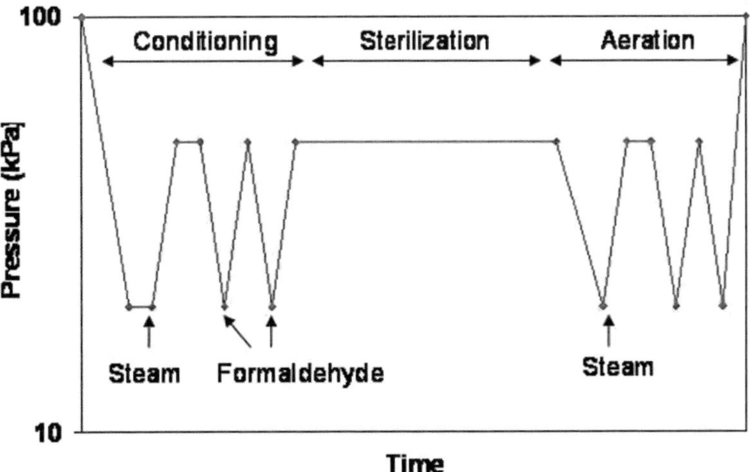

FIGURE 6.6 A typical LTSF sterilization cycle.

polymerization on storage). When the desired formaldehyde concentration (typically in the 5 to 50 mg/liter range), humidity (75 to 100%), and temperature (50 to 80°C) set points are achieved, the load is considered conditioned and is held under these conditions for a given sterilization time at subatmospheric pressure. During aeration (and/or desorption), formaldehyde residuals are then removed from the chamber and load by a series of vacuum and steam pulses, followed by vacuum and air pulses to cool and dry the load (if required). The formaldehyde residues removed from the sterilizer can be condensed, diluted, and discarded down the drain. Post-process aeration, to remove residues, outside of the chamber may also be required depending on the load being sterilized (e.g., porous materials or fabrics). Formaldehyde residues can be deabsorbed by heating over time.

LTSF designs and cycle conditions vary from manufacturer to manufacturer. Some systems do not require steam for conditioning but use the temperature-controlled, jacketed walls of the sterilizer chamber alone to heat the load, and use the water present during the evaporation of the formalin solution as the source of humidity for the sterilization phase of the cycle. The concentration of formalin used for different systems also varies from 40% formaldehyde to as low as 2%. Dual-sterilizer designs can be used for high-temperature (steam) and low-temperature (LTSF) sterilization within the same chamber, which is an advantage where space for equipment installation is limited.

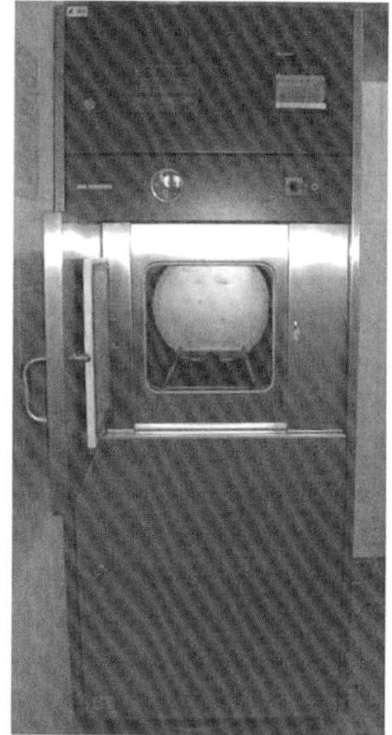

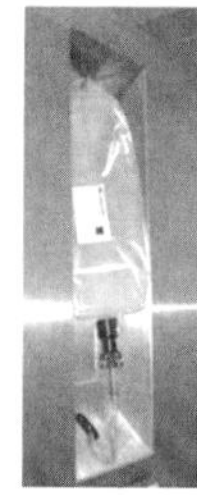

FIGURE 6.7 An LTSF sterilizer. The sterilizer (with open door) is shown on the left, with the liquid formalin delivery system on the right.

Other single-chamber designs have been described that can be used alternately for LTSF or EO sterilization (section 6.2).

LTFS systems are used for medical, dental, and some industrial sterilization processes. The most widely used application is for sterilization of reusable medical devices in health care facilities (Fig. 6.7). Overall, these systems are not widely utilized, although they do have particular applications in Scandinavia, some other European countries, and South America.

Examples of various standards and guidelines for formaldehyde sterilization applications are given in Table 6.3.

TABLE 6.3 Examples of standards and guidelines for LTSF sterilization applications

Reference[a]	Title	Summary
EN 14180	Sterilizers for medical purposes - low temperature steam and formaldehyde sterilizers - requirements and testing	Requirements and test methods for sterilizers using LTSF processes
ISO 11138-5	Sterilization of health care products - biological indicators - part 5: biological indicators for low-temperature steam and formaldehyde sterilization processes	Requirements for the manufacture of biological indicators used in validation and monitoring of LTSF sterilization processes
AAMI ST58	Chemical sterilization and high-level disinfection in health care facilities	Guidelines on the selection and use of chemical sterilization methods in health care facilities

6.3.2 Spectrum of Activity

When under the optimal process conditions of biocide concentration, temperature, and humidity, formaldehyde gas is rapidly biocidal. Formaldehyde sterilization processes are virucidal, bactericidal, mycobactericidal, fungicidal, and sporicidal. The activity of formaldehyde is significantly less effective in the presence of contaminating soil or in the presence of microbial clumping (particularly described with viruses). Formaldehyde sterilization has been shown to be ineffective against prions, presumably due to its protein cross-linking mechanism of action (see chapter 8, section 8.9). For further discussion on the spectrum of activity of formaldehyde see chapter 3, section 3.4.

6.3.3 Advantages

Formaldehyde is a broad-spectrum biocide. Recent developments in the understanding of formaldehyde sterilization processes and the availability of modern equipment have minimized the disadvantages previously associated with formaldehyde sterilization, in particular, the risks of exposure to low levels of the biocide over time. These sterilization systems are generally cost-effective, and some can be used as both low-temperature (LTSF) and high-temperature (steam) sterilizers, which can be an advantage when space is restricted in a facility. Formaldehyde has a good compatibility profile with many plastics and metals, although some processes may be restricted due to temperature conditions (>65°C) and cross-linking activity, which may be incompatible with some plastics and elastomers. Formaldehyde is less stable than EO, breaking down into carbon dioxide and water (typically, a decrease of 2 mg/liter is observed per hour), which is an advantage for more rapid and controlled aeration over time. Further advantages of formaldehyde are discussed in chapter 3, section 3.4.

6.3.4 Disadvantages

As with EO, there remains significant concern about the safe use of formaldehyde gas, which is toxic, irritating, and considered mutagenic and carcinogenic. Adequate equipment design and ventilation can minimize these risks. Formaldehyde can polymerize to form less active paraformaldehyde, which can precipitate onto surfaces. Polymerization can be limited when exposure temperatures are maintained at >65°C. Similarly, tight control of humidity levels between 75 and 100% should be maintained for optimal activity, and care should be taken to ensure that steam condensation does not occur, which can lead to a loss of process effectiveness. Although formaldehyde breaks down into carbon dioxide and water, the presence of carbon dioxide, like the presence of air in a sterilizer load, can reduce penetration of humidity and formaldehyde, which are required for activity. Despite the optimization of the aeration cycles of new LTSF systems, certain material types (e.g., porous materials and fabrics) can absorb formaldehyde and require postprocess aeration in special heated chambers. Formaldehyde penetration into these materials is considered low and can increase the risk of polymerization. Processes with temperature >65°C may be restrictive for some materials (including some polymers and elastomers). LTSF cannot be used for liquid sterilization.

6.3.5 Mode of Action

Formaldehyde is a cross-linking agent that interacts with and inactivates proteins and nucleic acids (including DNA and RNA). The mode of action is discussed in more detail in chapter 3, section 3.4, and chapter 7, section 7.4.3.

6.4 HIGH-TEMPERATURE FORMALDEHYDE-ALCOHOL

H—C(H)=O $CH_3.CH_2.OH$

Formaldehyde Ethanol

6.4.1 Type and Application

High-temperature formaldehyde-alcohol sterilization is a process that combines the biocidal activities of heat (chapter 5, section 5.2) with formaldehyde (chapter 3, section 3.4) and alcohol (section 3.5). A unique mixture of formaldehyde (0.23%), alcohols (72% ethanol and <4% methanol), and distilled water (known as Vapo-Steril) is vaporized under pressure (138 kPa) by heating to 132°C in a dedicated sterilizer (e.g., a Harvey® Chemiclave).

A typical sterilization cycle includes the chamber warm-up, pressurization to 138 kPa and vaporization of the sterilizing agents, exposure for 20 minutes at 132°C, depressurization, and purging (at 48 kPa) to remove formaldehyde residuals through an emission filter. Older systems may not contain emission filters and should be used under venting hoods to reduce noxious and toxic odors. A typical cycle time is ~20 to 40 minutes, with optional shorter (flash or immediate use) cycles with exposure times of 7 minutes available in some models. Sterilizers are generally small tabletop sizes (to accommodate smaller loads) and have had limited use in dental and medical clinics for reusable device sterilization.

6.4.2 Spectrum of Activity

The process has been shown to have broad-spectrum antimicrobial activity, including rapid sporicidal activity. The antimicrobial activity is primarily due to formaldehyde (chapter 3, section 3.4) and the high sterilization temperature (132°C; chapter 5, section 5.2); the contribution of ethanol (section 3.5) in the antimicrobial process is unknown. Overall, the antimicrobial efficacy of this process has not been widely studied.

6.4.3 Advantages

As a low-humidity process, high-temperature formaldehyde-alcohol sterilization demonstrates greater material compatibility than steam sterilization, including minimal rusting, corrosion, or staining. There is no drying phase required poststerilization, and the process is considered rapid. The process demonstrates broad-spectrum antimicrobial activity.

6.4.4 Disadvantages

The primary disadvantage is due to the toxic nature of formaldehyde, which is a known sensitizer and carcinogen. The risks of toxicity have limited impact with this technology. To minimize exposure, adequate (even dedicated) ventilation is recommended in the use of these sterilizers. Ventilation is also recommended due to the offensive odor of the sterilizing agents. Relatively low exposure limits are proposed (as low as 0.75 ppm for a typical 8-hour working day). Short-term exposure to formaldehyde-alcohol causes damage to the eyes and skin irritation. The sterilizing agent is flammable (due to the presence of alcohol). The sterilizers in benchtop sizes have limited capacity and should not be used to sterilize liquids, textiles, nylon, polycarbonate, or sealed containers. Since it is a high-temperature process, temperature-sensitive materials are incompatible with this sterilization process.

6.4.5 Mode of Action

The mode of action of the combination of biocides used in high-temperature formaldehyde-alcohol sterilization has not been particularly investigated. It is considered that the primary mode of action is due to formaldehyde (as a potent aldehyde, which is discussed in chapter 3, section 3.4), but the effects of heat (at 132°C) are also significant (being an effective sterilant in its own right). The modes of action of heat (chapter 2, section 2.2, and chapter 5, 5.2) and alcohol (section 3.5) are discussed in other sections.

6.5 HYDROGEN PEROXIDE

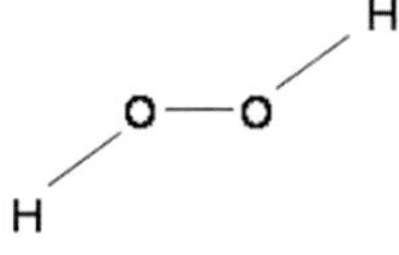

Hydrogen Peroxide

6.5.1 Types

Hydrogen peroxide (H_2O_2) is a powerful oxidizing agent with broad-spectrum activity and a reasonably good safety profile in comparison to other sterilants. Peroxide solutions, or formulations, and gas-based processes are widely used for antisepsis, disinfection, and fumigation applications (see chapter 3, section

3.13). Although low solution concentrations are sufficient for bactericidal and fungicidal activity, much higher concentrations (generally in the 25 to 60% range) are required for sporicidal activity. These required concentrations have restricted use due to safety and surface compatibility concerns. In some cases heated peroxide (30 to 59% solutions in water) has been used for sterilization (e.g., for liquid food containers), and some formulations in combination with other oxidizing agents (e.g., peracetic acid [PAA]) can provide rapid sporicidal activity (e.g., fumigation or direct surface treatments in high-risk areas such as clean rooms); however, hydrogen peroxide solutions are not widely used in sterilization processes. In contrast, gaseous hydrogen peroxide is rapidly sporicidal at much lower concentrations (≥0.1 mg/liter) and, depending on the process application, is considered significantly less damaging to surfaces (see section 3.13). The sporicidal effectiveness depends on the concentration of hydrogen peroxide gas (Fig. 6.8).

Gaseous hydrogen peroxide can be generated by evaporation or vaporization. Evaporation is a slow process in which a peroxide solution is allowed to generate a gas over time in an enclosed environment. This may be enhanced by heating the peroxide solution, but due to the vapor pressure differences between peroxide and water, the final gas mixture at saturation is predominantly water with a relatively low concentration of peroxide, with little practical value. Note that saturation is defined as the point at which the air cannot hold further peroxide and/or water, which is dependent on the concentration of each gas (water and peroxide vapor) and the temperature. In contrast, vaporization of liquid peroxide solutions instantaneously forms a peroxide and water gas mixture at the same proportion as the starting liquid concentration. Flash vaporization is achieved by dropping small volumes of liquid peroxide onto a heated surface (at >100°C), e.g., a simple hot plate, passing it through a heated cylinder, or by another direct heating mechanism (e.g., using a plasma [see below] or another high-energy source) to produce the gas in a chamber. Alternatively, the peroxide-water solution can be introduced directly into a preheated and evacuated chamber, generally under a deep vacuum (e.g., <1.5 kPa), to be instantaneously vaporized into a gas.

Low-temperature sterilization processes have been developed with gaseous peroxide alone

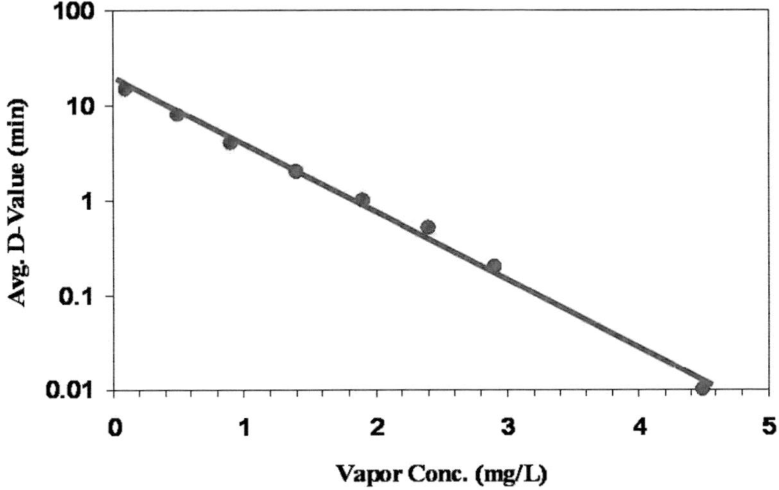

FIGURE 6.8 An example of the effect of hydrogen peroxide gas concentration on sporicidal activity. Various gas concentrations were tested under atmospheric pressure with *Geobacillus stearothermophilus* spores.

or in combination with plasma. Plasma may be considered the "fourth" state of matter (with solids, liquids, and gases), where the molecules of a gas are excited and produce a highly excited mixture of charged nuclei and free electrons (chapter 5, section 5.6.1). A true plasma is considered to consist of positively and negatively charged particles at approximately equal concentrations. Plasmas can be generated by the application of sufficient energy, in the form of temperature or an electromagnetic field, to a gas, including hydrogen peroxide. Alternatively, plasma has also been used to generate hydrogen peroxide gas (at a low energy and therefore not sufficient to generate a true plasma) or to aid in the removal of peroxide residuals in loads during aeration (following peroxide gas exposure for sterilization).

6.5.2 Applications

Liquid-based processes have had limited use, in particular, for food applications. Examples include validated processes for the sterilization of containers used in high-speed, aseptic filling lines and consist of 30 to 60% hydrogen peroxide (minimally at food grade chemical quality) applied to the surface for a given amount of time, which depends on the application. Increased temperature can dramatically decrease the minimum exposure time for the accepted level of sterilization. Peroxide residuals may be removed by rinsing with sterile water, heating, or simply tolerated by contact with the contents of the packaging (which can react with the peroxide, causing it to degrade into water and oxygen).

Peroxide gas-based processes have more widespread applications. Atmospheric-pressure processes have been developed for various applications, including as an alternative to the liquid sterilization aseptic filling line applications. A typical high-speed application may use 4.5 mg/liter of hydrogen peroxide at 40 to 45°C directly on a surface for less than 10 seconds of exposure time and has the further advantage of producing minimal residues in comparison to liquid sterilization applications. To ensure the sterilization of packaged materials (such as medical devices), porous materials, or more complicated instruments (such as those containing lumens, mated surfaces, or dead-ends), it is necessary to remove air, similar to the requirement in other sterilization processes such as steam (see chapter 5, section 5.2) or EO (see section 6.2) sterilization. The simplest way to achieve this is by sterilization under vacuum. At least two types of vacuum-gas peroxide sterilization processes have been developed, which use simple peroxide gas systems or gas in combination with plasma during their exposure conditions. A typical sterilizer design is shown in Fig. 6.9.

A hydrogen peroxide gas sterilizer consists of an aluminum (or other nonreactive material) chamber capable of withstanding and maintaining pressure levels of typically <0.02 kPa. The chamber walls may be heated and/or insulated, if required, to maintain the load at ambient temperature during the sterilization cycle. The chamber can be evacuated by a vacuum pump, which may have an associated destroyer module capable of degrading peroxide before it enters the pump or is released into the environment. Liquid hydrogen peroxide is provided in aqueous solution at 35 to 59%, which is either metered as a predetermined volume onto a heated vaporizer and introduced into the chamber or provided in a single-unit-dose cartridge which is punctured and pulled into the evacuated chamber when required during the process. In some sterilizer designs, the peroxide gas is formed in a smaller, evacuated prechamber and then introduced into the load exposure chamber. Such prechamber designs (specifically those used in the STERRAD NX series of sterilizer) are also used to concentrate hydrogen peroxide by preferentially reducing the temperature in the chamber to allow for the condensation of peroxide alone (due to the vapor pressure differences between water and peroxide gas), removing the water (remaining in gas form), and producing a gas from the remaining concentrated peroxide solution (typically in the 85 to 95% range). An air vent (HEPA filtered or similar) is used to vent the chamber during

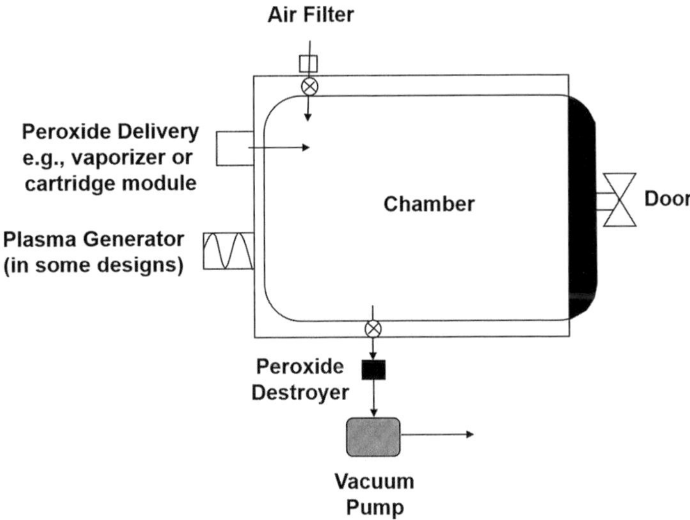

FIGURE 6.9 Typical gas hydrogen peroxide sterilizer.

or at the end of the cycle. The most widely used processes (e.g., the STERRAD range of sterilizers) contain a plasma generator associated with the chamber, which can be activated at various stages during the process, but other sterilizer designs do not specifically use plasma as part of the sterilization process (Fig. 6.10).

Typical examples of peroxide gas sterilization processes are shown in Fig. 6.11. Overall, these processes are relatively similar. In both cases a simple gas cycle includes multiple phases including a leak test (not shown), conditioning, sterilization, and aeration. During a leak test, the chamber is held under vacuum for a preset time and the pressure is monitored to ensure that the chamber is leakproof. During the conditioning phase, the vacuum system can be used to dry the chamber and load and to condition the load temperature for sterilization (generally in the range of 25 to 55°C). Note that although the chamber wall temperature

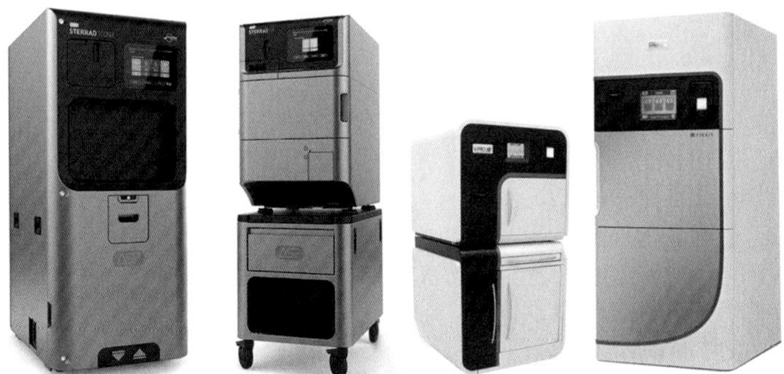

FIGURE 6.10 Examples of hydrogen peroxide gas sterilizers. The examples on the left are the STERRAD hydrogen peroxide gas plasma sterilizers (far left image: STERRAD® Systems with ALLClear™ Technology and second from left STERRAD VELOCITY™ Biological Indicator System). Examples on the right are the STERIS V-Pro Low Temperature Sterilization Systems (smaller V-PRO 60 and larger V-PRO maX). Images courtesy of STERIS Corporation and Advanced Sterilization Products, with permission. ASP and the ASP logo are trademarks of Advanced Sterilization Products Division of Ethicon, Inc.

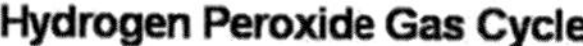

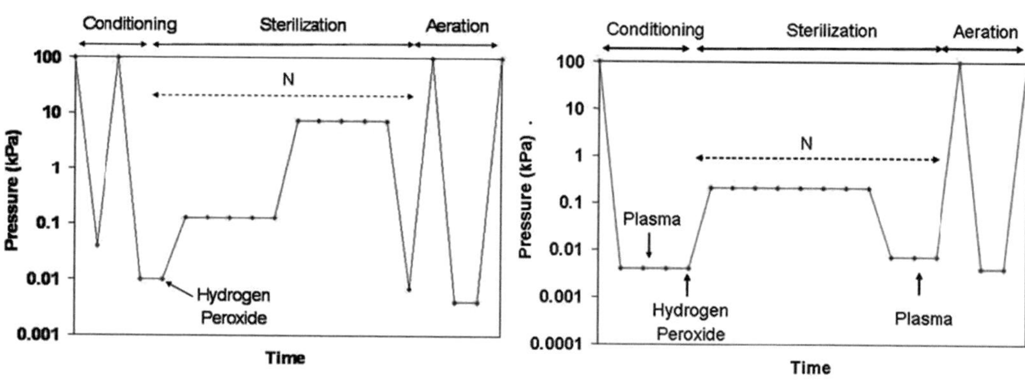

FIGURE 6.11 Typical hydrogen peroxide gas sterilization processes. In the cycle on the right, only single conditioning, sterilization, and aeration pulses, which can vary in number (*N*) depending on the application, are shown. Similarly, the gas-plasma cycles can have multiple-stage pulses (only a single pulse is shown); for example, the most widely used health care application (the STERRAD 100S) consists of two (*N* = 2) peroxide injections.

may be relatively high in some designs (up to 55°C), the actual load temperature is generally ambient (20 to 35°C) during the sterilization cycle, depending on the specific process used. Peroxide gas is then generated from 35 to 59% liquid peroxide in the evacuated chamber by flash vaporization (heating at >100°C) or direct introduction under vacuum, and allowed to diffuse. In some situations, dry air or nitrogen gas may be introduced (which is shown as an increase in pressure in Fig. 6.12, below) to improve the penetration of the gas. Single or multiple peroxide pulses may be introduced into the chamber, because peroxide will break down on contact with the load in the chamber over time. The number of peroxide pulses depends on the application (e.g., device design, materials of construction, load size, etc.) and

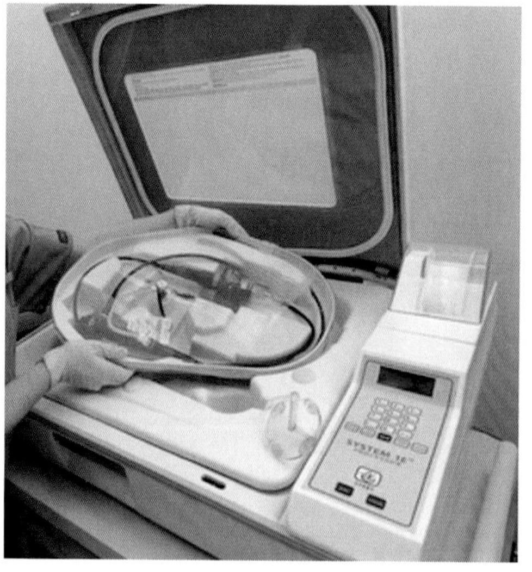

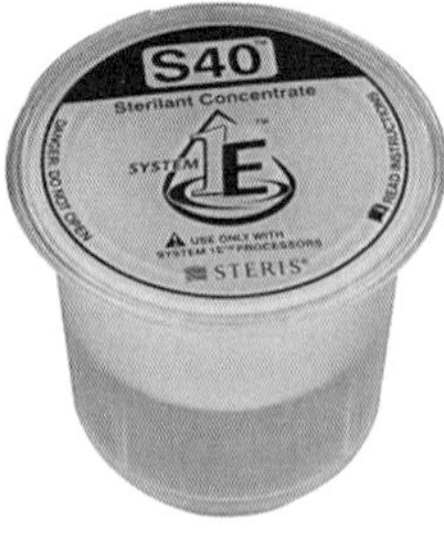

FIGURE 6.12 SYSTEM 1E Liquid Chemical Sterilant Processing Systems with S40 Sterilant Concentrate. Images courtesy of STERIS, with permission.

given validated process, varying from 1 to 12 pulses under some conditions. Typical peroxide gas concentrations range from 4 to 9 mg/liter, although lower and higher concentrations may be used to achieve sterilization. As noted above (for the NX processes), the peroxide solution used to generate the gas during the process can be concentrated to reduce the water content and improve the available concentration of peroxide gas for load penetration. Finally, during aeration the vacuum system is used to rapidly remove peroxide from the chamber and load by a series of vacuum and HEPA-filtered air introduction pulses.

In the most common plasma-based systems, following exposure to hydrogen peroxide gas, a plasma is created in the chamber. In these applications, the plasma may also be triggered during the conditioning phase as a heating or drying mechanism, which can decrease the conditioning time. The use and generation of plasmas is considered further in chapter 5, section 5.6.1; in the STERRAD sterilizers discussed above, the plasma is typically produced by applying 400-W radio frequency energy to create an electrical field, which generates the plasma from surrounding peroxide and water molecules. This reaction creates ozone and other radicals (including ·OH and ·OOH) on reaction with residual water and peroxide. These effects may contribute (although minimally) to the overall antimicrobial efficacy, but they also increase the degradation of peroxide, thereby reducing aeration time. In some cycles, the plasma pulse is sufficient to aerate the load, removing the need for subsequent aeration cycles. Many variations of plasma-peroxide systems have been described that combine these processes during the whole exposure phase, thereby increasing the generation of active oxygenated species during the sterilization phase. For these processes, no further extended aeration time was reported to be required in comparison to EO sterilization, minimizing the overall time and cost for product availability. Although the cycle time may vary depending on the application, the overall total cycle time can generally be 3 hours or less. Other, similar processes have been described in specially constructed exposure containers that coupled with the sterilizer peroxide gas generation system to allow for the directed, repeated flow of peroxide gas under vacuum through lumens and over the other device surfaces. A previously commercialized example was the AMSCO VHP100 sterilization process for flexible endoscope and dental devices, which operated at 35 to 49°C and 6 to 8 mg/liter of peroxide for a total cycle time of 30 to 45 minutes. Sterilizers that use combinations of hydrogen peroxide and other biocides in gas form have also been patented and developed, including the STERIZONE VP4 sterilizer that used hydrogen peroxide and ozone gas. In this example, the sterilization process is similar to the hydrogen peroxide gas cycle (in Fig. 6.11), but peroxide gas is introduced into the chamber at a fixed rate until the desired pressure is achieved, to accommodate variations in the load capacity and temperature; following this phase, ozone is introduced (produced from oxygen; see section 6.6.4) and mixed with peroxide to achieve sterilization. In this case, two pulses of peroxide and ozone gas exposure are used for sterilization, followed by aeration of the chamber and load by two vacuum pulses.

Sterilization applications with hydrogen peroxide gas include medical device, material, and equipment sterilization (e.g., for freeze-dryer chambers and electron microscopes). A range of hydrogen peroxide gas systems (examples given in Table 6.4) have become widely used for low-temperature sterilization of reusable medical devices in hospitals as alternatives to EO and formaldehyde sterilizers (see sections 6.2 and 6.3, respectively). The chamber sizes and sterilization cycles of peroxide gas sterilizers vary in cycle times ranging from 25 to 80 minutes and in chamber temperatures from 20 to 55°C. The applications with these systems can include the sterilization of rigid and flexible lumen instruments (including flexible endoscopes), which are a particular challenge for sterilization. The specific use of the sterilizer, which can include single or multiple

TABLE 6.4 A comparison of hydrogen peroxide gas sterilization systems used in health care and industrial applications.[a] Chamber sizes are shown in parentheses for each sterilizer type but may not indicate the actual total load capacity

Cycle	STERRAD 100S (100 liters)	STERRAD 200 (150 liters)	STERRAD NX[b] (50 liters)	V-Pro maX (136 liters)	ES 1400 (142 liters)	STERIZONE VP4 (125 liters)	HMTS-80 (80 liters)
Cycle time (mins)	54–72	75 (and load specific)	28–38	28–55	28–50	46–70	35–40
Conditioning	Vacuum, plasma	Vacuum, plasma	Vacuum	Vacuum	Vacuum	Vacuum	Vacuum
Sterilization	Peroxide gas, plasma	Peroxide gas, plasma	Peroxide gas, plasma	Peroxide gas	Peroxide gas	Peroxide gas, ozone	Peroxide gas, plasma
Aeration	Vacuum, plasma	Vacuum, plasma	Vacuum, plasma	Vacuum	Vacuum	Vacuum	Vacuum

[a]Health care applications provide fixed cycle conditions, while industrial cycles can be specifically customized for each application.
[b]Uses the removal of water from the hydrogen peroxide solution to give a higher concentration of 85 to 95% versus 59%.

sterilization cycles, varies depending on the load to be sterilized. Cycle claims can vary from manufacturer to manufacturer, depending on registration requirements in different countries. Examples include nonlumened devices up to a weight of ~9 kg and particular restrictions for loads containing lumened devices based on their lumen lengths, diameters, and construction materials (e.g., multiple-lumened rigid [stainless steel] devices at ≥0.7 mm internal lumen diameter and ≤500 mm in length, or a flexible [plastic] lumened device ≥1 mm diameter and ≤1,000 mm lumen length). In some cases, as for longer lumened devices such as endoscopes, a "booster" device extends lumen length claims; this device contains a volume of 59% liquid hydrogen peroxide that is attached externally onto the device lumen and is vaporized during the cycle to allow the vapor to flow through the lumen for sterilization. Overall, cycle times are dramatically less than alternative gas sterilization processes, particularly EO sterilizers. Similar peroxide gas or gas-plasma systems are used for industrial device and material sterilization, with cycles specific for the given application. These cycles can range from 0.1 to 10 mg/liter peroxide and from 4 to 80°C, although most temperature-sensitive materials are sterilized at <65°C. Hydrogen peroxide gas systems are not practically used for textile or liquid sterilization.

6.5.3 Spectrum of Activity

The broad-spectrum efficacy of hydrogen peroxide was discussed in chapter 3, section 3.13. *G. stearothermophilus* spores are generally accepted as being the most resistant organism to gaseous peroxide, with *B. atrophaeus* spores being more resistant to liquid peroxide. *G. stearothermophilus* spores are typically used to validate and confirm the antimicrobial efficacy of the hydrogen peroxide (including gas-plasma) sterilization process. Biocide penetration is less efficient under atmospheric gas or in liquid-based processes, with applications generally limited to direct application to exposed surfaces. Hydrogen peroxide gas is more penetrating under vacuum conditions, due to the removal of air. Vacuum-based cycles demonstrate broad-spectrum antimicrobial activity to provide a sterility assurance level (SAL) of 10^{-6} or as required by the process. Gaseous peroxide has been confirmed as effective against adult and dormant stages of protozoa such as *Cryptosporidium*, *Giardia*, and *Acanthameoba* and nematodes (*Enterobius*, *Caenorhabditis*, and *Sphacia*). Studies on the efficacy of hydrogen peroxide gas vacuum cycles against prions have shown mixed results; hydrogen peroxide gas is effective in comparison to liquid peroxide, but efficacy appears to be cycle- or process-dependent. Gaseous peroxide has also been used to reduce surface contamination with endotoxin, protein exotoxins (e.g., anthrax and botulinum toxins), and some cytotoxic drugs.

6.5.4 Advantages

Hydrogen peroxide is a broad-spectrum antimicrobial with a good environmental profile (chapter 3, section 3.13). Liquid peroxide is easy to use, but preferred sterilization applications with gas use less peroxide and demonstrate greater material compatibility, including with electrical equipment. Peroxide gas rapidly breaks down into water and oxygen in the environment. Low-temperature sterilization cycles are rapid in comparison to alternative gas processes (e.g., EO, which can take ~12 hours, depending on the application) or, in some cases steam, e.g., larger equipment sterilization due to the time required for the equipment to cool down. The ability to sterilize at low temperatures is clearly a benefit to the reprocessing of temperature-sensitive devices and materials. An advantage over steam sterilization is that peroxide gas has been shown under certain conditions to have activity against endotoxins, which are not degraded by steam. Combined processes with plasma may provide greater efficacy in some cases and shorter aeration times, in particular, for certain porous plastic materials. Improved efficacy in combination with other oxidizing agents including PAA and ozone has been cited, but little evidence of any synergistic benefit has been shown. Low- and high-concentration peroxide gas sensors can be used to monitor sterilization processes and detect gas leaks if present in an environment. Peroxide sterilizers have minimal utility requirements (electricity only) in comparison to steam, EO, and formaldehyde sterilizers.

6.5.5 Disadvantages

Certain materials absorb and break down peroxide, which can lead to inefficient sterilization processes and/or elongated aeration times. In general, peroxide (particularly the gaseous form) is not suitable for the sterilization of large amounts of cellulosics or other protein-based materials. For liquid applications, higher concentrations are required, which can pose some safety and handling risks. Also, peroxide residues should be removed by rinsing with water or using energy sources such as dry heat; this is an important consideration in, for example, high-speed food-packaging lines, where residuals can lead to spoilage. Although these effects are less of a concern in gaseous processes, some aeration may be required depending on the material type. Highly adsorbent or porous loads require special cycle development to ensure adequate sterilization, due to residuals. Hydrogen peroxide gas is less stable and therefore considered less penetrating than EO. With gaseous sterilization, only certain synthetic packaging materials or containers can be used that allow penetration of peroxide (e.g., one- or two-sided Tyvek packaging); paper packaging cannot be used, which may increase costs. Peroxide gas can cause bleaching (or dulling) of colored anodized aluminum; although the plasma process itself does not damage surfaces, the generation of active radicals on reaction with water/peroxide residues can be damaging to some surfaces over time. Widely used solutions of 35% and 59% peroxide cause burns on the skin with direct contact, although these risks have been reduced with the design of single-use, noncontact delivery systems. Low-concentration gas leaks cause short-term health effects, which subside on evacuation of the area. Higher concentrations pose a greater risk, such as inhalation and lung damage. Peroxide vapor cannot be used to sterilize liquids.

6.5.6 Mode of Action

The mode of action of liquid and gaseous hydrogen peroxide, as powerful oxidizing agents, is discussed in chapter 3, section 3.13, and in further detail in chapter 7, section 7.4.2.

6.6 OTHER OXIDIZING AGENT-BASED PROCESSES

This section discusses other oxidizing agent-based sterilization processes that have been described or that are widely used. These include some specific applications with hydrogen peroxide, chlorine dioxide, PAA, and mixed oxidants (chapter 3, section 3.13). It should be remembered that although all of these active agents can be sporicidal, their use in sterilization processes is somewhat limited to date. A sterilization process is required to be validated (and, in most countries, approved) to render a product free from viable microorganisms. In a typical process, the rate of microbiological death can be expressed as an exponential function to be able to give a probability of survival. A key component of this is the demonstration of an SAL (typically at 10^{-6}) that is described in more detail in chapter 1, section 1.4.3, and section 6.1. Processes that have described the demonstration of an SAL are discussed in this section.

6.6.1 Liquid PAA

The most widely used liquid processes to date are systems for low-temperature sterilization of reusable, immersible medical devices such as flexible endoscopes (e.g., the SYSTEM 1 and SYSTEM 1E processes; Fig. 6.12).

The process is conducted in a tabletop, compact machine in combination with a single-use cartridge (STERIS 20 or S40 Sterilant Concentrate) containing the sterilant concentrate of liquid PAA, separated from a dry mixture of surfactants, buffers, anticorrosives, and surfactants. During the process, the devices and components of the cartridge are immersed in water and automatically mixed. In addition, the sterilant is allowed to contact all internal surfaces of the processor liquid-handling system during sterilization, up to and including the sterile water filter. Liquid connectors are also supplied and specifically validated to ensure the flow of sterilant through specific device designs and lumens, as well as around connector sites on devices. The sterilization portion of the cycle is 6 to12 minutes at ~46 to 56°C and is followed by 2 to 4 water rinses (depending on the specific process). In one system, rinse water is provided through a 0.2-μ sterile water filter for a total cycle time of ~30 minutes. In a more recently developed design, the water is extensively treated to include the removal of bacteria and protozoa by filtration through a 0.1-μ filter, UV treatment to reduce any potential virus contamination, and an air purge—in a total cycle time of ~23 minutes.

The sporicidal activity of PAA in formulation can be dramatically increased at higher temperatures, up to 60°C, but this causes a decrease in the half-life of PAA (see discussion in chapter 3, section 3.13 [Figure 3.26]). For example, an average *D* value in the STERIS 20 formulation at 30°C is ~1.4 minutes, compared to <10 seconds at 55°C. Following sterilization and rinsing, devices are recommended to be used directly, because there is no sterile maintenance on removal from the processor. The advantages of the system include a rapid cycle time, broad-spectrum antimicrobial activity (including a validated SAL of at least 10^{-6}, biofilm removal, efficacy against vegetative and dormant forms of *Cryptosporidium* and *Giardia*, and endotoxin reduction), residual soil removal (due to flow over surfaces), no toxic residues, and a reasonably good safety and environmental profile. Disadvantages include the lack of sterile packaging or storage, and for lumened instruments, all channels should be confirmed as being clear of blockages prior to processing (as part of cleaning). The system utility requirements include potable or greater microbial quality water for processing. Further consideration of PAA as a biocide is discussed in section 3.13.

6.6.2 Electrolyzed Water

6.6.2.1 Types. The use of electrolyzed water has been described for sanitization, disinfection, and liquid sterilization applications. These processes are based on the electrolysis of water, in which water is passed through an electrolysis device to generate a biocidal solution (Fig. 6.13). Applications can include tap water alone or, more commonly, water with a small concentration of a salt (for example, 0.1 to 0.5% NaCl or KCl) or other electricity-conducting agents added.

A variety of generator designs have been described, but they all operate on a similar principle. A generator consists of an electrolytic

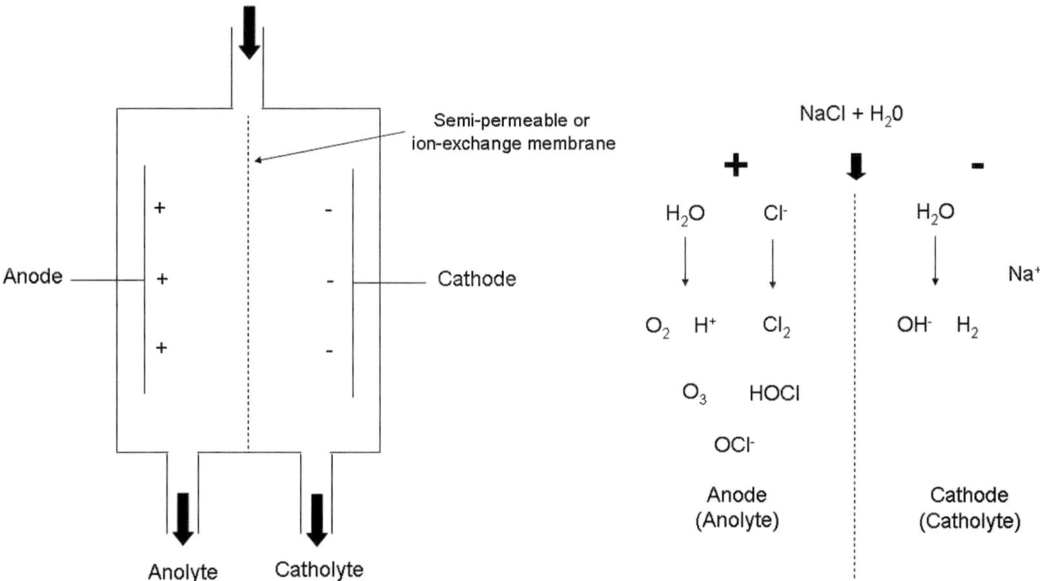

FIGURE 6.13 Electrolyzed water system. (Left) A representation of a typical electrolyzed water generator. (Right) Generation of electrolyzed water, with a simple depiction of the active species formed.

cell, with an anode and cathode separated by an ion-permeable membrane (Fig. 6.13). The membranes can be charged (e.g., an ion exchange resin) or noncharged, consisting of some porous structure (e.g., ceramic filters). When a voltage is applied to the electrodes, the water ions that are present are separated based on their respective charges into a reduced, or alkaline (pH 9 to 13), solution at the cathode (referred to as a catholyte) and into an oxidized, or acidic (pH 2 to 4), solution at the anode (the anolyte), separated by the membrane (Fig. 6.13). In some designs, in addition to the application of a voltage to the chamber, other forms of energy may be applied. This may include electromagnetic radiation sources within the radio frequency and microwave wavelength ranges (see chapter 2, section 2.4), which also act to charge the feed water, with the formation of free radicals and other active species. The anolyte has a high oxidizing potential, with an oxidation-reduction potential (which is measured by an electrode and electronic meter) of ~1,100 mV, and is highly antimicrobial. The antimicrobial effect is primarily due to the generation of available chlorine, mostly hypochlorous acid (for further discussion of the chemistry and antimicrobial effects of chlorine, see chapter 3, section 3.11). Anolytes can therefore have a slight to negligible chlorine odor. Other oxygenated and antimicrobial species may also be formed, including dissolved oxygen, ozone, and superoxide radicals (see section 3.13), which also contribute to the overall microbicidal efficacy of the anolyte. Generators can be sized to be able to produce electrolyzed water at the required volumes, e.g., up to 12,000 liters/hour or higher.

The anolyte itself can be essentially sterilized, because it is rapidly effective against bacteria, fungi, viruses, and waterborne parasites, with slower efficacy against spores (including bacterial spores) over time. The anolyte can also be directly applied to surfaces for disinfection and sterilization applications. The solution is not stable and is therefore generated on-site, close to the time of use, and is not stored for long times. In addition to the direct use of the anolyte, it can be combined with a portion of the catholyte (for neutralization or pH adjustment) or used in combination as part of a cleaning-disinfection process. An example of an electrolyzed-water process, the Sterilox Maxigen system controls the pH to between 5.75 and 6.75 by recirculating a portion of the catholyte into the anode chamber to give a typical range of 180 to 220 mg/liter of available free chlorine at pH 5 to 7. In this case, the pH, temperature, conductivity, and water flow rate of the generator system were tightly controlled to ensure consistent quality. The system required potable feed water (at <100 CFU/ml and hardness level at <30 mg/liter as $CaCO_3$) and had a constant capacity of 200 liters/hour of disinfectant water and 750 liters/hour of rinse water, which is recommended posttreatment. Corrosion inhibitors could be added to the water generator to improve the material compatibility of the anolyte. Water generated from this system was recommended for use for medical device reprocessing applications. Similar systems have been developed for other applications, including food or food-contact surfaces. Some systems recommend the use of other salts or minerals (e.g., organic acids such as ascorbic acid and gallic acid) during the generation process to control the pH or to remove available free chlorine, which can be overaggressive for some surface applications. In all cases, the antimicrobial solution produced can be referred to as "oxidized," "superoxidized," or "activated" water.

In addition to the use of the anolyte for antimicrobial purposes, the catholyte, a strong alkaline solution that is composed mostly of metal hydroxides, has been found to have cleaning abilities. Alkaline solutions are particularly used for the removal and breakdown of proteins and potentially other organic materials on surfaces.

6.6.2.2 Applications. Electrolyzed-water generators can be used to sanitize, disinfect, and in some cases, sterilize water for various applications, including drinking water, wastewater, and other feed-water applications (e.g., rinsing). In addition to antimicrobial activity, systems have been used for odor control. The use for routine water line disinfection or sterilization is of particular interest due to the ability of electrolyzed water to remove and disinfect surfaces contaminated with biofilm (including for *Legionella* and *Pseudomonas* control) (see chapter 8, section 8.3.8, for a detailed discussion of biofilms). Applications have included the use of electrolyzed water for surface rinsing following a chemical disinfection process, to remove residues of the disinfection chemistry. In other uses, the anolyte can be used as a hard-surface disinfectant and may not require any rinsing postdisinfection due to the short-lived nature of active species. Surface applications have included food-contact, veterinary, industrial, dental, and medical applications. For example, electrolyzed-water systems have been recommended for chemical disinfection of temperature-sensitive devices, including flexible endoscopes. Examples of such systems for these applications are the STERILOX generators (Fig. 6.14).

In these systems, the water generator could be located as a central supply unit that is plumbed to multiple washer-disinfectors in a facility. Electrolyzed water could be generated and stored for up to 24 hours prior to use. The sporicidal disinfectant anolyte was rapidly antimicrobial, within a typical exposure time of 5 to 10 minutes. Some applications have described the use of electrolyzed water at controlled temperature conditions (up to 50 to 60°C) for greater sporicidal activity. Some combined cleaning-disinfection applications (e.g., for routine decontamination of dialysis systems, dental units, or other systems containing reusable water or fluid lines), refrigerated storage of the anolyte for up to 14 days, and direct use of the low (<3) pH anolyte for device reprocessing. Systems have been described that use normal water for precleaning of surfaces, catholyte cleaning for 2 to 3 minutes, rinsing (to remove residual catholyte), and disinfection or sterilization with the anolyte for the required level of antimicrobial efficacy (generally 5 to 15 minutes). In these applications, the anolyte can remain *in situ* (as a preservative) until the next use of the device, or residual anolyte can be flushed away with air;

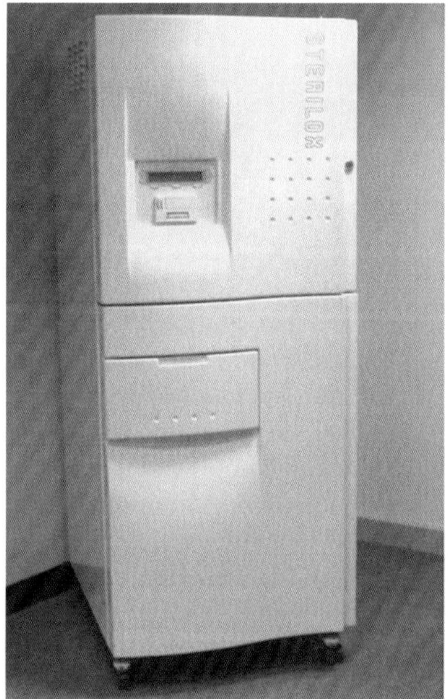

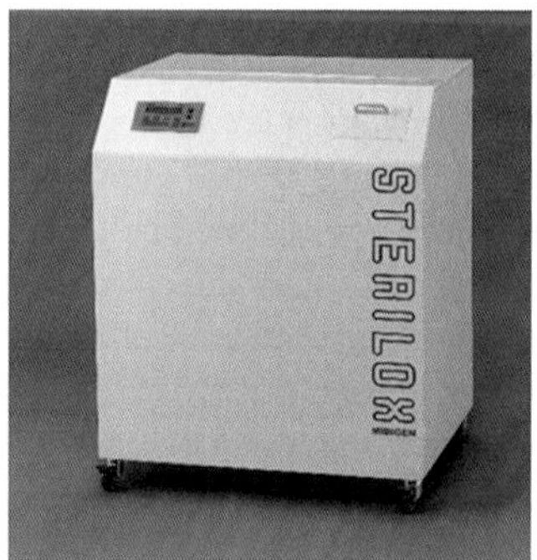

FIGURE 6.14 Examples of electrolyzed-water generators. ©2016 Mar Cor Purification, Inc.

under some use conditions, no further rinsing is required due to the low concentrations of biocidal species and the fact that they are generally short-lived, posing no toxic risk on subsequent reuse of the system.

Electrolyzed-water systems have been developed for a wider range of applications. These include the economical production of drinking water, wound or skin rinsing (as a nontoxic antiseptic), food rinsing and disinfection (e.g., tofu and fruits), and horticulture.

6.6.2.3 Spectrum of Activity. Given the range of antimicrobial effects observed with anolytes, it is not surprising that they are rapidly bactericidal and fungicidal. Rapid efficacy has been reported in both low-pH (<3) and mid-pH (5 to 7) ranges against Gram-positive and -negative bacteria, molds, yeasts, and mycobacteria. Virucidal efficacy has been confirmed against enveloped (including hepatitis B virus) and nonenveloped viruses, depending on the concentration and exposure time. Typical exposure conditions with anolytes for efficacy against these organisms are 100 to 250 mg/liter of available free chlorine for 2 minutes. Lower levels (as low at 100 mg/liter of chlorine solutions) have been claimed to be effective for the sanitization of cleaned surfaces against vegetative bacteria. Longer exposure times, between 5 and 10 minutes, or higher concentrations are generally required for sporicidal activity, although sterility assurance levels have not yet been widely published with electrolyzed water solutions. The presence of organic soil dramatically reduces the observed antimicrobial effects. Electrolyzed-water solutions have shown little to no effect against prions, although this has not been investigated in detail.

6.6.2.4 Advantages. Electrolyzed water (anolyte) demonstrates broad-spectrum antimicrobial, including sporicidal, activity but is nonirritating and presents minor toxicity concerns. Solutions have not been found to be sensitizing and can be safely disposed following use or expiration. The lower- and higher-pH solutions generated can cause damage on direct exposure to the skin, mucous membranes, and eyes; for generators that mix and control the pH of the water produced, this may be less of a concern. In addition to the anolyte biocidal activity, the high-pH catholyte also acts as a cleaner for surfaces, including for biofilm removal. Water generators can be low-cost, with few operational costs (energy and low concentrations of salts or minerals). Electrolyzed water has been shown to react with some undesirable, dissolved organic and inorganic water contaminants, causing them to coagulate and/or precipitate; these can then be removed from the water by simple filtration. Some activity has been reported against bacterial toxins and endotoxins, which can be present in water due to the presence of Gram-negative bacteria. Further, the anolyte can also cause the breakdown of toxic substances (for example, sulfides) into nontoxic compounds.

6.6.2.5 Disadvantages. Electrolyzed water can be damaging to some surface materials; for example, it can promote corrosion on metals such as stainless steel and damage to polyurethane over multiple applications. Material compatibility concerns have limited the widespread use of these systems. In some applications (e.g., flexible endoscope reprocessing), it was recommended that the device surface be coated with an oxidation-resistant, protective barrier (e.g., polytetrafluoroethylene), which could reduce these effects. Incompatibility on surfaces could be minimized by formulation effects (e.g., the addition of corrosion inhibitors such as phosphates and sulfates), which are added to the anolyte on production, or by controlling the pH at near-neutral by addition of catholyte. Equally, the catholyte is incompatible with soft metals, including aluminum. The activity, and damage to surfaces, varies depending on the quality of water used for generation. For example, when the feed water is chlorinated, high levels of chlorinated compounds may be produced, which can be aggressive on sensitive plastic and metal surfaces. Degassing from generated solutions should be controlled to ensure that these compounds do not accumulate to toxic levels. Further, other compounds may be formed in the anolyte or catholyte that can remain on a surface following treatment or be harmful when present in treated water. Examples include chlorinated by-products, as discussed in chapter 3, section 3.11. It is therefore recommended that the chloride levels and pH produced are controlled during use of the anolyte for antimicrobial applications. Other concerns can be the buildup of deposits on the electrodes and in the generators over time due to scaling, etc., which may be controlled by pretreatment of the water (ranging from water softening to the supply of reverse-osmosis water). These deposits or precipitates may be a concern on subsequent release from the generator but can be prevented by using filtration.

The antimicrobial effect of anolyte water is dramatically affected by the presence of contaminating soils. Surfaces are recommended to be adequately cleaned prior to application to ensure the required level of efficacy. Solutions are unstable, which also depends on the redox potential and pH; stability times are shorter at higher temperatures.

6.6.2.6 Mode of Action. Electrolyzed water, given as a mixture of antimicrobial agents, has multiple modes of action on microorganisms. Overall, these active agents (in particular, in the anolyte) cause damage to the cell wall, membrane, and intracellular components, as well as to the surfaces of spores and viruses. These targets are likely to include proteins, lipids, and nucleic acids. Specific effects observed in bacteria have included enzyme inactivation, outer and inner membrane structural changes, cytoplasmic leakage, DNA fragmentation, and cell wall damage. pH effects alone (both high- and low-pH solutions) are, at a minimum, restrictive to the growth of microorganisms but also cause bactericidal and fungicidal loss of structure and function. Vegetative organisms are particularly sensitive due to the delicate balance between the organism and its environment, as dictated by the cell wall-cell membrane structure, including osmotic pressure and the role of porins (chapter 8, section 8.3.4). In general, bacteria and fungi (depending on the genus and species) show a great variability in their ability to tolerate high or low pH and redox potential effects. In general, for pH this can range between 4 and 11, with some extremophiles (see sections 8.3.9 and 8.3.10) surviving at the extremes of this range; however, these highly pH-tolerant microorganisms are generally restricted to extreme environments and are not routinely identified in most environments. With a typical pH of <3 for a directly produced anolyte, little resistance of the solution to the multiple effects of pH is expected, although the mode of action of pH-controlled solution in the pH 5 to 7 range is primarily due to the presence of available free chlorine, in particular, as hypochlorous acid. The mode of action of hypochlorous acid and hypochlorite ions, as a major source of the antimicrobial activity, was discussed in chapter 3, section 3.11. In addition, the combined effects of oxygenated species, including ozone (section 3.13), also contribute to the overall microbicidal activity.

6.6.3 Gaseous PAA

Similar to the hydrogen peroxide gas systems, sterilization processes have been developed based on gaseous PAA and in combination with plasma (Fig. 6.15).

PAA is a broad-spectrum antimicrobial at relatively low concentrations and has been primarily used in liquid formulations for disinfection and sterilization (see chapter 3, section 3.13, and section 6.6.1). PAA gas can be produced by vaporization of liquid PAA-water solutions such as at 35 to 45% by heating or heating under vacuum. PAA solutions are supplied in solution with water, hydrogen peroxide, and acetic acid, so vaporization of these solutions can provide a mixture of PAA and peroxide gases (both powerful biocides). Some sterilization processes have described the use of vaporized PAA under vacuum, in cycles similar to those described for hydrogen peroxide (section 6.5) for reusable or single-use medical device and industrial sterilization applications. Gaseous PAA sterilization processes consist of the vaporization of PAA-water solutions into an evacuated chamber, exposure for a required exposure time, and aeration of the chamber by evacuation through a catalytic converter to break down the gas to water and acetic acid. The water content of the PAA solution can be sufficient to provide the necessary humidity for optimal antimicrobial activity (generally 20 to <100% relative humidity) or

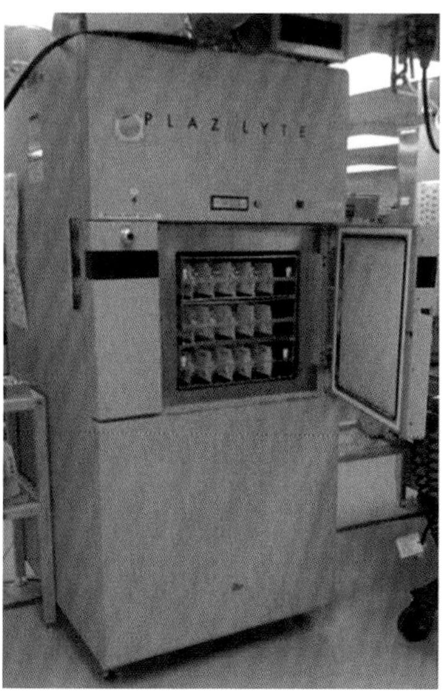

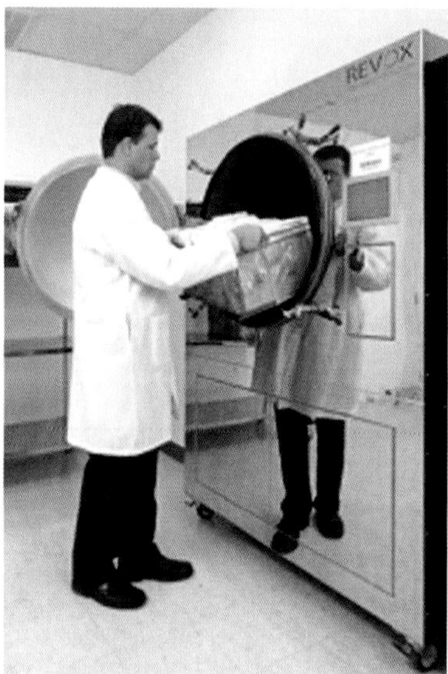

FIGURE 6.15 Examples of PAA gas sterilizers. (Left) Image courtesy of Johnson & Johnson, with permission. (Right) ©2016 Mar Cor Purification, Inc.

supplemented by further humidification (during the conditioning and/or sterilization phases) with low-temperature steam. PAA gas demonstrates optimal antimicrobial activity under humidified conditions. Exposures may be controlled at ambient temperatures or up to 40 to 55°C, with increased efficacy at higher concentrations and temperatures; higher temperatures may also cause the rapid breakdown of the gas and loss of efficacy. Proposed sterilization cycles include 10 mg/liter at 45°C for 60 minutes and ranges of cycles at 4 to 20 mg/liter at 20 to 30°C for 5 to 60 minutes of exposure to PAA gas (with a total cycle time ranging from 0.5 to 4 hours). Some systems have described the use of plasma generation (chapter 5, section 5.6.1) during or following PAA gas exposure during sterilization. As in hydrogen peroxide-plasma systems, this causes the production of antimicrobial radicals and other species on reaction with water and PAA gas and also can aid in rapid aeration of the chamber and load postexposure.

A PAA-plasma sterilization process (PLAZLYTE) was marketed in the United States for health care and industrial use, and although no longer commercially available, remains in industrial use. During the process, the load was treated with PAA gas at ~0.5 mg/liter, generated by direct vaporization in an evacuated chamber, which was followed by exposure to the gas, evacuation, and then introduction of a low-temperature plasma. The pulses could be repeated for the desired sterilization time, and then the chamber and load would be aerated by repeated vacuum applications. Similar processes to those described for hydrogen peroxide gas sterilization (see section 6.5 and Fig. 6.11) with PAA gas have been described for industrial sterilization applications in larger chambers (REVOX 417- to 3,000-liter chambers) under vacuum or atmospheric pressure conditions. Other processes have included atmospheric pressure applications (or a slight pressure differential), which allows the directed flow of gaseous PAA through and over the device or load surfaces. This can be achieved by directed flow under pressure or by creating a pressure differential between a two-component container system. Special containers to allow exposure and subsequent sterile storage of a load have been described for these purposes but are not commercially available.

Similar to hydrogen peroxide gas, gaseous PAA is a broad-spectrum antimicrobial with efficacy at lower concentrations than required for liquid formulations. PAA gas has been claimed to have greater stability and penetration into loads than other gaseous oxidizing agents, with some penetration of paper and porous materials. As with other gaseous sterilization processes, liquids cannot be treated and surfaces should be dry prior to treatment. PAA (as an acid and powerful oxidizing agent) can be corrosive to surfaces, although it is less so in gas form. Although these effects can be minimized in liquid formulation, PAA gas can be aggressive on many polymers and metals (depending on the concentration used and in particular on polyurethane and metals such as aluminum, brass, and copper). PAA gas is also irritating and sensitizing at low concentrations, with higher concentrations being toxic and damaging to the eyes, skin, and mucous membranes. Care should be taken to ensure that PAA and other toxic residuals that can form on surfaces during sterilization are adequately aerated to remove the risks of adverse reactions, particularly for critical surgical devices.

6.6.4 Ozone

Many systems have been proposed and designed based on the use of ozone in low-temperature sterilization processes. Ozone has been widely used for drinking water disinfection and area deodorization applications (chapter 3, section 3.13) and has some key advantages: it can be generated from water or in the presence of oxygen, demonstrates broad-spectrum antimicrobial efficacy, and rapidly breaks down in the environment to nontoxic residues (water and oxygen). However, although ozone is effective at low concentrations against vegetative bacteria and other pathogens, much higher, sustainable concentrations are required for sporicidal activity and to allow the development of validated sterilization processes. Some limited applications for food surfaces have been described, where ozone is directly produced and applied to surfaces for disinfection/sterilization. These processes have been difficult to apply to sterilization of defined loads, including medical devices, due to the higher humidity (>70%) and ozone concentrations required to achieve the required sterility assurance levels. Processes that combine PAA or hydrogen peroxide gas with ozone have also been described, with the recent development of a combined hydrogen peroxide gas-ozone sterilizer (although the primary antimicrobial activity appears to be due to hydrogen peroxide gas [see section 6.5]).

A humidified, low-temperature ozone gas sterilization system has been described for the sterilization of reusable medical devices and accessories (marketed as the STER-O_3-Zone 100) but has seen little practical application. The devices were placed into a rigid aluminum chamber module which was directly coupled to an ozone generator. The process consisted of preconditioning the load to a relative humidity of 75 to 95% and sterilization with ozone for 40 to 60 minutes at 25 to 30°C. The chamber was then aerated by passing residual ozone through a catalytic converter, and the container was used for subsequent sterile storage. Another approved system (TSO_3 125L ozone sterilizer) used humidified ozone under vacuum at 85 mg/liter for 15 minutes at a temperature of ~31°C to 36°C for low-temperature sterilization of medical devices (including metals, plastics, and restricted lumened devices) and other industrial applications (Fig. 6.16).

The sterilizer had minimal utility requirements, requiring high-quality water (which is provided as prepackaged purified water), medical grade oxygen, and electricity. The 125L sterilizer was a simple design consisting of a chamber, a humidifier, an ozone generator, and a vacuum pump. Similar to other gaseous sterilization methods, the process consisted of preconditioning, sterilization, and ventilation phases. During preconditioning the chamber was evacuated and the load humidified. The sterilization phase was conducted with two identical stages consisting of evacuation to ~0.01 kPa, humidification, ozone injection, and diffusion. Humidity was controlled at 85 to 100% while avoiding condensation of water/ozone. Antimicrobial efficacy with ozone is claimed to be optimal with humidity at ~95%. Ozone was generated from medical-grade oxygen by passing through a corona discharge, which was cooled to prevent decomposition, and introduced into the chamber to give an effective dose of 85 mg/liter. Humidified ozone was allowed to diffuse into the load for the required exposure time, was evacuated, and the load was exposed to an additional sterilization stage. The sterilization temperature was

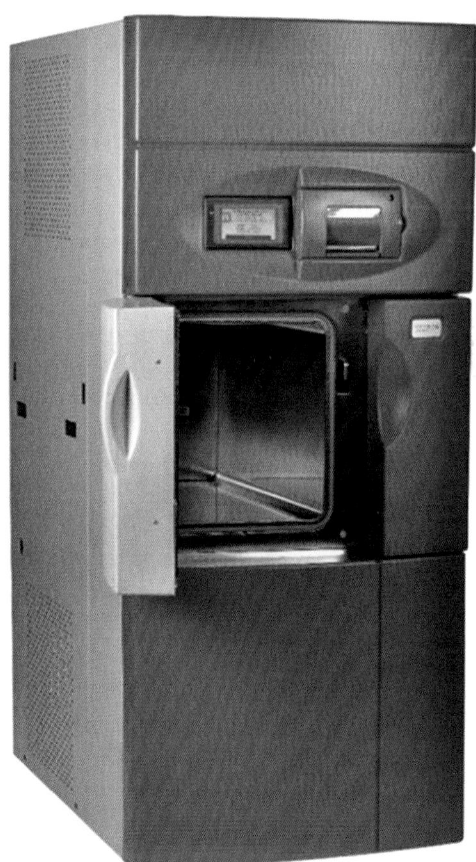

FIGURE 6.16 An ozone sterilizer. Image courtesy of TSO3, with permission.

maintained at 30 to 36°C. The chamber was then ventilated by evacuating the gas it through the ozone destroyer (catalytic converter), and then it was returned to atmospheric pressure to allow for load access. Approximately 700 to 880 liters of oxygen and a few milliliters of water were used during the process for a typical total cycle time of ~4.5 hours. The ventilation stage was short due to the rapid degradation of ozone, with no requirement for special venting or subsequent aeration. Overall cycle costs were claimed to be low, but this system had little commercial success due to material compatibility concerns and was subsequently discontinued.

Humidified ozone is a powerful antimicrobial but can be reactive or damaging to some plastic and metal surfaces over repeated applications. Incompatibility with ozone treatment has previously been observed with aluminum, brass, polyurethanes, and rubber materials. Woven textiles and liquids cannot be reprocessed with ozone.

6.6.5 Chlorine Dioxide

Although not widely commercialized, chlorine dioxide gas-based sterilization systems have also been described, which are not dissimilar to EO, ozone, and LTSF systems. Chlorine dioxide (ClO_2) is a gas at room temperature and, due to its reactive nature, is generated at the site of use (see chapter 3, section 3.13). Sterilization processes were conducted under vacuum in an evacuated chamber. A deep vacuum was drawn to <5 kPa, and the load was humidified by the introduction of low-temperature steam. This was important, because humidity should be maintained during the process at >65% for optimal ClO_2 sporicidal activity. ClO_2 can be generated by a variety of methods (including the use of chlorine gas passed through a column of sodium chlorite) to ~10 to 50 mg/liter and, by the addition of nitrogen gas, maintained at 80 kPa for the desired contact time. Multiple pulses of ClO_2 may be required to ensure the required load penetration and sterility assurance level. Sterilization processes have been described at 10 mg/liter, 25 to 30°C, and 70 to 80% relative humidity for up to 1.5 hours of total cycle time. A series of vacuum pulses are then used to remove residual ClO_2 (or breakdown products that include Cl_2 and O_2) from the chamber, usually by passage through a converter column. Aeration times are generally considered short, due to the rapid breakdown of the gas. Chlorine dioxide is a well-established broad-spectrum antimicrobial, including rapid sporicidal activity. It is a gas that rapidly breaks down on contact with surfaces; therefore, short sterilization cycles can be developed. A key consideration is the development of optimal ClO_2 generation technology to prevent the contamination of the load with chlorine gas (which is more destructive to surfaces) and other gases, as well as to minimize the presence of breakdown or generated residuals (including chlorine and NaCl) on critical surfaces. A further consideration is that chlorine dioxide itself can be damaging to some materials over time and has the same restrictions on penetration into complex loads as other gaseous oxidizing agents, in particular, with porous loads. Chlorine dioxide is considered toxic at high concentrations, with a recommended exposure rate of 0.1 ppm over a typical 8-hour work day and a short-term exposure safety risk of as low as 0.3 ppm for 15 minutes; gas sensors are available to monitor the presence of the gas in work environments.

6.6.6 Nitrogen Dioxide

Nitrogen dioxide gas disinfection and sterilization systems have been recently described but have as yet not been widely commercialized. Nitrogen dioxide (NO_2) is a gas at room temperature (specifically, >21°C [70°F]) and a potent oxidizing agent. Its main application to date has been industrial sterilization, but it has also been under investigation as a gaseous disinfection system for enclosed areas such as aseptic filling lines and isolators, similar to hydrogen peroxide and chlorine dioxide gas systems (chapter 3, section 3.13). Sterilization applications have been proposed as an alternative to EO and other low-temperature processes, in particular, for combination products such as bio-resorbable implantable devices, collagen scaffolds, and prefilled syringes. Disinfection and sterilization can be conducted under atmospheric and vacuum conditions, depending on the particular application need; but like other gaseous sterilization processes, this process can be more efficient under vacuum conditions due to the removal of air and efficient gas flow/penetration rates.

An example of a nitrogen dioxide-based sterilizer design is shown in Fig. 6.17. The load is placed in the sterilization chamber, which has been designed for exposure under vacuum conditions. The source of NO_2 is a liquefied gas (under pressure) of NO_2 and, predominantly, its dimer nitrogen tetroxide (N_2O_4). In the design shown, the liquid evaporates into a gas as a valve is opened into a smaller evacuated prechamber to prepare the gas and measure the concentration for dosing into the load chamber. The NO_2 dose, typically containing 90% NO_2 and about 10% N_2O_4, is then evacuated in the main sterilization chamber. Filtered air and humidity (water) can also be added during the process. Because NO_2 is a toxic gas, following exposure, the gas can be evacuated through a destroyer (catalytic converter) and out through a vacuum pump. NO_2 gas concentrations can also be monitored during the process or, as a safety precaution, in the evacuated air from the chamber through the destroyer.

Nitrogen dioxide gas has demonstrated broad-spectrum antimicrobial activity, including against bacteria, fungi, viruses, and bacterial spores. Viruses, in particular nonenveloped viruses, and bacterial spores are considered to be the most resistant, based on the reports published to date, with *G. stearothermophilus* spores being considered the organism most resistant to inactivation. Optimal antimicrobial activity is dependent on the gas concentration and humidity, similar to other gaseous sterilants such as EO, ozone, and chlorine dioxide. Sterilization applications can range from 500 ppm (~0.05%) to 10,000 ppm (~1%), ranging in *D* value against bacterial spores from ~50 minutes and 0.2 minutes, respectively. Although NO_2 has shown sporicidal activity over a wide range of humidity (e.g., 30 to 80%), optimal antimicrobial activity for the gas has been dem-

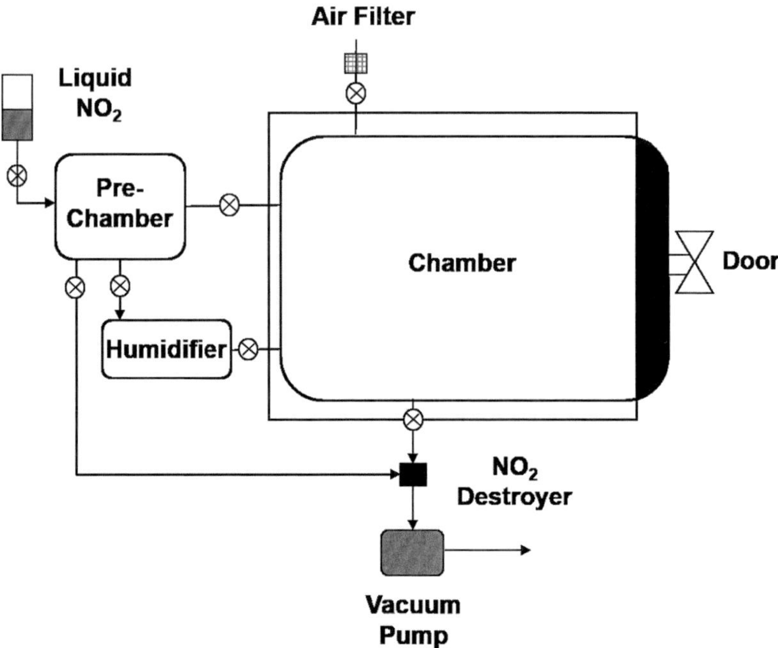

FIGURE 6.17 A representation of a nitrogen dioxide gas sterilizer.

onstrated at >70%. Overall, the antimicrobial activity can be optimized depending on the gas concentration, desired humidity, and exposure time. For example, in bacterial spore studies, at 75% humidity and for 3 minutes of exposure, little activity was observed at 4 mg/liter NO_2, but rapid activity was shown at ≥5 mg/liter. Equally, at 10 mg/liter and 1.5 minutes of exposure, the gas demonstrated ineffective activity at <65% humidity but was rapidly effective at ≥70%. Overall, by studying the sporicidal activity under different conditions, log-linear kinetics for antimicrobial activity can be demonstrated as the prerequisite for a given sterilization process.

A typical sterilization process with NO_2 gas is shown in Fig. 6.18. The air is evacuated from the chamber and load by pulling a vacuum, and this can be optimized by the depth of vacuum and by pulsing mechanisms as described for other processes. During this phase the load can be subjected to further conditioning, such as prehumidification, if desired. NO_2 gas and then humidity are added to the chamber to equilibrate and are then held for a specified contact time for sterilization. Depending on the load configuration and requirements for sterilization, this phase may be repeated multiple times (two gas exposure pulses are shown in Fig. 6.18). The gas is then removed from the chamber and load by pulling a vacuum multiple times to meet the required gas concentration safety levels for the chamber to be evacuated to atmospheric pressure and the load recovered.

Although studies and applications are limited, NO_2 has some important advantages as a disinfectant and sterilant. Notably, it has broad-spectrum antimicrobial activity that can be optimized over a range of gas concentrations, times, and humidity levels, allowing it to be adaptable to a variety of potential applications. The process can be effective and does not appear to be affected over a wide temperature range, allowing for room temperature applications, which is an important benefit over processes such as EO (see chapter 2, section 6.2) for temperature-sensitive products. Because it is a true gas over 21°C (70°F), the risk of liquid condensation is lower than for oxidizing agents such as hydrogen peroxide. Equally, the shorter sterilization process times and potential lack of any extended aeration associated with EO are also benefits in some applications. The overall environmental impact is considered low, and the gas is not considered carcinogenic (unlike traditional gases such as EO and formaldehyde). NO_2 has also been re-

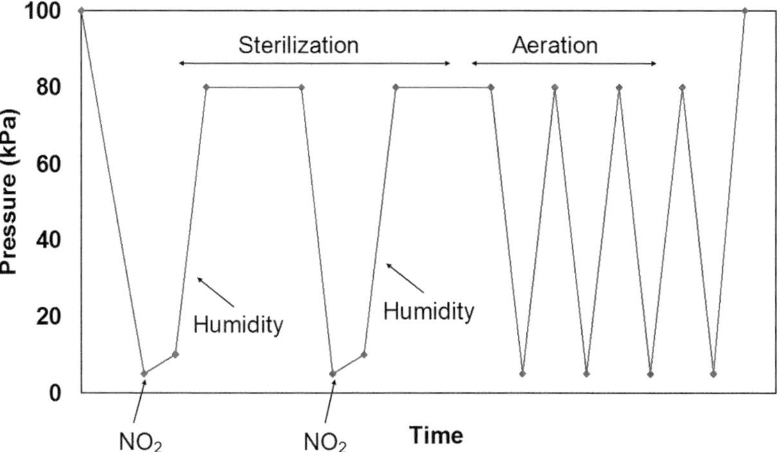

FIGURE 6.18 Typical nitrogen dioxide gas sterilization process.

ported to have a reasonable material compatibility and biocompatibility profile; however, this varies depending on the material and sterilization process. Polymeric materials such as polyethylene, polycarbonate, and polypropylene have been shown to be compatible, but others such as nylon, polyurethane, and polyacetate are less compatible. Some of these materials (such as polyurethane and polyvinylcarbonate) may require longer aeration times due to gas adsorption. Similar to other oxidizing agents, cellulosic materials (including paper) are not generally compatible because they react with and adsorb these gases. The use of NO_2 for the sterilization of metals may also require special consideration. Although stainless steel is considered compatible, it can act as a gas catalyst depending on the material quality and finishing; other metals require special cycle development such as with copper and anodized aluminum (in the latter case due to surface damage and bleaching of colors often incorporated during the anodization process).

NO_2 is a well-described pollutant (as a byproduct of combustion) and toxic substance. Health effects can range from minor at 10 to 20 ppm gas concentrations to life-threatening at 100 ppm. At lower concentrations (5 to 20 ppm) the gas can demonstrate delayed effects by causing inflammation of the mucous membranes and other tissues including the skin, eyes, and particularly, the lung epithelial levels. Exposure to lower concentrations can be reversed by moving to fresh air. At certain concentrations NO_2 can lead to skin burns and eye irritation, but early effects include dizziness and headaches, leading to delayed effects such as shortness of breath (due to bronchoconstriction) and, over time, reduced immune response and other effects on the lungs. The recommended exposure rate is 0.2 ppm over a typical 8-hour work day, and the short-term exposure safety risk is 1.0 ppm for 15 minutes; gas sensors are available to monitor the presence of the gas in work environments. A further consideration during safety evaluations is that NO_2 can react with water to form nitric acid and nitric oxide, which can pose an additional toxicity risk.

Initial studies of the mode of action of NO_2 have shown particular effects of DNA single-stranded breaks and fragmentation. The effects of humidity on the antimicrobial activity against bacterial spores is likely due to the hydration of the outer protective spore structures (section 8.3.11) that allow for greater gas penetration into the core nucleic acid. It is likely that due to its potent oxidizing agent activity, other mechanisms will include specific effects on protein and lipid structures, but similar to hydrogen peroxide gas (section 6.5), the primary mechanism of action is DNA (or nucleic acid) damage.

MECHANISMS OF ACTION

7

7.1 INTRODUCTION

Many compounds and processes have been identified as antimicrobial agents. For the purpose of this review, they are classified as being anti-infectives or biocides (chapter 1, section 1.2). Anti-infectives are substances (or drugs) capable of inhibiting or inactivating microorganisms (particularly pathogens) that are associated with various infections within animals, plants, and humans. This term is used to encompass drugs that specifically act on certain types of microorganisms, including antibacterials (i.e., antibiotics), antifungals, antivirals, and antiprotozoal agents. In contrast, biocides are chemical or physical agents that are used on inanimate surfaces or the skin and mucous membranes. Biocides demonstrate a much wider range of antimicrobial activity than anti-infectives and are applied in a wider range of applications. A comparison of the characteristics of anti-infectives and biocides is shown in Table 7.1.

Anti-infectives have been identified and developed for their specific use in the control of microbial infections while having limited to no toxic effect on the host. Examples include the antifungal drugs known as the azoles and polyenes, which specifically inhibit the biosynthesis or disrupt the structure of ergosterol. Ergosterol is a unique molecule found in many fungal cell membranes (chapter 1, section 1.3.3.2, and chapter 8, section 8.10) and is distinct from other sterols found in human cell membranes. Specific activity against ergosterol therefore allows greater activity against the target fungal infection, with limited damage to the host cells; however, ergosterol is not found in bacterial cell membranes, and therefore azoles and polyenes have a limited spectrum of activity against certain fungi. Similarly, reverse transcriptase (a viral enzyme required for the replication) is a unique anti-infective target for retroviruses, including HIV, because the enzyme is not found in other eukaryotic or prokaryotic cells; equally, anti-infectives that target reverse transcriptases are only effective against viruses that express those enzymes. Overall, most anti-infectives have specific modes of action and limited spectra of activity. Biocides have multiple modes of action and a broader range of antimicrobial activity; however, their toxic effects have limited their use to liquids, materials, and surfaces, including inanimate materials and, in a limited number of cases, on the skin or mucous membranes (see chapter 4).

This chapter only briefly considers, for comparison, the modes of activity of various anti-infectives, which are discussed as antibacterials

TABLE 7.1 A general comparison of anti-infectives and biocides

Criteria	Description: Anti-infectives	Description: Biocides
Spectrum of activity	Generally narrow, e.g., antibiotics can be effective against certain types of vegetative bacteria; efficacy can depend on the specific genus or species	Broader spectrum of activity, depending on the biocide and exposure conditions; can be effective against vegetative (actively metabolizing forms) and "dormant" (including viruses and spores) microbial forms
Effects on humans, animals, plants	Minimal toxicity, being one of the criteria for successful use	Generally toxic
Mechanism of action	Single or, in some cases, a number of specific targets	Generally multiple targets that can include proteins, carbohydrates, nucleic acids, and lipids
Stability	Notably stable to permit uptake and effectiveness at the site of infection	Most (although not all) unstable in the environment or on contact with organic/inorganic material
Target use	Usually internal to the host, e.g., within the bloodstream or plant structure	Directly on or at the contaminated surface, liquid, or area
Potentiation ability	Generally none or limited to the presence of the active agent at the correct concentration at the site of infection and susceptibility of the target microorganism	Can be substantially affected by a variety of factors including concentration, pH, temperature, formulation, state of the biocide, and presence of interfering substances
Potential of resistance development	High	Limited

(antibiotics), antivirals, antifungals, and antiprotozoal agents. The mode of action of biocides is discussed under four main classifications based on their primary mechanisms of action: oxidizing agents, cross-linking or coagulating agents, transfer-of-energy agents, and other structure-disrupting agents. Considerable progress has been made in understanding the mechanisms of action of some biocides on bacteria, including vegetative bacteria and endospores. In contrast, studies of their modes of action against fungi, viruses, protozoa, algae, and prions have been limited and may be postulated based on known antibacterial mechanisms. Because the targets of biocides often include at least one or all of the four major types of macromolecules (proteins, lipids, carbohydrate, and nucleic acids) that make up the range of microbial structures and functions, these are also briefly introduced.

7.2 ANTI-INFECTIVES

Before considering the broad-spectrum activity of biocides, some discussion is warranted on the mode of action of specific anti-infectives. Examples include the relatively narrower spectrum of activity reported for penicillin, tetracyclines, and some sulfonamides against bacteria, although in some cases activity has also been demonstrated against some protozoa. In contrast, other antibiotics demonstrate more restricted spectra of activity; they include the glycopeptides that are only effective against Gram-positive bacteria. Many applications using these anti-infectives are restricted by the balance that must be struck between obtaining a minimum concentration of the active agent at the site of infection required for efficacy and avoiding any adverse effects on the host. Despite this, most antibiotics demonstrate some toxicity or adverse effects; for example, oral penicillin doses can result in diarrhea, allergic skin rashes, and in rare cases, anaphylaxis in some individuals. The narrower spectra of activity of anti-infectives are related to their specific modes of action.

7.2.1 Antibacterials (Antibiotics)

Antibiotics have been indispensable for their use for the treatment and control of bacterial infections since their discovery and first use in the 20th century. Summaries of some of the major antibiotics and their modes of action are given in Fig. 7.1 and Table 7.2. Many antibiotics specifically interact with certain cellular targets that are involved in key bacterial processes, including DNA replication, transcription, translation, and formation of cell components (Fig. 7.1). These act by specifically binding to ribosomes (which are required for protein biosynthesis), proteins (in particular, key enzymes), protein-DNA complexes, and cell wall components (Table 7.2). In addition, some antibiotics specifically interact with the Gram-negative cell membrane (e.g., the polymyxins), not unlike the mode of action of some biocides such as the surfactants, which disrupt structure and function (see chapter 3, section 3.16, and section 7.4.5).

Given the specific mechanisms of action of antibiotics, it is not surprising, considering their widespread use and often misuse, that bacterial resistance has developed. Resistance can be a natural attribute of bacteria due to the lack or inaccessibility of a specific target or other natural resistance mechanisms that they express. Bacteria, originally sensitive to antibiotics, have also demonstrated great resilience to develop acquired resistance to antibiotics through mutations or acquisition of genetic material (plasmids and transposons; chapter 8, section 8.7.3). Acquired resistance mechanisms include reduced uptake, drug inactivation, and specific loss or alteration of key cellular targets.

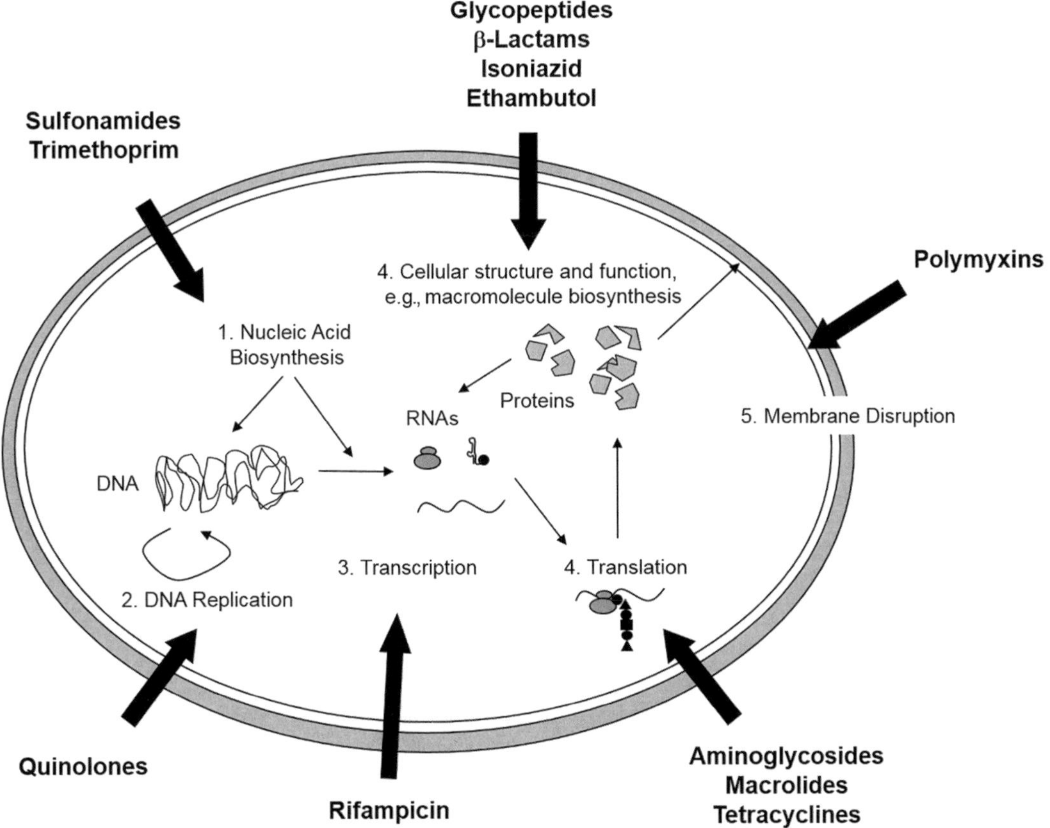

FIGURE 7.1 Primary bacterial targets of key antibiotics.

TABLE 7.2 Widely used antibiotics (antibacterials) and their mechanisms of action

Class	Example	Spectrum of activity	Mechanism of action
Aminoglycosides	Streptomycin	Gram-positive and Gram-negative bacteria, including *Mycobacterium* spp.	Inhibit protein synthesis; bind to ribosomal RNA to inhibit initiation, misreading of mRNA, and prevent translocation
β-lactams	Penicillin	Generally more effective against Gram-positive than Gram-negative bacteria, but also some activity against actinomycetes and protozoa (e.g., *Treponema* spp.)	Inhibit cell wall synthesis; bind to enzymes involved in peptidoglycan cross-linking
Chloramphenicol	Chloramphenicol	Inhibitory against Gram-positive and Gram-negative bacteria including mycoplasma	Inhibits protein synthesis; binds to ribosomal RNA
Glycopeptides	Vancomycin	Gram-positive bacteria, but not mycobacteria	Inhibit cell wall biosynthesis; bind to peptidoglycan precursors to prevent cell wall formation
Isoniazid	Isoniazid	Mycobacteria	Inhibits mycolic acid biosynthesis in mycobacteria
Macrolides	Erythromycin	Broad-spectrum activity against Gram-positive and Gram-negative bacteria (generally inhibitory), including *Mycobacterium*	Inhibit protein synthesis; bind to ribosomal RNA
Polymyxins	Polymyxin B	Gram-negative bacteria, including *Pseudomonas* spp.	Cell membrane insertion and disorganization
Quinolones	Ciprofloxacin	Gram-positive and Gram-negative bacteria, including *Mycobacterium* and *Mycoplasma*	Inhibit DNA replication by inhibiting DNA gyrase
Sulfonamides	Sulfapyridine	Broad-spectrum inhibitory activity against Gram-positive and Gram-negative bacteria, as well as some actinomycetes and protozoans (e.g., *Plasmodium* and *Toxoplasma* spp.)	Inhibit nucleotide biosynthesis by binding to bacterium-specific enzymes (involved in folic acid synthesis)
Tetracyclines	Tetracycline	Gram-positive and Gram-negative bacteria, including *Mycobacterium* and some protozoans (e.g., *Plasmodium* spp.)	Inhibit protein synthesis; bind to ribosomal RNA

Bacterial resistance to antibiotics is a major concern and highlights the importance of the safe and prudent use of antibiotics.

7.2.2 Antifungals

Similar to antibiotics, antifungals specifically target key biosynthetic or structural targets in fungi (Table 7.3). The structure of ergosterol and its biosynthetic process are an important target for many anti-infectives, which cause disruption of the structure and function of the fungal cell membrane. Most of the important fungal pathogens, including molds (*Aspergillus* spp. and the dermatophytes) and yeasts (*Candida* and *Cryptococcus* spp.), contain ergosterol and are generally sensitive to these anti-infectives, although this can vary depending on the species and specific drug (primarily due to variable intracellular accumulation). As with bacteria, fungal resistance can easily develop due to various adaptations, including changes in sterol structure and levels in the cell membrane and in specific enzymes involved in biosynthetic pathways. Other antifungal targets include inhibition of 1-3-β-D-glucan and, therefore, cell wall biosynthesis (Table 7.3).

7.2.3 Antivirals

Anti-infectives that target viruses have been identified or specifically developed to inhibit key stages in viral infection and replication within cells (Table 7.4). Some antivirals can specifically block penetration into target cells, while others inhibit various stages of intracellular virus multiplication. An important class of antiviral drugs, the interferons, primarily act to induce the host immune system to target the viral infection; however, some specific inhibitory effects on virus multiplication, including penetration, virion release, and nucleic acid translation, have been reported.

7.2.4 Antiparasitic Drugs

Various antiparasitic drugs have been widely used for protozoal or helminth infections or as preventative drugs. These have also been shown to be somewhat tolerated by the host and to have specific mechanisms of action (Table 7.5). Some are also well-known antibiotics, including tetracyclines and sulfonamides (section 7.2.1).

7.3 MACROMOLECULAR STRUCTURE

The basic structures of microorganisms are described in chapter 1. Although they present with a variety of different sizes, structures, and arrangements, they are essentially composed of four basic macromolecules, which give them structure and function: nucleic acids, proteins, carbohydrates, and lipids. These macromolecules combine to form complex and balanced structures, including cell walls, envelopes, capsids, cell membranes, nucleic acids, and cytoplasmic constituents, which are required for the growth and/or proliferation of the micro-

TABLE 7.3 Widely used antifungal drugs and their mechanisms of action

Class	Example	Spectrum of activity	Mechanism of action
Polyenes	Amphotericin B	Broad antifungal activity, including against *Candida*, *Cryptococcus*, and *Aspergillus* spp.	Disruption of cell membrane synthesis; bind to ergosterol
Azoles	Ketoconazole	Broad antifungal activity, including against *Candida*, *Cryptococcus*, and *Aspergillus* spp.	Inhibition of ergosterol biosynthesis, required for cell membrane structure
Allylamines	Terbinafine	Dermatophytes, but also other fungi, including *Candida* spp.	Inhibition of ergosterol biosynthesis, required for cell membrane structure
Antimetabolites	Flucytosine	Broad antifungal activity, including against *Candida*, *Cryptococcus*, and *Aspergillus* spp.	Integration into fungal RNA and inhibition of DNA synthesis
Glucan synthesis inhibition	Capsofungin	Broad antifungal activity, including against *Candida*, *Cryptococcus*, and *Aspergillus* spp.	Inhibition of cell wall synthesis; blocks synthesis of 1-3-β-D-glucan

TABLE 7.4 Widely used antiviral drugs and their mechanisms of action

Class	Example	Spectrum of activity	Mechanism of action
Nucleoside analogues	Acyclovir	Herpes simplex viruses	Inhibit genome replication; viral-DNA polymerase inhibition
Virus penetration inhibitors	Amantadine	Influenza viruses	Block a cellular membrane channel, which prevents membrane-virus fusion
Mutagens	Ribavirin	Broad-spectrum activity against RNA viruses including hepatitis C virus, herpes simplex virus, measles virus, and mumps virus	Inhibit viral RNA synthesis
Assembly, maturation, release inhibition	Oseltamivir (Tamiflu)	Influenza virus	Prevent virus budding from the cell; neuraminidase inhibitors
Cell defense promoters	α, β, and γ interferons	Hepatitis B and C viruses	Activation of host cell (immune) defense mechanisms

organism. Brief descriptions of each of these are given as background for the discussion on specific modes of action of biocidal processes.

Macromolecules are composed of the same major elements: carbon, hydrogen, oxygen, nitrogen, phosphorus, and sulfur. These elements are linked to form the basic building blocks of macromolecules, which are amino acids (proteins); sugars (polysaccharides); fatty acids or, in some cases, phytanes (lipids); and nucleotides (nucleic acids). The linkages between these building blocks can be considered as covalent or noncovalent bonds. Covalent bonds are strong bonds between elements and include peptide (in proteins), glycosidic (in polysaccharides), and phosphodiester (in nucleic acids) bonds. Noncovalent bonds are considered weaker associations but have an essential role in dictating the structure and function of macromolecules; these include hydrogen bonding, van der Waals forces, and hydrophobic interactions.

Proteins (or polypeptides) are composed of repeating units (or polymers) of amino acids. There are 21 main amino acid types commonly found in microorganisms. The basic amino acid structure is shown in Fig. 7.2. Amino acids are covalently linked by peptide (or amide) bonds to give the primary structure (or amino acid sequence) of the protein.

It is the sequence and types of amino acids present that dictate the structure and function of proteins. This is achieved by folding of the primary sequence to give the protein secondary and tertiary structures. The amino acids interact by hydrogen bonding with adjacent and distant residues in the primary structure to produce the secondary structure of the protein, consisting of local formations known as α-helixes and β-sheets. These arrangements allow for further interactions between amino acids (by covalent bonding, hydrogen bonding, and other interactions) to produce the protein tertiary structure. In many cases, the tertiary form is the final

TABLE 7.5 Widely used antiparasitic drugs and their mechanisms of action

Class	Example	Spectrum of activity	Mechanism of action
Macrolide endectins	Ivermectin	Arthropods and nematodes	Inhibit a neurotransmitter in the parasite
Benzimidazoles	Mebendazole	Nematodes, cestodes, helminths, and protozoa	Inhibit cytoplasmic functions; bind to microtubules (tubulin)
Pyrazinoisoquinoline	Praziquantel	Nematodes and trematodes	Affect cell membrane permeability and cause tegument disintegration
Tetracyclines	Doxycycline	Protozoa and bacteria	Block protein synthesis
Sulfonamides	Sulfadimethoxine	Protozoa, including *Isospora* spp., and bacteria	Inhibit nucleotide and folic acid synthesis
Quinine-related	Chloroquine	*Plasmodium* spp.	Multiple effects related to the malarial parasite infection of red blood cells

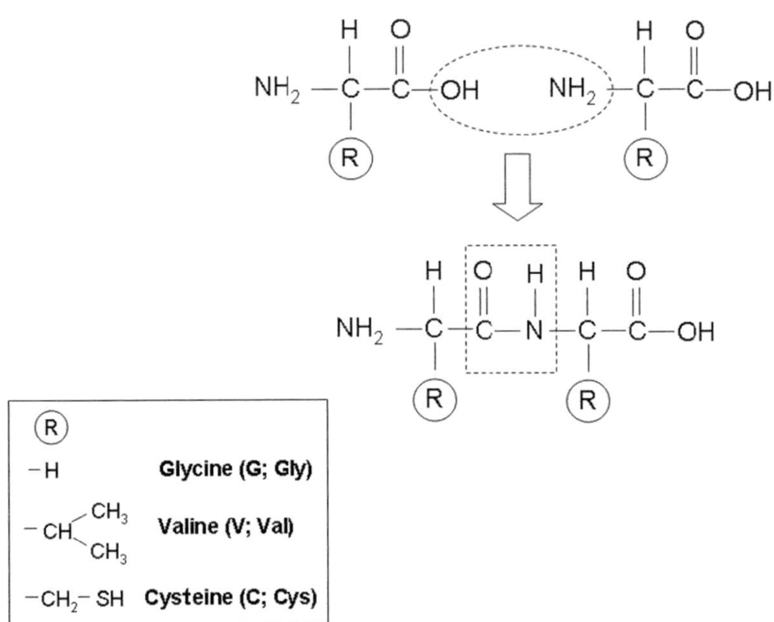

FIGURE 7.2 The structure of amino acids and peptide bonding. Representations of two amino acids are shown condensing to form a dipeptide linked by a peptide bond. Examples of the various side groups (R) that define the different amino acids are shown.

structural and functional form of the protein; however, in some cases, a quaternary structure is also formed by similar covalent and/or noncovalent interactions between different proteins (or polypeptides) to give a larger functional assembly. Tertiary and quaternary forms can change their conformation as part of their biological function or relative to various environmental conditions. The functions of proteins can be considered as structural and/or enzymatic, therefore playing an essential role in the growth and survival of microorganisms.

Polysaccharides are polymers that consist of multiple subunits of monosaccharides (or "simple" sugars). Sugars have a simple structure consisting of carbon, hydrogen, and oxygen (Fig. 7.3).

Sugars can be classified according to the number of carbon units, for example, pentoses (five carbon units such as ribose and deoxyribose, which are the building blocks of nucleic acid backbone structures) and hexoses (six carbon units, including glucose). Polysaccharides, including starch, glycogen, cellulose, and peptidoglycan, are formed by monomeric sugars linked together by various types of glycosidic bonds. For example, starch, glycogen, and cellulose are all polymers of glucose but are linked by different glycosidic bonds (Fig. 7.3). Peptidoglycan is a more complex polysaccharide consisting of two repeating sugars, *N*-acetylglucosamine and *N*-acetylmuramic acid, linked by β-1,4 glycosidic bonds to form the glycan chains, which are cross-linked by peptides; peptidoglycan is a major component of bacterial cell walls (chapter 1, section 1.3.4.1). Polysaccharides play important roles in the structure and energy storage of microorganisms.

Lipids are a structurally diverse group of organic compounds that are typically insoluble in water. They include various types of fats, oils, and waxes. The major components of microbial lipids are fatty acids, which are long hydrocarbon chains with a hydrophobic and hydrophilic region (Fig. 7.4).

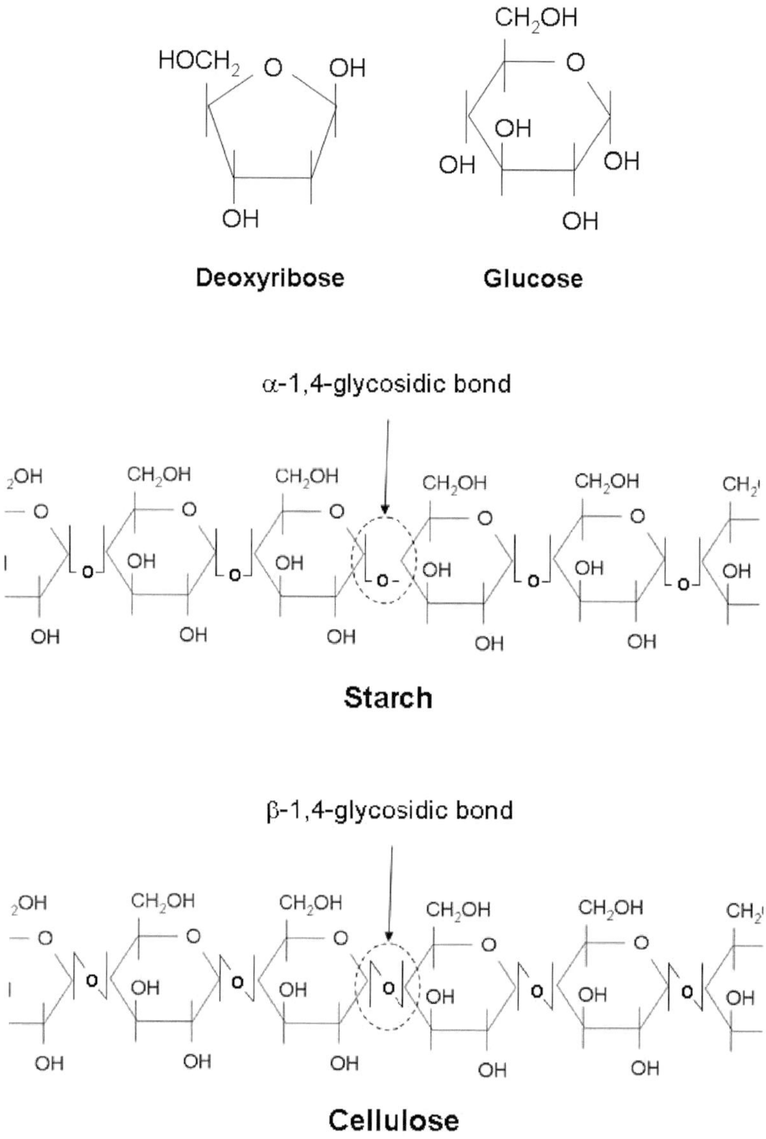

FIGURE 7.3 Examples of sugars, polysaccharides, and glycosidic bonds. The polysaccharides shown are both polymers of glucose but vary in the structure of the glycosidic bond linkages.

Fatty acids can be classified based on the number of carbons and the presence or absence of double bonds within the hydrocarbon chain, with those containing double bonds referred to as being unsaturated and those not as saturated (e.g., palmitoleic acid is a $C_{16:1}$ monounsaturated fatty acid, and stearic acid is a C_{18} saturated fatty acid). Examples of lipid structures are shown in Fig. 7.5. Simple lipids commonly found in microorganisms include the triglycerides (fats), which are composed of three fatty acids linked by ester bonds to glycerol (a type of alcohol). Lipids that are more complex include phospholipids (which contain a phosphate group) and glycolipids (which are linked to various sugars). The phospholipids and sterols are an

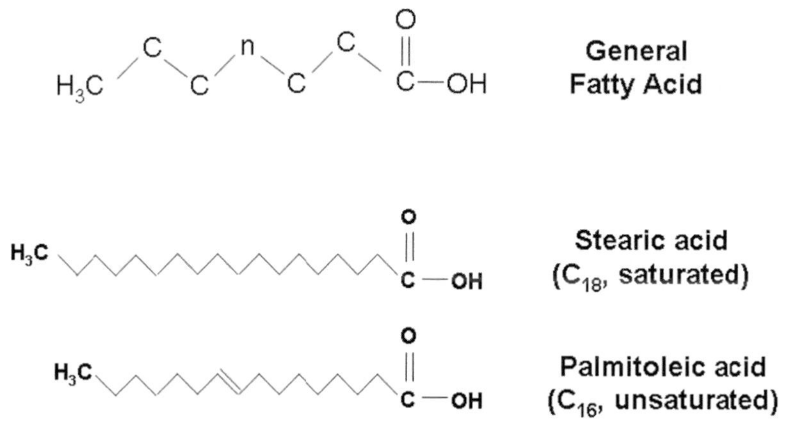

FIGURE 7.4 The basic structure of fatty acids. The number of carbons in the fatty acid structure can vary. Examples of stearic acid (C_{18}) and palmitoleic acid (C_{16}) are shown.

important part of the structure and function of membranes (e.g., see chapter 1, section 1.3.4.1). Overall, lipids play key roles in the microbial structure and as energy reserves.

Nucleic acids are polymers of nucleotides (and therefore also known as "polynucleotides"), which are molecules consisting of three components: a sugar, a nitrogen-containing base, and a phosphate group (Fig. 7.6). The five carbon sugars can be either ribose or deoxyribose (Fig. 7.3), with attached bases (purines, adenine, and guanine or pyrimidines, thymine, cytosine, and uracil) and phosphate groups.

Polynucleotides are formed by nucleotides covalently linked via their phosphate groups to form sugar-phosphate ("phosphodiester") bonds. Polynucleotides include deoxyribonucleic acid (DNA) and ribonucleic acid (RNA), which are the genetic materials found in microorganisms. DNA is a double-stranded polynucleotide in a double-helix structure and is the inherited, genetic material in most organisms (Fig. 7.7). In addition to the covalently linked nucleotides within each DNA strand, the individual bases of the strands are also linked by noncovalent hydrogen bonding between complementary purine and pyrimidine bases (A:T and G:C), which keeps the strands in the double-helix structure together. DNA contains only deoxyribose sugars and adenine, guanine, thymine, and cytosine bases; RNA contains ribose sugars and contains uracil bases instead of thymine. RNA is generally single-stranded (e.g., messenger-RNA), although it can assume various secondary structures by folding and base-pairing between complementary sequences (as in the case of transfer- and ribosomal-RNA, which are involved in protein translation; Fig. 7.7). It should be noted that the inherited (genetic) material found in viruses can include double- or single-stranded DNA or RNA (see chapter 1, section 1.3.5). Monomeric nucleotides are also found which play important roles in cellular metabolism (e.g., adenosine triphosphate [ATP] is a source of energy [Fig. 7.7]).

7.4 GENERAL MECHANISMS OF ACTION

7.4.1 Introduction

Unlike the anti-infectives discussed in section 7.2, the antimicrobial effects of most biocides and biocidal processes are generally broad-spectrum, with multiple effects on target microorganisms and their associated macromolecules. The following discussion considers

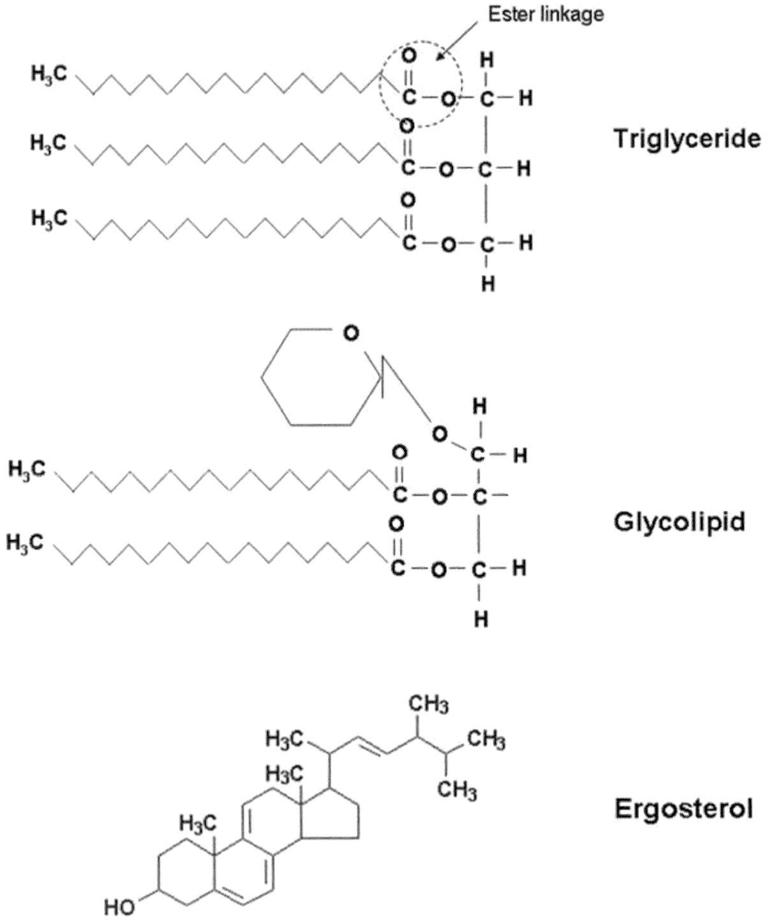

FIGURE 7.5 Examples of various types of lipids. The general structures of a triglyceride, a glycolipid (with one sugar linked to two fatty acids), and a sterol (ergosterol) are shown.

the known major targets or effects of certain groups of biocides, but in many cases secondary and, in some cases, multiple chemical effects have been observed. The effects of ionizing radiation on a target cell can be taken as an example. It is clear that the major targets of action of radiation are the nucleic acids; however, the reaction of radiation with water, with other cellular molecules, and even with the associated surface or liquid where the microorganism is found also lead to the localized production of free radicals. These radicals include hydroxyl radicals, which are powerful oxidizing agents that can have multiple destructive effects on nucleic acids, proteins, lipids, and other molecules. Further, in some cases, specific key targets for some biocides have been identified and are known targets for some antibacterial antibiotics (e.g., triclosan, which is discussed in further detail below).

Overall, biocides are microbial poisons, and what is known about their effects on microorganisms has been discussed for each active agent in chapters 2 to 6. They are covered in more detail in this section. It is convenient to consider the major modes of action of biocides in four groups: oxidizing agents, transfer of energy, cross-linking agents, and agents that specifically bind to and disrupt the structure of certain macromolecules.

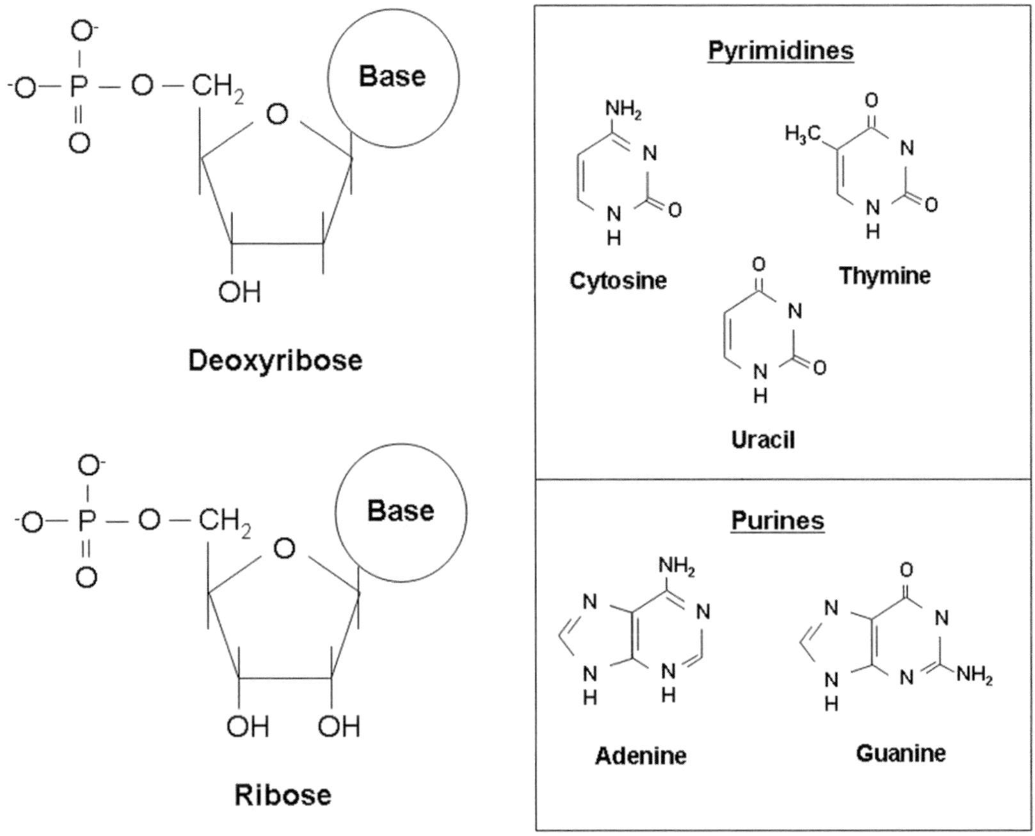

FIGURE 7.6 The basic structure of nucleotides. The structure consists of a sugar (ribose or deoxyribose) linked to phosphate (only one monophosphate group is indicated) and various bases (pyrimidines and purines).

7.4.2 Oxidizing Agents

Chemically, oxidizing agents remove electrons (oxidation) from a substance, thereby gaining electrons themselves (Table 7.6). Biocides that possess oxidizing agent ability are widely used and include the halogens (chlorine, bromine, and iodine) and peroxygens (peracetic acid [PAA] and hydrogen peroxide).

Although the exact mode of action of these biocides is often unknown and difficult to study, studies of microorganisms have shown some common effects. Effects observed on whole cells have included loss of structure and integrity, leaking of cytoplasmic components, inhibition of multiplication, etc. Further investigations have been conducted into their specific effects on macromolecules, with a particular focus on nucleic acids at lower concentrations of oxidizing agents. These studies have focused on the effects of oxidizing agents on cells that have been associated with cell aging and some diseases (in particular, those associated with aging) and the associated defense (including repair) mechanisms that can protect the cell from damage. Oxidizing agents are naturally formed in prokaryotic and eukaryotic cells that use oxygen during respiration and/or metabolism. These include hydrogen peroxide and short-lived radicals (such as the hydroxyl radical, $^{\cdot}OH$, and the superoxide anion radical, O_2^-). The significance of the presence of these reactive species as antimicrobial agents has been discussed (chapter 3, section 3.13). Specific effects of these agents have been investigated and found to have four major targets: nucleic acids, lipids, proteins, and carbohydrates.

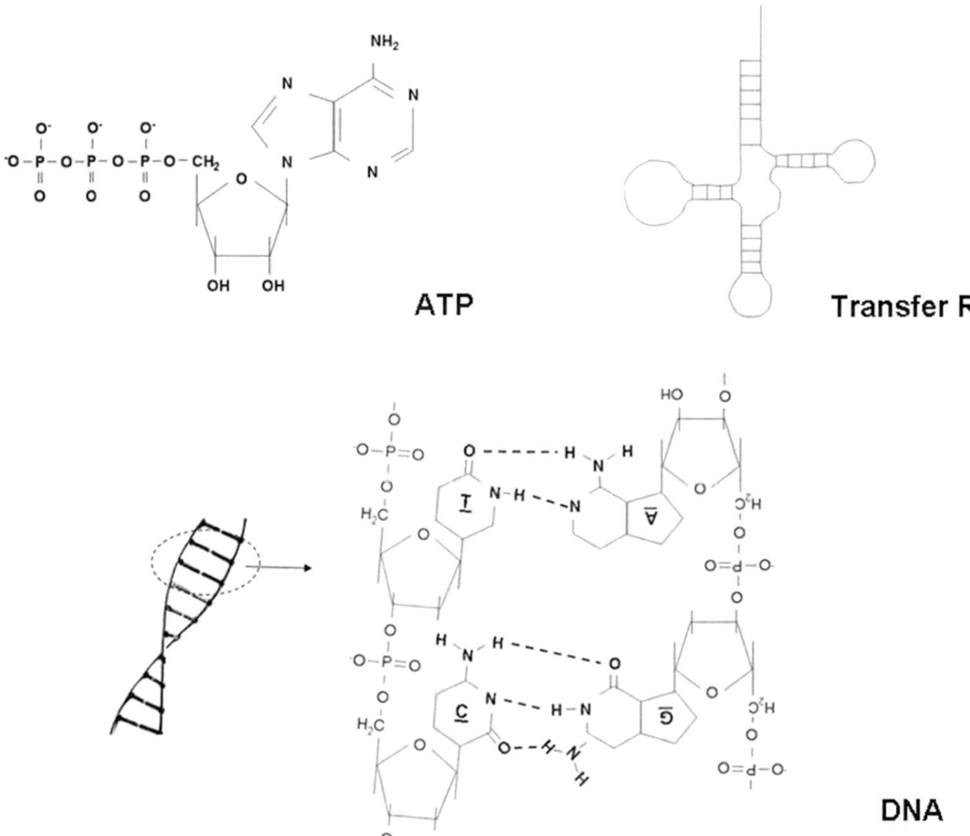

FIGURE 7.7 Nucleotide structures. ATP (top left) is a mononucleotide, while DNA (bottom) and RNA (top right; simple structure shown) are polynucleotides. DNA is a double-stranded polynucleotide (with hydrogen bonding holding together the two parallel strands); the representation of a transfer RNA polynucleotide shows single- and double-stranded sections (with hydrogen bonded bases shown as lines between the strands).

TABLE 7.6 Biocides with an oxidizing agent-based mode of action

Halogens and halogen-releasing agents	Peroxygens and other forms of oxygen
Iodine	Hydrogen peroxide
Iodophors, e.g., PVPI	Peracetic acid
Chlorine	Chlorine dioxide
Hypochlorites	Ozone
Chloramines, e.g., sodium dichloroisocyanurate	
Bromine	
Bromine-releasing agents, e.g., Bronopol	

Oxidizing agents have a dramatic effect on DNA and RNA structures. They readily attack both the nucleotide bases and the sugar-phosphate backbone (Fig. 7.8). These effects cause strand breakage and can cause reactions between converted bases/sugars and other molecules associated with the nucleic acid, including the formation of adducts. Such damage disrupts the function of polynucleotides, including DNA, RNA, and other similar nucleotide monomeric structures (including ATP, which is a source of chemical energy required for cellular activities). Specific effects on polynucleotides can not only lead to mutations

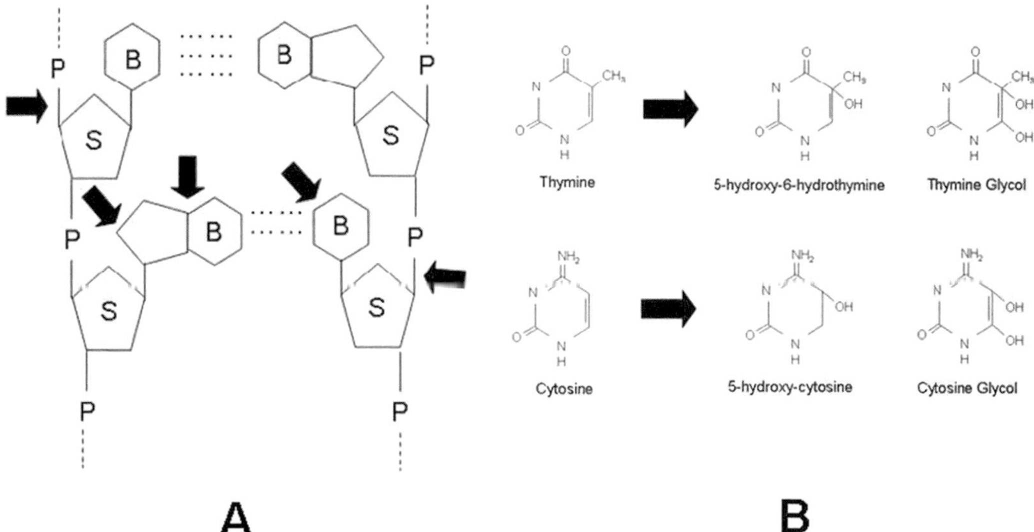

FIGURE 7.8 The major target sites for oxidizing agents on the structure of **(A)** DNA and, specifically, on **(B)** the nucleotide bases, with examples of the pyrimidine bases thymine and cytosine.

but can also disrupt cellular processes such as replication, transcription, and translation which are required for multiplication and microbial survival. This has been particularly studied with hydrogen peroxide, which shows these effects in both liquid and gas form, PAA, chlorine dioxide, chlorine solutions, and nitrogen dioxide. Some studies have suggested a role of iron (as a catalyst) in these reactions, presumably due to Fenton reactions causing the localized generation of short-lived hydroxyl radicals that react with the nucleic acid. The sporicidal activity of both hydrogen peroxide and PAA (as is likely for other oxidizing agents) has been shown to be particularly dependent on the penetration of these biocides into and reacting with the spore core DNA; these biocides also have effects on various other components on the spores to allow for penetration over time (see section 8.3.11).

Specific effects on lipids, in particular, the fatty acids associated with the cell membrane, have also been studied. Reactions of lipids with oxidizing agents can cause changes in their structure and degradation into smaller-chain fatty acids. Unsaturated fatty acids, which contain double bonds within long carbon chain structures, are considered to be particularly sensitive due to specific reactions at these double bonds. Some of these reactions can lead to the production of other toxic substances (for example, aldehydes such as 4-hydroxyalkenals and malonaldehydes) that contribute to cell damage. The reactions cause lipid peroxidation, which can lead to changes in fatty acid structure and degradation into other reactive agents, which, as radicals themselves, can react with other cellular components, in particular, other fatty acids and proteins within the cell membranes. The overall effects on the cell membrane can be dramatic, particularly leading to a loss in fluidity that disrupts the overall structure and function (including permeability) of the membrane. These include the disruption of embedded proteins, as the membrane increases in hydrophilicity, and ultimately lead to leakage of cytoplasmic constituents as the membrane loses its structure. Given the importance of the cell membrane for a variety of cellular functions, it is clear that these effects have a dramatic effect on the viability of bacteria, fungi, and some enveloped viruses.

Further investigations have focused on the specific reactions of oxidizing agents on amino acids and proteins. For example, the accumulation of protein damage due to oxidizing agents has been observed in certain diseases including neurodegenerative diseases. As in the discussion on the effects on polynucleotides, oxidizing agents can specifically affect the primary and higher-order (e.g., secondary and tertiary) structures of proteins. Oxidizing agents have multiple effects on proteins, including changes in amino acid structure, peptide bond breakage (leading to protein fragmentation), interruption of metal binding sites (which are required for some catalytic protein functions), and specific reactions with other amino acid bonds (for example, the disulfide bond between cysteine amino acids). These effects cause the loss of enzymatic activities and the loss of protein structure. On the primary sequence of proteins, oxidizing agents can specifically modify the side chains of amino acids, which can lead to changes in the amino acid sequence. Such effects have been shown with liquid hydrogen peroxide and with the halogens, including chlorine. Chlorine has been shown to directly oxidize and form chloro-derivatives of amino acids such as on reaction to glycine, serine, cysteine, lysine, and arginine. With some amino acids such as glycine these effects were shown to be more prominent at higher concentrations and under alkaline pH conditions. Notable effects with oxidizing agents generally include the formation of carbonyl groups and an increase in acidity. Because the primary sequence dictates the folding and overall protein structure, these reactions lead to disruption in the protein structure and therefore loss of function. Some of the specific reactions that have been described are given in Table 7.7. These can include changes in the amino acid structure, as well as the production of reactive side chains that can readily react with other structures to cause cross-linkages.

Of note is the effect of oxidizing agents on the amino acid cysteine (with its associated thio or sulfhydryl [-SH] groups that are particularly sensitive to oxidation). As well as their role in the amino acid primary structure of many proteins, cysteine residues can play an important part in the folding of certain proteins, in particular, those that are excreted from the cytoplasm and associated with the cell wall or membrane. Two cysteine residues within the primary structure of a protein can interact to form disulfide bonds, due to reactions between the sulfurous side chains. These bonds not only play an important role in the overall structure of some proteins but also play an important regulatory role in the proteins' activity. For example, *Escherichia coli* cells can react to oxidative stress within their environment (as in the case of the presence of oxidizing agents) by a specific response mediated by a transcriptional activator protein (OxyR), which causes the cell to express specific protecting and repair mechanisms that can help it survive. OxyR is specifically activated by the formation of a disulfide bond between two cysteine residues due to the presence of oxidizing agents. This so-called oxidative response is discussed in further detail in chapter 8, section 8.3.3 as a specific adaptive response mechanism to increase bacterial resistance to oxidizing agent damage. Because the formation of disulfide bonds is a benefit in this case, the opposite is true for other proteins, in particular, intracellular proteins, which do not normally contain disulfide linkages between cysteine residues. The effect of oxidizing agents to cause the formation of disulfide bonds leads to the loss of structure and function of many enzymes and proteins, thus also contributing to the overall mode of action.

TABLE 7.7 Examples of products observed on reaction of oxidizing agents on amino acids

Target amino acids	Products observed
Arginine	Glutamic semialdehyde
Cysteine	Cysteic acid, disulfides
Histidine	Asparagine, aspartic acid
Lysine	2-Aminoadipic semialdehyde
Tyrosine	3,4-Dihydroxyphenylalanine, cross-linkages or adducts between tyrosine residues

Some oxidizing agents have also been shown to cause peptide bond breakage, including PAA, gas hydrogen peroxide, and chlorine. Peptide bonds are covalent bonds that connect amino acids together to form peptides and proteins (section 7.3). These effects are postulated to be due to specific reactions with hydrogen atoms in the amino acids, which become reactive and cause bond disruption. These structures are known cellular targets for proteolysis, including attachment by intracellular proteases, which cause further degradation via the cells' natural enzymatic activities. Additional effects can be speculated on due to reaction of these amino acids with other biomolecules, including other associated amino acids, which can cause adducts to or within the protein structure. In contrast to the sensitivity of proteins that have been damaged by disruption of peptide bonds by proteases, some of these protein-protein interactions are proposed to be less sensitive to proteases and lead to toxic accumulations with the target cell. The subtle difference in these effects may be an important factor in the optimization of the effects of oxidizing agents on prions, which are proposed infectious peptides. In one case, the optimization of the peptide bond breakage may enhance the activity against prions, but in contrast, the increased cross-linking may increase the overall resistance of this entity. These effects may be responsible for the differences observed between different oxidizing agents, in combination with other liquid formulation properties or in various states (e.g., liquid or gas), in their activity against prions.

An example of the subtle differences in the activity of oxidizing agents against proteins has been shown in the activity of hydrogen peroxide in gas or liquid form. Gaseous hydrogen peroxide is known to be more reactive and effective at lower available concentrations than when in liquid form (see chapter 3, section 3.13 and Table 3.4). These differences may be partially due to the increased reactivity of the gas in comparison to the liquid, but subtle differences in their effects on proteins have been described. Liquid hydrogen peroxide solutions in water were shown to specifically oxidize the side chains of various amino acids, including cysteine, methionine, lysine, histidine, and glycine. These effects will clearly have a direct impact on the structure and function of proteins, as well allowing for further reactions (e.g., cross-linking) with other amino acids in the same or adjacent protein structures to cause cell or virus death. Studies with a range of enzymes have shown a greater impact in some protein types than others in causing the loss of enzymatic activity. Overall, these effects appear to depend on the particular protein structure (see section 7.3) and availability of various amino acids to be oxidized. Further, in studies with different hydrogen peroxide- and PAA-based disinfectants, protein cross-linking was observed with some formulations and not with others; with some formulations, protein fragmentation was specifically noted, presumably due to breakdown of peptide bonds. Interestingly, amino acid oxidation was not observed in experiments with gas hydrogen peroxide, but the gas form did show peptide and protein fragmentation. Therefore, peroxide gas appeared to target peptide bonds, and this also varied depending on the protein types, presumably due to the accessibility of the protein structure to oxidation.

It is speculated that these differences in mechanisms of action may explain inconsistencies in the reported effectiveness of hydrogen peroxide against prions, particularly in gas form. Hydrogen peroxide gas has been shown to be effective, but in some disinfection and sterilization systems if the gas is allowed to condense during the process, the presence of liquid peroxide may lead to protein cross-linking and persistent prion infectivity. These effects may also explain the differences in antimicrobial activity of condensed and noncondensed peroxide processes when interfering soils (such as blood or food proteins) are present and the persistence of microorganism under these conditions over time; studies with condensed systems have shown that low concentrations of viruses may persist even over extended contact time, in contrast to the noncondensing process, which showed complete viral inactivation.

Another example of differences in the direct effects of oxidizing agents has been shown in bacterial spore penetration studies with liquid hydrogen peroxide and PAA. Liquid hydrogen peroxide was shown to have poor penetration into the spore over time but did rapidly react with the spore coat proteins (outer protective layers in bacterial spore structure; see chapter 8, section 8.3.11 and Figure 8.18). Although this did not appear to cause more rapid penetration of peroxide into the spore, it did appear to act synergistically to allow greater penetration of PAA to elicit rapid sporicidal activity. In contrast, pretreatment of spores with PAA did not significantly change the sporicidal activity of hydrogen peroxide. In other reports, gaseous peroxide appeared to have little effect in the penetration through bacterial spore structures but needed to directly reach and degrade the nucleic acid in the spore core to elicit its sporicidal activity. Similar to studies with hydrogen peroxide, the activity of liquid PAA varies depending on its formulation and exposure conditions. For example, in some formulations cross-linking of proteins was observed, while in others the mechanism was protein fragmentation, which was enhanced at increased temperatures (40 to 55°C).

Similar to the effects described for heavy metals (such as iron) increasing the effects of hydrogen peroxide and other oxidizing agents against nucleic acids (as described above), both amino acid oxidation and protein fragmentation are also enhanced with hydrogen peroxide in the presence of heavy metals. Because many cellular or viral proteins have bound metals required for their enzymatic activities, their structures, or the safe transport of toxic metals (for example, iron) within the cell, the disruption of these proteins by oxidizing agents may also cause the release of these metals into or around the microorganism, which adds to the observed toxic effects. The toxic effects of heavy metals are discussed further in section 7.4.5.

Some studies have suggested that certain bacterial and yeast proteins are clearly major targets for the effects of oxidizing agents. For example, studies of *E. coli* have shown specific inactivation of many key bacterial proteins and enzymes associated with essential bacterial metabolic functions. These include glucose metabolism (enolase), protein biosynthesis and folding (e.g., EF-G, an elongation factor involved in protein translation from mRNA, and DnaK, a protein chaperone which is involved in the folding of newly synthesized proteins into their correct secondary structure), and outer membrane structure (e.g., OmpA, a major structural protein in the *E. coli* cell wall). These proteins may not be particularly more sensitive to the effects of oxidizing agents, but damage to them clearly has greater consequences for cell survival. Further, the reaction of oxidizing agents with peptides and proteins can lead to the generation of toxic molecules in the cell, such as in the case of the generation of chloramines on reaction of chlorine with protein amine groups and by peptide bond breakage. It is clear that further investigations into the effects of oxidizing agents on cellular targets may identify other key targets in microorganisms that are more central to cell survival or pathogenesis.

The exact reactions of oxidizing agents on carbohydrates have been less studied, but overall, reactions similar to those on proteins are expected. Simple sugars such as glucose can be readily oxidized, and more complex carbohydrates have been shown to degrade by a variety of reactions (including Fenton reactions). These have been studied with hydrogen peroxide. Hydrogen atoms are specifically targeted on carbohydrate molecules, leading to reactive species, which are proposed to cause chain breakage (such as glycosidic-bond disruption), polysaccharide breakage, and reactions with other cellular targets. These effects likely contribute to the overall loss of structure and function of key carbohydrate and carbohydrate-linked (e.g., glycoprotein) molecules, as well as disruption of other functions by cross-reactions.

Overall, oxidizing agents have multiple effects on proteins, lipids, carbohydrates, and nucleic acids, which lead to loss of their structures and functions. Specific effects include changes in structure, breakdown of these macromolecules into smaller constituents, transformation of structural and functional groups, as well as some effects leading to cross-linking within and between these molecules. These effects culminate in the loss of viability of the microbial target. They are clearly significant on vegetative and actively metabolizing microorganisms, including bacteria and fungi. The overall damage to dormant structures such as spores, cysts, and viruses also appears to cause a loss in viability, presumably due to specific effects on surface proteins and lipids, but also on penetration to and effects directly on the nucleic acid. The antimicrobial effects can be modified based on the biocide state (e.g., liquid or gas), formulation, and exposure conditions, which may be important considerations in certain applications.

7.4.3 Cross-linking, or Coagulating, Agents

Cross-linking, or coagulating, agents cause interactions between macromolecules, particularly proteins and nucleic acids, that lead to loss of structure and function (Table 7.8). Many biocides and biocidal processes can cause the clumping or coagulation of macromolecules at higher concentrations due to their modes of action. Notably, these can include some oxidizing agents depending on their formulation or process exposure conditions, which in addition to their oxidation mode of action discussed in section 7.4.2, can also cause the production of aldehydes, leading to cross-linking under certain conditions. These coagulating reactions are also seen with other types of biocides, such as quaternary ammonium compounds (QACs), heat, and alcohols. However, some biocides demonstrate specific interactions with macromolecules that suggest a primary mode of action as cross-linking, or coagulation, agents. Of particular note are the aldehydes and alkylating agents, although some discussion of the phenolics and alcohols, which are considered general coagulating biocides, is also appropriate.

TABLE 7.8 Biocides with cross-linking or coagulation-based modes of action

Aldehydes (cross-linking agents)
Formaldehyde
Glutaraldehyde
Ortho-phthaldehyde
Alkylating agents (epoxides)
Ethylene oxide
Propylene oxide
Phenolics
Phenols
Cresols
Bisphenols
Alcohols
Ethanol
Isopropanol

Alkylating agents are highly reactive chemical compounds which can react with amino, carboxyl, sulfhydryl, and hydroxyl groups, particularly in protein amino acids or within nucleic acids. "Alkylating" refers to their ability to introduce alkyl (methyl or ethyl) groups into macromolecules. Many alkylating agents are specifically used as anticancer agents (e.g., mitomycin C and cyclophosphamide), because they are toxic to eukaryotic cells. The major mechanism of action of many of these drugs is the DNA molecule, in particular, the cross-linking of guanine bases that inhibit the unraveling and separation of DNA, which is required for its replication and transcription. Ethylene oxide is the most widely used alkylating agent for disinfection and sterilization. Like other alkylating agents, it specifically targets proteins and nucleic acids. Three principal effects of alkylating agents have been described against nucleic acids:

1. They react to guanine (and to a lesser extent adenine) nucleotide bases, which causes the addition of alkyl (or ethyl in the case of ethylene oxide) groups (Fig. 7.9). These structural changes can promote cellular repair mechanisms, which can cause DNA strand breakage and can culminate in cell death. Further, the presence of alkyl groups also inhibits

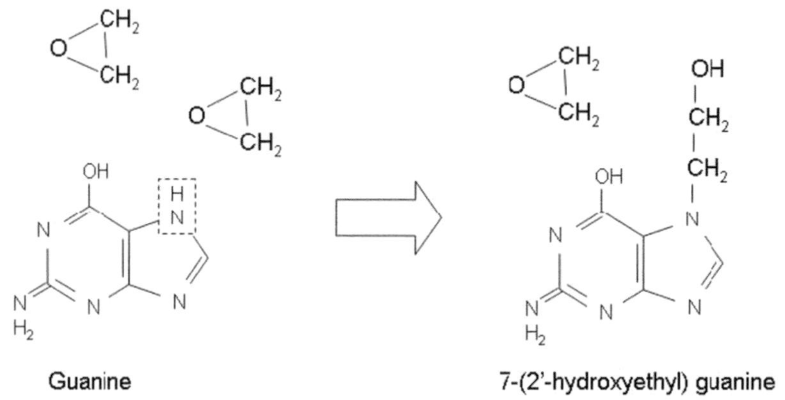

Guanine

7-(2'-hydroxyethyl) guanine

FIGURE 7.9 Reaction of ethylene oxide with guanine.

the replication and transcription of DNA, as well as functional changes to cellular RNA molecules.

2. The presence of alkylated guanine bases can cause mispairing of nucleotide bases in DNA and RNA structures, due to pairing with thymine and uracil residues in place of the normal cytosine pairing. Mispairing causes changes in RNA folded structures and may also cause point mutations in DNA over time.
3. The presence of the alkyl groups promotes the formation of cross-linkages between other adjacent nucleotide bases via the terminal hydroxyl group. These cross-linkages can occur within the same or parallel DNA strands or with other associated macromolecules (in particular, proteins). The formation of cross-linkages also inhibits DNA and RNA functions, specifically DNA unwinding and RNA translation.

Overall, these effects on nucleic acids cause mutations, arrest of essential cellular functions (replication, transcription, and translation), loss of cell viability, and viral infectivity.

Similar introduction of alkyl groups is observed in reactions with amino, carboxyl, sulfhydryl, and hydroxyl groups of amino acids (Fig. 7.10).

The alkylation of amino acids disrupts the structure and function of proteins, including essential enzymes. In addition, similar to the reactions described for nucleic acids, epoxide bridge cross-links can form due to further reactions with adjacent amino acid side chains, which will also disrupt protein structures and cause precipitation. Certain exposed amino acids appear to be particularly targeted, including cysteine, histidine, and valine. These are probably key in the initial attacks on the surfaces of microorganisms, including dramatic effects on the structure of peptidoglycan and other surface glycans due to cross-linking of peptides that link the polysaccharide chains. Reactions of alkylating agents most likely occur with other macromolecules but have not been studied.

Aldehydes are typical cross-linking agents and are widely used for a variety of biochemical and industrial purposes due to their mode of action of fixing materials, including attachment of materials to surfaces (chapter 3, section 3.4). An example is the use of glutaraldehyde as a fixative to stabilize the structure of cells for electron microscopy analysis. Aldehydes widely used for biocidal purposes include formaldehyde, which is used for fumigation, and glutaraldehyde and ortho-phthaldehyde, which are used as low-temperature hard-surface disinfectants. The primary targets for aldehydes are proteins and, to a lesser extent, other macromolecules such as nucleic acids, but the mode of action is more specific than that described for alkylating agents. Although aldehydes have a dramatic effect on intracellular components

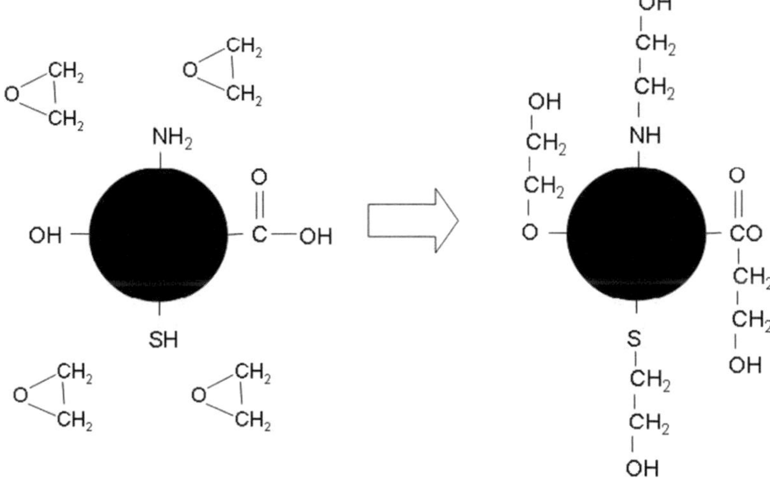

FIGURE 7.10 Reaction of ethylene oxide with amino acid side chains.

and processes, the primary mode of action is the surface of microorganisms and therefore exposed proteins and peptides, including peptidoglycan.

Aldehydes cause cross-linkages to form between amino acids within or between proteins, specifically, the amine group of lysine or hydroxylysine. Free amine groups, at terminal amino acids within a peptide or protein or as side chains on some amino acids, are particularly sensitive to cross-linking with aldehydes (Fig. 7.11).

The formation of these covalent bonds causes changes in the structure and function of

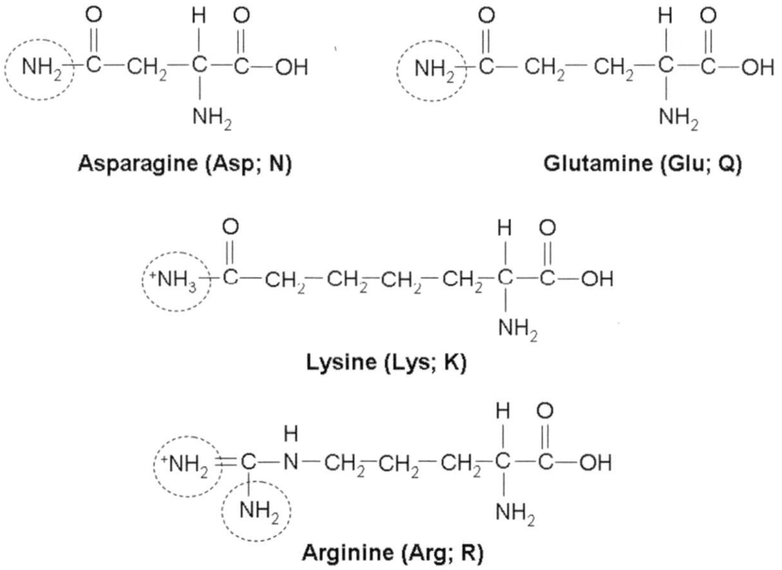

NH_2—C(=O)—CH_2—CH(NH_2)—C(=O)—OH

Asparagine (Asp; N)

NH_2—C(=O)—CH_2—CH_2—CH(NH_2)—C(=O)—OH

Glutamine (Glu; Q)

$^+NH_3$—C(=O)—CH_2—CH_2—CH_2—CH_2—CH(NH_2)—C(=O)—OH

Lysine (Lys; K)

$^+NH_2$=C(NH_2)—NH—CH_2—CH_2—CH_2—CH(NH_2)—C(=O)—OH

Arginine (Arg; R)

FIGURE 7.11 Amino acids that are susceptible to cross-linking by aldehydes. The side chain amino group of lysine is particularly sensitive; in addition, other amino groups that are not associated with peptide bonds and therefore are at the ends of proteins/peptides are also susceptible.

proteins and enzymes and allows for protein aggregation. Access of lysine or other sensitive amino groups is an important factor in protein susceptibility to cross-linking; clearly, if the amino group is exposed on the protein surface, it will be at greater risk of cross-linking, in contrast to groups protected due to protein folding. Accessibility of these groups may be an important factor in the development of high-level resistance to aldehyde-based disinfectants in mycobacteria (see section 8.4). Further, proteins with a higher proportion of lysine residues are also more susceptible to cross-linking. Examples include specific studies of the sensitivity of exposed lysine residues within the capsid proteins on the surface of non-enveloped viruses, which appear to be primary targets leading to the loss of viral infectivity. The number and accessibility of lysine residues within a given surface protein type appear to be an important consideration in the sensitivity of nonenveloped viruses to glutaraldehyde. Direct crystallography examination of glutaraldehyde-treated viruses has indicated a loss of capsid flexibility and an increased surface rigidity, which is proposed to disrupt the release of the viral genome on contact with the host cell. Cross-linking can occur between the nitrogen atoms of free amino groups and another atom within or adjacent to the protein; the most common cross-link with formaldehyde is between lysine residues and adjacent peptide bonds to form methylene (-CH_2-) bridges (Fig. 7.12).

Reactions with formaldehyde and proteins may also cause the entrapment of associated nucleic acids (intracellularly) and lipids or carbohydrates (at the cell membrane or cell wall); however, reports have suggested that there are no direct effects on the chemical structures of these molecules. The normal functions of these macromolecules are clearly disrupted, which affects the overall viability of the microorganism.

The glutaraldehyde molecule is more flexible in its cross-linking ability than formaldehyde, presumably due to its structure, which consists of three flexible methylene bridges and two terminal aldehyde groups (chapter 3, section 3.4). This is in comparison to a single aldehyde group in formaldehyde and allows for the interaction of the aldehyde groups over a wider access range. In addition to reactions with free glutaraldehyde, aldehyde polymers can also be present, which can cross-link amino acids over a greater distance, both with nitrogen atoms within the same protein and with adjacent proteins. At the same time, glutaraldehyde monomers demonstrate greater penetration than aldehyde polymers. In addition to cross-linking free amino groups, glutaralde-

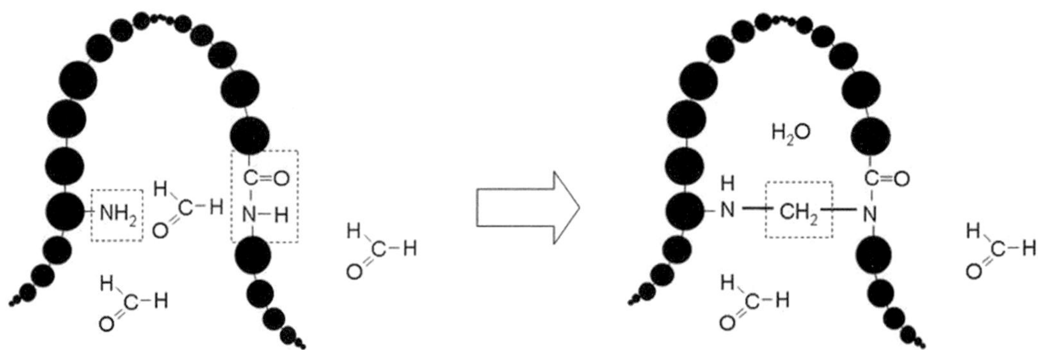

FIGURE 7.12 A typical cross-linking reaction with formaldehyde between a lysine amino acid side chain and an adjacent peptide bond. The sensitive amino group (NH_2) of the lysine residue is shown, as well as reaction with the N atom of the peptide bond with formaldehyde, to form a methylene bridge.

hyde may also form cross-linkages between other nitrogen atoms within the amino acid structure (Fig. 7.13).

The bactericidal activity of glutaraldehyde has been particularly well studied. Early reports demonstrated the following:

- Strong binding of glutaraldehyde to the outer layers of Gram-positive (*Staphylococcus aureus*) and Gram-negative (*E. coli*) bacteria
- Inhibition of solute transport in Gram-negative bacteria
- Inhibition of the activity of surface and periplasmic enzymes
- Prevention of lysis with other agents such as lysostaphin in *S. aureus* and sodium dodecyl sulfate in *E. coli*
- Increased cell membrane resistance to lysis (in spheroplast and protoplast studies)
- Direct inhibition of RNA, DNA, and protein synthesis

It is clear that the mechanism of action of glutaraldehyde is strongly due to cross-linking within the outer layers of bacterial cells, specifically with exposed amino groups on the cell surface. These effects cause dramatic inhibition of the activities of key surface proteins involved in transport into and out of the cell and, directly, on enzyme systems, where access of the substrate to the enzyme is prohibited. In studies in which the bacterial cell wall is partially or completely removed to produce spheroplasts or protoplasts, glutaraldehyde appeared to react specifically with the cell membrane proteins to increase the membrane's resistance to lysis when placed into a hypotonic environment; this "tightening," or increase in rigidity, would make the membrane less sensitive to direct disruption. Studies of *Micrococcus lysodeikticus* supported this conclusion, because treatment with glutaraldehyde prevented the release of some membrane-bound enzymes.

Other studies have investigated the activity of glutaraldehyde against bacterial spores. Clearly, bacterial spores demonstrate greater resistance to aldehydes than do vegetative bacteria. This may be related to the sensitivity and uptake of the biocide or availability of reactive sites. The bacterial spore presents several sites (including the spore coats) at which interaction with glutaraldehyde is possible, although in contrast to vegetative bacteria, interaction with particular surface sites does not necessarily have an effect on spore inactivation. *E. coli*, *S. aureus*, and vegetative cells of *Bacillus atrophaeus* bind more glutaraldehyde than do resting spores of *B. atrophaeus*. Spores are more susceptible

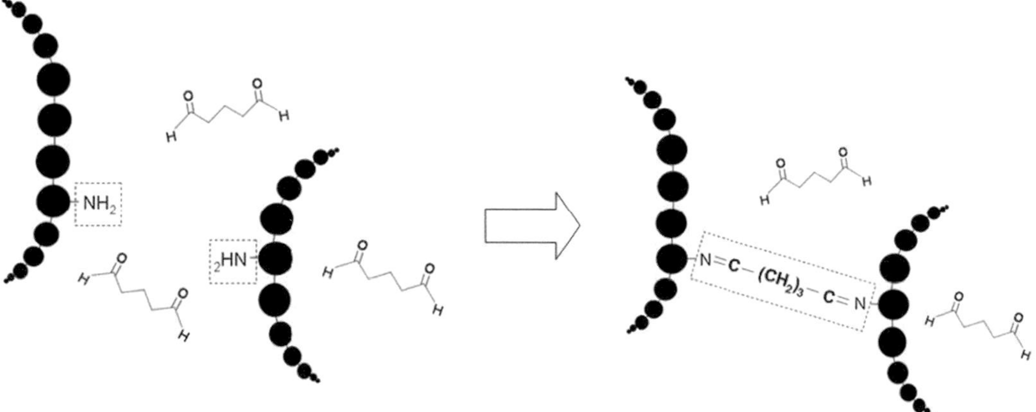

FIGURE 7.13 A typical cross-linked reaction by glutaraldehyde between two amino acids in adjacent proteins. The reactive amino group in each amino acid reacts with the aldehyde group on each end of the glutaraldehyde molecule, leading to the formation of a flexible, methylene bridge.

during their development (sporulation) and activation to a vegetative state (germination and outgrowth; chapter 8, section 8.3.11). During sporulation, the bacterial cell becomes less susceptible to glutaraldehyde (see section 8.3.11). By contrast, germinating and outgrowing cells reacquire sensitivity. Uptake of glutaraldehyde is greater during germination and outgrowth than with mature spores but still much less than with vegetative cells. Low concentrations of glutaraldehyde (0.1%) inhibit germination, in contrast to the typical 2% concentration used for sporicidal activity. Glutaraldehyde exerts an early effect on the germination process. L-alanine is considered to play an important role during bacterial spore germination by binding to a specific receptor on the spore coat, which triggers germination and the irreversible loss of the spore's dormant properties. Glutaraldehyde at high concentrations has been shown to inhibit the uptake of radioactive alanine to *Bacillus subtilis* spores by an unknown mechanism, but this is possibly the result of a sealing effect of the aldehyde on the cell surface. Direct interaction with the proteinaceous outer spore layers has been described. The resulting cross-linked structure inhibits the germination of the spore and even, as with vegetative bacteria, increases the resistance to other sporicidal methods. Low concentrations of glutaraldehyde increase the surface hydrophobicity of spores, again indicative of an effect at the outermost regions of the spore; binding seems to be greater under alkaline pH, suggesting that increased surface cross-linking and not spore penetration is responsible for increased activity under alkaline conditions.

A limited number of studies have investigated the effects of glutaraldehyde on other microorganisms. A similar mode of action to bacteria is expected against fungi, with the fungal cell wall observed as a major target site, especially the major wall component, chitin, which is analogous to the peptidoglycan found in bacterial cell walls. Glutaraldehyde is also a potent virucidal agent with effects on viral envelope and capsid proteins, in particular, cross-linking of available lysine residues, which is expected to reduce viral infectivity and cause loss of structure. Low concentrations (<0.1%) of alkaline glutaraldehyde have been shown to be effective against whole, purified nonenveloped polioviruses but had little effect on poliovirus RNA up to 1% at pH 7.2 and only slowly inactivated the nucleic acid at pH 8.3. These results support the major mode of activity against viruses associated with capsid damage or cross-linking. Viruses do demonstrate varying levels of resistance to low concentrations of glutaraldehyde, presumably reflecting major structural differences in the exposed, sensitive amino acid amino group in their external envelope and capsid structures. For example, echoviruses are much more sensitive than polioviruses to glutaraldehyde. It should be noted that, like the differing abilities of aldehydes to form cross-links, which explains their varying effects on bacteria, aldehydes have also shown differences in their ability to form protein-nucleic acid cross-links in viruses. In studies with viral DNA synthesis *in vitro*, some aldehydes (including the less used glyoxal, furfural, and acetaldehyde) did not show significant cross-linking abilities and had no effect on viral DNA synthesis; this was in contrast to inhibition of DNA synthesis observed with aldehydes that did form such cross-links, including glutaraldehyde and formaldehyde.

Overall, aldehydes have a similar mode of action, but it is difficult to pinpoint accurately any one specific target responsible for microbial inactivation. Their interactive and cross-linking properties certainly play considerable roles in their activities, but they vary. For example, formaldehyde and, even more the case, *o*-phthalaldehyde (OPA) are much slower sporicidal agents than glutaraldehyde, although both glutaraldehyde and OPA are rapidly effective against vegetative bacteria and fungi. The difference between the activities of dialdehydes (glutaraldehyde and OPA) and monoaldehydes (formaldehyde) may be related to the distance between the two aldehyde groups in glutaraldehyde (and possibly in OPA) for optimal interaction between sensitive protein and nucleic acid groups. OPA appears to demonstrate greater penetration through bacterial cell walls and membranes than does glutaraldehyde, but as a dialdehyde, it is less cross-reactive than glutaraldehyde. OPA only appears to react with the free amino groups at terminal amino acids and at arginine or lysine residues; in contrast, glutaraldehyde reacts with other nitrogen atoms within amino acid structures. Further, the OPA molecule is structurally less flexible than glutaraldehyde due to the greater rigidity of the benzene ring (chapter 3, section 3.4) and restrictive interaction with other available amino groups. It is proposed that the greater penetration of OPA through bacterial cell surfaces may be due to differences in the structure of the biocide under different conditions. Under hydrophilic environments, which are observed at the external surface of the cell, the biocide may adopt a "locked" structure (1,3-phthalandiol) with unexposed, unreactive aldehyde groups, allowing penetration of the bacterial cell. Under hydrophobic conditions, typical in the cell wall and membrane, the open, active dialdehyde structure is proposed to be prevalent and therefore cross-reactive.

The mode of action of phenolics was discussed briefly in chapter 3, section 3.14. Phenolics particularly target surface and internal proteins. They physically bind to proteins by a variety of interactions, including covalent binding, hydrogen bonding, and ionic and hydrophobic interactions. These interactions cause the protein along with other associated macromolecules to lose their structure (denature), coagulate, and precipitate. Many phenolics are used for their protein precipitation and inactivation activities in biochemical or molecular biological manipulations. The reactive form of the phenolic is the free hydroxyl (-OH) group, with other substitutions of groups to the phenol ring having multiple effects that could increase antimicrobial efficacy. For example, certain substitutions either increase or decrease the relative hydrophobicity of the molecule, which can be important in improving the penetration of the phenolic through Gram-positive or mycobacterial lipophilic cell walls (chapter 1, section 1.3.4.1). Others increase the toxicity of the phenolic molecules. These substitutions include the addition of alkyl (methyl or ethyl) groups with up to six carbons to improve solubility in lipids without decreasing solubility in water, halogenation (in particular, the addition of chlorine atoms, called "chlorophenols"), and nitration (called "nitrophenols"). However, some chemical modifications cause a decrease in antimicrobial activity, as observed with the condensed bisphenols that are particularly effective against Gram-positive bacteria but less so against Gram-negative bacteria and have little to no activity against mycobacteria.

As the phenolic biocide approaches the microbial surface, it interacts with any available proteins. These effects have been particularly studied in bacteria, with the major target being the cell wall and membrane proteins. Initial effects are observed on surface or surface-associated proteins, including disruption of energy metabolism, lipid and other macromolecule (e.g., peptidoglycan) synthesis, motility and chemotaxis, and secretion or transport proteins. For example, phenolics at low concentrations (particularly as described with chlorophenols) have been shown to specifically interfere with the membrane-associated electron transport carrier proteins; these are involved in the generation of electrical energy across the membrane (the proton motive force; see section 8.3.4), which is used for many cellular functions including ion transport, ATP formation (oxidative phosphorylation), and bacterial motility (chemotaxis and flagella rotation). These interactions fundamentally change the structure of the bacterial surface, resulting in a rapid increase in cell wall and membrane permeability. The effects on the cell wall allow greater penetration to intracellular constituents and further damage on the cell membrane proteins. Most phenolics can diffuse into the membrane, causing disruption of the phospholipids and interaction with embedded proteins. At low concentrations of phenolics, this disruption of the cell membrane rapidly leads to leakage of intracellular components as the membrane structure is destabilized. Further penetration of the biocide into the cytoplasm also disrupts the structure and function of proteins and enzymes, which culminates in the loss of cellular activities and precipitation of cytoplasm components. Specific effects on proteins and lipid membranes have been studied with the bisphenols (which are further discussed in chapter 3, section 3.15).

It is likely that similar effects are also seen with other microorganisms, in particular, molds and yeast. Phenolics are not effective against bacterial spores, except in some cases with extended incubation, but they have activity against less resistant fungal spores. These effects are considered to be due to direct interaction with surface proteins. Studies have investigated the mode of action against viruses, which varies depending on the viral structure. Some phenolics (including phenol itself, which is now rarely if at all used as a biocide due to human toxicity concerns) demonstrated activity against enveloped and nonenveloped viruses; however, other phenolics (including *o*-phenylphenol, OPP) are only effective against the more sensitive enveloped viruses. Enveloped viruses are more sensitive to phenolics due to the accessibility of key surface protein and lipid targets that are required for virus infectivity. OPP is particularly effective against enveloped viruses due to its greater lipophilicity, thereby penetrating the lipid envelope. As with bacteria, halogenated and nitrated phenols are more effective against most viruses. Overall, phenols react with and cause precipitation of viruses due to interaction with surface proteins.

Chemically, phenolics are a class of alcohols. Other alcohols are simple compounds that possess a hydroxyl (-OH) group attached to a hydrocarbon chain. Shorter-chained alcohols, including isopropanol, *n*-propanol, and ethanol, are widely used and effective as antiseptics and disinfectants (chapter 3, section 3.5). Since these alcohols have both water and lipid solubility properties, they can also have rapid effects on surface and membrane-associated proteins. Alcohols cause lipid peroxidation, protein adducts, and lipid and protein denaturation, leading to coagulation and precipitation. As in the reactions described for phenolics, since the hydroxyl group can readily react with proteins to form or break hydrogen bonds, this leads to protein denaturation and coagulation. Alcohols can particularly denature the tertiary structures of proteins by disrupting hydrogen bonding between exposed amino acid side chains; in this reaction, the alcohol reacts with the side chain to form new hydrogen bonds with the amino acid. Direct inhibition of enzyme activity is observed at relatively lower concentrations of alcohol (~50% ethanol and 30% isopropanol). Overall, these effects are similar to those observed with phenols. Direct interaction with the various cell membrane, envelope, or specific cell wall lipids also causes membrane hydration, lipid extraction and disruption of structure and function. These effects play further roles in the rapid antimicrobial activities of alcohols.

7.4.4 Transfer of Energy

Macromolecules are dependent on their structures to perform their various biological functions, based on the close interactions of various atoms and molecules. These are particularly sensitive to the effects of the sudden transfer of energy (e.g., in the form of heat or radiation), causing disruption of these structures and therefore loss of their functions. Biocidal processes with the primary mechanism of action due to the transfer of energy are listed in Table 7.9.

Heat is a form of energy that is transferred from one system to another due to differences in their temperature. It is therefore not surprising, considering the importance of temperature in biological systems, that most common vegetative bacteria, fungi, viruses, and parasites are readily inactivated at temperature >60°C. Heat can be directly applied in moist or dry forms, which are widely used as disinfection and sterilization techniques (chapters 2 and 5). Heat transfer also plays an important role in the mode of action of radiation methods, particularly the lower energy, nonionization methods (infrared and microwaves). The effects of heat include

TABLE 7.9 Biocidal processes with transfer-of-energy-based modes of action

Heat
Moist heat
Dry heat
Nonionizing radiation
UV
Infrared
Microwaves
Ionizing radiation
X rays
γ rays
E beams

the denaturation of nucleic acids, lipids, and proteins; loss of structure and function; and coagulation of protein and other macromolecules. In particular, as the temperature increases, the molecules present in these structures become more disordered as they absorb heat energy, which disrupts their structures.

Temperature has a dramatic effect on the structure of nucleic acids, in particular, DNA and double-stranded RNA molecules (such as transfer RNAs in bacteria/fungi or the nucleic acid in some viral genomes). Temperature denaturation of nucleic acids has been investigated, for example, as an important method in molecular biology investigations; heat denaturation is used as part of the cyclic reaction to amplify sections of DNA in PCRs by causing the nucleic acid to unfold. Double-stranded nucleic acids are formed by hydrogen bonding between two complementary polynucleotide strands (see section 7.3 and Figure 7.7). These structures are quite resistant to the initial effects of heat but can be broken at ≥85°C to produce separated (or denatured) strands. The adsorption of heat by the linked molecules causes them to vibrate vigorously, leading to disruption of bonding (Fig. 7.14).

Nucleic acid denaturation can be further enhanced under alkaline conditions (pH >11). Ribosomal RNAs and other RNA molecules have been shown to degrade at relatively low temperatures (45 to 65°C). The rate at which DNA denatures (referred to as its melting temperature, T_m) varies depending on its guanine-cytosine content; greater hydrogen bonding (three in comparison to two hydrogen bonds) (section 7.3) is observed between these base pairs in comparison to adenine-thymine pairings (or adenine-uracil pairings in RNA molecules). Further, the topology (or rate of supercoiling) of the microbial DNA has also been suggested to cause heat and cold resistance, in particular in some thermophiles. Double-stranded polynucleotide denaturation is itself reversible, and if the temperature is lowered, the structure can readily re-form. However, at 85°C over time, or at higher temperatures, the polynucleotide strands are further damaged by specific breaks in the phosphodiester linkages between nucleotides in the sugar-phosphate backbone (known as "nicks"), causing nucleic acid fragmentation (Fig. 7.14). Single- and double-stranded breaks in the nucleotide backbone structure have also been observed at lower test temperatures. These effects can be repaired in bacteria and fungi but are also recognized by endogenous nucleases, which can lead to further enzymatic degradation by the cell; the overall effect on the target microorganism ultimately depends on the extent of damage and the organism's ability to repair damage. Clearly, viral nucleic acids are particularly sensitive to the effects of heat, because unlike bacteria and fungi, they are unable to repair any such damage.

The enzymatic and structural properties of proteins are also affected by heat (Fig. 7.14). As hydrogen bonding is disrupted in nucleic acid structures, so are similar bonds and other nonpolar hydrophobic interactions in the secondary, tertiary, and quaternary structures of proteins. Increased heat directly affects the various interactions that allow the biological functions of proteins in their tertiary and quaternary forms, including hydrogen bonding, salt bridges, disulfide bonds, and nonpolar interactions. Further denaturation of the specific protein secondary structure also occurs, due to the disruption of α-helices and β-sheets that are primarily formed by the presence of hydrogen bonds between the amine groups of

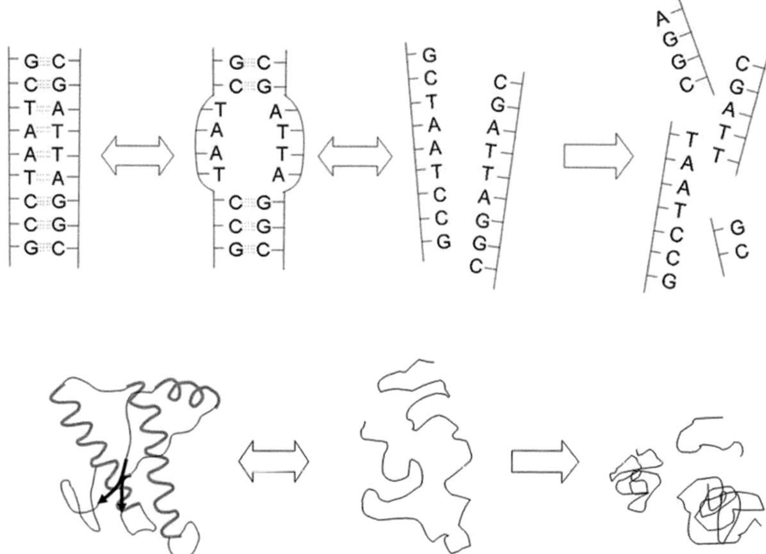

FIGURE 7.14 Heat denaturation of DNA (above) and protein (lower). As the temperature rises, the hydrogen bonding between the DNA nucleotides is broken, with adenine-thymine linkages being particularly sensitive. Above 85°C the strands are further denatured and eventually separated. On cooling, the DNA strands can reanneal, but fragmentation also occurs, due to breakages in the sugar-phosphate backbone. Similarly, the noncovalent interactions in proteins are disrupted, causing them to lose their functional structure and assume their primary structure. In some cases, on cooling, the protein may refold to its original structure, but most proteins reassemble into inactive forms and precipitate. Breakage of peptide bonds that link amino acids also occurs, leading to peptide fragmentation.

amino acids. The majority of the resulting protein primary structures do not re-form correctly on cooling, precipitate, and coagulate. The covalently linked amino acids (by peptide bonds) are more resistant to heat damage, but higher temperatures cause peptide bond disruption and peptide fragmentation.

In addition to the direct effects on amino acid bonds, subtle effects on protein hydration (or the degree of the absence or presence of water) also affect their structure and function. Water is required for the correct folding and maintenance of protein structure. It allows the formation (and at higher temperature, the disruption) of hydrogen bonds and other interactions, but it also affects the degree of flexibility of the protein structure, which is also important to biological functions. Therefore, as the temperature changes to a colder or hotter environment, the structure of the protein changes to eventually lead to denaturation. Under dry-heat conditions, the water is both removed and heated, which interferes with protein functions prior to the denaturating effects at higher temperatures. The opposite effect is initially seen with the application of moist heat with increased hydration of the protein structure but is quickly followed by denaturation.

Specific effects are observed with the hydration of hydrophilic amino acids (including lysine, serine, and aspartic acid), leading to protein denaturation under cold conditions; however, these effects are often reversible except under freezing conditions, when the formation of ice crystals can disrupt and denature the protein structure. Heat denaturation appears to primarily affect hydrophobic amino acids (including leucine, tyrosine, and valine), causing an increase in the degree of disorder within these molecules. For example, in studies with viruses, differences in their heat stability appeared to be due to the sensitivities of the viral capsid proteins to heat denaturation and precipitation; some were easily denatured at <50°C, while others required higher temperatures. These effects aid proteins to withstand harsh environmental conditions, as observed with some viruses and hyperthermophilic bacteria (chapter 8, section 8.3.10). Many proteins from thermophilic bacteria are found to have greater hydrophobicity and have more internal bonding between amino acids, which demonstrates greater resistance to unfolding and denaturation due to heat. Similar effects of hydration and hydrogen bonding have also been observed with some polysaccharide structures; the presence or absence of water affects polysaccharide flexibility and conformation, and increased heat leads to denaturation and polysaccharide fragmentation. Overall, these mechanisms are similar to the effects discussed on nucleic acid heat denaturation, with the disruption of these key macromolecules upon both changes in water activity and breakdown of the various bonding interactions that are responsible for their biological functions.

Lipids are also affected by extremes of cold or hot temperatures. Heat, as a form of energy, causes the oxidation of fatty acids, in particular, unsaturated fatty acids, in which the degree of oxidation increases with the degree of unsaturation. Fatty acid oxidation causes the production of free radicals, which lead to further deterioration and breakdown of these structures. Various reactive breakdown components can be formed, including ketones, alcohols, and aldehydes, which also react with proteins, causing cross-linking and other reactions. Considering the effects of temperature fluctuations on proteins alone, lipid structures such as membranes are indirectly affected by the disruption of integrated and associated proteins. The phospholipid membrane structure is also directly affected by the degree of hydration, with colder temperatures leading to less flexibility of membrane fluidity and higher temperatures eventually causing the bilayer to separate. The phospholipid bilayer is held together by hydrophobic interactions (including van der Waals forces), which stabilize the membrane structure; with an increase in temperature, these interactions are disrupted, and the membrane changes from a highly ordered structure to a disordered state. The effects on the lipid bilayer may play a role in the mode of action of heat against microorganisms. This can be proposed based on the lack of membrane bilayers in some hyperthermophilic bacteria; in these cases, specific lipid monolayers that would not be prone to separation in the presence of higher temperatures have been identified. Effects on bacterial membranes have been observed, including increased leakage of cytoplasmic constituents at the temperature increases, suggesting membrane disruption. Similar effects are expected on fungal, viral, and parasite lipid structures.

The overall effects of cold or freezing temperature conditions have been less studied than those of higher temperatures. Clearly, the removal of heat (or energy) also has an effect on various macromolecular structures. In general, these effects initially arrest the functions of enzymes and change the structure and function of various other proteins, lipids, and nucleic acids. The effects on lipids prevent the correct functioning of lipid membranes. Overall, cold temperatures appear to be more preservative (microbiostatic) to microorganisms, which can be revived following cooling and heating cycles; however, single or multiple freeze-thaw cycles cause macromolecules to degrade and vegetative bacteria, fungi, and parasites to lyse. The formation of ice crystals, especially large ice crystals formed during slow freezing, plays a role in the disruption of structure and function.

The mode of action of radiation is also due to the direct transfer of energy to target molecules. Radiation is energy in the form of particles or electromagnetic waves (chapter 2, section 2.4). The specific modes of action vary depending on the respective energies applied to the target microorganism and can be conveniently considered as nonionizing or ionizing radiation effects (Fig. 7.15). The lower-energy

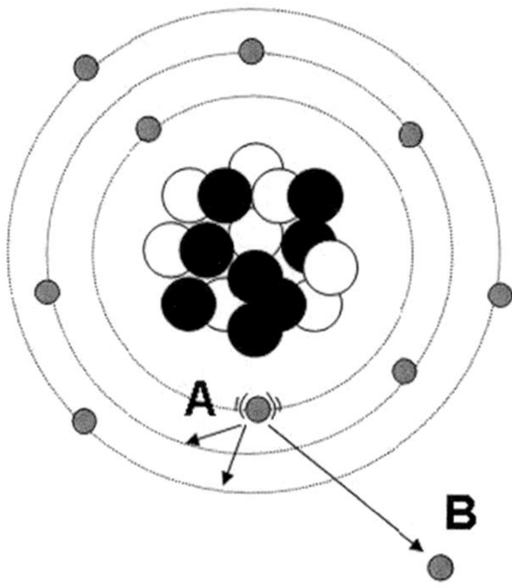

FIGURE 7.15 The effects of ionizing and nonionizing radiation on a target atom. **(A)** Nonionization causes the excitement of electrons due to adsorption of energy, which if sufficient causes electrons to move to a higher, outer energy orbital. **(B)** In the case of ionization, sufficient energy is adsorbed to expel the electron from the atom entirely. In both cases, these effects destabilize the individual atoms, the molecules they are part of, and interactions between those molecules.

sources (including microwaves, infrared, and increased heat leads to light) are nonionizing and cause the excitement of electrons within the atom structure. The higher-energy radiation sources (including γ rays, E beams, and X rays) transfer so much energy to target electrons that they are ejected from the atom structure (and are therefore ionizing), leading to further irreversible destruction of target molecules.

The energy transmitted by microwaves and infrared radiation is absorbed by water and other molecules to cause an increase in heat, and their primary mode of action is believed to parallel those described for heat disinfection and sterilization methods. Direct adsorption of radiation by the target molecules also causes destabilization in their structure and function, in particular, due to disruption of hydrogen bonding and other noncovalent interactions. Further adsorption of heat by available water molecules also causes the localized production of moist heat, leading to additional disruption of noncovalent and covalent bonds (including peptide and phosphodiester bonds), denaturation, and fragmentation of macromolecules (section 7.3). Some studies have proposed that low-energy radiation doses may cause direct disruption of covalent bonds, in particular, within nucleic acids. Studies with microwave energy have suggested that, despite having sufficient direct energy to break covalent bonds, fragmentation of DNA was observed, in contrast to heating to the same temperature alone. These effects may simply be due to localized higher production of heat within the cell (because microwaves heat from the inside out) in comparison to the application of "external" moist or dry heat. But this may also be due to the production of oxygen radicals on reaction with water, which act as oxidizing agents to cause fragmentation (section 7.4.2). The specific effects of heat on microbial macromolecules were discussed in detail above.

Disruption of specific molecular bonding and of molecules themselves is increased as higher-energy sources, such as UV radiation, are applied. The effects of UV radiation on nucleic acids have been well studied, and they are considered its primary microbial targets. Many lines of evidence suggest this; for example, the most effective antimicrobial wavelength for UV radiation is at 265 nm, at which DNA and RNA demonstrate maximal adsorption. UV radiation not only initiates a certain amount of DNA unraveling, due to disruption of hydrogen bonding between nucleotides, but specifically causes photochemical reactions between adjacent pyrimidine bases within the same nucleic acid strand. These reactions lead to the production of cyclobutane pyrimidine dimers, particularly thymine dimers (Fig. 7.16). Other, similar dimers are also observed, but at a lower frequency, including thymine-cytosine and cytosine-cytosine dimers. Additional photoreactive products, including thymine radicals (thyminyl and thymyl radicals) and pyrimidines, also contribute to the toxic effects within microorganisms. One such product, 5-thyminyl-5,6-dihydrothymine, has been observed in UV-treated bacterial spores.

Overall, dimer formation causes distortion of nucleic acid structures, limiting the access

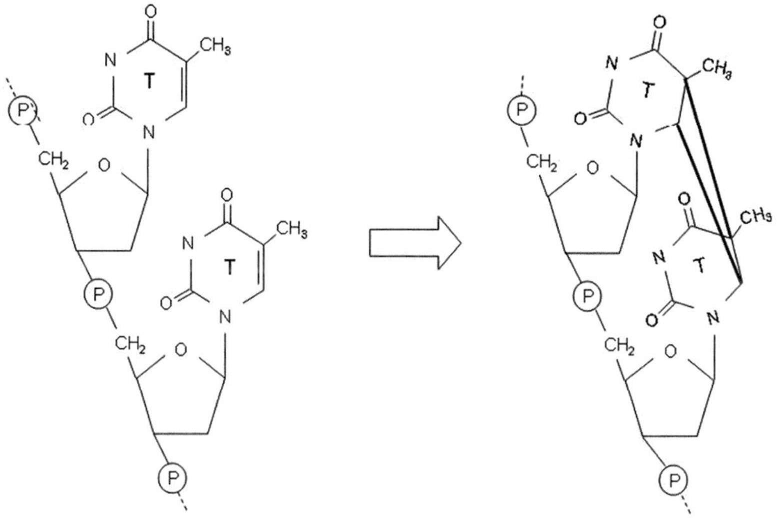

FIGURE 7.16 The production of thymine dimers between adjacent thymine bases in DNA.

of key polymerase enzymes and preventing the unraveling of DNA for replication and transcription and RNA-related functions within a target cell. Damage to viral nucleic acid can also prevent its injection on virus attachment to a cell and, indeed, infectivity if introduced into a cell. Other macromolecules are also affected by the presence of UV radiation, but these may be indirectly due to the production of radicals within microbial structures. The aromatic amino acids within proteins, including tyrosine, tryptophan, and phenylalanine, have been reported to be particularly sensitive to the effects of UV radiation. Effects on the structures and functions of cell membranes have also been reported.

The biocidal effects on the transfer of energy to microorganisms are particularly rapid and destructive in the presence of ionizing radiation (chapter 5, section 5.4). These can be considered as direct, on macromolecules, as well as indirect effects. As ionizing radiation interacts with various molecules, high energy is transferred, depending on the atomic composition and density of the material. This leads to both excitation and ionization of electrons within the atomic structure to various degrees. The most destructive is the highest-energy source, γ irradiation. Direct effects on lipids, carbohydrates, nucleic acids. and proteins cause disruption of covalent and noncovalent bonds, leading to rapid loss of structure and precipitation. The resulting charging of atoms and molecules also leads to reactions between adjacent atoms and molecules to cause cross-linking and precipitation. Nucleic acids appear to be the primary targets, in particular, due to fragmentation (single- and double-strand breaks). In a study comparing genetically simple microorganisms, such as viruses, to more complicated organisms with complex and multiple chromosomes (animals and plants), the organisms with greater nucleic acid volume were predictably more sensitive to the effects of ionizing radiation. Further, specific resistance to ionizing radiation has been partly linked to efficient DNA repair mechanisms, which can remediate the effects of some radiation damage (further discussed in chapter 8). Loss of protein structure and cell membrane damage have also been reported as important effects of the biocidal activity of ionizing radiation methods. The effects of heat transfer in these cases may also be important, but these may be considered minimal depending on the process application.

Similar to other biocidal processes, the transfer of energy, in the form of heat or radiation, causes other secondary or indirect effects on microbial structure and function. An important example is the localized production of oxidizing and reducing agents due to interactions with water and other chemicals around or within the microorganism. These agents also affect macromolecular structures. In particular, the effects of the localized oxidizing agents that are produced have been described, including the production of hydrogen peroxide and hydroxyl radicals due to radiation interactions with water, leading to further damage (section 7.4.2). The effects of oxidizing agents have been linked to mutagenic effects on DNA. Direct oxidation of proteins and other structures (such as lipids) is also believed to play a role in the modes of action of dry-heat processes.

7.4.5 Other Structure-Disrupting Agents

Biocides that specifically disrupt the arrangement and function of certain macromolecular structures are listed in Table 7.10.

TABLE 7.10 Biocides that act by disrupting the structures and functions of specific macromolecules

Acridines
Proflavine
Aminacrine
Anilides
Triclocarban
Surfactants
Quaternary ammonium compounds
Nonionic/anionic surfactants
Diamidines
Biguanides
Chlorhexidine
Organic acids/esters
Acetic acid
Benzoic acid
Parabens
Metals
Copper
Silver

The acridines are a typical example of biocides whose primary mode of action is direct interference with the structure of macromolecules, in this case, double-stranded nucleic acids. Their exact mode of action has been studied in some detail, because acridine derivatives have been proposed as potent chemotherapeutic agents. Acridines have a central fused aromatic ring structure that has an overall flattened structure, which can easily intercalate between the nucleotide base pairs of a double-stranded nucleic acid structure (chapter 3, section 3.7; Fig. 7.17).

The dye, which is positively charged, is initially attracted to the negatively charged DNA molecule and then can slot in between adjacent nucleotide base pairs. This causes a distortion in DNA structure but also disrupts DNA-enzyme interactions, which are essential to replication and transcription. Further interaction with the DNA, and associated proteins, further destabilizes and prevents vital functions. Some acridines have been shown to prevent or disrupt the interactions of key enzymes, including topoisomerases, which are involved in the supercoiling (or higher-ordered structure) of DNA. The exact interaction varies depending on the acridine molecule. For example, the intercalation of proflavine appears to follow two mechanisms, depending on the biocide concentration and time. The first mechanism is rapid, intercalating and binding between every four to five nucleotides; some reports have suggested a greater affinity for adjacent purine residues, which may be simply related to accessibility of the biocide at these sites. Not only does the actual proflavine molecule slot into the DNA structure, but the two amine (NH_2) groups form ionic linkages with phosphate residues in the DNA backbone structure. Other parts of the molecule are also held in place by further interactions (particularly van der Waals forces) with the purine and pyrimidine rings in the nucleotides. The second mechanism has molecular binding similar to the first, but at a lower

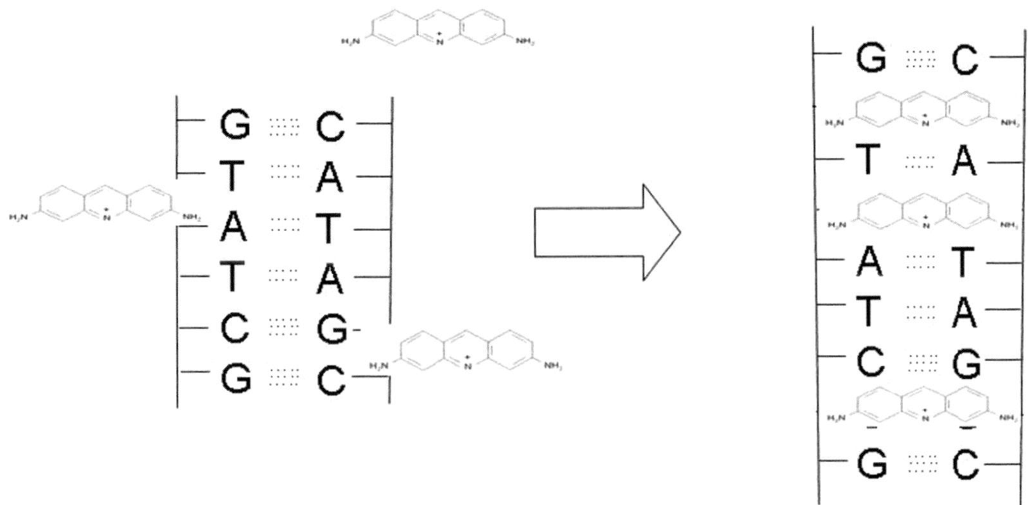

FIGURE 7.17 The mode of action of acridine dyes. The acridine molecules shown (proflavine) intercalate between the nucleotide bases in the DNA molecule, causing disruption of structure and function.

rate and intercalating more frequently between all adjacent nucleotides. The acridines are also photosensitive and therefore adsorb light energy, causing photochemical reactions. These reactions have been shown to lead to guanine base damage, strand unraveling (due to breakages in hydrogen bonds), single- and double-stranded nucleic acid breaks (due to breakage of phosphodiester bonds), and DNA-protein cross-links. These effects are not dissimilar to those of other biocides or biocidal processes described in other sections. Therefore, although the primary effects are due to intercalation, multiple effects, including nucleic acid fragmentation, enzyme inhibition, and surface interactions, also contribute to the mode of action of the acridines (chapter 3, section 3.7).

Further disruption of microbial macromolecular structures has been described with antimicrobial metals. Many metals, including iron, sodium, potassium, and calcium, are required for microbial life, with varied structural and functional roles. Removal of these key metals leads to inhibition of growth, and equally, higher concentrations lead to a variety of toxic effects on the cell. For example, calcium and magnesium play an important role in the structure of the bacterial cell wall and cell membrane. Magnesium is also involved in the stabilization of ribosomes, cell membranes, and nucleic acids, as well as being required for the activity of various enzymes. The activities of chelating agents on bacteria and fungi demonstrate the importance of these divalent ions in their structures and functions. Chelating agents, such as EDTA, remove these cations from macromolecules, which can inhibit their activity and cause structural changes. An often cited example is the effect of EDTA on the Gram-negative bacteria cell wall structure; EDTA increases the permeability of the cell wall to allow the penetration of other biocides. The general Gram-negative cell wall structure differs from the Gram-positive bacteria wall, particularly in having an outer membrane that is somewhat similar in structure to the inner, cytoplasmic membrane but contains lipopolysaccharide (LPS) in addition to phospholipids and integral or associated proteins (chapter 1, section 1.3.4.1). LPS contains a lipid portion that forms part of the external surface of the outer membrane, which is linked to a polysaccharide portion extending toward the outside of the cell (Fig. 1.15; see section 1.3.7).

Similar to the inner membrane, proteins can be found associated through or at the periplasmic or external surface of the outer membrane. Magnesium ions play an important role in maintaining the integrity of these LPS interactions by interacting with the negatively charged polysaccharide (core) portion. When magnesium is chelated (or removed) from these interactions, it causes disruption and release of LPS from the outer membrane structure. This destabilization leads to increased permeability of the outer membrane and disruption of key associated proteins or other functions. It is clear that as divalent cations are required for other functional and structural roles in microorganisms, the effects of chelating agents also disrupt their activities over time.

The biocidal metals include silver and copper (see chapter 3, section 3.12); others, such as mercury and arsenic, are less used due to toxicity concerns but demonstrate similar disruption of structure. As positively charged ions in solution, they all have affinity for negatively charged microbial surfaces. This affinity causes some disruption of the proton motive force and cell membrane-associated activities, including energy generation and mobility. Surface proteins are particularly targeted by metals. Specific protein binding has been reported with silver, mercury, and other cations, with exposed sulfhydryl groups being particularly sensitive. Sulfhydryl groups, present on cysteine amino acids, play an important role in the enzymatic activity and functional activity of many proteins; for example, sulfhydryl groups are important in the tertiary structure of proteins due to the formation of disulfide bonds to give them the correct folded structure (see section

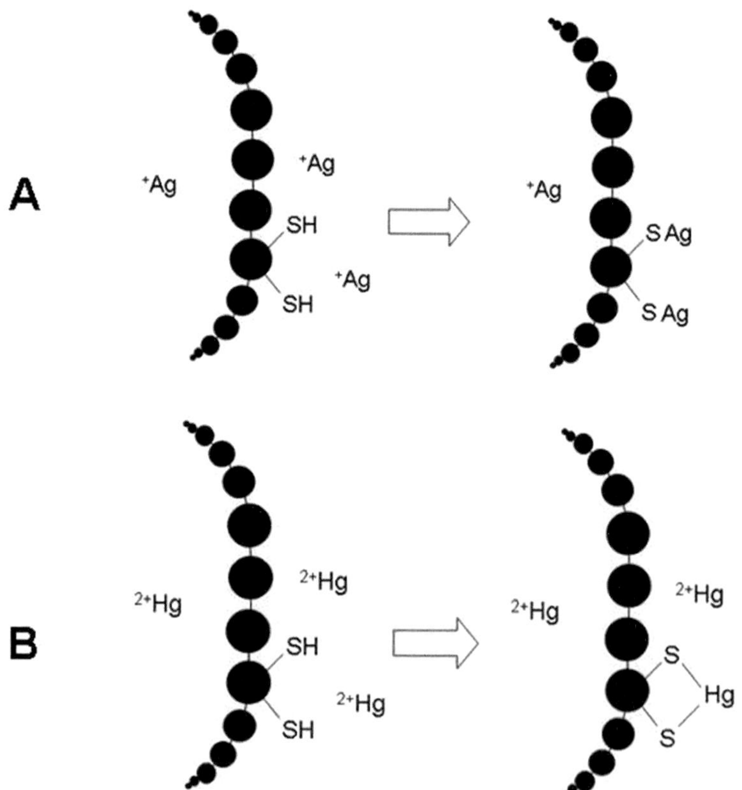

FIGURE 7.18 The reaction of metal ions on exposed sulfhydryl groups on cysteine amino acid within a peptide.

7.3). Typical metal reactions reported with sulfhydryl groups are shown in Fig. 7.18. These reactions change not only the structure of some proteins, but also their activity.

Specific interactions with nucleic acids, particularly those causing pyrimidine dimers, disrupt the function and structure of DNA, with reports of prevention of DNA replication. Indirect effects, such as the production of hydrogen peroxide and superoxide radicals during oxidative stress in the cell, lead to further nucleic acid, lipid, and protein damage. DNA appears to clump and disintegrate on exposure to copper over time. The inhibition of key cytoplasmic enzymes involved in bacterial and fungal respiration may also play a role in the indirect accumulation of reactive oxygen species, which also cause oxidation of macromolecules. Metals have also been shown to cause structural changes in the cell envelope, with detachment of the bacterial cell membrane from the cell wall and leakage of cell wall components.

Many biocides target microbial surfaces, membranes in particular, as a primary mode of action, with a variety of subsequent effects noted due to disruption of the structure and function of the membrane and associated proteins and enzymes (Fig. 7.19).

Microbial membranes are complex structures consisting of lipids (particularly phos-

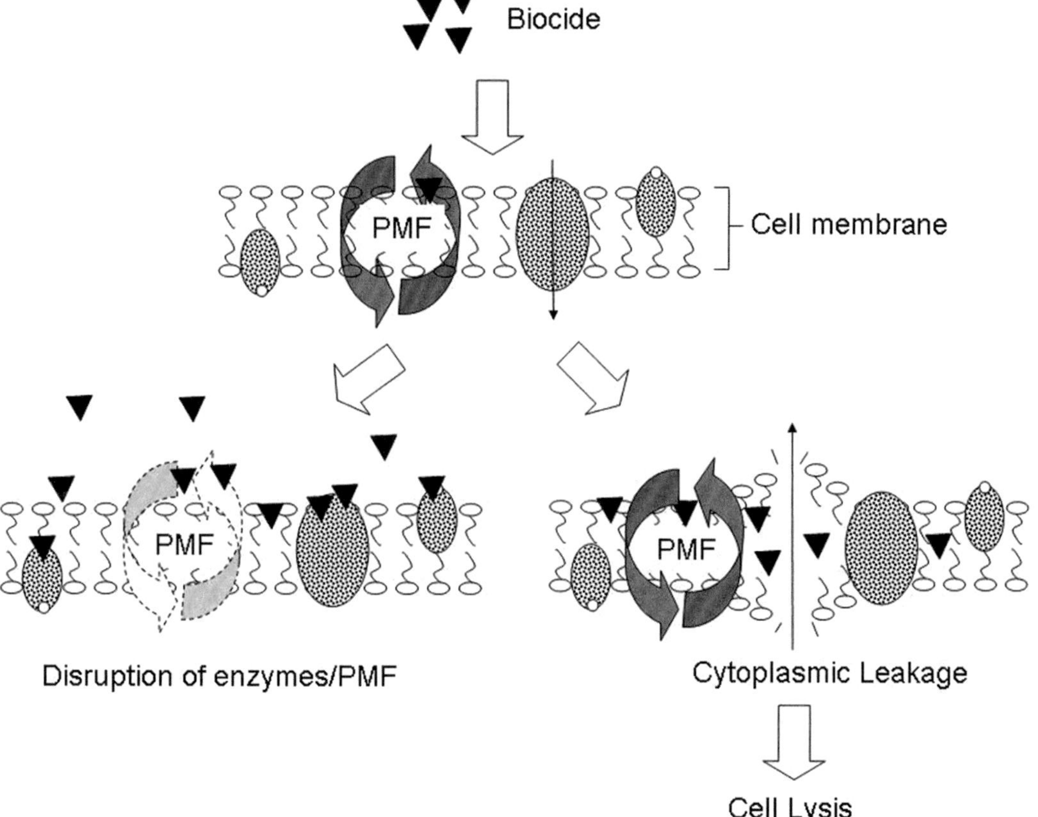

FIGURE 7.19 The effects of biocides on cytoplasmic membranes. The biocide can have subtle effects on membrane functions including surface or membrane-associated proteins (involved in substrate transport across the membrane or other enzymatic reactions) and disruption of the proton motive force. The biocide can also have more drastic effects on lipid membrane structure, leading to an increase in permeability and cytoplasmic leakage; further damage can eventually lead to cell lysis.

pholipid bilayers and, in some archaea, lipid monolayers) and associated proteins (chapter 1, section 1.3.4). The cytoplasmic membranes of bacteria and fungi provide a permeability barrier to the external environment and to contain the internal cytoplasm. The basic structure in many microorganisms consists of a phospholipid bilayer. The phospholipids are further stabilized by the presence of divalent cations such as Ca^{+2} and Mg^{+2}, but in general it is a fluid structure. Fungi and other eukaryotes may also contain other lipids such as sterols, which can add further stability to the membrane in comparison to bacterial membranes.

Membrane and membrane associated proteins play important roles in cellular processes, including enzymes involved in cell wall biosynthesis, nutrient transport into the cell, export of molecules out of the cell, and energy generation. A key example of these is the membrane-associated electron transport carrier proteins that are involved in the generation of electrical energy across the membrane that is known as the proton motive force. As a source of energy, the proton motive force is required for key cellular processes including energy (in the form of ATP) synthesis ("oxidative phosphorylation"), active ion transport, and cellular motility and chemotaxis. Similar lipid membrane structures are also seen in the outer membranes of Gram-negative bacteria (chapter 1, section 1.3.4.1) and enveloped viruses (section 1.3.5). Direct damage to the structure and function of lipid membranes has been described for various types of active agents. The biocides discussed here have been described as having the disruption of the structure and function of lipid membranes as their primary mode of action. These membrane-active biocides include surfactants (including the cationic QACs), the biguanides, organic acids and esters, and the anilides. Direct damage to the membrane can cause subtle effects on the protein-related functions, which are observed as enzyme inhibition and disruption of the proton motive force, including the various associated metabolic processes. More dramatic effects include an increase in permeability, leakage of cytoplasmic materials, and cell lysis (Fig. 7.19).

The surfactants (or "surface-active agents") have been shown to particularly disrupt the structure of bacterial membranes, which leads to leakage of cytoplasmic components. They have two regions in their molecular structures, one a water-repellent (hydrophobic) hydrocarbon group and the other a water-attracting (hydrophilic or polar) group (chapter 3, section 3.16). Their overall structure therefore allows them to react with and penetrate into lipid membranes. The most effective are those with a greater positive charge in solution, including the cationics (such as the QACs) and the amphotherics (which have both detergency and antimicrobial attributes). The anionics and nonionics are less effective as microbicides, but they increase the permeability of cell wall and membrane structures and, at higher concentrations, can be biocidal. The QACs have been particularly studied against bacteria (section 3.16); they have been shown to rapidly adsorb to and penetrate the cell wall and then react with the membrane lipids and proteins to cause loss of integrity and cytoplasm leakage at relatively low concentrations. Indications of cytoplasmic leakage include the extracellular detection of typical intracellular components such as potassium, inorganic phosphate, amino acids, and even nucleic acids following treatment with surfactants. It has been known for many years that QACs are membrane-active agents, with target sites predominantly at the cytoplasmic (inner) membrane in bacteria or the plasma membrane in yeasts.

The following sequence of events is proposed with microorganisms exposed to cationic agents: (i) adsorption and penetration of the agent into the cell wall; (ii) reaction with the cytoplasmic membrane (lipid and/or protein) followed by membrane disorganization; (iii) leakage of intracellular low-molecular-weight material; (iv) degradation of proteins and nucleic acids; and (v) wall lysis caused by autolytic enzymes. There is thus a loss of structural organization and integrity of the cytoplasmic membrane in bacteria, together with other damaging effects to the bacterial cell. Evidence suggests that the main effects are due to insertion into the lipid bilayer, but direct effects on the protein structure have also been reported. For example, the QAC cetrimide has been shown to interfere with the proton motive force. The QACs have been specifically shown to interact with phospholipids, while the anionic surfactants appear to be more active against cell surface proteins. The initial toxic effect of QACs on yeast cells has also been shown to be due to a disorganization of fungal plasma membranes. Similar effects are expected to be responsible for the loss of infectivity observed with enveloped viruses. Further effects on intracellular proteins and nucleic acids culminate in cell lysis. Because the diamidines are considered similar to cationic surfactants (chapter 3, section 3.9), their mode of action is also related to disruption of the cell membrane, leading to inhibition of transport systems and cytoplasmic leakage.

The biguanides and polymeric biguanides demonstrate effects similar to those of QACs, and their interactions with the bacteria and yeast cell membranes have been investigated in some detail. Initial displacement of Ca^{+2} and Mg^{+2} cations that are associated with phospholipids has been observed, followed by direct binding to surface phospholipids and attraction of adjacent molecules to disrupt the membrane structure, leading to cytoplasm leakage. The mode of action of chlorhexidine has been particularly well described in bacteria and yeast. In studies with bacteria, the uptake of chlorhexidine was found to be very rapid in both Gram-negative (*E. coli*) and Gram-positive (*S. aureus*) bacteria and depended on the biocide concentration and pH. Insertion and interaction with the cell wall were reported to cause damage but were insufficient to induce cell lysis or death. Similar results were observed with yeasts. After passing through the cell wall or outer membrane, presumably by passive diffusion, the biocide subsequently attacks the bacterial cytoplasmic/inner membrane or the yeast plasma membrane as the major mode of activity. Direct damage to the semipermeable membrane has been shown to induce leakage of intracellular constituents but may be an indirect consequence of further cellular damage and cell death. The exact interactions that affect the structure and function of the cell membrane are not known but appear to be due to insertion into the membrane, resulting in disruption of structure and function. At lower concentrations, chlorhexidine collapses the membrane potential by disruption. The mode of action of alexidine and the polymeric biguanides may differ slightly in the disruption of the cell membrane.

Alexidine is more rapidly bactericidal and produces a significantly faster alteration in bactericidal permeability than chlorhexidine. This biocide differs chemically from chlorhexidine in possessing ethylhexyl end groups (chapter 3, section 3.8). It has been suggested that the nature of the ethylhexyl end group in alexidine, as opposed to the chlorophenol end group in chlorhexidine, may influence the ability of a biguanide to interact with membrane lipids to produce lipid domains in the cytoplasmic membrane. Similarly, PHMB (polyhexamethylbiguanide) causes domain formation of the acidic phospholipids of the cytoplasmic membrane. Permeability changes and altered function of some membrane-associated enzymes ensue. Membrane damage has also been shown to be the major mode of action of chlorhexidine in other microorganisms, including mycobacteria, protozoa, and enveloped viruses. Other effects are observed at higher biguanide concentrations. For example, high concentrations have been shown to be an inhibitor of both membrane-bound and soluble adenosine triphosphatase (ATPase) as well as uptake of potassium in *Enterococcus faecalis*; these and other effects on enzymatic and transport protein functions appear to be secondary lethal effects. In bacteria and yeasts, chlorhexidine also penetrates into the cytoplasm of cells. High concentrations of chlorhexidine cause coagulation of intracellular constituents. It has been noted that an initial high rate of cytoplasm leakage rises as the concentration of chlorhexidine increases, but at higher biocide concentrations leakage is reduced because of the coagulation of the cytoplasm components.

The acids and esters have subtler effects, as investigated in bacteria and fungi, to disrupt the proton motive force and therefore associated functions. In the case of some acids, the change in pH alone is sufficient to disrupt the function and structure of surface proteins and enzymes and other macromolecules. Therefore, the overall effects appear to disrupt membrane enzymes but without disrupting the overall structure of the membrane, as indicated by the lack of observed leakage. The paraben esters appear to have a greater overall disruptive effect on membrane enzymes than the acids. The more hydrophobic acids and esters are also expected to interact and disrupt the membrane structure due to integration. The anilides have also been shown to disrupt the proton motive force across the bacterial surface and to interrupt key membrane functions, including active transport and energy metabolism. Trichlorocarbanilide and trichlorosalicylanide have more specific effects on the cell membrane, as indicated in protoplast (artificial cell wall-free bacteria) experiments. This action is more likely due to direct adsorption and destruction of the semipermeable character of the cytoplasmic membrane, but without loss of integrity. Increased halogenation of anilides appears to cause increased reactions with membrane constituents and an increase in bactericidal activity.

Many biocides have been described that cause direct changes in the structure and function of proteins. These include the effects of oxidizing agents leading to oxidation, changes in structure and fragmentation, cross-linking of amino acid side chains, transfer of energy leading to denaturation and coagulation, and disruption of structure, as described above with the interactions of metal ions and surfactants. These effects may also be considered nonspecific protein interactions, although some proteins may be more sensitive to these effects than others, depending on their respective structures and localizations. Until recently it was widely considered that biocides had more nonspecific modes of action, in contrast to antibiotics and other anti-infective drugs. These include interruption of cellular protein transcription machinery (e.g., the aminoglycosides and chloramphenicol), direct inhibition of specific enzymes (e.g., the quinolones against DNA gyrase), and interference with other functions required for multiplication of the microorganism (e.g., nucleoside analogue inhibitors of viral replication; section 7.2.3). Further analysis of the mode of action of some more selective biocides has, surprisingly, shown preferred inhibition of specific enzymes; these include studies of the mode of action of the bisphenols. Phenols, which have already been discussed, target surface and internal proteins by binding to proteins by a variety of interactions including covalent binding, hydrogen bonding, and ionic and hydrophobic interactions (section 7.4.3). These interactions cause proteins, along with other associated macromolecules, to lose their structure (denature), coagulate, and precipitate. At low concentrations, the bisphenols have been shown to specifically inhibit enoyl reductases (see discussion in chapter 3, section 3.15). Triclosan interacts with the substrate binding site (in particular, tyrosine residues) on the enzyme, simulating the enzyme's natural substrate, and the associated nicotinamide ring of the enzyme cofactor (NADH or NADPH), which allows for the tighter, irreversible binding of the biocide. X-ray crystallography has shown that these interactions are noncovalent and are formed by hydrogen bonding, van der Waals forces, and other hydrophobic interactions.

The enoyl reductases play a key role in the biosynthesis of fatty acids (thus affecting cell membrane structure) and therefore inhibit the growth of bacteria and some protozoa. In the case of triclosan, the interaction is initially reversible but over time causes a conformation change and precipitation of the protein/coenzyme structure that is irreversible. These effects remove the enzyme from its key role in fatty acid biosynthesis and cause complex precipitation. Another bisphenol, hexachlorophene, forms noncovalent interactions comparable to triclosan but does not form the irreversible complex with the enzyme-cofactor. A similar mode of action has been shown for the antimycobacterial antibiotic isoniazid; however, isoniazid forms covalent bonds with the cofactors at the enzyme active site. Triclosan and hexachlorophene, like other phenols, have been shown to specifically inhibit other enzymes and affect the structure of the cell membrane. It was therefore not surprising to find that various mutations or overexpression of enoyl reductases in bacteria can increase the minimal inhibitory concentration of bisphenols but not necessarily the minimal biocidal concentration. However, the identification of an identical bacterial target for an antibiotic and a biocide, even at low concentrations, is of some concern, especially if the use of the biocide in the environment could be a factor in the development of cross-resistance to antibiotics that are more restricted in their modes of activity and therapeutic concentrations. The results with bisphenols suggest that this could potentially be the case, although the significance of this continues to be debated (chapter 8, section 8.7.2).

MECHANISMS OF MICROBIAL RESISTANCE

8

8.1 INTRODUCTION

Different types of microorganisms vary in their response to antiseptics, disinfectants, and sterilants. This is hardly surprising, in view of their different cellular and viral structures, compositions, and physiologies (chapter 1). Traditionally, susceptibility to biocides has been classified based on microbial structural differences and overall sensitivities to biocides (Fig. 8.1).

This classification can be used only as a general reference for biocidal products and processes; the relative resistance of various microorganisms can vary, depending on the microorganism itself, the biocide under investigation, process or application conditions, and any formulation effects (in the case of liquid biocide preparations) (as discussed in chapter 1, sections 1.4.6 and 1.4.7). Therefore, although this hierarchy of resistance can be a useful guide, it may not reflect the true resistance profile of each biocide type. As examples, certain nonenveloped viruses show equivalent resistance profiles as bacterial spores to dry-heat inactivation, and fungal spores are more resistant to UV radiation than mycobacteria are.

This chapter discusses the various mechanisms of biocide resistance described in microorganisms. Because diverse types of organisms can react differently, it is convenient to consider bacteria, fungi, viruses, protozoa, and prions separately. Although resistance mechanisms in all of these microorganisms have been identified and described, research has focused on certain bacteria due to their ease of cultivation and manipulation in the laboratory. In contrast, there is only limited research on viruses and other microorganisms such as protozoa, which are potential areas for further investigations.

8.2 BIOCIDE-MICROORGANISM INTERACTION

Whatever the type of microbial cell (or entity), there is a common sequence of events in the interaction with a biocide (Fig. 8.2).

This can be envisaged as (i) interaction of the biocide with the microbial surface, followed by (ii) penetration into the microorganism and (iii) action at the target site(s), which can include the cell wall, the viral envelope and/or capsid, the cell membrane, and the various cytoplasmic constituents. This progression of events depends on the biocide type and the target microorganisms.

The biocide should be at a sufficient level (either in intensity or concentration) to interact with and penetrate into the microbial surface (or at least to a site of antimicrobial action).

	Microorganism	Examples
More Resistant	Prions	Scrapie, Creutzfeld-Jacob Disease, Chronic Wasting Disease
	Bacterial Spores	*Bacillus, Geobacillus, Clostridium*
	Protozoal Oocysts	*Cryptosporidium*
	Helminth Eggs	*Ascaris, Enterobius*
	Mycobacteria	*Mycobacterium tuberculosis, M. terrae, M. chelonae*
	Small, Non-Enveloped Viruses	Poliovirus, Parvoviruses, Papilloma Viruses
	Protozoal Cysts	*Giardia, Acanthamoeba*
	Fungal Spores	*Aspergillus, Penicillium*
	Gram Negative Bacteria	*Pseudomonas, Providencia, Escherichia*
	Vegetative Fungi and Algae	*Aspergillus, Trichophyton, Candida, Chlamydomonas*
	Vegetative Helminths and Protozoa	*Ascaris, Cryptosporidium, Giardia*
	Large, Non-Enveloped Viruses	Adenoviruses, Rotaviruses
	Gram Positive Bacteria	*Staphylococcus, Streptococcus, Enterococcus*
Less Resistant	Enveloped Viruses	HIV, Hepatitis B Virus, Herpes Simplex Virus

FIGURE 8.1 General microbial resistance to biocides and biocidal processes.

Important variables can include the biocide mode of action (see chapter 7), concentration or dose, process conditions (e.g., temperature), formulation effects, and environmental conditions. The biocide concentration or dose is a particularly important variable and must at least be at the minimum inhibitory or, preferably, at the minimum biocidal concentration to have a significant effect. Various formulation effects can assist in the penetration of liquid biocides to and into target microorganisms (as is in the case of enhanced triclosan penetration into Gram-negative bacteria in the presence of EDTA and other chelating agents; see chapter 1, section 1.4.6). Process effects such as the presence of liquid or gas-phase biocides, pressure, and temperature also play important roles. In addition to direct biocidal-product effects, the presence of interfering substances can limit interactions with microbial surfaces. Two important, and often associated variables, are the nature of the contaminated surface or liquid and the presence of soils. Microorganisms can circumvent the activity of a biocide by protection within a given surface or liquid. Examples include the survival of microorganisms in the skin during antisepsis (chapter 4) and within surface imperfections (e.g., cracks, crevices, or porous materials) on inanimate surfaces during disinfection and/or sterilization. Other variables can be due to phase separation in liquid formulations, with the microorganisms being present and allowed to multiply in one phase, and the biocide being separated into another. The contaminated surface or liquid itself can also be reactive with the biocide, as is the case with cellulose-based materials (e.g., paper) and many oxidizing agent biocides,

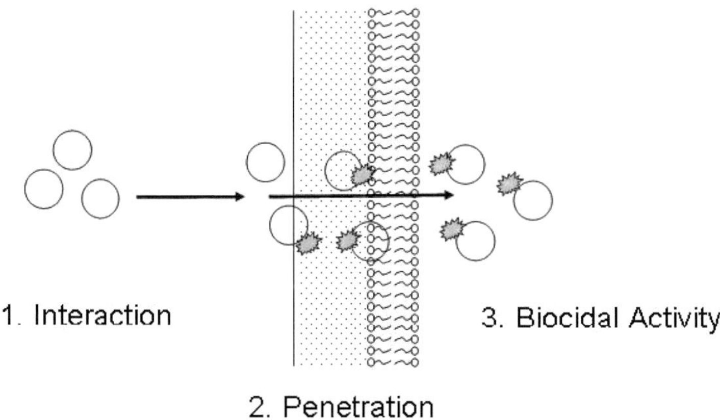

FIGURE 8.2 Initial sequence of events on biocide-microorganism interaction.

which limits their ability to contact the target microorganisms within these materials. Various types of organic and inorganic soils, including blood, serum, water hardness, and the presence of salts, can significantly reduce the penetration (by reaction or sequestration) of a biocide and interaction with microbial targets; these effects highlight the importance of cleaning as a prerequisite to surface disinfection or sterilization, or at least considering the impact of the extent of soiling present during any surface biocidal treatment (section 1.4.8). Other similar interfering effects depend on the nature of the application. As a simple example, the suspension of microorganisms in water can inhibit the penetration of gaseous chemical biocides.

The natures and compositions of the different types of microbial surfaces vary from one cell (or entity) to another but can also alter because of changes in the environment. These alterations are considered in more detail as mechanisms of intrinsic resistance. Biocide interaction at the cell surface itself can produce a significant effect on viability (e.g., with glutaraldehyde, surfactants, and oxidizing agents), but most antimicrobial agents appear to have significant biocidal effects intracellularly or on the internal structures of viruses. The outermost layers of microbial cells can thus have a significant effect on their susceptibility (or insusceptibility) to biocides. These can range from the relatively sensitive envelopes of enveloped viruses to the highly resistant spore coats associated with endospore structure (see chapter 1, section 1.3, and section 8.3.11). Overall, it is disappointing to note how little is known about the mode of entry of many of these antimicrobial agents into different types of microorganisms.

8.3 INTRINSIC BACTERIAL RESISTANCE MECHANISMS

In recent years, considerable progress has been made in more fully understanding the response of different types of bacteria (mycobacteria, nonsporulating bacteria, and bacterial spores) to antibacterial agents. Resistance can be either a natural property of a microorganism (intrinsic) or acquired over time, such as by mutation in its chromosomal (nucleic acid) structure or by the acquisition of plasmids (self-replicating, extrachromosomal DNA) or transposons (transmissible DNA cassettes that can be chromosomal or plasmid-integrated). Examples of resistance mechanisms are given in Table 8.1.

Mechanisms of intrinsic resistance in bacteria are described in this section, with further consideration of the various types of bacteria in sections 8.4 to 8.6. Acquired resistance mechanisms in bacteria are discussed in section 8.7.

TABLE 8.1 Examples of intrinsic and acquired mechanisms of resistance to biocides in bacteria

Mechanism	Resistance	Examples
Impermeability	Intrinsic	Bacterial spores, with various internal protective layers, act as an efficient barrier to the entry of biocides
		Mycobacteria, among all vegetative bacteria, demonstrate notable resistance to biocide penetration due to their unique, lipophilic cell wall structure
		The outer membrane of Gram-negative bacteria, in many cases, presents a more efficient barrier to prevent uptake or penetration of the biocide than that of Gram-positive bacteria
		Capsules and other extracellular matrices (including biofilm development) can act as effective barriers to biocide penetration
	Acquired	High glutaraldehyde resistance of some mutant strains of *Mycobacterium chelonae* is most likely due to decreased uptake due to acquired resistance mechanism(s), particularly cell wall structure changes
		The presence of some plasmids can change the expression of outer membrane proteins in Gram-negative bacteria and increase the resistance to biocides such as formaldehyde
Efflux	Intrinsic	Extrusion of the biocide from the cytoplasm due to active efflux mechanisms (e.g., with chlorhexidine, antimicrobial dyes, and triclosan)
	Acquired	Plasmid-mediated and/or mutations leading to upregulation of efflux mechanisms
Decreased target susceptibility	Acquired	Specific mutations that decrease the affinity of some biocides (e.g., triclosan) to key cellular targets
Inactivation	Intrinsic	Production of enzymes and chemicals that neutralize biocides (e.g., formaldehyde dehydrogenase and peroxidases)
	Acquired	Expression of plasmid-associated enzymes and other proteins (such as those that sequester the biocide) intolerance to metals (such as mercury, silver, and copper) and oxidizing agents

8.3.1 General Stationary Phase Phenomena

Bacteria multiply by binary fission, an asexual reproductive process in which one cell replicates its DNA and separates into two distinct, genetically identical cells. The growth of bacteria in laboratory culture and at optimal environmental conditions follows a similar trend that can be plotted (Fig. 8.3).

Four phases can be generally recognized, depending on the environmental conditions. During the initial lag phase, the bacterial cells

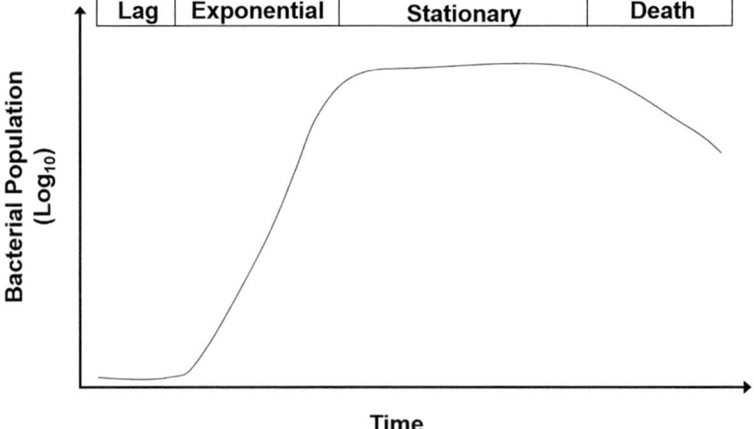

FIGURE 8.3 A typical bacterial growth curve, showing the four phases of population growth.

are actively metabolizing but not multiplying; the length of this stage depends on the nature and type of bacteria present, as well as the presence or absence of various environmental conditions (including availability of nutrients, tolerated temperatures, presence or absence of oxygen, etc.). As the cells begin to multiply by binary fission, a maximal rate is attained at which the number of bacteria doubles within an optimum time interval, referred to as the generation time. The actual generation time varies, depending on the bacterial species and growth conditions; under optimal laboratory conditions, *Escherichia coli* strains can demonstrate rapid generation times as short as 15 minutes, in contrast to the slower-growing *Mycobacterium tuberculosis* (~900 minutes) and *Treponema palladium* (~2,000 minutes). These initial phases of growth are generally the most sensitive to the effects of biocides on the growth and survival of bacteria. Under optimal conditions, where the bacterial culture has a continual source of nutrients and a lack of any inhibitory substance, the bacteria can continue to grow exponentially (see Fig. 8.3); however, when nutrients become limiting, toxic by-products of metabolism accumulate, and in the presence of other adverse environmental conditions (including deviations in temperature and the presence of biocides) the bacterial culture enters into stationary phase. During this phase, bacteria demonstrate various morphological and physiological response mechanisms to survive in a more competitive environment; many of these responses intrinsically cause an increase in tolerance to various biocides and biocidal processes. These include the heat shock and oxidative stress responses (section 8.3.3). The length of this phase depends on the severity of the environmental conditions. For example, strains of *E. coli* may survive for up to 3 to 4 days. As adverse conditions continue to develop, the rate of bacterial death (including cell lysis) will be greater than multiplication, with an overall decrease in the bacterial population over time (death phase). In addition to the various physiological cellular responses during the stationary/death phases of growth, some bacterial species can enter into more dramatic developmental stages to assume dormant forms of life. These include sporulation (section 8.3.11) and other low or nonmetabolizing dormant stages, which allow bacteria to resist adverse conditions. The various stationary-phase responses and development of dormant forms, which allow bacteria to resist the effects of biocides and biocidal processes, are discussed further below.

8.3.2 Motility and Chemotaxis

Late in the exponential or early in the stationary phases of bacterial growth, many bacteria can adapt specifically to allow them to be motile. These mechanisms include flagella expression, gliding motility, and chemotaxis. Flagella are thin appendages that are attached to the bacterial surface but freely rotate to allow for bacterial movement (chapter 1, section 1.3.4.1). The presence, location on the bacterial surface, and number (single or multiple) of flagella vary. Examples of bacteria that produce flagella are species of *Escherichia*, *Salmonella*, and *Bacillus*. In comparison, gliding refers to a process of motility on a surface but in the absence of flagella; the exact mechanisms of gliding are not exactly known, but in some bacteria it has been linked to the production of polysaccharide slime. Examples of gliding bacteria include *Myxococcus* and filamentous cyanobacteria. The production of slime or protective capsules can also provide an efficient barrier for the penetration of some biocides, which will be further considered in section 8.3.7. Nonmotile bacteria also demonstrate the ability to move away from the presence of various chemical agents by chemotaxis. These are considered indirect mechanisms of biocide tolerance only, in that they allow bacteria to relocate to a less adverse environment and permit the circumvention of biocide attack under limited circumstances.

8.3.3 Stress Responses

During the transition between the exponential and stationary phases of growth, bacteria have been shown to demonstrate structural and chemical changes in their structure in reaction to the restricted availability of nutrients required for growth. This has been particularly studied in *E. coli*, which demonstrates an overall reduction in cell size, changes in cell structure, increased rigidity of the cell wall peptidoglycan, and changes in the types and lengths of fatty acids in the cell membrane. In general, cells at this stage show increased, although limited, tolerance to biocides due to reduced uptake and decreased cellular metabolism. Initially, this appears to be due to an imbalance in the production of macromolecules and cell division. In some cases, the slowdown in macromolecular synthesis is restricted, but cells continue to divide, resulting in a population of smaller cells, which may also include multiple copies of the bacterial DNA molecules in the same cell. With *E. coli*, these smaller cells appear more coccoid than the typical rod-shaped cells for that species (chapter 1, section 1.3.4.1). These effects become more dramatic as the cell reacts to the lack of nutrients: the cells continue to become smaller and more compact, which is referred to as "dwarfism."

In *E. coli* this is due to the degradation of parts of the cell membrane and the cell wall (peptidoglycan), but not the outer membrane, with a resulting increase in the size of the periplasmic space. The reduction in size is also observed in other bacteria, although in the case of *Pseudomonas*, sections of the outer membrane are also lost, with no subsequent increase in the periplasm size. The components of the outer cell structure that are removed may be used as nutrient sources by the cell but also allow it to assume a more compact structure. Specific changes in the control of fatty acid synthetic and degradative processes have been described. The increased transcription of the *fad* (for fatty acid degradative) enzymes in *E. coli* and *Salmonella* allows restricted degradation of the cell membrane-associated and other fatty acids in the cell as carbon sources; however, degradation also appears to be more specific for short- and medium-chained fatty acids, with an observed increase in longer-chained fatty acids in the cell membrane. The increase in longer-chained fatty acids leads to increased hydrophobicity of the membrane and less penetration of some biocides. In combination, these changes in the cell structure and function may allow greater tolerance of the presence of biocides at lower concentrations; this can be significant when the biocide is used at bacteriostatic or preservative concentrations but has little benefit for cell survival at typical disinfection and sterilization conditions.

Bacteria have been shown to have specific responses to various environmental challenges or stresses, particularly during stationary phase or low-nutrient conditions, that can also contribute to intrinsic resistance to biocides, either directly or indirectly (Table 8.2). These have been particularly well studied in the Gram-negative bacteria *E. coli* and the Gram-positive *Bacillus atrophaeus* because they present interesting mechanisms of control in their cells. Some of these responses are discussed briefly below as potential mechanisms of intrinsic conditions.

The stringent response is a specific example of a stress response that results from the lack of nutrients, in particular, as first described

TABLE 8.2 Examples of bacterial responses to environmental stress

Environmental stress	Response
Lack of essential nutrients	General nutrient restriction or starvation
Amino acid and other (e.g., fatty acid) starvation	Stringent response
DNA damage (increase in single-stranded DNA)	SOS response
Increases in heat or presence of biocides that denature proteins (e.g., alcohols)	Heat shock
Changes in pH, acidification	pH or acid tolerance
Presence of reactive oxygen species	Oxidative stress
Changes in osmolarity	Osmotic stress

for amino acid starvation, and is closely linked to the transition of a cell from exponential to stationary growth. In addition to amino acid starvation, the stringent response can also be induced by fatty acid, carbon, and nitrogen limitations, as well as in response to sublethal UV light. During the response, the level of nucleotide molecules such as guanosine 3′,5′ tetraphosphate (ppGpp) that are known as alarmones rises in the cell cytoplasm and inhibits the synthesis of ribosomal and transfer RNA. The subsequent restriction of protein synthesis (transcription) causes a decrease in the various cellular metabolic and structural functions, including cell division and membrane transport, which are typical of transition into stationary phase. The presence of alarmones also appears to promote the transcription of certain genes such as those involved in amino acid biosynthesis and virulence. The stringent response has been particularly well described in *E. coli* but is also known to be a basic phenomenon in bacteria, fungi, and plants, including *Bacillus*, *Vibrio*, *Mycobacterium*, and *Streptomyces*. In mycobacteria it is proposed that the stringent response could trigger the developmental adaptation of low-metabolic or dormant stages of growth that are a hallmark of persistence of these bacteria in cases of infection.

The SOS response has been described in bacteria as a response to a variety of environmental factors including transition to stationary phase, starvation, and the presence of biocides. These events are all linked to the detection of DNA damage by the cell. The response can be induced in reaction to low-dose radiation (such as UV light) and reactive oxygen species, which both damage DNA by dimer formation and oxidation of susceptible bonds (chapter 7, sections 7.4.4. and 7.4.2, respectively). DNA damage or the inhibition of DNA replication causes an increase in the presence of single-stranded DNA. A specific bacterial protein, RecA, binds to single-stranded DNA, which activates the protein to promote the autocleavage of LexA, a repressor protein. LexA represses (negatively regulates) the transcription of a variety of genes and the expression of cellular proteins that are involved with DNA repair and inhibition of cell division; cleavage of LexA therefore removes the repressor and allows these proteins to be expressed. Inhibition of cell division gives the cell time to repair any damage, mediated by the various DNA repair enzymes. When the level of single-stranded DNA eventually decreases, the process can revert to repression of the SOS genes. The SOS response may afford some intrinsic resistance to biocides and biocidal processes (such as radiation) by the inhibition of cell division (lowering the sensitivity of the bacteria), but also by repairing damage, particularly sublethal damage, to the cell.

As discussed in chapter 7, section 7.4.2, various active oxygen species have dramatic effects on the structure and function of nucleic acids, proteins, and lipids. These oxygen species (including the superoxide ion, hydrogen peroxide, and the hydroxyl radical) are produced during normal cell metabolism, particularly in aerobic or facultative anaerobic bacteria, and need to be controlled to prevent damage within the cell. Bacteria (and other microorganisms such as fungi and protozoa) have a variety of enzymatic and nonenzymatic processes that can neutralize these species, and their expression can offer some advantage as mechanisms for increased tolerance to biocides. An increase in the intracellular or extracellular concentration of oxidants triggers the production of these antioxidative processes in the "oxidative stress" response in bacteria. At least two distinct but often overlapping oxidative stress responses have been described in bacteria as being specifically induced by hydrogen peroxide or the superoxide ion. These responses are usually observed to be activated during the stationary phase of growth, at which stage bacteria are generally more resistant to the effects of oxidants. They are considered separate responses, because they demonstrate differences in the enzymatic and nonenzymatic proteins or other antioxidants that are produced during induction; examples of the differences observed in protein expression in these responses are given in Table 8.3. Various

TABLE 8.3 Differences observed in the expression of proteins during the hydrogen peroxide- or superoxide ion-induced oxidative stress response in *E. coli*

Protein/enzyme	H_2O_2-induced[a]	O_2^--induced[a]	Function
Catalases	+	–	Enzymatic degradation of hydrogen peroxide
Superoxide dismutases	–/+	+	Enzymatic conversion of O_2^-
GroES	+	+	Chaperone[b]
GroEL	–	+	Chaperone[b]
DnaK	+	–	Chaperone[b]

[a]+, induced; –, not induced; ±, sometimes induced.
[b]Chaperones are proteins that assist other proteins to fold correctly to assume their structure/function.

response mechanisms have been described, but all contribute to the protection of the cell from oxidative damage.

The peroxide stress response is modulated by a specific cellular protein, OxyR. OxyR is both a sensor protein and a transcriptional activator. It is present in an inactive form that is activated by the formation of disulfide bonds between adjacent sulfur groups of cysteine residues in the protein structure, by the same processes by which oxidants damage proteins (chapter 7, section 7.4.2). Most cytosolic proteins that contain cysteine residues in their sequence are found to be in the reduced (-SH) form, unlike secreted or membrane-associated proteins, which are more often in their oxidized form as disulfide (S-S) bonds. Therefore, the presence of oxidants induces the formation of disulfide bonds, with a dramatic effect on the structure and function of proteins (section 7.4.2). In the case of OxyR, the formation of disulfide bonds allows the protein to act as an activator to promote the transcription and translation of about 30 to 40 proteins associated with the response. These include enzymes such as catalases, peroxidases, and reductases that are involved in oxidant neutralization or repair (DNA, protein, and lipid) mechanisms. This reaction is also reversible when there is a reduction in the presence of oxidants and the antioxidants expressed during the stress response reverse the effect on OxyR, thereby allowing the cell to return to its nonstressed state (Fig. 8.4).

The superoxide stress response is similarly induced by increasing levels of the superoxide ion and is coordinated by two regulatory proteins, SoxR and SoxS. The response has been particularly well studied in *E. coli*. SoxR is a sensing protein that becomes activated due to oxidation in the presence of the superoxide ion, which stimulates the transcription of SoxS. SoxS is a transcriptional activator protein that directly or indirectly promotes the transcription of about 30 to 40 proteins that are involved in antioxidant repair and metabolic

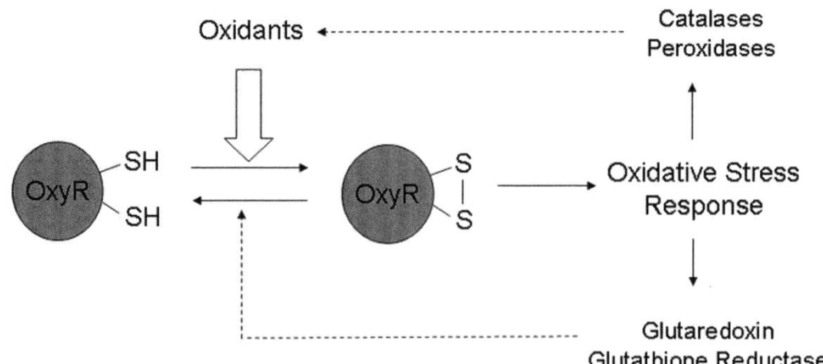

FIGURE 8.4 The activation and deactivation of the OxyR protein, as an activator in the peroxide-induced oxidative stress response.

functions. The expression of superoxide dismutase, which enzymatically promotes the formation of hydrogen peroxide from available superoxide ions, may also be involved in the activation of the peroxide response in the cell.

In both responses, a variety of enzymatic and nonenzymatic components are expressed that counteract the presence of oxidants. Some examples of enzymatic reactions are given in Fig. 8.5.

The presence of catalases and peroxidases neutralizes hydrogen peroxide. Their expression in various aerobic and facultative anaerobic bacteria has been shown to cause a marginal increase in their tolerance to the presence of hydrogen peroxide as a biocide, although this depends on the concentration of the biocide present; these effects allow the survival of these bacteria under lower concentrations (generally around the minimum bactericidal concentration) of hydrogen peroxide. For example, *B. atrophaeus* was shown to be inhibited by 10 mM hydrogen peroxide during exponential but not during stationary phase. The expression of antioxidants (including glutathione, thioredoxin, and the membrane-associated menaquinone) plays a similar role in tolerance to oxidizing agents in bacteria, due to the reaction with the antioxidant and the protection of sensitive macromolecules. Glutathione reacts directly with and neutralizes the various oxidants, as well as reversing the formation of disulfide bonds in proteins (by reduction).

Other protective mechanisms expressed during oxidative stress include chaperone proteins such as DnaK and GroEL; chaperones are proteins that assist other proteins to fold correctly to assume their appropriate folded structures and functions and that assist when proteins have been partially denatured to allow them to refold into their normal structure. These proteins also play roles to protect the cell against sublethal conditions that specifically denature proteins, including heat treatment (as in the heat shock response). Additional repair mechanisms expressed are various DNA repair enzymes (endonucleases and exonucleases) and other protein repair enzymes (e.g., for the reduction of disulfide bonds). Finally, the production of metal chelators such as metallothionein (in protozoa and yeasts) reduces the effects of metal-associated reactions with oxidizing agents (such as the Fenton reaction with iron as a catalyst), as well as protects against the antimicrobial effects of heavy metals such as iron, copper, and silver. Differences have been described in the specific oxidative responses in Gram-positive and Gram-negative bacteria,

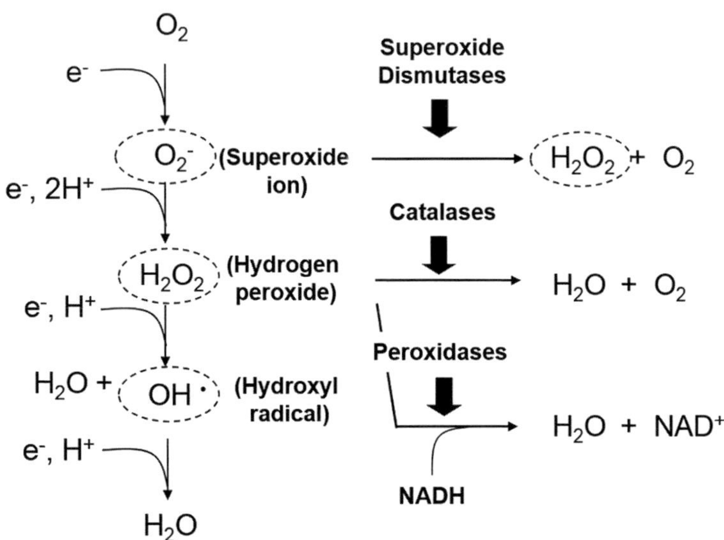

FIGURE 8.5 The function of various enzymes induced during oxidative stress.

but with the same overall effect of protecting the cell against damage. Interestingly, these protection mechanisms are seen not only in aerobic and facultative bacteria, but also in anaerobes; examples include flavoproteins that reduce oxygen to form water and superoxide reductases. Similar responses have been described in yeasts and other fungi. Overall, the oxidative stress response allows the cell to tolerate some amount of damage in the presence of many biocides and biocidal processes, particularly at bacteriostatic and minimal bactericidal conditions.

Another response that has been described in prokaryotes and eukaryotes is the heat shock response, which has been particularly well studied in *E. coli*, other bacteria, and yeasts. Bacteria can grow over a wide range of temperatures, but *E. coli*, as an example, is a mesophilic organism with an optimum temperature for growth at ~37°C. When the temperature is increased to 42 to 45°C, the bacterium reacts to shift transcription away from normal housekeeping functions to the production of a series of heat shock proteins (~40 proteins), which aid the cell to survive at these restrictive temperatures. The response has also been shown to be triggered by some biocides, such as alcohol, presumably due to a similar denaturing mode of action seen with increased heating (section 7.4.4). This response is controlled at the transcriptional level by an increase in the translation of the sigma factor σ^{32} (encoded by the *rpoH* gene in *E. coli*). Sigma factors are proteins that allow RNA polymerase to recognize and initiate the transcription (production of mRNA) of specific genes by promoter recognition in the bacterial DNA. *E. coli*, for example, has been found to have at least seven sigma factors, including σ^{70} for controlling gene transcription involved in general housekeeping (or primary) functions, σ^{32} used during starvation or stationary phase responses, and σ^{32} for controlling the heat shock response. Many of the proteins upregulated during the heat shock response are chaperones and proteases.

Proteins, including GroES, GroEL, and DnaK, are chaperones involved in the correct folding of proteins and are expressed during heat shock and other stress responses. The mode of action of heat involves the denaturation and precipitation of proteins (see chapter 2, section 2.2); therefore, the presence of chaperones allows the proteins to maintain or resume their correct structures and functions under restrictive conditions. DnaK is further involved in controlling the levels of σ^{32} itself, because the heat shock response can be reversed as the temperature falls to an optimum level required for growth. Other enzymes that are expressed include proteases (in the cytoplasm, but also in the periplasm of Gram-negative bacteria), which degrade denatured proteins that have lost their structure and function. The heat shock response only allows for the partial tolerance of heat changes in the environment and is thought to have little benefit for survival of vegetative bacteria at typical disinfection and, especially, sterilization conditions.

Other responses to environmental stress have been studied in *E. coli*, other bacteria, and yeasts. These include responses to pH, in particular, acid tolerance and osmotic stress. The acid tolerance response demonstrates the expression of up to 50 proteins, including the activation of proton pumps to allow the bacteria to re-establish the normal proton motive force and other functions associated with the cell membrane. Upregulation of the proton motive force also affects bacterial resistance to certain biocides, which have also been shown to disrupt this process (section 8.3.4). Similar stress responses have been described in *Streptomyces*, during particular stages of growth and development, in which the stringent response is coupled to stationary phase adaptation (formation of aerial mycelia leading to spore production) and the production of secondary metabolites (including hydrolytic enzymes and antimicrobial agents).

In conclusion, these responses have evolved in bacteria to tolerate various environmental stresses experienced during normal growth and survival. Their overall practical contribution to biocidal resistance is minimal, considering typically used concentrations or conditions of disinfection and sterilization processes; however, these effects may allow survival of bacteria under sublethal or preservative conditions, where low concentrations or doses of biocides are used, and could afford them some protection from biostatic effects. Despite this, these considerations can play a contributory role in the accumulation of higher-level resistance mechanisms observed in certain types of microorganisms (e.g., *Deinococcus* resistance to radiation; see section 8.3.9) and during biofilm development (see section 8.3.8).

8.3.4 Efflux Mechanisms

A major function of the bacterial membrane is to control the exchange and transport of various chemicals and substances between the cell and its environment. The lipophilicity of the membrane acts as an effective barrier for most compounds. A variety of specific mechanisms have been identified that allow for the exchange of materials either into (influx) or out of (efflux) the cell. These can be considered passive diffusion, facilitated diffusion, and active transport mechanisms (Fig. 8.6).

Passive diffusion is the movement of water, gases, or some small, uncharged polar molecules across the membrane driven by a concentration gradient from an area of high to an area of low concentration. Examples include oxygen, carbon dioxide, ethanol, and water; the passive diffusion of water from a high to a low concentration area is known as osmosis. These processes can be facilitated in some cases by membrane-associated transporter proteins, such as in the case of water by proteins known as aquaporins. Other molecules that can be facilitated include larger and/or lipophilic molecules. These facilitated processes are still directed by diffusion but can be assisted by energy generated from the proton motive force. In cytoplasmic or membrane-associated electron transport systems, electrons are passed from one carrier to another in a sequence of oxidation-reduction reactions with a simultaneous release of energy. This energy can be used to transport (or pump) protons (H^+) across the cell membrane into the space between the cell membrane and cell wall. This results in an overall positive charge on the external surface of the membrane and an overall negative charge on the internal surface (Fig. 8.7). This electrochemical gradient is known as the proton motive force and is used as a source of energy by the cell for the synthesis of ATP (or metabolic energy, which is the major source of energy for various cellular processes on hydrolysis to ADP and phosphate), rotation of flagella, and transport of materials across the membrane.

The establishment and maintenance of the proton motive force become important when active transport is considered. Active transport uses energy sources to transport substances against their concentration gradients and is

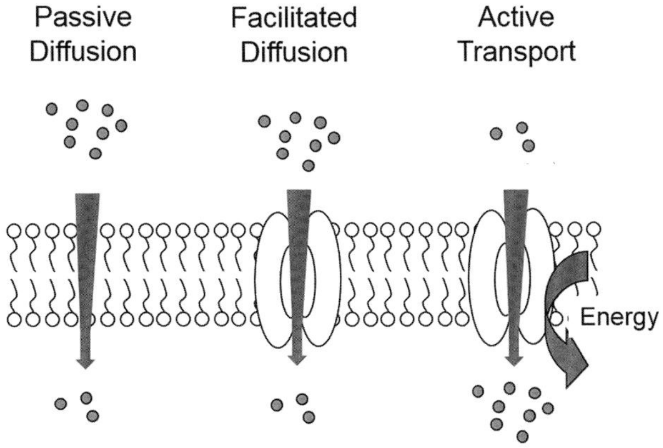

FIGURE 8.6 Transport systems in bacteria across a typical cell membrane.

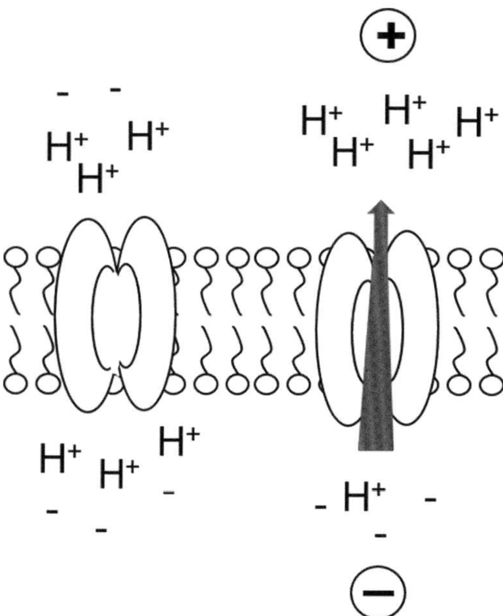

FIGURE 8.7 Establishment of the proton motive force.

particularly important to consider during the attack of a cell by a biocide at high concentrations from the external environment. Sources of energy include the proton motive force and the hydrolysis of ATP or other high-energy compounds. A variety of active transporters have been identified in the influx and efflux of nutrients, ions, and antimicrobial agents. A summary of the major classes is given in Table 8.4.

It is clear that many biocides directly affect these processes by disrupting the cell membrane (and associated protein) structures and functions, including disruption of the proton motive force (section 7.4.5). The prevention of the influx and efflux of various molecules has multiple effects on cell metabolism and survival. However, bacteria have also been shown to specifically efflux or pump out low concentrations of various biocides (as well as antibiotics, heavy metals, and other toxic substances), which can reduce the accumulation of the biocide and other substances in the cytoplasm. This may be particularly important in cases where the biocide has limited penetration through the cell wall, as in many Gram-negative bacteria. Active efflux has been shown to be a concern in antibiotic and biocide resistance in bacteria and has been particularly well studied in *E. coli* and *Pseudomonas* spp., although they are present in all types of cells including bacteria, protozoa, and fungi. Many of these play a significant role in biocide resistance because the outer membrane in Gram-negative bacteria (in particular, *Pseudomonas*) presents a much lower permeability barrier to biocides than the cell walls of Gram-positive bacteria, and active-efflux systems can therefore provide a further advantage to biocide survival.

For the purpose of this discussion, three major groups of efflux systems have been associated with increased antimicrobial tolerance in bacteria (including Gram-positive and Gram-negative bacteria). These are the following families:

TABLE 8.4 Examples of active transporter systems

Types	Description	Examples
Uniporters, symporters	Transport of molecules across the membrane in the same direction as another substance; driven by the proton motive force. Uniporters transport one type of molecule, while symporters transport multiple molecules	Ions (HSO_4^-, HPO_4^-, and H^+), glucose, and some amino acids
Antiporters	Transport of molecules across the membrane in parallel to another substance in the other direction; driven by the proton motive force	Ions (Na^+ and H^+), glucose, and some amino acids; some antibiotics and biocides
ATP-binding cassette (ABC) systems	Examples of protein-assisted transfer through the periplasm and active protein-mediated transport through the membrane in an ATP-dependent manner; driven by hydrolysis of ATP	Sugars and amino acids; some antibiotics, chloroquine, some biocides
Group translocation	Substance is chemically modified for unidirectional transport across the membrane	Glucose and other sugars

- Major facilitator superfamily (MFS). For this discussion, this group includes two similar yet distinct families: the small multidrug resistance (SMR) family and the multidrug and toxic compound extrusion family. These families are often considered as separate groups of efflux systems from the MFS.
- Resistance-nodulation-division (RND) family, which is unique in Gram-negative bacteria.
- ATP-binding cassette (ABC) family.

Although the exact modes of action of each efflux system can be different, they at least consist of single cytoplasmic proteins that can operate on their own (as in the case of Gram-positive bacteria such as NorA in *Staphylococcus aureus* and PmrA in *Streptococcus pneumoniae*) or, particularly in Gram-negative bacteria, in combination with other periplasmic- and outer membrane-associated proteins (Fig. 8.8 and Table 8.5). The MFS and RND systems consist of a cytoplasmic membrane antiporter protein which uses the proton motive force as an energy source to drive the biocide out of the cytoplasm in exchange for protons; however, although examples of MFS systems have been shown to require only the cytoplasmic antiporter protein for efflux, the RND family has been shown to require associated periplasmic and outer membrane components for effective biocide efflux (Fig. 8.8). The ABC family uses ATP as an energy source to pump the active agent out of the cell.

The RND-type pumps have been identified and well-studied in Gram-negative bacteria, particularly in *Pseudomonas* spp. They have been particularly associated with antibiotic/biocide extrusion as mechanisms of multidrug resistance (MDR). They are usually associated as a three-component system consisting of a

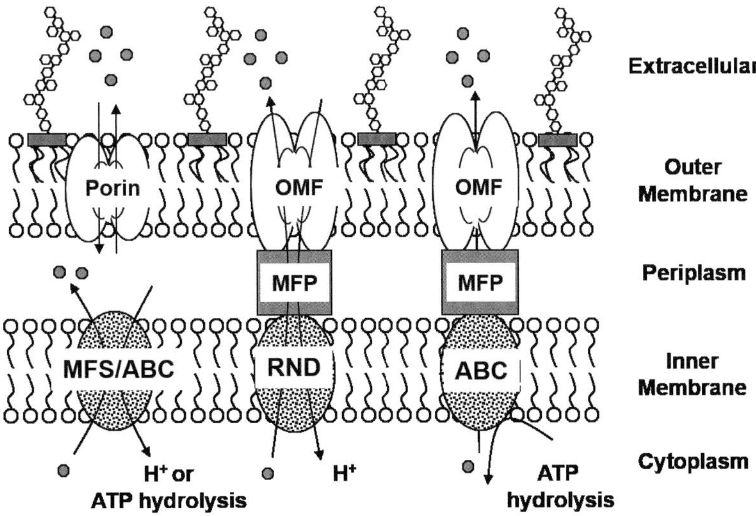

FIGURE 8.8 Summary of the various types of efflux pumps associated with antimicrobial resistance identified in bacteria. A typical Gram-negative bacteria cell wall is shown with associated cytoplasmic and outer membrane (see chapter 1, section 1.3.4.1) proteins. Note that similar cytoplasmic-membrane-associated efflux pumps (MFS and ABC) have been identified in Gram-positive bacteria (which do not have an outer membrane; section 1.3.4.1). Efflux is energy-dependent, derived from the proton motive force (antiporter efflux with H+) or ATP hydrolysis (to ADP and inorganic phosphate). Abbreviations: MFS, major facilitator superfamily; RND, resistance-nodulation-division family; MFP, membrane fusion protein (periplasmic); OMF, outer membrane factor; ABC, ATP-binding cassette family.

cytoplasmic membrane-associated transporter, a periplasmic-associated protein (known as a membrane fusion protein [MFP]), and an outer-membrane-associated protein (the outer membrane factor). They all use energy from the proton motive force to pump the compound out of the cell. In many cases their exact physiological function may not be fully understood, although they do play a role in reacting to adverse environmental conditions such as controlling divalent metal ion concentrations (CzrAB-OpmD systems in *Pseudomonas aeruginosa*) and solvent (toluene) resistance (the SrpABC and MepABC systems in *Pseudomonas putida*). Solvent resistance in *P. putida* is due to multiple factors. Solvents have been shown to accumulate and disrupt the structure and function of the cytoplasmic membrane. *P. putida* strains can survive the presence of solvents such as toluene by varying the structure and type of phospholipids in the cell membrane (with an increase in trans-unsaturated fatty acids, which changes the membrane fluidity) and the rate of membrane turnover, by changes in the outer membrane lipopolysaccharide (LPS) and protein composition, and by the presence of normal and inducible efflux pumps. The SrpABC mechanism is a three-component system consisting of a membrane-associated RND pump (SrpB), a periplasmic MFP (SrpA), and an outer membrane factor (SrpC). This system appears to be inducible by and unique to toluene efflux; in contrast, the MepABC system allows for efflux of toluene and other compounds such as the β-lactam antibiotics and antimicrobial dyes. It has been suggested that these RND systems may operate in three modes, depending on the type of drug being extruded: the membrane-associated RND pump alone (which drives hydrophilic drugs into the periplasm), the RND pump combined with the periplasmic MFP (to efflux amphiphilic molecules), and the three-component RND/MFP/outer membrane factor (for the extrusion of amphiphilic and lipophilic drugs).

The presence or activation of these efflux pump mechanisms can affect the overall influx and concentration of some biocides within the cytoplasm and (in Gram-negative bacteria) periplasmic space; however, similar to other physiological responses to biocides, they only afford partial survival under MIC or minimum bactericidal concentration (MBC) values of the biocide, which can be an important consideration at preservative or residual levels of the active agent. In some cases, the presence of the biocide has been shown to induce the expression of efflux-related proteins in bacteria, while in others the efflux pumps are present due to normal vegetative growth functions. Examples of pumps that have been linked to the efflux of biocides from bacteria are listed in Table 8.5. Efflux mechanisms also play a further role in acquired resistance to biocides (including both

TABLE 8.5 Examples of bacterial efflux systems that have been shown to efflux biocides and antibiotics

Efflux proteins	Family	Bacteria examples	Antimicrobials extruded[a]
NorA	MFS	*S. aureus*	Fluoroquinolones, antimicrobial dyes, quaternary ammonium compounds [QACs], tetraphenylphophonium, rhodamine
BmrR	MFS	*B. atrophaeus*	Fluoroquinolones, antimicrobial dyes, QACs, tetraphenylphophonium, rhodamine
PmrA	MFS	*S. pneumoniae*	Fluoroquinolones, acriflavines, antimicrobial dyes
LmrA	ABC	*Lactobacillus lactis*	Fluoroquinolones, acriflavines, antimicrobial dyes
EfrAB	ABC	*Enterococcus faecalis*	Fluoroquinolones, acriflavines, antimicrobial dyes
AcrAB-TolC	RND	*E. coli*	β-lactams, fluoroquinolones, tetracycline, acriflavines, antimicrobial dyes, SDS, pine oil (phenolics), triclosan, chlorhexidine, QACs
MexAB-OprM	RND	*P. aeruginosa*	β-lactams, fluoroquinolones, acriflavines, triclosan, SDS, toluene, antimicrobial dyes (e.g., crystal violet), QACs
MexCD-OprJ	RND	*P. aeruginosa*	β-lactams, fluoroquinolones, acriflavines, triclosan, SDS, toluene
CzrAB-OpmN	RND	*P. aeruginosa*	Cadmium, zinc

[a]The full spectrum of biocides that may be extruded due to efflux remains to be determined.

mutation and plasmid-acquired mechanisms which are further discussed in section 8.7); the activation, upregulation, or acquisition of efflux mechanisms due to treatment with biocides has been suggested as an important consideration in the development of antibiotic resistance, where increased MIC/MBC levels present a greater therapeutic challenge. Recent examples have demonstrated the induction of the MexAB-OprM efflux system in *P. aeruginosa* and the SmeDEF efflux system in *Stenotrophomonas maltophilia* by triclosan. In both cases, triclosan was found to specifically bind to key regulation proteins of the efflux genes, causing their overexpression and parallel increased resistance to antibiotics (e.g., fluroquinolones).

8.3.5 Enzymatic and Chemical Protection

Various enzymes and chemicals that neutralize and allow tolerance to the presence of biocides have been identified in bacteria and yeast (in addition to those described in the various stress responses in section 8.3.3). In some cases, microorganisms can use biocides as a carbon source under appropriate conditions, as described for phenols, cresols, QACs, and chlorhexidine. *Pseudomonas* spp. are particularly implicated in these cases because they present a wide metabolic diversity, using a range of compounds as carbon sources for growth; however, the levels of tolerance tend to be within the normal inhibitory and sometimes bactericidal range observed with pseudomonads, with higher concentrations of the biocide generally being effective against these isolates because they overwhelm the tolerance factors.

The advances in genome sequencing and proteomics have allowed more detailed studies of mechanisms of resistance in bacteria such as *Pseudomonas* and *Burkholderia*. For example, the main mechanisms of intrinsic resistance in *Burkholderia cepacia* to the QAC benzalkonium chloride have been shown to be increased efflux activity (see section 8.3.4) and enzymatic degradation, which are associated with the activity of many enzymes such as dealkylases and other catabolic enzymes. Many of these strains are industrially beneficial, because they are used for the biodegradation of toxic compounds in the environment. Degradation of cresol and phenol as carbon sources has been demonstrated in strains of *P. putida* and *Pseudomonas pickettii*, due to the presence of various metabolic enzymes such as dehydrogenases and hydroxylases. Enzymatic degradation of triclosan has been specifically demonstrated in *P. putida* and *Alcaligenes xylosoxidans*. Similarly, inactivation of formaldehyde has been reported with *P. aeruginosa*, *P. putida*, and *Pseudomonas syringae* and is mediated by the production of glutathione-dependent formaldehyde dehydrogenases. Various formaldehyde dehydrogenases and transketolases are involved in the metabolism of formaldehyde in methanotrophs such as *Methylococcus*. The degradation of formaldehyde by *E. coli* has been studied in some detail; glutathione reacts with formaldehyde to form hydroxymethylglutathione, which is then oxidized by the dehydrogenase to S-formylglutathione and subsequently metabolized by the cell.

Similar alcohol dehydrogenases in *E. coli* and yeasts facilitate the conversion between alcohols and aldehydes; for example, ethanol is oxidized by a dehydrogenase to form acetaldehyde, which is rapidly converted into acetyl-coA for use by the cell. Other enzymes are directly involved in neutralizing biocides in a cellular response to their presence. Various oxidases and reductases have been identified in bacterial tolerance to toxic metals, including arsenate reductase, mercuric reductase, and copper oxidases (section 8.3.6). Catalases and peroxidases are known to degrade hydrogen peroxide (section 8.3.3). Other enzymes (such as DNA gyrases) are involved in increasing the tolerance of bacteria to heat damage and repairing biocidal damage to the cell, including endonucleases, exonucleases, and proteases.

Glutathione reductase plays an important role in the reduction of oxidized glutathione (formed on reaction with an oxidant) to form reduced glutathione. Reduced glutathione is an example of a chemical antioxidant that can afford some tolerance to low levels of oxidizing agents by direct oxidant neutralization and reversal of disulfide bond formation in proteins. Other chemical antioxidants produced by microorganisms include ascorbic acid, the flavonoids and carotenoids, and some amino acids such as proline. Cytochromes (cell cofactors involved in enzymatic reactions) have been shown in *E. coli* and *Geobacter* spp. to cause the reduction of heavy metals and oxidizing agents. Polypeptide-induced heavy metal sequestration has been described in *E. coli* (see section 8.3.6); the release of the polypeptide AgBP2 into the periplasm is involved in binding to silver and forming nanoparticles to sequester the biocidal activity.

8.3.6 Intrinsic Resistance to Heavy Metals

Metal ions play an important role in many cellular functions, including macromolecular structure, as cofactors in enzymatic reactions, and as cellular catalysts. Relatively low concentrations are required for these essential roles, while increased cellular concentrations have toxic effects, as exemplified by their use as biocides (chapter 3, section 3.12). Those most widely utilized as biocides are copper and silver. Intrinsic resistance mechanisms to various heavy metals in *Bacteria* and *Archaea* have been described. These are considered in more detail because they represent typical mechanisms of intrinsic (and in some cases acquired) resistance mechanisms to biocides and other antimicrobials. Many of these mechanisms have evolved to allow microorganisms to survive under restrictive concentrations of heavy metals. However, further investigations of the potentials of these mechanisms to induce cross-resistance to other antimicrobial agents are required.

At least five intrinsic mechanisms of heavy-metal tolerance have been described (Fig. 8.9), and examples of each are considered below.

The first mechanism is exclusion from the cell. This can be due to the effects of various surface structures, including the cell wall structure and the presence of capsules, slime layers, or S-layers (section 8.3.7) that can entrap or

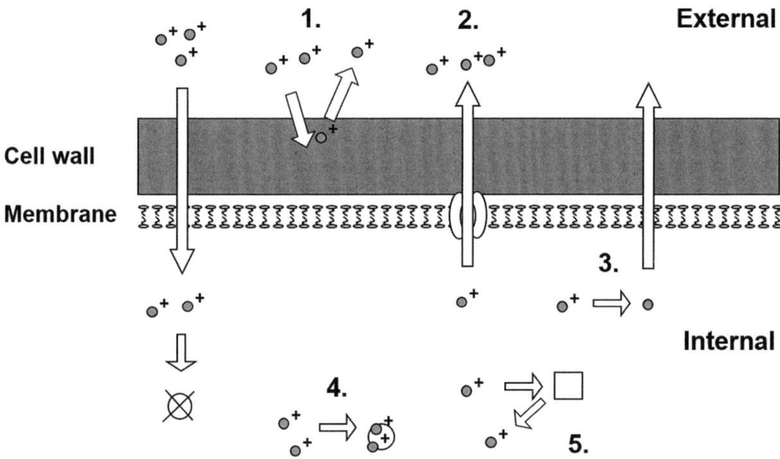

FIGURE 8.9 Intrinsic mechanisms of microbial resistance to heavy metals. The heavy metal ions can pass through the cell wall and membrane with a subsequent intracellular increase in concentration and inhibitory/biocidal effects (shown on the far left). Mechanisms of resistance are **(1)** exclusion, due to the presence of various surface structure or more subtle changes in porin or pump specificity to allow the uptake of essential but not biocidal ions; **(2)** active efflux out of the cell, against a concentration gradient; **(3)** enzymatic conversion of the ion to a different form, which is less toxic and can be released from the cell; **(4)** sequestration, in which macromolecules can absorb the biocide, thereby reducing the available concentration; and **(5)** changes in the structure of target molecules, which reduces their susceptibility to biocidal action.

repel their penetration. An example has been described with silver (and other heavy metals) in Gram-negative bacteria such as *E. coli* and *Geobacter* spp. Various cytochromes and polypeptides associated with the cell wall have been shown to reduce (essentially neutralize) or sequester heavy metals in the periplasm. Reducing mechanisms also allow for increased tolerance to oxidizing agents. In *E. coli*, the release of the polypeptide AgBP2 into the periplasm has been shown to be involved in binding to silver and forming nanoparticles to sequester the biocidal activity. Subtler mechanisms have been described that limit arsenic uptake. Arsenate ions (As^{+5}) can permeate into the cell or, in Gram-negative bacteria, are actively transported into the cell across the outer membrane by the same protein transport mechanism as for phosphate influx. In *E. coli* the outer membrane porin PhoE mediates this mechanism and is induced on phosphate limitation. Therefore, strains underexpressing PhoE are less sensitive to phosphate and therefore arsenic uptake. Similar transport across the cell membrane is mediated by two further mechanisms: the transmembrane Pit protein, which transports both phosphate and arsenate, and the Pst system, which demonstrates greater specificity for phosphate and exclusion of As^{+5}. The Pst system is an inner membrane, ATPase-coupled uptake system induced during phosphate starvation, which demonstrates a link between starvation responses and increased metal resistance. It should also be noted that specific mutations within the *Pit* gene have been shown to allow for greater specificity for phosphates over arsenic as a mechanism of acquired resistance (section 8.7).

Efflux plays an important role in intrinsic and acquired resistance to heavy metal ions. In another example of arsenic tolerance in *E. coli*, the chromosomally encoded ArsB protein is a transmembrane efflux pump (ABC-type; section 8.3.4) that uses energy to transport arsenic ions against a concentration gradient. In some bacteria, but also described in archaea and yeasts, ArsB-like proteins are coupled with an ATPase (ArsA) that uses ATP hydrolysis as a source of energy for transport; ArsA-associated operons are commonly found to be acquired (plasmid-encoded) mechanisms of resistance. Other acquired mechanisms have been described in bacteria (particularly Gram-negative, but also in Gram-positive bacteria) and archaea for a variety of toxic metals including silver (Ag^{+}), copper (Cu^{+2}), mercury (Hg^{+2}), and lead (Pb^{+2}). Similar to arsenic efflux, these include proton motive force and ATP-driven mechanisms (section 8.3.4). Specificity of various ATP-driven pump families has been reported for monovalent (e.g., Cu^{+1}, Ag^{+1}) and divalent (e.g., Hg^{+2}, Zn^{+2}, and Pb^{+2}) ions in bacteria (Gram-positive and Gram-negative) and other microorganisms.

The next mechanism (mechanism 3 in Fig. 8.9) involves enzymatic conversion (reduction) of the toxic ion followed by active or passive expulsion from the cell. Arsenic may be present in two ionic forms: As^{+5} (arsenate) and As^{+3} (arsenite). Arsenate demonstrates intracellular toxicity similar to other heavy metals (see chapter 7, section 7.4.5), including As^{+5} replacing phosphate in various metabolic processes, the affinity of As^{+3} for protein thiol groups (thereby disrupting protein structures), and promoting the formation of DNA-DNA and DNA-protein cross-links. ArsC is an arsenate reductase expressed in *E. coli* in response to increased levels of arsenic. The *ars* operon consists of three proteins: ArsC, ArsB (the efflux pump), and ArsR, a regulator protein which controls expression of the operon. ArsC reduces As^{+5} to As^{+3}, which can then be effluxed from the cell. This enzyme is also associated with the ArsA-based plasmid-encoded operons described above. Similar arsenate reductases have been described as metal-tolerance mechanisms in yeast (*Saccharomyces*) and algae. The reduction of the pentavalent to trivalent ion may seem unusual, considering that As^{+3} is more toxic to the cell than As^{+5} is; this appears to be due to the greater specificity for arsenite efflux from the cell. In other cases, including *Pseudomonas* strains and the acidophilic archaea of the genus *Thiomonas*, arsenate oxidases that convert As^{+3} to As^{+5} as tolerance mechanisms have been described; these examples represent interesting mechanisms of bioremediation of environmental arsenic contamination. Further examples of enzymatic conversion have been described for mercury resistance with the chromosomal or plasmid-mediated expression of mercuric reductases. In this case, ionic mercury (Hg^{+2}) is reduced by the enzyme to its elemental form (Hg), which then volatizes from the cell. Other enzymes (hydrolases) also play a role in the tolerance of toxic mercuric compounds, causing the hydrolysis and release of the Hg^{+2}, which can then be neutralized.

Two further mechanisms of toxic metal resistance, which can also be intrinsic or acquired, have been described. Sequestration involves binding the metal to macromolecules (known as metallochaperones), thereby reducing accessibility to key intracellular targets. This may simply be due to unspecific interaction with external proteins or other macromolecules to reduce the penetration through the cell wall and/or membrane or be caused by a more specific mechanism. A particular example has been described with copper resistance, including the expression of intracellular, periplasmic, and extracellular copper-binding proteins. CutC is a chromosomally encoded cytoplasmic protein in *E. coli* that binds and transports copper to efflux-associated proteins, although the exact mechanisms of action remain to be elucidated. A similar protein (CopZ) in *Enterococcus* also has a metallochaperonic function associated with CopB, an ATPase-associated efflux pump. Similar detoxification proteins have been described in *Acinetobacter* that are expressed in the stationary phase of growth and on exposure to elevated levels of copper. Further, the *P. syringae* plasmid-encoded CopA and CopC are periplasmic proteins that bind Cu^{+1} and Cu^{+2} to reduce influx into the cytoplasm and transport to the outer membrane efflux pump, CopB; Cu^{+1} is particularly toxic to the cell, and oxidase activity to the less toxic Cu^{+2} ion has been associated with CopC/CopA in *Pseudomonas* and the periplasmic CueO oxidase in *E. coli* and in other bacteria. Finally, particularly in extremophiles (sections 8.3.9 and 8.3.10), various intracellular proteins have been identified that are overall less sensitive to the effects of toxic metals. For example, mercury has been described to interfere with cellular oxidase systems; in *Thiobacillus* strains, cytochrome C oxidases have been shown to be less sensitive to mercury, although the exact mechanism is currently unknown.

Overall, these resistance mechanisms can allow the cell to survive in the presence of inhibitory or microbicidal concentrations of toxic metals. The most efficient appear to be Gram-negative bacteria (e.g., *E. coli* can survive up to 4 mM As^{+3} and 1 mM Cu^{+2}) and *Archaea* including *Acidiphilium* and *Thiobacillus* (up to 30 mM As^{+3} and 10 mM Cu^{+2}).

8.3.7 Capsule and Slime Layer Formation and S-Layers

In addition to the protective cell wall structure, many bacteria (and yeasts such as *Cryptococcus* and *Candida* spp.) also produce material on the outside of the cell wall (chapter 1, section 1.3.4.1). These include S (surface) layers, capsules, and slime layers (Table 8.6).

Capsules and slime layers are also referred to as glycocalyx structures and generally consist of insoluble polysaccharide materials present on the cell surface. Bacterial capsules are well-defined layers of polysaccharide that are tightly associated with the cell wall. In some cases, the capsule may also be protein-based. Slime layers

TABLE 8.6 Protective cell surface structures external to the bacterial cell wall

Structure	Constituents	Examples
S-layers	Protein, glycoprotein	*Bacteria* (*Bacillus*, *Geobacillus*, *Aeromonas*) and *Archaea* (*Halobacterium*)
Capsules	Polysaccharide, protein	*Bacillus*, *Acinetobacter*, *Escherichia coli*, *Streptococcus*, *Pseudomonas*, *Staphylococcus*
Slime layers	Polysaccharide, protein	*Myxococcus*, *Azotobacter*, *Staphylococcus*, *Streptococcus*

are generally much thinner and easily deformed or removed layers of partially soluble material on the cell surface. A major function of these layers is protection from drying, bacterial viruses, immune systems, and adverse environmental conditions. The exact composition of the glycocalyx varies depending on the bacterial species and its environment, although the main components are typically polysaccharides. The polysaccharide may consist of a single sugar polymer or more complex polymers of different sugars. Examples include the streptococcal dextran capsule, which is enzymatically generated from glucose and allows *Streptococcus mutans* to effectively bind to the surface of teeth, while other glycan polysaccharides allow the binding of *Staphylococcus epidermidis* strains to inanimate surfaces. Many proteins and other components such as lipids are often found associated with the glycocalyx. Only in rare cases is the capsule found to be primarily composed of protein, with a notable example being the poly-D-glutamic acid capsule of *Bacillus anthracis* and the polypeptide slime on *Staphylococcus epidermidis*; in the case of *B. anthracis*, the genes required for capsule formation are plasmid-based.

The extent to which the presence of a capsule or slime layer can contribute to bacterial tolerance of biocides is currently unknown, but at a minimum it can present a barrier to biocide penetration. An example is the increased resistance to chlorine reported for *Vibrio cholerae*, which expresses an amorphous exopolysaccharide causing cell aggregation ("rugose" morphology), without any loss in pathogenicity. Capsule formation is believed to play an important role in the unique and varied intrinsic tolerance of *Pseudomonas* strains to various biocides, which is further considered in the resistance of microorganisms in biofilms (section 8.3.8). Studies of *Pseudomonas* spp. have shown that the presence of a capsule specifically inactivated active chlorine but also limited the penetration of chloramines into the cell membrane and cytoplasm; interestingly, the chloramines were found to have low reactivity with the capsule, in comparison to chlorine, but retarded chloramine access to the cell. *S. aureus* strains can present as nonmucoid or mucoid forms, with the mucoid cells surrounded by a slime layer. In a comparison between mucoid and nonmucoid cells, the mucoid cells demonstrated greater tolerance to certain biocides, such as to chloroxylenol, QACs, and chlorhexidine, but little to no difference with phenols or chlorinated phenols; removal of slime by washing rendered the cells sensitive. However, in other investigations with *S. aureus*, no increase in biocide tolerance was observed between capsular and noncapsular strains. A disinfectant-tolerant *Klebsiella* strain has also been linked to the expression of a mucoid capsule.

Overall, the capsule or slime can have a protective role, either as a physical barrier to disinfectant penetration or as a loose layer reacting with or absorbing the biocide molecules. Variations in biocide tolerance are related to greater penetration of some biocides (e.g., phenolics) over others (QACs) and to the nature of the capsule or slime, including the specific bacterial strain, stage of growth or stress response, and types or extents of polysaccharides or other materials present. It should be noted that the capsule can also afford protection to a microorganism by aiding attachment to a surface, which can indirectly protect the target cell. The development of a capsule may also be considered the initial step in the development of a biofilm, which will provide further resistance to the effect of biocides (section 8.3.8).

S-layers are found in Gram-positive and Gram-negative bacteria as well as in many *Archaea*. They consist of proteins or glycoproteins in a regular crystalline array. The functions of the S-layer are similar to those described for capsules. The specific contribution of the S-layer to biocide tolerance is not well studied, although in some cases the S-layer is known to provide tolerance to changes in pH, some enzymes (such as proteases), and other environmental stresses. S-layers may also play a role by allowing for aggregation and coaggregation of yeasts and bacteria to protect cells in clumps from biocide penetration in comparison to free cells.

8.3.8 Biofilm Development

Vegetative microorganisms, like bacteria and fungi, are often considered to be planktonic, or "free-growing" cells, but this is certainly not the case in their natural environments, where they can associate, multiply, and survive on surfaces or at surface interfaces. Microbial growth in their natural environments may more accurately be considered "biofilms," which are defined as communities of microorganisms (either single or multiple species) developed on or associated with surfaces (Fig. 8.10). These surfaces include solid inanimate surfaces, foods, soft tissues, and liquid/air or liquid/liquid interfaces. Biofilms can consist of monocultures or mixed cultures either actively growing (such as bacteria and fungi) or associated with the community (including viruses and protozoa). Bacterial (Gram-positive and Gram-negative) and fungal (particularly yeasts) biofilms have been described in some detail, and some of the more prevalent microorganisms associated with problematic biofilms are shown in Table 8.7.

Biofilms are important for several reasons, notably due to their association with biocorrosion, biofouling, and reduced water quality and their acting as foci for contamination of products, including foods, devices, waterlines, and manufactured drugs. The control of biofilm development and proliferation is therefore an important clinical and industrial challenge. In other cases, biofilms may be beneficial, for example, in the intestine, where the various associated microorganisms play protective (to prevent invasion of pathogenic organisms) and nutritional (producing some amino acids and vitamins) roles. The roles of such complex communities of microorganisms in their various ecosystems (referred to as microbiota

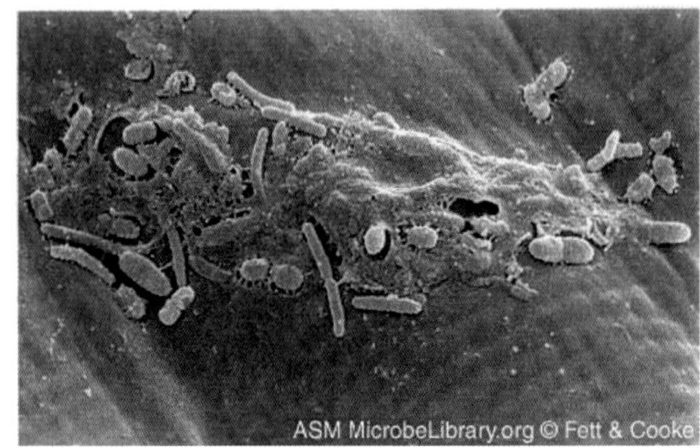

FIGURE 8.10 A *P. aeruginosa* biofilm on a surface. Individual rod-shaped bacteria can be seen developed in a polysaccharide matrix. Image courtesy of ASM MicrobeLibrary, ©Fett & Cooke, with permission.

TABLE 8.7 Typical bacteria and fungi associated with biofilm formation

Microorganism	Associated biofilms
Streptococcus mutans, *Streptococcus sobrinus*	Cause tooth plaque and periodontal disease; consist of layers of bacteria and polysaccharide growing on the teeth, which can cause damage to the teeth and gums over time; one of the first types of biofilms to be described
P. aeruginosa and other pseudomonads including *B. cepacia*	Most prevalent biofilms associated with water surfaces and systems, including water pipes, washing machines, and water circulation systems; often associated with industrial biofouling (including corrosion and clogging) and nosocomial infections (related to devices such as implants, washer-disinfectors, and contaminated water lines); *P. aeruginosa* also forms biofilms in the lungs of patients with cystic fibrosis, leading to persistent infections
Legionella pneumophila	Legionnaires' disease associated with contaminated aerosolized moisture from air and heating/cooling water distribution systems
S. aureus, *S. epidermidis*	Skin and device-related infections
Mycobacterium fortuitum, *M. chelonae*	Biofouling and waterborne persistent infections or "pseudo" infections (e.g., misdiagnosed as pathogenic mycobacteria)
Propionibacterium acnes	Often considered the cause of acne; a persistent skin infection, in particular, in young adults
Deinococcus geothermalis	Biofouling of paper machines, impairing operation and product defects
Candida albicans	Most prevalent fungal-type biofilms; has been reported in device-related infections and root canal or endodontic infections

or microbiome to include their associated genetic material) are an area of research, particularly due to human and plant health. For example, the human microbiome has been associated with impacted body weight and various diseases such as oral, cancer, diabetes, and Parkinson's disease.

The formation of a biofilm may be considered as a series of stages (Fig. 8.11).

The initial step is the association of the microorganism with the surface (adsorption). Individual bacteria have been found to use a variety of mechanisms to aid in preliminary attachment to the surface, including electrostatic attraction, physical forces (including van der Waals forces), fimbriae, pili, and surface capsules/slime layers (section 8.3.7). The presence of carbohydrate or other organic molecules on a surface, which is known as "conditioning," can provide sites for adhesion and may enhance these mechanisms. In some bacteria, an initial reversible attachment to the surface is observed, which develops into a more permanent adsorption, for example, due to the production of and affinity with capsules. The adsorbed cells begin to multiply and produce various extracellular polymeric materials, in particular, various polysaccharides of mannose, glucose, *N*-acetylglucosamine, and other sugars. The associated polysaccharides assist in maintaining the cells in close contact and trap nutrients from the environment. As the biofilm continues to develop, the individual cells within the community are at various stages of growth and metabolism in response to their environment. For example, facultative bacteria require less oxygen and nutrients in the depths of the biofilm, with

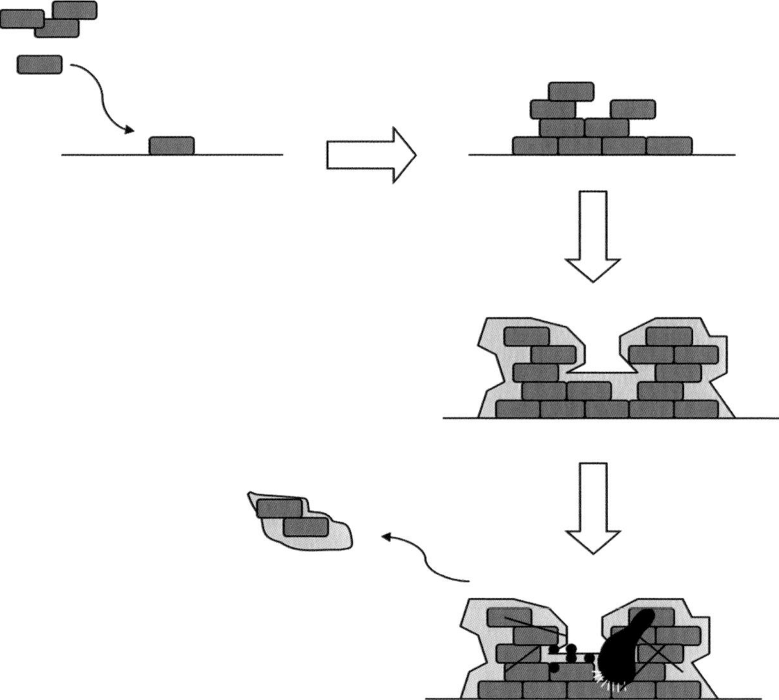

FIGURE 8.11 The development of a biofilm. Initial attachment (adsorption) of a microorganism may be reversible or permanent, leading to proliferation and extracellular polysaccharide production. This matrix develops over time, allowing the entrapment of nutrients and other microorganisms, which can also proliferate to produce a mature biofilm. Sections of the biofilm can slough off over time, bind to other surfaces, and subsequently develop further biofilms.

cells growing anaerobically in comparison to the surface layers, where cells grow aerobically. These stresses surrounding the cell are sensed by the microorganism with the initiation of the various responses described in section 8.3.3.

There is also some evidence of complex interactions between cells; for example, "quorum sensing" as a response to population density with a bacterial community has been described in many bacteria, including *S. aureus* and *P. aeruginosa*. The extracellular matrix development plays an important role in the protection of the cells from various environmental challenges, including penetration and contact with biocides and biocidal processes. In most cases the matrix is predominantly composed of polysaccharides and water, with various other associated proteins (including enzymes), and organic and inorganic materials that are excreted from the cells or entrapped from the environment. This also acts as a trap for various other microorganisms (including bacteria, fungi, viruses, protozoa, and algae), many of which also proliferate within the matrix. Therefore, the mature biofilm can vary considerably depending on the environment, but it clearly is a complex and cooperative interaction. Sections of the biofilm can also slough off over time, with subsequent binding to other surfaces and further biofilm formation (Fig. 8.11).

Biofilms present a significant challenge to disinfection and sterilization processes, as well as to the activity of other chemical antimicrobial agents. Several reasons account for the reduced sensitivity of bacteria and other microorganisms within a biofilm (Table 8.8).

A major factor in biofilm resistance is reduced access to the cells within the biofilm. It is known that binding to a surface alone affords some protection, because planktonic cells are more sensitive to the effects of biocides in comparison to cells on a surface (chapter 1, section 1.4.2.2); this may be partially due to the surface itself interfering with the biocide or bacteria being shielded from these effects within various microscopic imperfections at the surface. More significantly, the biofilm consists of cells at various depths within a thick polysaccharide matrix that the biocide needs to penetrate to elicit its effects. The biocide (e.g., with oxidizing agents such as chlorine and peracetic acid) can attack the various polysaccharides and proteins of the biofilm, because they are often themselves key targets, and reduce the concentration available for action against the microorganism. Organic and inorganic components of the biofilm also directly neutralize the activity of biocides. An example is the presence of enzymes such as peroxidases and catalases that reduce the available concentration of biocides such as hydrogen peroxide (section

TABLE 8.8 Biofilm and microbial responses to antimicrobial agents

Mechanism of resistance associated with biofilms	Comment
Exclusion or reduced access of the biocide to underlying cells	Depends on: Nature of biocide or biocidal process Nature of the surface Binding capacity and reaction of glycocalyx toward biocide Rate of growth of biofilm relative to diffusion rate of the biocide
Sensitivity of the individual cell	Associated with: Stress responses Growth rate/phase Metabolic activity
Increased production of degradative enzymes and other neutralizing agents	Enzymes decrease the available concentration of some biocides; neutralizing agents can include organic and inorganic materials
Increased genetic exchange between or mutations within cells	The close interaction between cells may potentially enhance exchange of genetic material and associated acquired tolerance to biocides

8.3.3). The direct chemical interaction between the disinfectant and biofilm can be important for other reasons. Cross-linking agents (such as aldehydes) may allow for the formation of polymeric surface barriers that can inhibit penetration of the biocide to bacteria deeper within the biofilm; in contrast, other biocides (such as peracetic acid and other oxidizing agents) can be formulated to allow degradation of the biofilm structure and its removal from the surface and therefore greater penetration.

Because penetration can be reduced within a biofilm, many of the other intrinsic resistance mechanisms may play greater roles cumulatively in protecting the cell at lower concentrations of the biocide. These mechanisms include the various responses to environmental stress (section 8.3.3), a decreased growth rate (section 8.3.1), and allowing the cells time to develop into their dormant stages (section 8.3.11). Bacteria in different parts of a biofilm have been shown to experience different nutrient environments, so that their physiological properties are affected. Slowly growing bacteria are known to be less sensitive than more actively metabolizing cells. Similarly, the presence of biocides can induce cells to increase the production of polysaccharide and other agents as defense mechanisms.

In most cases, bacteria removed from a biofilm, isolated, and recultured under laboratory conditions are generally no more resistant than the original planktonic cells of that species; however, it has been suggested that under biofilm growth conditions, the microorganism can mutate or acquire extrinsic genetic material to allow greater resistance to biocides and antibiotics (as acquired resistance mechanisms; see section 8.7). These mechanisms can be retained by the bacteria on subculturing. For this reason, it is often suggested (in particular, in industrial applications) that periodic rotation of different disinfectant types may be more efficient for microbial control, e.g., routine biocidal treatment with frequent temperature disinfection or rotation of biocidal treatments with different modes of action. There is mixed evidence of the advantages of such practices.

Biofilms are a constant challenge to control in various manufacturing, commercial, health care, and food processing facilities (Table 8.7). Several instances of the contamination of antiseptic or disinfectant solutions by bacteria have been described, although when subcultured, the bacteria appeared to be rapidly sensitive to the formulations. Examples include the prolonged survival of *Serratia marcescens* and *B. cepacia* in chlorhexidine solutions and contamination of iodophor antiseptics with *Pseudomonas* spp. These cases were attributed to the embedding of these organisms within thick biofilm matrices that adhered to the walls of storage containers or were associated with other interfaces within a formulated product, thereby allowing the bacteria to survive. In one of these cases with *Pseudomonas*, the source of the biofilm was found to be the interior surfaces of polyvinyl chloride water pipes used during the manufacture of providone-iodine antiseptics. Pseudomonads and other Gram-negative bacteria are often cited as causes of industrial water pipe or tank contamination, which over time can lead to corrosion of surfaces and cross-contamination of manufactured products. Filters are particularly sensitive to biofilm proliferation, because by their nature they entrap microorganisms and nutrients, allowing their proliferation over time. In some extreme cases, bacteria have been shown to be capable of "growing through" the filter over time, thereby allowing downstream contamination; theoretically, this may be due to gradual damage to the filter by chemicals or by the biofilm itself, reducing its retentive capabilities. For this reason, the integrity of filters in critical applications should be periodically verified, and they should be frequently disinfected (by biocides or heat) during use (see chapter 2, section 2.5). Another example of biofilm contamination is with *Legionella pneumophila*, which is often found in health care and commercial water distribution systems, including cooling towers. Chlorination, in combination with continuous heating (≥60°C) of incoming water, is usually the most appropriate disinfection measure; however, because of biofilm production, the contaminating organisms are often less susceptible to this treatment than expected.

Incidences of biofilm contamination with various medical devices, particularly with indwelling devices, have been well described. Indwelling devices, including contact lenses (on the eye), intravenous or urinary catheters, and various prosthetic devices, are placed within or on the body for a variety of medical applications. Many of these devices are provided sterile but can become contaminated by contact with the skin (from the patient during insertion or during handling), with other surfaces, or from the air (e.g., by aerosolization). Contamination can lead to overgrowth, biofilm formation, and protection of the microorganisms from the host's immune system. Contamination and biofilm formation on devices with Gram-positive bacteria (*Staphylococcus* and *Enterococcus* spp.), Gram-negative bacteria (*Escherichia* and *Pseudomonas* spp.), atypical mycobacteria (e.g., *Mycobacterium chimaera*), and fungal (*Candida* spp.) pathogens have been reported. These biofilms invariably resist the antimicrobial effects of integrated or applied biocides and antibiotics used to control bacterial growth; further, release of a high concentration of endotoxins from Gram-negative bacterial biofilms can lead to more complications and, potentially, death.

A further consideration is with multiple-use surgical or investigational devices, which require reprocessing (cleaning, disinfection, and/or sterilization) between uses. Recent advances in noninvasive procedures (including minimum invasive surgery and flexible endoscope interventions) offer significant advantages but pose cleaning and disinfection challenges. Many of these devices are designed with lumens (to allow access during surgery) or other complex design features, which can be difficult to clean and disinfect. This can be a particular challenge with devices made of heat-sensitive materials (e.g., flexible endoscopes) that are dependent on chemical disinfection or sterilization, which can be especially impacted by the presence of biofilms. Biofilm or pseudo-biofilm contamination is often cited as a cause of infections related to these devices, primarily due to inadequate reprocessing and/or recontamination following reprocessing. Inadequate reprocessing can be due to the device design restricting penetration of cleaning and disinfection processes or inadequate removal or disinfection of patient material, allowing subsequent overgrowth of microorganisms. Health care-acquired infection outbreaks due to a variety of microorganisms such as *P. aeruginosa*, *M. chelonae*, *M. tuberculosis*, HIV, and hepatitis C (the viruses being associated and protected by the presence of residual material or within a biofilm) underscore the importance of biofilm formation in the contamination of flexible fiberoptic scopes. Many of these outbreaks were associated with inadequate cleaning of endoscopes, which compromised subsequent disinfection with high-level chemical disinfectants and allowed bacterial overgrowth over time (e.g., device storage prior to patient use). The use of cross-linking agents such as glutaraldehyde following inadequate cleaning can cause a buildup of insoluble residues and associated microorganisms in endoscopes and associated automated reprocessing (washer-disinfector) machines. Recontamination is a further concern due to water rinsing of devices following chemical disinfection. Biofilm formation within the reprocessing machine or in the water lines used to rinse devices can recontaminate the device and allow for biofilm development during subsequent storage.

An effective treatment against biofilms is a continuous process that includes an antimicrobial component and physical disruption, with removal of the extracellular matrix. For this reason, liquid oxidizing agents and detergent formulations are used due to their physical removal and structure-disrupting mode of action (chapter 7, section 7.4.2). Chlorine, as sodium hypochlorite, is particularly used for this purpose, but at much higher concentrations than those required for normal biocidal activity. Such concentrations can be damaging to water lines and components, in particular, metals such as stainless steel and copper, and some plastics. Similar effects have been shown for other oxidizing agents, including ozone, chlorine dioxide, and peracetic acid, although the activities of these biocides can be dramatically influenced by various formulation effects (see section 7.4.2). Nonoxidizing agents that are often recommended include the QACs, due to their surfactant and physical removal and cleaning activities. Other chemical biocides are less attractive due to their modes of action. Examples are the aldehydes and heat. Aldehydes such as glutaraldehyde are used to remediate biofilms that build up in oil and other industrial pipelines. But in these cases, aldehyde use can allow entrapment of viable bacteria within the biofilm and, by fixing material on a surface, provide enhanced sites for subsequent bacterial attachment.

Despite this, successful biofilm control depends on the physical and chemical properties of the biocide, its formulation, and the field of application. In the pharmaceutical and medical device industries, where the quality of water used is maintained at a high standard (e.g., water for injection), the water is kept at high temperatures (often ≥80°C), which significantly decreases (if it does not remove) the risk of bacterial and fungal survival and proliferation within these systems. Other physical methods such as nonionizing radiation (in particular, UV treatment) and/or the use of microbial retentive filters only allow for the reduction or removal of microbial contamination within the water stream at their site of use but do not prevent biofilm development up- or downstream of such interventions. Overall, the frequent use of antimicrobial processes is only one consideration in the control of biofilms. Other control mechanisms can include the integration or generation of biocides and/or antibiotics onto surfaces to prevent or reduce attachment, the use of materials with reduced surface attachment properties (e.g., as is claimed for Teflon), nutrient restriction, and design of water systems (e.g., no standing water or inaccessible areas such as dead-legs or crevices).

Although biofilms have been particularly well described in water and other liquid-based systems, they can also allow for environmental persistence under dry conditions. These have been recently studied with *Pseudomonas* and *Staphylococcus* spp. The impact of dry biofilms has been described for two conditions. The first is the attachment and development of micro- or macrocolonies of bacteria on surfaces and, by the production of protective mechanisms such as capsule formation, the persistence of microorganisms on environmental surfaces even under extended dried conditions. This is considered to provide a major persistence mechanism for bacteria to survive on environmental surfaces such as in health care and food-manufacturing surfaces. As an example, some strains of *S. aureus* have been shown to survive on dry surfaces for many months, therefore posing a cross-contamination risk. The second condition has been shown by allowing repeated biofilm development in liquid culture and then subjecting the biofilm to extended dehydration. Some experiments have studied the effectiveness of disinfection with sodium hypochlorite on such dehydrated biofilms. By traditional surface disinfection and bacterial culturing techniques, high levels of bacterial inactivation were observed, but live (yet nonviable) bacteria could be detected using live-dead staining techniques. These techniques use specific dyes (typically fluorescent dyes that bind to nucleic acids, such as SYTO 9 and propidium iodide) and can differentiate bacteria based on their ability to penetrate the cell membrane (damage to the cell membrane being indicative of a lack of cell viability). Viable cells detected by using these techniques could be subsequently revived following prolonged culturing. The mechanisms of resistance were clearly an intrinsic property of the bacteria, because subsequent culturing and testing of biocide activity against these isolates had the same result as the starting bacteria cultures. In both cases, the protective effects of the biofilm structure appear to allow bacteria to survive under adverse environmental conditions, including drying.

8.3.9 Bacteria with Extreme Intrinsic Resistance

Many of the intrinsic mechanisms of resistance discussed so far allow some survival of bacteria under various adverse conditions, although in most cases the bacterial cells are still considered relatively sensitive to various biocides at typical concentrations and/or conditions. There are a number of notable exceptions that demonstrate more extreme intrinsic resistance to various adverse conditions. Examples of these are given in Table 8.9.

The extremophiles, including thermophiles (which grow under different temperature extremes) and acidophiles (which grow in acidic environments) are considered in more detail in section 8.3.10. These have been isolated from various extreme environments, although it should be noted that these bacteria have unique growth requirements that allow them to grow under what we may consider extreme (e.g., high or low temperature and high or low pH). These conditions are often required for their normal growth and survival. They are interesting to study for considering their unique intrinsic resistance mechanisms to these conditions. Unlike the extremophiles, some bacterial species (including *Geobacillus*, *Bacillus*, and *Clostridium*) grow optimally under conditions similar to those for many other bacteria and can be pathogenic; however, under adverse conditions, they can develop into dormant spores, which are protected from adverse environmental stresses until suitable conditions are available for normal vegetative growth. These spores demonstrate tremendous intrinsic resistance to physical and chemical disinfection and sterilization processes and are discussed in further detail with other dormancy mechanisms of resistance in section 8.3.11.

Deinococcus spp. are notable examples of vegetative bacteria with dramatic intrinsic resistance to radiation (including ionizing and nonionizing radiation, chapter 2, section 2.4), even in comparison to bacterial spores (Fig. 8.12).

D. radiodurans, a Gram-positive staining bacterium with a cell wall structure more similar to Gram-negative bacteria, was first identified in canned meat products that had been irradiated and led to food spoilage. The microorganisms were subsequently found to survive typical disinfection and sterilization doses of γ irradiation, ranging from 5 to 20 kGy doses; as a reference point, a radiation dose of 5 kGy is sufficient to kill a human, and vegetative bacteria are typically inactivated at the 0.2 to 0.8 kGy range (see chapter 5, section 5.4). These results were initially considered unusual since *D. radiodurans* and other deinococcal isolates were shown to be nonsporulating, Gram-positive, nonmobile, aerobic bacteria (Fig. 8.13). However, the intrinsic resistance of these strains was confirmed, and similar radiation-resistant strains were soon

TABLE 8.9 Examples of known extreme resistance to biocides and biocidal processes

Bacteria	Resistance	Mechanisms of resistance
Thermophiles, including *Thermococcus* and *Pyrococcus*	Heat and salt conditions	Multiple, including unique cell wall structures, heat-resistant proteins and lipids/lipid membranes, and protein/DNA protective/repair mechanisms
Acidophiles, including *Thiobacillus* and *Thermoplasma*	Acids and heat (some)	Multiple, including unique cell wall structures, active efflux, and exclusions methods
Bacterial endospores, including *Geobacillus* and *Clostridium*	Heat, biocides (including gases and liquids), radiation, desiccation	Dormant spore production with various intrinsic resistance mechanisms
Deinococcus	Radiation, oxidizing agents, and desiccation	Multiple, including efficient repair mechanisms and unique cell wall structure
P. domesticum	Radiation and ethylene oxide gas sterilization	Fungi associated with the production of sclerotia (hard masses of hyphae) and development of ascospores (in fruiting bodies known as apothecia) (see section 8.10)

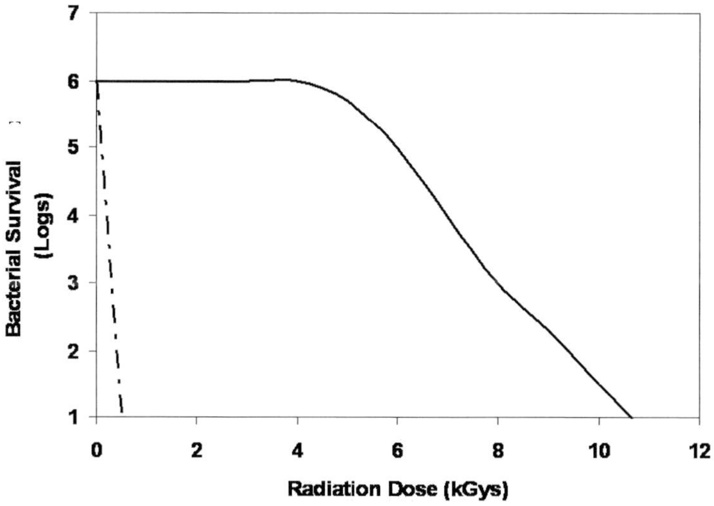

FIGURE 8.12 An example of *Deinococcus radiodurans* survival of radiation. The survival of *D. radiodurans* (solid line) is compared to a typical radiation-sensitive bacterial strain (dotted line) when exposed to increasing doses of γ irradiation (measured in kilograys; chapter 5, section 5.4).

identified. These included the *Deinobacter* spp., which were similar to *Deinococcus* but stained as Gram-negative bacteria. *Deinococcus* and *Deinobacter* spp. have subsequently been found to be widely distributed in the environment and have been isolated from soil and dust and associated with nuclear waste. Other bacteria with unusual resistance profiles to radiation have included strains of *Geodermatophilus*, *Rubrobacter*, *Acinetobacter*, *Methylobacterium*, and *Kocuria*. Although *Deinococcus* strains have not been described as being pathogenic (although they have been implicated in food spoilage), the Gram-positive *Kocuria* and Gram-negative *Methylobacterium* spp. have been associated with infection in immunocompromised patients; they are also ubiquitous in the environment, with *Kocuria* found on the skin, in dust, and in contaminated meat, while *Methylobacterium* spp. (often presenting as pink colony forms) are found in soil and associated with foods (e.g., rice) and water. *Methylobacterium* spp. are often found to be cross-resistant to chlorine (being found to survive in treated tap water), glutaraldehyde, and heavy metals (such as zinc) and to demonstrate higher than expected tolerance to heat and dehydration. High levels of γ radiation resistance have also been described in many archaea, such as *Thermococcus gammatolerans* (with resistance described up to 30 kGy) and *Pyrococcus*. These archaea can also demonstrate high-level cross-resistance to heat (see section 8.3.10).

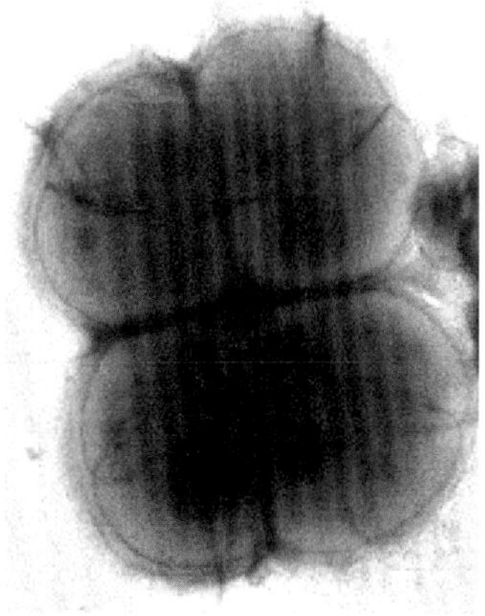

FIGURE 8.13 Micrograph of *D. radiodurans* cells, in a typical tetrad formation. Image courtesy of Max-Planck-Institute for Molecular Genetics.

In addition to radiation resistance, many of these bacteria and archaea have been shown to be cross-resistant to oxidative damage (e.g., effects of oxidizing agents) and dehydration. In these cases, damage to bacterial DNA is considered to be a major part of their modes of action. It is therefore not surprising to find that one of the key mechanisms of resistance in these microorganisms is efficient DNA repair activity. The mechanisms of resistance have been particularly well described in *Deinococcus* spp. such as *D. radiodurans*. Although less studied, other bacteria and archaea appear to share similar mechanisms of resistance. Many bacteria and fungi have been shown to tolerate minor DNA damage by the induction of response mechanisms (such as the SOS response; see section 8.3.3), but *Deinococcus* spp. are capable of tolerating a significantly greater extent of DNA strand breakage (in the case of ionizing radiation exposure) and the presence of other photoproducts (such as thymine and other base dimers on exposure to UV light; section 7.4.4).

Similar to other bacterial stress responses, various repair mechanisms are induced (mediated by a RecA homolog; section 8.3.3), including increased DNA repair and recombination, DNA replication, cell wall metabolism, and other increases in metabolic functions. Multiple DNA lesions are efficiently repaired by two major processes within 12 to 24 hours following radiation exposure: single-strand annealing and homologous recombination. During recombination, the RecA protein facilitates the repair of double-stranded DNA breakages by cutting out a section of the molecule and replacing it with a similar section of DNA. This procedure is enhanced in radiation-resistant strains by the presence of multiple (sometimes 4 to 10) copies of the bacterial genome; alignment of these copies allows for the efficient recovery of a viable genome. Other significant defense mechanisms have been identified, including protection and repair mechanisms. *D. radiodurans* growth has a typical pink or red colonial color due to the presence of carotenoid pigments that act as free-radical scavengers and can protect the cell from hydroxyl radicals, which are formed on contact with various oxidizing agents. In addition, high levels of defense enzymes such as catalase and superoxide dismutase confer some protection against biocides such as ozone and hydrogen peroxide (section 8.3.3). Studies of strain desiccation have shown a buildup of internal manganese levels, which may act as antioxidants to protect against oxidation from oxidizing agents and radiation.

Finally, the deinococcal cell wall structure is considered unique among Gram-positive bacteria (chapter 1, section 1.3.4.1). The cell wall has an unusual thickness (50 to 60 nm) and consists of an inner, substantial layer of peptidoglycan, an outer membrane, and an external S-layer, which varies in thickness. The peptidoglycan structure is similar to other Gram-positive bacteria but has the amino acid ornithine instead of diaminopimelic acid in the various peptide cross-linkages. The outer membrane is a lipid bilayer but does not contain LPS, as in Gram-negative bacteria; overall differences in phospholipid and fatty acid profiles have been reported, which may also contribute to the intrinsic resistance. Although less studied, strains of *Deinobacter* appear to have a similar cell wall structure in comparison to *Deinococcus* but stain Gram-negative, presumably due to their thinner peptidoglycan layer.

8.3.10 Extremophiles

Microorganisms are found in diverse environments and vary considerably in their growth requirements. Research into various extremophiles has identified unique and multiple intrinsic mechanisms of resistance or tolerance to extreme conditions. The term "extremophilic" is taken from the original Greek word *philein*, "to love," and can be further subdivided into descriptive groups based on the major requirement(s) for growth: temperature, pH, water or salt concentrations, and oxygen. For example, thermophiles (or thermophilic microorganisms) can survive at higher temperatures (with many *Archaea* described as hyperthermophiles, which multiply at even more extreme temperature conditions), while their opposites, psychrophiles, grow in cold environments, halophiles survive extreme salt conditions, and acido- or alkaliphiles are found in low- or high-pH environments, respectively. It should be noted that these growth conditions are generally not extreme for the microorganism in question and in many cases are actually required for growth. For example, the hyperthermophilic *Pyrolobus fumarii* cannot grow at temperatures less than 85°C.

The optimum temperatures for microbial growth vary considerably, in particular, with fungi, bacteria, and archaea. The microorganisms can be grouped into three temperature ranges: psychrophiles (which grow optimally under lower temperatures), mesophiles (which grow within an ambient or mid-temperature range), and thermophiles (which grow preferably at higher temperatures) (Fig. 8.14).

Within the mesophilic group, many bacteria and fungi can tolerate lower or higher temperatures within a given range but show slower metabolism at lower temperatures and specific protective responses such as the heat shock response (section 8.3.3) at higher temperatures. These responses allow some protection and survival to the cells under less optimal temperature conditions. The psychrophiles and thermophiles are different in that they have modified microbial structures and processes that allow them to thrive under cold or hot growth conditions. Overall, the mechanisms of heat or cold tolerance are similar yet distinct. In particular, they include specific protein-enzyme and lipid structures that are more tolerant to specific growth conditions. Enzymes in mesophilic bacteria have significantly less activity at lower temperatures and are generally denatured at higher temperatures (chapter 7, section 7.4.4).

In the psychrophilic bacteria that have been studied, a drop in temperature has been shown to be detected by proteins in a two-component, cell membrane-associated signal transduction system that leads to the initiation of a cold shock response and the expression of cold-tolerance mechanisms. These can include nucleic acid compaction, cell membrane lipid changes, protein association, production of cryoprotectants, cold shock proteins and antifreeze proteins, and the expression of cold-functioning enzymes. Many of these cold-associated mechanisms have been particularly described in the hyper-psychrophilic bacteria that can survive and grow in temperatures as low as −15 to −20°C, such as in salt water arctic or antarctic conditions. These include species of *Arthrobacter*, *Phychrobacter*, *Halomonas*, and *Pseudomonas*. In psychrophiles, many of the key metabolic enzymes and structural proteins show a greater proportion of α-helix secondary structure and increased polar (hydrophilic) amino acids (with decreased hydrophobic residues), which appear to allow proteins greater flexibility at lower temperatures; however, the exact contributions of

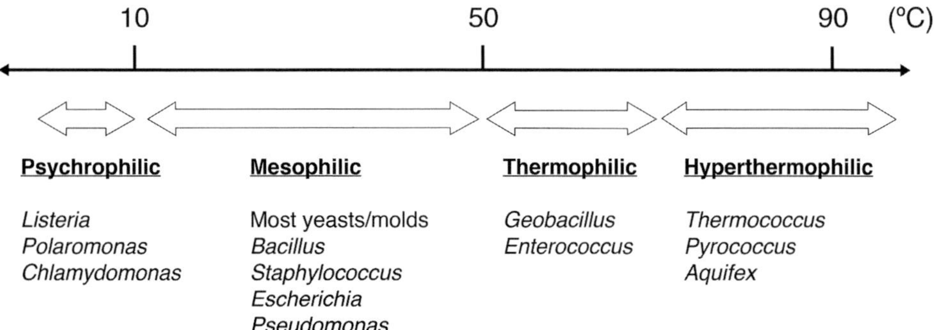

FIGURE 8.14 Microbial growth and optimum temperature conditions. Examples of various vegetative microorganisms are shown, although the sensitivities of specific species to heat vary. *Geobacillus* spores may be considered hyperthermophilic but are dormant in comparison to their vegetative forms (see section 8.3.11).

protein primary and secondary structures to cold tolerance are not fully known. Some of these appear to be associated with chaperone (causing the refolding of damaged proteins) and antifreeze activity, in combination with the cryoprotectants such as glycine betaine (involved in stabilizing the cell membrane). Another difference is the increased occurrence of unsaturated fatty acids and carotenoids, particularly associated with the cell membrane to provide greater fluidity and stability at low temperatures than saturated fatty acids. Higher concentrations of polyunsaturated, long-chained lipids in the cytoplasm have also been described in some psychrophiles. Psychrophiles in soil, by association, have been shown to provide some level of cold temperature tolerance to plants.

The opposite effects are observed in thermophiles and hyperthermophiles. Proteins in these bacteria are often found to have greater heat stability, particularly due to increased chemical (ionic) bonds between amino acid residues in their secondary and tertiary structures and to some minor changes in their primary structures, which overall resist unfolding at elevated temperatures. The primary structures of proteins were generally found to have significantly higher proportions of charged amino acids (such as glutamic acid, arginine, and lysine) and fewer uncharged amino acids (such as glutamine and serine). In some cases, proteins were found to have a greater proportion of disulfide bonds (between cysteine residues) that further increases their stability, where a specific enzyme (protein disulfide oxidoreductase) was found to be important in bond formation. Overall, these structural differences provide proteins with greater resistance to the effects of heat by preventing unfolding and loss of structure and/or function. A further difference is the presence of various proteins or other molecules that protect the proteins from heat-inactivation; these also include chaperones (which are discussed under heat shock responses in section 8.3.3) and sugars such as diglycerol phosphate and mannosylglycerate. There are also many repair or protective mechanisms to reduce the effects of heat on DNA, including DNA gyrases that increase the supercoiling to prevent unraveling and DNA-binding proteins that insulate the DNA molecule. Increased proportions of G:C base pairing in the DNA structure (see chapter 7, section 7.3) also afford greater resistance to unraveling on heat exposure. In contrast to the lipids prevalent in psychrophiles, thermophiles are found to have a larger proportion of saturated fatty acids, which allow greater membrane stability and resistance to phospholipid bilayer separation at higher temperatures. Lipids have also been found to have ether linkages, in comparison to the more common ester linkages in bacterial lipids (see section 7.3). In some hyperthermophiles among the *Archaea*, heat-resistant membrane lipids are formed in monolayers of long-chained fatty acids that are more resistant to disruption; many thermophilic archaea are also acidophiles, growing at low pH ranges (pH 1 to 5).

Microorganisms can also be separated on the basis of their pH requirements or tolerance (Fig. 8.15).

The concentration of hydrogen ions (H^+) in solution is expressed as pH, which is a logarithmic scale ranging from acidic through neutral to basic, or alkaline, conditions. Microorganisms have been isolated at the extremes of this range, from acidophiles, which can tolerate low-pH conditions, to alkaliphiles, which prefer high-pH conditions. It should be noted that although these extreme pHs can be tolerated and even required for growth, cells have typically developed mechanisms to maintain the internal cytoplasm close to neutral pH, allowing the various internal metabolic functions. This is primarily maintained by efficient membrane-associated efflux pumps that pump hydrogen ions in either direction across the membrane to maintain internal neutral conditions (see section 8.3.4). Acidophiles, which generally survive at pH levels less than 5, pump H^+ ions out of the cell at a constant high rate to maintain internal pH levels between 6.5 and 7. The internal pH levels in alkaliphiles are generally within the pH 7 to 8 range and are

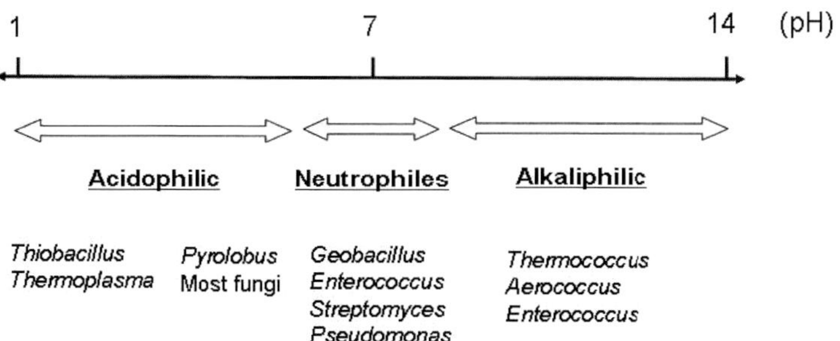

FIGURE 8.15 Microbial growth and optimum pH conditions. Examples of various microorganisms are shown, although specific species vary in their sensitivity to pH.

maintained by pumping H^+ into the cytoplasm. A well-studied acid-tolerant bacterium is *Helicobacter pylori*, which can survive in the stomach (pH ~1 to 2) and is the causative agent of peptic ulcers. *H. pylori* is a neutrophilic organism, but a variety of acid-tolerating mechanisms have been identified. An interesting mechanism comes from studies of the dependence on the presence of urea for growth at pH <4. Urea is transported into the Gram-negative periplasm under acidic conditions, where the presence of urease causes the formation of NH_3, allowing neutralization of the periplasm, the generation of a proton motive force, and active efflux of H^+ from the cell. Further, an exclusion mechanism involving specific inner and outer membrane proteins of *H. pylori* that reduce the overall proton permeability of the cell has been described. Many acidophiles also present tolerance to various toxic heavy metals, which can be due to intrinsic (section 8.3.6) and/or acquired (section 8.7) resistance mechanisms.

Similar effects have been described regarding the tolerance of various salt concentrations by microorganisms; an example of tolerances to sodium chloride (NaCl) is shown in Fig. 8.16. The concentration of salt surrounding a microorganism affects its survival due to the diffusion of water into or out of the cell. Water is required for metabolism, but an increase in cytoplasmic water content can lead to cell lysis, and equally, a loss of water can lead to loss of cell viability. The diffusion of water naturally occurs from an area of low solute (or salt) concentration to a high concentration in a process known as osmosis. These effects have been studied to some extent in bacteria and fungi, with some isolates (known as nonhalophilic) growing under high-water-activity (or low-solute) conditions and others (halophiles) requiring much lower water (and therefore

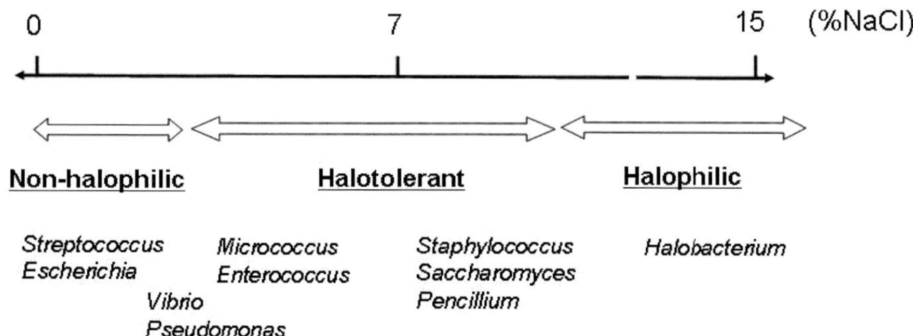

FIGURE 8.16 Microbial growth and optimum salt conditions. Examples of various microorganisms are given, although specific species vary in their sensitivity to salt concentrations.

higher solute) activity for growth. In some cases, extreme halophiles have been described that require a concentration of >10% NaCl, including the *Halobacterium* archaea. A wide range of organisms also grow within an intermediate salt range and are known as halotolerant; for example, *Vibrio* spp. can survive in seawater (~3% salt; Fig. 8.16).

Various adaptations in *Bacteria* and *Archaea* that allow them to survive extreme osmotic effects have been described. Intracellular water loss in bacteria can be controlled by increasing the cytoplasmic salt (or solute) concentration to inhibit the loss of intracellular water, which effectively reduces the osmotic effect. This is achieved by a combination of the activity of influx pumps (to pump inorganic ions such as K^+ into the cell) and by the synthesis of intracellular organic solutes, which are compatible with metabolic processes (including glycerol, glutamate, and amino acids). An example has been described in *S. aureus* strains, which can grow in up to ~7.5% NaCl by increasing the internal concentration of proline (an amino acid) as a solute. Other mechanisms have been studied in extreme halophiles. Cytoplasmic proteins have a higher level of acidic amino acids (e.g., aspartic acid and glutamic acid), with much lower levels of basic (e.g., arginine and lysine) and hydrophobic (glycine, alanine, and proline) residues; these proteins appear to be less sensitive to higher concentrations of salts. Exclusion is also a key mechanism. *Halobacterium* spp. and other halophiles among the *Archaea* have unique cell wall structures in comparison to bacteria. These include thick polysaccharide or protein and glycoprotein cell walls (instead of the bacterial peptidoglycan) and paracrystalline S-layers (section 8.3.7), which appear to assist in preventing water loss to the environment. *Halobacterium*, in particular, has a predominantly glycoprotein-based cell wall (also with a high proportion of acidic amino acids), which is further stabilized by the presence of a high concentration of sodium ions.

Another example of microbial survival under extreme conditions is different oxygen requirements (Table 8.10). Microorganisms can be classified based on their requirements for oxygen for growth. Aerobes require oxygen at the typical concentrations in air (~21%), while strict anaerobes require the absence of oxygen for growth. Within these extremes are bacteria that specifically require reduced oxygen levels (microaerophilic), can grow under aerobic and anaerobic conditions (facultative), or can tolerate the presence of oxygen but do not use it (aerotolerant anaerobes). These requirements reflect differences in metabolic activity. Aerobes metabolize using oxygen by aerobic respiration, while anaerobes metabolize by fermentation or anaerobic respiration. In some cases, for example *Clostridium*, the presence of oxygen can lead to cell death that may be linked to the lack of protective response mechanisms to active oxygen species in these bacteria (sections 8.3.4 and 8.3.5). With the exception that strict anaerobes may be more sensitive to the effects of peroxgyens and other forms of oxygen, the various oxygen requirements for growth do not appear to affect biocide sensitivity.

8.3.11 Dormancy

Bacteria display a variety of adaptive processes that allow them to survive limiting environmental conditions, including the presence of

TABLE 8.10 Examples of oxygen requirements for microbial growth. Examples of microorganisms are given, although specific species may vary in their oxygen requirements

Type	Requirement or ability to grow	Examples
Aerobic	~21% oxygen (typical in air)	*Micrococcus, Bacillus, Pseudomonas, Neisseria, Legionella*
Microaerophilic	Reduced (<20%) levels of oxygen	*Spirillium, Helicobacter*
Facultative	Can grow under aerobic and anaerobic conditions	*Escherichia, Haemophilus, Staphylococcus, Streptococcus*
Anaerobic	Require or tolerate the absence of oxygen	*Clostridium, Methanobacterium*

biocides and restricted nutrient availability (as discussed earlier in this chapter). In some cases, they can become dormant with very low levels of metabolism; examples include pathogenic *Mycobacterium* spp., which can remain dormant within the body, and *Vibrio* spp. in water. Others include "persister" cells that remain dormant in the presence of antibiotics and can be associated with chronic infections. The dormant forms of these bacteria (often associated with biofilms [see section 8.3.8] or cells under stress response [see section 8.3.3]) can be less sensitive to various antibiotics and biocides due to lower metabolic rates or other stationary-phase phenomena (see section 8.3.1), but overall, they have not been difficult to study in detail due to simulating these forms under laboratory conditions. The most dramatic dormant adaptation is displayed by certain bacteria known generally as the Gram-positive endospore-forming rods and cocci (chapter 1, section 1.3.4.1). Examples of bacteria in this group include *Geobacillus*, *Bacillus*, and *Clostridium* spp., with examples given in Table 8.11; they are widely isolated from various environments (including soil, air, foods, and environmental surfaces), and many are known pathogens (primarily due to the production of toxins; section 1.3.7).

These bacteria undergo a remarkable change in their normal vegetative growth processes in response to environmental stress to produce dormant and resilient forms of themselves, known as bacterial spores or "endospores." They are referred to as endospores because they are developed within the "mother" cell in a coordinated process known as sporulation (Fig. 8.17).

The sporulation process has been particularly well studied in *B. atrophaeus* (previously known as *B. subtilis*) and involves a coordinated adaptation in the transcription and translation machinery of a cell to become dedicated to the development of an endospore. The resulting endospores are invariably some of the most resistant of all types of bacteria, if not all microorganisms, to antiseptics, disinfectants, and sterilants (with the exception of some extremophiles discussed in section 8.3.10). For this reason, they are used in the development and routine monitoring of various sterilization processes (chapter 1, section 1.4.2.3). Many biocides are bacteriostatic or even bactericidal at low concentrations for nonsporulating bacteria,

TABLE 8.11 Spore-forming bacteria and their significance

Bacteria	Significance
Geobacillus	Aerobic, Gram-positive rods; thermophilic; previously defined under the genus *Bacillus*
Geobacillus stearothermophilus	Often cited as the microorganism most practically resistant to steam and other gaseous sterilization processes; used to test the efficacy of these processes, for example, in biological indicators (see chapter 1, section 1.4.2.4).
Bacillus	Aerobic, Gram-positive rods; generally mesophilic; diverse species; common environmental contaminants
B. anthracis	Pathogenic and has been used as a bioterrorism agent; causative agent in anthrax, a disease of animals and humans
B. atrophaeus	Regarded as the most practically resistant microorganism to ethylene oxide and other sterilization processes; therefore used to test the efficacy of these processes, for example, in biological indicators; formerly known as *Bacillus subtilis* var. *niger*
Bacillus cereus	Causative agent of food poisoning
Clostridium	Anaerobic, Gram-positive rods
Clostridium difficile	A common cause of institutional-related diarrhea
Clostridium perfringens	Used as a test organism to verify the sporicidal efficacy of biocides in the United States; commonly associated with decaying matter; pathogenic, including wound infections (gas gangrene) and food poisoning
Clostridium tetani	Causative agent of tetanus; linked to deep wound infections
Clostridium botulinum	Causative agent of botulism, a food poisoning disease

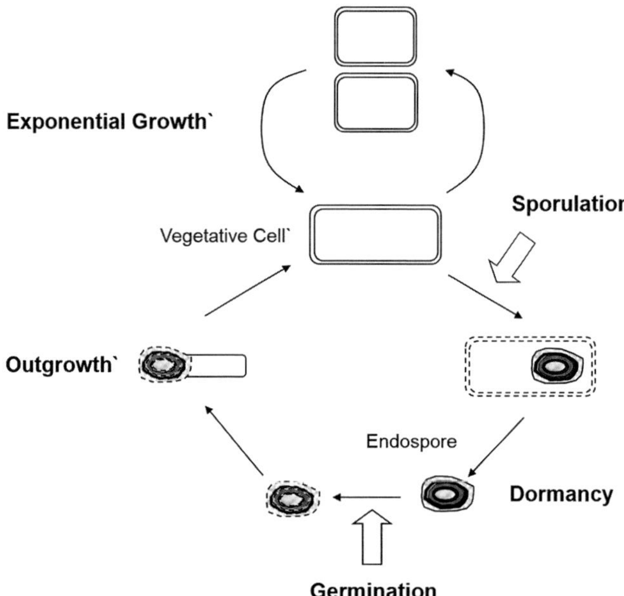

FIGURE 8.17 The basic life cycle of Gram-positive endospore-forming rods. The vegetative growth of the bacteria is limited due to the reduction of essential nutrients (for example, carbon or nitrogen sources) or other environmental factors, causing the initiation of the sporulation cascade, death of the mother cell, and release of the dormant spore. Under the right environmental conditions, conducive to bacterial growth, the spore becomes activated, germinates, and outgrows to produce a viable vegetative bacterial cell over time, which resumes metabolism and multiplication.

including the vegetative forms of *Bacillus* and *Clostridium* spp., but higher concentrations, doses, and/or temperatures with often longer contact times are necessary to achieve a sporicidal effect (e.g., with oxidizing agents, aldehydes, and steam) (Table 8.12).

Many biocides have little to no practical sporicidal activity, but a wider spectrum of biocides and exposure conditions are effective to prevent endospore germination (sporostatic activity). Examples include high concentrations of alcohol, phenolics, QACs, and chlorhexidine, which all lack any appreciable sporicidal effect, although in some cases this may be achieved when these compounds are used at elevated temperatures or in synergy with other biocides. Endospores, depending on the species, also show varying abilities to survive high temperatures (in particular, the thermophilic *Geobacillus* spp.) and drying, or desiccation; they can therefore survive in many environments for up to many years, depending on the genus, species, and environmental conditions.

TABLE 8.12 Sporistatic and sporicidal concentrations of biocides[a]

Biocide	Concentration (mg/liter)	
	Sporistatic	Sporicidal
Benzalkonium chloride	5	–[b]
Chlorhexidine	1	–
Ethanol	700	–
Sodium hypochlorite	1	100
Phenol	500	–
Hydrogen peroxide	500	50,000
Peracetic acid	10	100
Glutaraldehyde	50	10,000
Formaldehyde	500	20,000

[a]Concentrations are approximate and vary depending on the bacterial endospore type and test conditions. All biocides were tested as suspensions in water.

[b]Little to no sporicidal activity reported at maximum solubility, but this can vary depending on the endospores tested.

In spite of this, under the right environmental conditions for growth, including temperature and the presence of nutrients, the spore can become activated and germinate (Fig. 8.17). The germination process is quite rapid and irreversible and is the first indication of the dormant spore resuming vegetative metabolism. During this stage the protective spore coats are broken, with release of the spore core contents and breakdown of intrinsic, unique proteins to the spore core (the SASPs; see below). The germinated spores then move to a further regeneration stage known as outgrowth. During this stage, water is reabsorbed into the spore, and the normal cellular processes (including protein, lipid, carbohydrate, and nucleic acid synthesis and their respective activities) resume, allowing for the regeneration of a vegetative cell and normal growth and proliferation.

A closer understanding of endospore structure is of interest to understand their resilience in the environment and intrinsic resistance to biocides. A so-called typical endospore has a complex structure in comparison to the parent vegetative cell, consisting of an inner spore core that is surrounded by a series of protective spore layers (Fig. 8.18).

A comparison of endospores and their vegetative cell forms is given in Table 8.13. The innermost part of the endospore is the spore core (or "protoplast"), which contains the essential components for viability but differs substantially in its constituents in comparison to the mother cell (see Table 8.13). The spore core contains DNA, some RNAs, acidic proteins, and metal ions but demonstrates little to no metabolic activity. The first major difference is the degree of hydration. A typical endospore contains ≤30% of the normal water concentration found in a vegetative cell. This limits any macromolecular activity but also acts as a barrier to the penetration of liquids and gases, as well as being a poor conductor of heat, thereby protecting the nucleic acid from damage. The spore core contents are further protected by the presence of dipicolinic acid (DPA), which is chelated with a high concentration of calcium ions (calcium dipicolinate [Ca-DPA]), overall taking up approximately 10% of the dry weight of the endospore. The Ca-DPA appears to protect the spore core from heat, radiation, and chemicals by stabilization of the bacterial DNA and protecting essential proteins (presumably by reducing the water content in the spore core). Spore mutants that lack Ca-DPA are unstable (spontaneously germinating), suggesting that Ca-DPA has a stabilizing effect on spore dormancy. In addition to calcium, other chemicals are present at higher concentrations in the spore core, including potassium, manganese, and phosphorus, which may also play a role in protection of the nucleic acid. The protein component is predominantly made up of small acid-soluble spore proteins (SASPs), which are produced during the sporulation process and used as an energy or nutrient source during the germination and outgrowth of the spore. They appear to protect the viability of the spore by tight binding to the bacterial DNA and preventing biocide or other environmental damage to the nucleic acid. Spores lacking SASPs are more sensitive to oxidizing agents and radiation methods.

In addition to these protective mechanisms, the spore core is further protected from environmental stresses by a series of spore layers, including lipid and protein membranes, cell wall-type layers, the cortex, and spore coats (Fig. 8.18). The inner and outer membranes are similar in structure to (and derived from) the vegetative, mother cell membrane, consisting of a bilipid membrane and integrated proteins. During the development of the spore, they differentiate in the spore structures and are distinct from the vegetative cell membrane in their permeability functions. These differences appear to be due to differences in the compression of their structure to limit the mobility of the lipids and thereby restrict chemical permeability (particularly for the inner membrane structure).

The germ cell wall and cortex are similar in structure to the Gram-positive cell wall peptidoglycan. The inner germ cell wall, which is found to be present in some endospore types, consists of peptidoglycan, essentially the same as

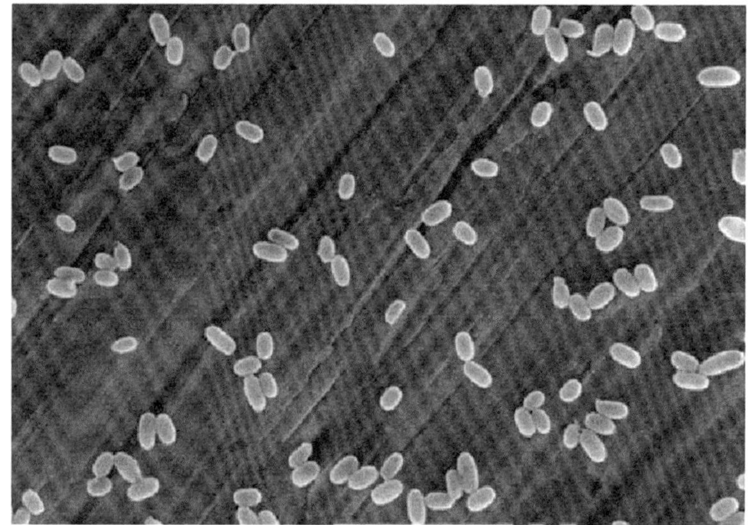

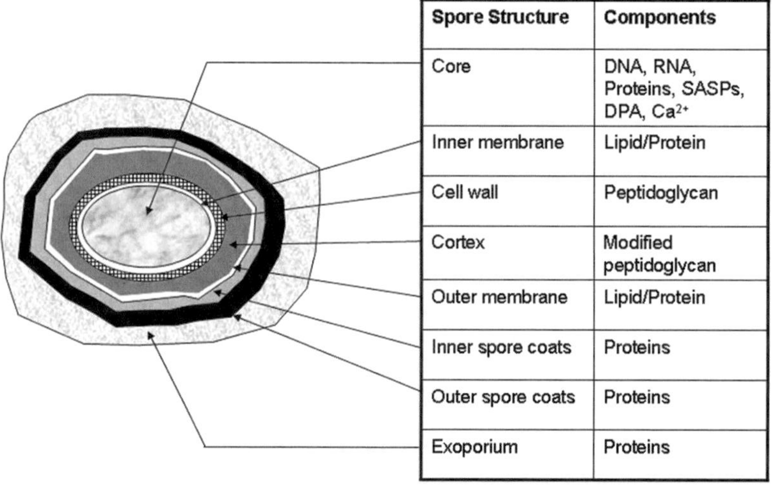

Spore Structure	Components
Core	DNA, RNA, Proteins, SASPs, DPA, Ca^{2+}
Inner membrane	Lipid/Protein
Cell wall	Peptidoglycan
Cortex	Modified peptidoglycan
Outer membrane	Lipid/Protein
Inner spore coats	Proteins
Outer spore coats	Proteins
Exoporium	Proteins

FIGURE 8.18 Typical bacterial endospore structure. A micrograph of endospores on a surface is shown, with a representation of the various spore layers shown below (not to scale). The shapes of the spores vary depending on the bacterial genus and species.

in the vegetative cell wall. Although the structure of peptidoglycan can vary depending on the bacterial genus and species, its basic structure is a polysaccharide of two repeating sugars, *N*-acetylglucosamine and *N*-acetylmuramic acid, cross-linked by glycosidic (sugar-sugar) bonds (see chapter 1, section 1.3.4 and Figure 1.8). The cortex has subtle differences from vegetative cell peptidoglycan. In *B. atrophaeus*, these include increased cross-linking between the *N*-acetylglucosamine residues, the formation of *N*-acetylmuramic acid cyclic structures (muramic-D-lactam, consisting of the sugars with muramic lactam-*N*-acetylglutamic linkages), and lower concentrations of associated teichoic acids. Overall, the cortex appears to provide greater rigidity to the spore structure and resistance to biocide penetration. The cortex also appears to play a role in regulating the water content of the inner core.

TABLE 8.13 Structure, components, and activities of endospores and their vegetative cells

Characteristic	Endospore	Vegetative cell
Internal pH	~6	~7
Heat resistance	High; some strains can survive at >100°C	Low, although some thermophiles grow optimally at ~55°C
Chemical resistance	High	Low, with the exception of some extremophiles
Structure	Various protective layers surrounding an inner spore core	Typical Gram-positive cell wall structure
Water content (%)	<30	~80
Calcium level	High	Low
Macromolecular synthesis	Low to none	Active
Dipicolinic acid	Present	Absent
Small acid-soluble proteins	Present	Absent
Typical life span	Years in some cases	Days depending on environment

The inner and outer spore coats comprise a major part of the overall spore content. These structures consist largely of protein, with an alkali-soluble fraction made up of acidic polypeptides found in the inner coat and an alkali-resistant fraction associated with the presence of disulfide-rich bonds in the outer coat. At least 70 spore coat proteins have been identified in *B. atrophaeus*, and many of these are similar in structure to other *Bacillus*, *Geobacillus*, and *Clostridium* spp. Various carbohydrates and lipids are also found to be associated with spore coat structures. Finally, where present, the exosporium provides a further penetration challenge to biocides and predominantly consists of proteins, often loosely associated with the spore surface. Exosporia have been particularly studied in *B. cereus* and can be found to consist of ~50% of the dry weight of spores. The exosporium is hydrophobic, which may have a minor contribution to the resistance profile of the spore but also increases the adherence potential to surfaces. Overall, the observed layers and structure of endospores vary from species to species; for example, the exosporium is only present in some species, while the spores of others are more simply surrounded by just one spore coat layer. These aspects, especially the roles of the spore coat(s) and cortex, are all relevant to the cumulative mechanism(s) of resistance presented by bacterial spores to biocides and biocidal processes.

As mentioned above, the endospore structure is developed in a sequential and controlled manner over approximately 8 hours (Fig. 8.19). The sporulation process has been particularly well studied in *B. atrophaeus* as a primitive yet instructive and complex example of how cells are capable of differentiating during their life cycles. The control of the transcriptional and translational machinery of the cell is coordinated by a series of RNA polymerase-associated sigma (σ) factors that specifically direct the translation of specific genes at different phases of the sporulation cascade, and therefore direct production of proteins away from normal housekeeping functions to those required for the development of the spore. The overall process has been defined as a series of at least seven integrated yet definitive stages, termed stages 0 to VI (Fig. 8.19).

During this process, the vegetative cell (stage 0) undergoes a series of morphological changes that culminate in the release of a mature spore (stage VII). A cell undergoing the first stages of sporulation demonstrates a change from normal binary fission to asymmetric cell division (stages I and II), followed by engulfment of the forespore (stage III). The forespore then develops the cortex (stage IV) and spore coats (stages V and VI), in parallel with dehydration of the spore core and accumulation of calcium, DPA, and the SASPs. The final stage (VII) demonstrates further maturation of the spore structure and lysis of the mother cell to release the mature endospore.

Studies with a normal *B. atrophaeus* strain (in particular, strain 168) and various sporulation

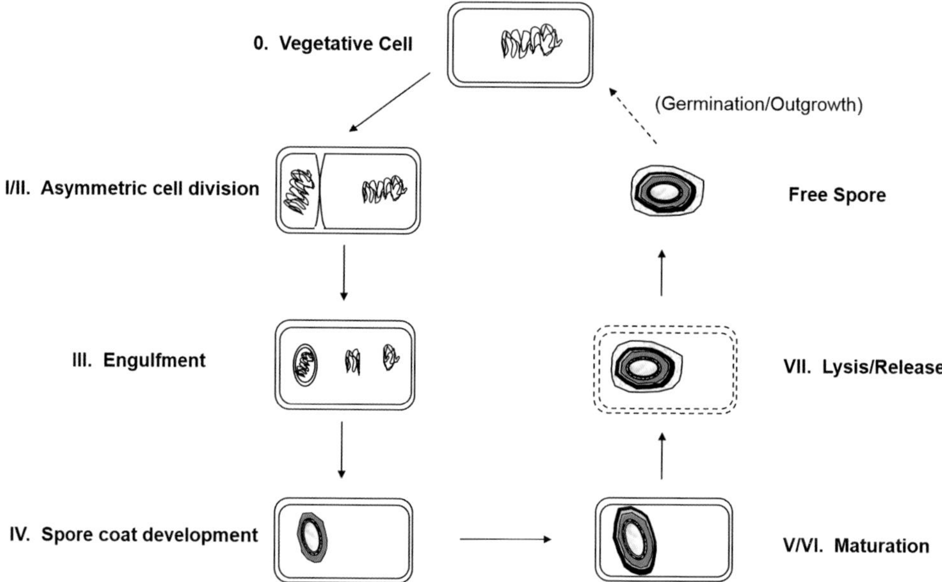

FIGURE 8.19 A representation of a typical sporulation process, with the key (seven) stages identified.

(Spo$^-$) mutants that develop only to a certain stage in the cascade have been used to understand the genetic and biochemical nature of each stage and to study at which stage biocide resistance is observed. In particular, stages IV to VII (cortex development, maturation, and release) have been identified as the most important stages in the development of resistance (Fig. 8.20). The timing of specific resistance development has been found to depend on the nature of the biocide and can be defined as being either an early, intermediate, late, or very late event. Useful biocidal markers for monitoring these phases of

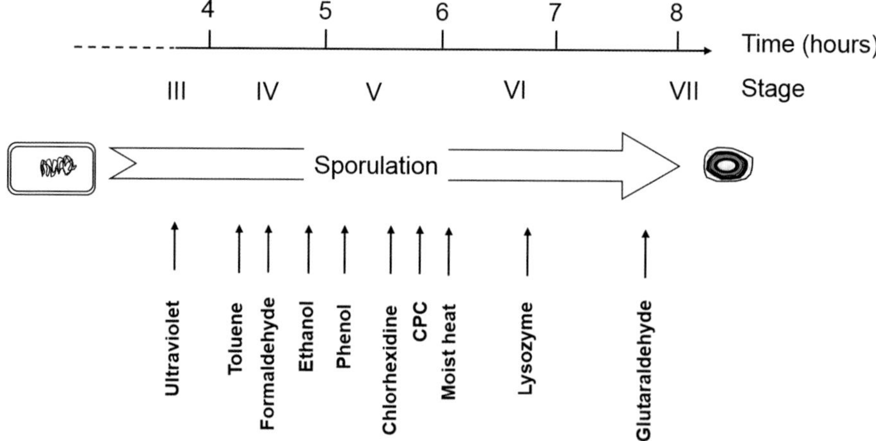

FIGURE 8.20 The development of resistance of bacterial endospores to biocides and biocidal processes. The defined stages of sporulation are given from stage III (engulfment of the forespore) to stage VII (release of the mature spore), as described in Fig. 8.19. The point at which the developing spore demonstrates resistance to each biocide or biocidal process is indicated.

resistance are toluene (resistance to which is an early event), heat (intermediate), and lysozyme (an enzyme effective against the normal bacterial cell wall peptidoglycan, to which spores become resistant late in sporulation). From these studies (Fig. 8.20), the order of development of resistance was found to be toluene (marker), formaldehyde, sodium lauryl sulfate, phenol, cresols, chlorhexidine gluconate, QACs (such as cetylpyridinium chloride), moist heat (marker), sodium dichloroisocyanurate, sodium hypochlorite, lysozyme (marker), and glutaraldehyde.

Development of resistance to formaldehyde during sporulation was found to be an early event but depended on the concentration (1 to 5% vol/vol) of formaldehyde employed. This appears to be at odds with the extremely late development of resistance to the dialdehyde glutaraldehyde. Because glutaraldehyde and the monoaldehyde formaldehyde contain an aldehyde group(s) and are alkylating agents (chapter 7, section 7.4.3), it would be plausible to assume that they have a similar mode of sporicidal action, even though the dialdehyde is a more powerful alkylating agent. If this were true, then it could also be assumed that spores exhibit the same resistance mechanisms for these disinfectants. In aqueous solution, formaldehyde forms a glycol in equilibrium; thus, formaldehyde in aqueous form could act poorly as an alcohol-type disinfectant rather than an aldehyde. Alkaline glutaraldehyde does not readily form glycols in aqueous solution. This chemical difference may be responsible for the differences observed in the development of resistance in spores. Overall, resistance to formaldehyde may then be more linked to cortex maturation and glutaraldehyde to coat formation.

As spores develop resistance to biocides during sporulation, they also lose resistance as they germinate and outgrow to reinitiate normal metabolism and growth (Fig. 8.21).

The activation of the endospore is a key stage to dedicate the spore to develop into a vegetative cell. Activation alone allows the spore to be more sensitive to heat and other biocides such as phenolics and normally sporistatic concentrations of aldehydes. Further biocide access and damage to the inner spore membrane and spore core following germination clearly play roles in inhibiting further outgrowth of the spore; during germination the protective barriers of the spore coats are lost and the integrity of the cortex and spore core is broken as indicated by the release of core constituents. As the outgrowth stage proceeds, biocides demonstrate their typical bacteristatic and bacteriocidal activities as observed in vegetative cells. It is interesting to note that

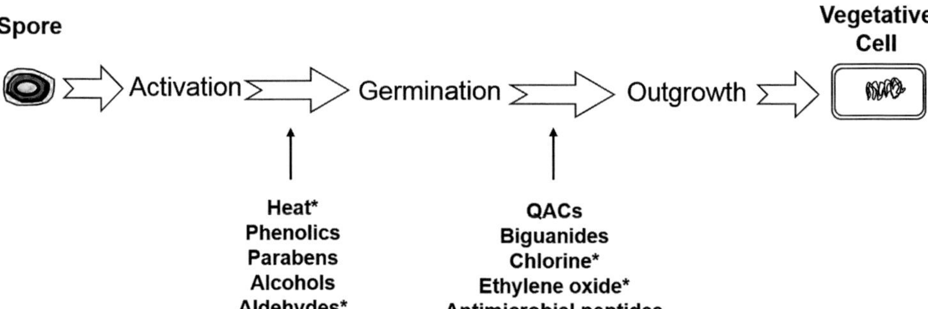

FIGURE 8.21 Loss of resistance to various biocides and heat during bacterial endospore germination and outgrowth. Many biocides inhibit the activation of endospores (sporistatic) and are bactericidal to vegetative cells. Others (marked by asterisks) are also sporicidal at higher concentrations and temperatures and longer exposure times. Biocides, at low concentrations and temperatures, have also been shown to specifically inhibit germination or outgrowth following activation of the spore.

biocide-treated spores may remain viable but difficult to revive.

Traditionally, heat shock and specific culture conditions have been cited as improving the efficiency of revival of endospores. In contrast, the revival of disinfectant-treated spores has been little studied. Experiments designed to distinguish between germination and outgrowth in the revival process have demonstrated that sodium hydroxide-induced revival increases the potential for germination. Some reports have suggested that *B. atrophaeus* and *G. stearothermophilis* spores treated with formaldehyde or glutaraldehyde could be revived following a subsequent heat shock proccss, but not with chlorine or iodine treatment. It is likely that this is not related to an intrinsic resistance mechanism of the endospore but may be related to the test method or mode of action of the biocide. Inadequate neutralization of the biocide (particularly when associated with the spore structure) during laboratory investigations inhibited the activation and germination of the endospore, even at low concentrations. It can also be suggested that the mode of action of aldehydes, where lack or penetration of the aldehydes may allow viable spores to be trapped in a cross-linked matrix, inhibits the germination of the spore, but it can be released and allowed to germinate following disruption by heat-shocking or other methods. This has been shown to be the case in a different situation with the use of aldehydes to treat viruses in vaccine preparations, where insufficient contact with the virus suspension allowed viable virus to survive normal virucidal treatment (section 8.8). Equally, the impact of spore revival may also be related to the efficiency of repair mechanisms (particularly DNA repair) on germination and outgrowth; if DNA damage can be repaired over time, then the spore may be able to fully develop into its vegetative form, although this process may be significantly delayed in comparison to normal untreated endospores.

Other techniques have been used to understand mechanisms of spore resistance to biocides. They include the specific removal of various layers (such as the spore coat and cortex), spore mutants that lack specific spore components, using growth techniques to achieve a highly synchronous population of spores at various stages in sporulation (where cellular changes can be accurately monitored), adding a biocide at the commencement of sporulation and determining how far the process can proceed, and examining the role of specific spore constituents such as the SASPs based on biochemical reactions and their genetic or protein structures. Further consideration is given to the layer removal techniques and the use of spore structure mutants.

The various layers of a spore can be removed, using chemical and/or enzymatic treatments, to study their roles in resistance. Spores without spore coats can be produced by the treatment of spores under alkaline conditions with urea, dithiothreitol, and sodium lauryl sulfate, while further treatment with the enzyme lysozyme can be used to remove the inner cortex structure. These tests can be difficult to perform to ensure that a uniform population of stripped spores is available for testing. Tests with pretreated spores have shown that both the spore coats and cortex play roles in conferring resistance, where the sensitivity of the spore increases as the various layers are removed. The initial development and maturity of the cortex correlate with the development of resistance to phenolics, chlorhexidine, and QACs; this resistance is further enhanced in developing spores by the initiation of spore coat synthesis.

A number of *B. atrophaeus* mutants have been developed that lack specific spore components but remain capable of sporulating and subsequently germinating; these have been useful tools in studying the resistance of spores to various biocides and biocidal processes. These have included *cotE* mutants that lack the CotE protein essential for generating the spore coats, *spoVD* and *spoVE* mutants that lack a full cortex structure, *sspA* and *sspB* mutants that lack the major SASPs (α and β types), *recA* mutants that have reduced ability to repair DNA damage, and strains that include mutations in *spoVF* that do not produce DPA. A comparison of the impact of these mutations on endospore resistance is given in Table 8.14. It is important to note that the specific effects of each biocide or biocidal process can vary, particularly depending on the concentration and formulation of the chemical biocides.

Overall, the various mechanisms of action and resistance factors vary depending on the antimicrobial process. It appears that the spore core and DNA protective mechanisms, including the presence of DPA and the SASPs, are important in heat resistance, but the cortex was also found to be an important factor. The role of the cortex is likely related to its association in establishing and maintaining the low water (and high mineral) content in the spore core. In contrast, the SASPs appear to play a greater role in resistance to oxidizing agents such as hydrogen peroxide. But care should be taken in correlating these results with other biocides, because the impact of the various resistance mechanisms in endospores can be complex. For example, it is interesting to note that some studies have found a resistance role for the SASPs and, to a lesser extent, DPA to UV light but not to γ radiation; these results are unusual given the mechanism of action (see chapter 7, section 7.4.4). Equally, subtle differences in the mechanisms of action and resistance with oxidizing agents have been described, such as those comparing hydrogen peroxide and peracetic acid. Liquid hydrogen peroxide had similar resistance profiles in wild type and spore coat mutants (with a minor decrease observed in the coat mutants), but SASP mutants were significantly more sensitive. In contrast, the wild type and SASP mutants had similar resistance profiles to peracetic acid, but the spore coat mutants were more sensitive. Similar resistant profiles to peracetic acid were reported in studies with sodium hypochlorite and glutaraldehyde. Further studies that investigated the pretreatment of spores with either hydrogen peroxide or peracetic acid found that pretreatment with hydrogen peroxide rendered the spore more sensitive to peracetic acid, but not the other way around. It was proposed that liquid hydrogen peroxide had specific synergistic effects on reducing the permeability barrier of the spore coats (e.g., by reacting with or extracting proteins) and allowing greater penetration of peracetic acid. These results may explain the increased sporicidal activity of peracetic acid formulations at low concentrations and in equilibrium with hydrogen peroxide (see chapter 3, section 3.13).

In addition to the bacterial species listed in Table 8.11, some actinomycetes also produce spores (exospores). Actinomycetes are true Gram-positive, generally facultative anaerobic bacteria that grow and appear to be more similar to fungi. They grow in long, branched filaments similar to fungal mycelia, and most can produce spores from aerial hyphae. Actinomycetes are classically prokaryotes in that they lack mitochondria and a nuclear membrane (chapter 1, section 1.3.4). They can be further classified into aerobic and anaerobic species. Aerobic species include the mycolic

TABLE 8.14 Biocide resistance impact in specific *B. atrophaeus* mutants that lack various components of their endospore structures

Biocide	Spore mutant and resistance impact[a]				
	DPA	SASPs	DNA repair limited	Cortex	Spore coats
Moist heat	↓	↓	↔	↓	↔
Dry heat	↓	↓	↓	↓	↔
Formaldehyde (liquid)	↔	↓	↓	?	↔
Hydrogen peroxide (liquid)	↔	↓	↔	?	
Sodium hypochlorite	?	↔	↔	?	↓
UV	↓	↓	↓	?	↓

[a]A downward arrow indicates a decrease in resistance in comparison to wild-type spores, a horizontal arrow indicates little to no impact on resistance, and a question mark indicates unknown.

acid-containing species (such as *Norcardia* and *Corynebacterium*), which are nonsporulating, and those without mycolic acids which form exospores (including *Streptomyces*). Facultative and anaerobic species, including *Actinomyces*, are also spore-forming bacteria; actinomycetes themselves can be mesophilic and thermophilic. The growth of *Streptomyces* (particularly *Streptomyces coelocolor*) has been well studied due to the various developments identified during its typical life cycle (Fig. 8.22). These include antibiotic synthesis, stress responses, and morphological differentiation; similar to bacteria, the coordinated control of these developments is primarily due to transcriptional control of various operons by specific sigma factors (>65 have been identified) in response to various environmental stresses.

Under the right environmental conditions for growth, *Streptomyces* cells initially grow as surface (or subsurface) hyphal groups. Over time, the cells differentiate (by the coordination of a specific set of genes) to form aerial hyphae and, subsequently, develop exospores. Similar to other spore-forming bacteria, this initiates on nutrient depletion of other environmental stresses to lead to a stationary-stage response, including the first stages of spore development. The first step is the production of aerial hyphae due to the protection of specific hydrophobic proteins known as chaplins and rodlins. Next, a modified type of cell division occurs to form long chains of prespore compartments, which then develop separation by septation. During this stage various proteins become associated with the nucleic acid. Finally, the spore wall matures by thickening (containing glycogen and trehalose), production of a spore pigment (gray polyketide), and spore desiccation. The overall sporulation cascade is controlled by gene expression, particularly the *whi* genes (e.g., *whiG* codes for an RNA polymerase sigma factor that coordinates the expression of sporulation-associated genes over normal vegetative genes, similar to that described in other bacteria). Different strains of *Streptomyces* demonstrate variable arrangements of spores, which have been used for classification.

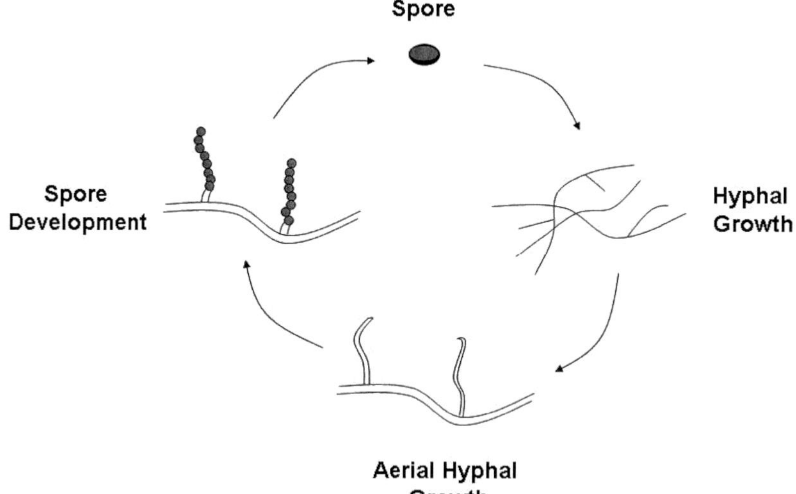

FIGURE 8.22 Typical life cycle of *Streptomyces*. A desiccated spore, under the right environmental conditions, will germinate and initiate hyphal growth. Under conditions of environmental stress and/or nutrient limitation, aerial hyphae develop in parallel with the production of secondary metabolites, including antibiotics and hydrolytic enzymes to assist in survival. The aerial filaments separate by simple cross-wall division to form prespore compartments and the development of desiccated spores, which can be released into the environment.

The purpose of sporulation is similar to bacterial endospores: the survival of cells under extreme nutrient depletion and harsh environmental conditions, but also dispersion to areas more conducive to vegetative growth. Exospores are particularly resistant to drying, surviving for extended periods, which aids in their dispersal; however, they are relatively easily destroyed by heat, chemicals (e.g., acid), and radiation processes in comparison to bacterial endospores but are clearly more resistant than their vegetative forms. Resistance of exospores to lysozyme, mild acid treatment, heating (moist and dry heat), and desiccation has been shown to be related to many factors. These include desiccation, increased calcium and magnesium concentrations, decreased membrane fluidity, and increased protein amino acids such as glutamic acid, alanine, and glycine. One of the most significant resistance factors is the internal concentration of the disaccharide trehalose. The levels of trehalose can be modified by increasing or decreasing the concentration of sugars (such as glucose) in growth media during spore development; higher concentrations of trehalose have been correlated with increased resistance to heating and chemicals. Overall, the mechanisms of resistance to biocides in exospores have not been investigated in much detail, although further investigations would be of interest.

8.3.12 Revival Mechanisms

Biocidal processes are applied under different situations and in many cases may not be sufficient to allow for the complete inactivation of various target microorganisms. Many of these situations have been described, including limited accessibility of the biocide through cell wall or other microbial surface structures (section 8.2), bacterial endospore development (8.3.11), and when the microorganisms are within biofilms (8.3.8). In many of these cases, damage to the target microorganism occurs but may not be sufficient to render them nonviable (Fig. 8.23).

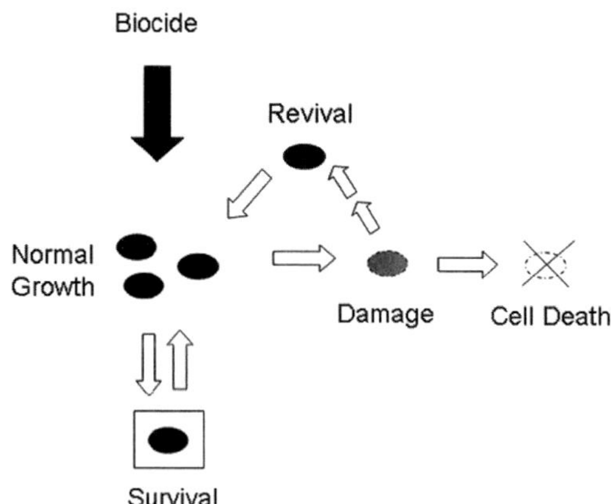

FIGURE 8.23 The potential revival of microorganisms after biocidal treatment. On exposure, microorganisms may survive due to lack of a contact or intrinsic resistance to the biocide. In other cases, the damaged microorganisms can be revived by active repair mechanisms and undergo subsequent growth or infectivity. Damaged microorganisms may therefore be initially uncultivable by normal laboratory methods but remain viable over time. Biocidal effects may also be sufficient to render the microorganism unviable (cell death or loss of infectivity).

Biocidal damage may be tolerated by the microorganism and in some cases repaired to allow for subsequent growth. These "revival" mechanisms can contribute to intrinsic resistance to biocides or biocidal processes because they allow microorganisms to recover over time. They are also important to consider in the evaluation of the efficacies of disinfection or sterilization processes (chapter 1, section 1.4.2), because injured microorganisms (particularly bacterial spores) may not initially grow on or in recovery media at the same rate as untreated cultures but can demonstrate growth over a greater time period or under the right environmental conditions. Examples of revival mechanisms are described in Table 8.15.

Revival mechanisms have been particularly studied in the recovery of bacterial endospores from moist-heat treatment, but also following radiation, dry-heat, and some chemical sporicidal methods (e.g., hydrogen peroxide). Studies have shown that the recovery of spores following these treatments can be increased by various growth medium factors and conditions. These include the composition of

TABLE 8.15 Examples of revival mechanisms that have been described following biocidal exposure

Revival mechanism	Comments
Cell wall/membrane regeneration	Described in fungi and bacteria, including known mechanisms of enterococcal resistance to antibiotics and in alcohol resistance in yeast and bacteria
Nucleic acid repair	Identified in all prokaryotes and eukaryotes in response to DNA damage by radiation and some chemical biocides; extremely efficient in some bacteria such as *Deinococcus* (section 8.3.9)
Heat shock response	Repair of damage to various cellular components in bacteria and fungi, including DNA repair mechanisms and macromolecular regeneration (section 8.3.3)
Growth medium or condition factors	Described in the recovery of endospores and some vegetative bacteria in the revival of heat, radiation, and chemical treatments
Viral reassociation or cooperation	Multiplicity reactivation in bacteriophages and other viruses, e.g., herpes simplex virus (demonstrated under laboratory conditions)

the recovery medium, pH, temperature, and incubation time. This was first described in the recovery of *Clostridium botulinum* spores, which were found to be more fastidious than untreated spores, requiring various medium supplements to support their recovery. This was subsequently found to be common to all bacteria sporeformers. Examples include the increased recovery of *B. atrophaeus* spores in media supplemented with amino acids (glycine, threonine, or homoserine) and sodium bicarbonate (a known germination stimulant) with *Clostridium* spores. The incubation temperature is another consideration. In one respect, the recovery of endospores and vegetative cells (including *E. coli* and *S. aureus*) has been shown to be greater when incubated at a temperature below the known optimal temperatures for the untreated bacterial culture. For example, in some studies with *Geobacillus stearothermophilus* endospores, greater survival was observed when cultures were grown at 45 to 50°C instead of the normal optimal temperature of ~55°C. In other reports, the heat shock of various heat- and chemically treated spores at 70 to 80°C for a number of minutes was also shown to increase recovery.

It is not known why these treatments aid in spore revival, but in the case of lower growth temperatures, this may be associated with a lower initial metabolic rate to allow for efficient repair of any damage. An alternative explanation of some of these findings has been proposed for aldehyde-treated spores. Increased revival of glutaraldehyde- and formaldehyde-treated spores has been shown by treatment with hydroxides (NaOH and KOH) and, in some cases, heat shock, but not with spores treated by iodine, chlorine, or hydrogen peroxide. Considering the cross-linking mode of action of aldehydes (chapter 7, section 7.4.3), it has been proposed that recovery may not be due to any true specific repair mechanism(s) but to the release of viable spores that are protected within cross-linked masses of spores and their associated debris. During exposure to aldehydes it is possible that viable spores become entrapped within these masses and are not released for growth until physical or chemical disruption occurs. Similar explanations may be considered for the recovery of heat- and chemically treated endospores. Mechanisms of revival have not been studied with fungal spores or other dormant microbial forms, which are generally less resistant than bacterial spores.

Exposure to sublethal concentrations of biocides damages bacteria and fungi but also activates various stress responses (section 8.3.3). These stress responses include repair mechanisms that allow injured cells to recover from biocide damage. Radiation, in particular UV, damage repair mechanisms have been described in some detail and have been identified in most prokaryotes and eukaryotes. Although these mechanisms are normally present in cells, they are upregulated in response to DNA damage, e.g., during the SOS response in *E. coli* (section 8.3.3). Two major repair mechanisms have been identified: excision repair and photoreactivation. Excision repair involves the removal of various DNA photoproducts (including pyrimidine dimers) that are formed on exposure to radiation by incisions on either side of the lesion, removal of the damage, and replacement of the DNA sequence. The mechanisms of repair are similar in prokaryotes and eukaryotes but involve different enzymes. Photoreactivation (which requires light) involves the repair of dimers via photolyase enzymes. The repair of DNA lesions affords some recovery of exposed cells, depending on the extent of damage, although it should be noted that radiation methods cause damage to other macromolecules in addition to DNA (see chapter 7, section 7.4.4). In addition to radiation, DNA repair mechanisms may also play a role in repairing damage in bacterial spores from certain oxidizing agents such as hydrogen peroxide gas, which appears to be particularly targeted against endospore core DNA (see section 7.4.2).

Another mechanism of revival, which has been observed in bacteria and fungi, concerns the regeneration of the cell wall and membrane. Because these structures are the front line in any biocide attack, a significant amount of damage can be observed even at sublethal concentrations of biocides. The ability to regenerate damaged cell walls has been shown by the generation of bacterial protoplasts (cell wall-deficient forms) under laboratory conditions; protoplasts have been found to be very sensitive to various biocides but subsequently increase their tolerance on redevelopment of the cell wall.

Because viruses are nonmetabolizing, they are not expected to directly express mechanisms of active repair to biocidal damage. Despite this, radiation-damaged DNA viruses (e.g., herpes simplex viruses and bacteriophages) have been shown to be repaired by host cell mechanisms following infection. Further studies have found that suspensions of damaged or disintegrated viruses or viral components can cooperate in a phenomenon known as "multiplicity reactivation" to allow for the infection of cells; this appears to occur at a high concentration of virus under laboratory conditions, and its environmental or clinical significance is unknown.

8.4 INTRINSIC RESISTANCE OF MYCOBACTERIA

Mycobacteria are well known to demonstrate resistance to biocides that is roughly intermediate between other nonsporulating bacteria and bacterial spores (see Fig. 8.1). This is particularly the case with chemical biocides, because mycobacteria do not present dramatically higher resistance to moist-heat inactivation in comparison to other vegetative bacteria (see chapter 2, section 2.2). For example, *Mycobacterium avium* is considered one of the more resistant strains but was readily inactivated by heat in the 60 to 70°C range, with efficacy increasing as the temperature increased (as described for other bacteria). As a note of caution, many reports in the literature suggest higher resistance levels of mycobacteria, but many of these studies on reinvestigation were found to be related to test methodology and not related to specific intrinsic tolerance of mycobacteria to heat. On the other hand, mycobacteria do demonstrate particular resistance to chemical biocides. The most likely mechanism for the high resistance of mycobacteria is their complex cell walls, which provide an effective barrier to the entry of biocides. The mycobacterial cell wall is a highly hydrophobic structure with a mycoylarabinogalactan-peptidoglycan skeleton (Fig. 8.24).

The peptidoglycan is covalently linked to a polysaccharide copolymer (arabinogalactan, made up of arabinose and galactose) and esterified to long-chain-length lipids known as mycolic acids (see chapter 1, section 1.3.4.1). The cell wall can also include various complex lipids, lipopolysaccharides, and proteins, including those that form porin channels through which hydrophilic molecules can diffuse into the cell. Similar cell wall structures exist in all the mycobacterial species examined to date, but they vary in structural components within species and strains. The cell wall composition of a particular species or strain is also found to be influenced by its environmental niche.

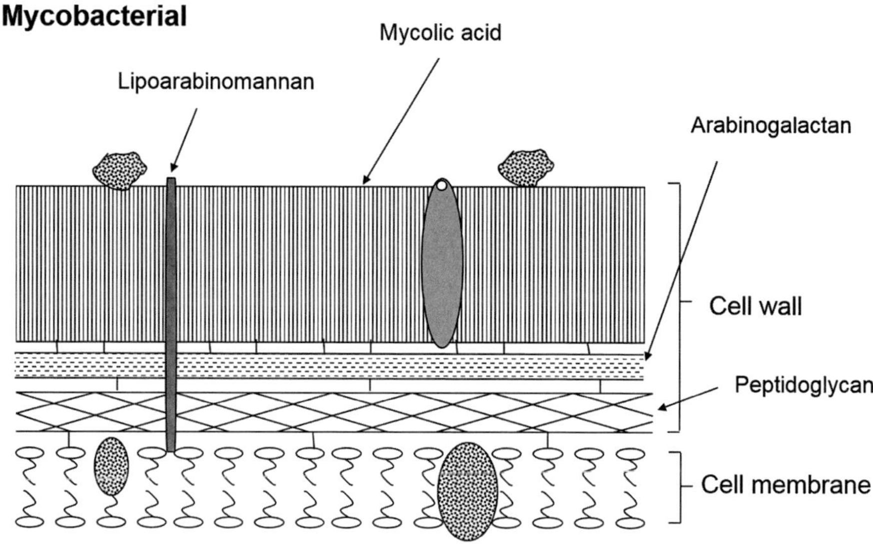

FIGURE 8.24 A representation of the mycobacterial cell wall structure.

More commonly described pathogenic bacteria such as *M. tuberculosis* and *M. bovis* have typically been studied in relatively nutrient-rich environments, whereas many atypical (or nontuberculosis) mycobacteria (e.g., *M. chelonae* and *M. fortuitum*) have been studied in often nutrient-poor conditions such as environmental surfaces or water and are often described to be more intrinsically resistant to anti-infective drugs and biocides.

Biocides that can exhibit mycobacterial activity include phenolics, peracetic acid, hydrogen peroxide, alcohols, and aldehydes. By contrast, other well-known bactericidal agents such as chlorhexidine and QACs are mycobacteristatic even when employed at high concentrations. However, their activities can be substantially increased by formulation effects. Thus, a number of QAC-based formulated products claim to have mycobacterial activity over time. Similarly, the activity of low concentrations of hydrogen peroxide can be significantly enhanced under acidic conditions, in comparison to neutral or alkaline formulations. It has been proposed that the resistance of mycobacteria to QACs was related to the unique lipid content of the cell wall. In support of this contention, *Mycobacterium phlei*, with a low total cell lipid content, was found to be more sensitive to QACs than *M. tuberculosis*, which has a higher lipid content. Others noted that the resistance of various species of mycobacteria correlated with the overall content of lipid material in their walls. It has been described that, because of the highly hydrophobic nature of the cell wall, hydrophilic-type biocides are generally unable to penetrate the mycobacterial cell wall in sufficiently high concentrations to produce a lethal effect. However, low concentrations of biocides such as chlorhexidine must presumably traverse this permeability barrier because minimal concentrations inhibiting growth (MIC values) are of the same order as those concentrations inhibiting the growth of nonmycobacterial strains such as *S. aureus*, although *Mycobacterium avium-intracellulare* is found to be particularly tolerant.

The other component(s) of the mycobacterial cell wall that contribute to high biocide resistance are largely unknown, although some information is available. Inhibitors of cell wall synthesis increase the susceptibility of *M. avium* to drugs; inhibition of glycolipids, arabinogalactan, and mycolic acid biosynthesis also enhances drug susceptibility. Treatment of this organism with *m*-fluoro-DL-phenylalanine (*m*-FL-phe), which inhibits glycolipid synthesis, produces significant alterations in the outer cell wall layers. Ethambutol, an antibiotic inhibitor of arabinogalactan and phospholipid synthesis, also disorganizes these layers. In addition, ethambutol induces the formation of dead cells without the dissolution of peptidoglycan ("ghost" cells). Methyl-4-(2-octadecylcyclopropen-1-yl) butanoate (MOCB) is a structural analogue of a key precursor in mycolic acid synthesis. Thus, effects of MOCB on mycolic acid synthesis and *m*-FL-phe and ethambutol on outer wall biosynthetic processes leading to changes in cell wall architecture appear to be responsible for increasing the intracellular concentration of chemotherapeutic drugs. These findings support the concept of the overall cell wall structure acting as a permeability barrier to various drugs. Fewer studies have been conducted of the mechanisms involved in the resistance of mycobacteria to biocides. However, the activity of chlorhexidine and of a QAC, cetylpyridinium chloride, against *M. avium* and *M. tuberculosis* can be potentiated in the presence of ethambutol. From these data it may be inferred that arabinogalactan is another cell wall component that acts as a permeability barrier to chlorhexidine and QACs.

Other general mechanisms of resistance have been described but have not been investigated in detail with a range of biocides. Mycobacteria, because of their hydrophobic nature, have a tendency to form clumps on surfaces due to cell aggregation; this is seen during human and animal infections with mycobacteria with the production on localized granulomas, consisting of cell clumps and other materials due to reactions with the immune system. These can often be difficult to treat with antibiotics due to lack of penetration and are equally more difficult for chemical biocides to penetrate. Environmental bacteria are commonly found in water systems and can produce persistent biofilms, with their associated intrinsic resistance profiles (see section 8.3.8). Recent research has focused on the impact of stationary-phase phenomena in resistance profiles. Mycobacteria have various stationary-phase effects that are known to contribute to partial tolerance to biocides. These include enzyme production (such as catalases and peroxidases), increased DNA repair, changes in structure, and reduced metabolism. In some studies, mycobacterial cultures that have entered into stationary phase are eventually reduced to a smaller population of persister cells that are in a low metabolic and nonreplicative state. These appear to be dormant forms and have been described to have greater heat tolerance (surviving 65°C). In some investigations with old cultures of *M. marinum*, *M. bovis*, and *M. avium*, it has been suggested that dormant forms have unique structures that allow greater tolerance to heat and enzymes, but their resistance profiles to a wider range of biocides have not been investigated in detail. Reports have suggested that these forms may be types of spores based on their heat resistance and microscopic structural analysis, but this proposal could not be verified by other investigators to date.

A final mechanism of resistance is the ability of mycobacteria to survive and sometimes multiply within amoeba such as *Acanthamoeba castellanii* and *Acanthamoeba polyphaga*. The successful relationship, from the mycobacterial point of view, to allow for survival and growth, depends on the specific species of mycobacteria and amoeba (or other protozoa). In addition to many strains of atypical mycobacteria that have been found to survive in amoebae (such as *M. avium*, *Mycobacterium kansasii*, and *Mycobacterium abscessus*), *Mycobacterium leprae* (the pathogen in leprosy and notoriously recalcitrant to laboratory manipulation) has been successfully cultured under laboratory conditions using amoebae. Survival within amoebae provides a mechanism of protection against biocides and other environmental stresses, where amoebae are considered the "Trojan horses" of microbial environments. This is a greater concern on vegetative amoebal development into dormant cysts, which are known to be highly resistant to many chemical biocides. Many of these mechanisms are not unique to mycobacteria and are further considered in section 8.11.

Certain strains of mycobacteria have been shown to have particularly high levels of resistance to aldehyde-based disinfectants, including glutaraldehyde and *o*-phthalaldehyde (OPA). Mycobacteria, due to their high level of intrinsic resistance to chemical disinfectants, are often used to verify high-level disinfection effectiveness for use in clinical practice (see chapter 1, section 1.4.4); high-level disinfectants are considered effective against all microbial pathogens, including mycobacteria, with the exception of large numbers of bacterial spores. Therefore, the identification of mycobacterial strains that were significantly resistant to high concentrations of aldehydes was not only surprising but also led to disinfection failure and the transmission of pathogenic mycobacteria from one patient to another. It is unknown if these strains are intrinsically resistant to these biocides or have developed resistance over time due to repeated exposure to aldehydes. The first of these strains was described in the 1990s as *Mycobacterium chelonae* isolates. They were found to be water-based and could be repeatedly isolated from flexible endoscopes and washer-disinfectors using glutaraldehyde-based chemical disinfectants to reprocess the endoscopes between patient uses. They were identified from investigations into the source of transmission to patients who had infections or were found to be contaminated with these bacteria. One such (presumably mutant) strain was remarkably not killed even after a 60-minute exposure to 2% alkaline glutaraldehyde; in contrast, a reference (wild type) strain showed an expected 5-$\log_{10}$ reduction after a contact time of 10 minutes. These glutaraldehyde-resistant *M. chelonae* strains had a slightly increased tolerance to peracetic acid, but not to sodium dichloroisocyanurate or to a phenolic disinfectant. Similar strains were subsequently identified from many countries. Other investigators have observed an above-average resistance of *M. chelonae* to glutaraldehyde and formaldehyde but not to peracetic acid. OPA, another aldehyde used for high-level chemical disinfection (see chapter 3, section 3.4), was also found to be less effective against these strains, but more effective than glutaraldehyde over time. Subsequent studies have shown that glutaraldehyde resistance can vary considerably, with some strains demonstrating cross-tolerance to OPA and others not. One stable glutaraldehyde-resistant strain of *M. chelonae* was found to be cross-resistant to many antibiotics used to treat atypical mycobacterial infections.

Although they are uncommon pathogens, atypical mycobacteria cause serious infections in immunocompromised patients or persistent infections when accidentally introduced into normally sterile tissues (e.g., during surgery). Anti-infective treatment of these infections is difficult due to these mycobacteria's intrinsic resistance to antibiotics, but the glutaraldehyde strains were even further resistant to some last-line antibiotics such as clarithromycin, tetracycline, and linezolid. In addition, this strain was found to have a slower growth rate and decreased glucose uptake compared to wild-type strains. These results suggested that resistance was related to changes in cell wall structure and potentially due to reduced uptake of glutaraldehyde by these *M. chelonae* strains. *M. chelonae* is also known to adhere strongly to smooth surfaces, which may render cells within a biofilm less susceptible to disinfectants, and this may increase the potential for development of tolerance by mutation at sublethal concentrations of biocides. Studies with a collection of *M. smegmatis* cell wall-associated mutants found that mutants with reduced mycolic acid content had an increased susceptibility to both glutaraldehyde and OPA, suggesting that the outer mycolic acid structure was a major resistance factor to these biocides. But mutants lacking the significant porin proteins (MspA and MspC) associated with outer cell wall structure were found to be highly resistant to the biocides. These results would also explain the decreased growth rates and glucose uptake in some resistant strains, including *M. chelonae*.

The analysis of porin genes in *M. chelonae*-resistant strains showed evidence of mutations in porin genes that would only produce truncated proteins, and the laboratory introduction of a plasmid containing a porin gene reversed the aldehyde-resistance phenotype. Overall, the lack or reduced expression of surface-associated porin genes is at least one of the major mechanisms of resistance to glutaraldehyde and OPA in mycobacteria. Because porins are involved in the influx and efflux of molecules (including biocide) from the cell, and efflux is a known mechanism of biocide resistance (see section 8.3.4), it may be that aldehyde resistance is also due to active efflux; however, this would seem unlikely given the protein cross-linking mechanism of action of aldehydes (see chapter 7, section 7.4.3). It is more probable that the lack of porin expression in mycobacteria, as a major protein component of the normal outer cell wall, causes a rearrangement of the cell wall structure (predominantly composed of mycolic acids) and a lack of protein-reactive sites for the aldehydes on the cell surface. This is also possible due to the increased sensitivity of mycobacteria to aldehydes in the presence of reduced mycolic acid concentrations on the cell wall surface.

Other species of environmental mycobacteria have subsequently been found to have higher than expected resistance profiles to glutaraldehyde (*Mycobacterium avium*, *Mycobacterium gordonae*, and *Mycobacterium massiliense*) and OPA (such as *M. abscessus* and *M. fortuitum* isolates). The *M. massiliense* isolates are a particular concern because they were associated with large health care-associated infection outbreaks (>1,000 patients at multiple health care facilities) related to the use of contaminated flexible endoscopes. The endoscopes had been disinfected with glutaraldehyde between patient uses and were linked to the sources of the outbreak. Investigators found that these isolates were highly resistant to glutaraldehyde solutions but varied in resistance profiles over time, with some strains demonstrating little to no efficacy in up to 7% glutaraldehyde solutions. These strains also had slower growth rates, reduced glucose update, and increased resistance to antibiotics in comparison to reference strains. The outbreak strains were found to have greater persistence in tissues such as the lungs and spleen in comparison to a reference strain when introduced into an experimental animal model, suggesting increased virulence. There was no evidence of cross-resistance to OPA or oxidizing agents, but attempts to understand the mechanism of resistance in these strains have been unsuccessful to date. Biochemical analysis of their cell walls did not identify any obvious changes in their component structures, and sequence analysis of their porin genes did not show any obvious signs of mutation. These results suggest that other mechanisms of resistance remain to be elucidated. There is some speculation that the mechanisms may be plasmid-mediated. To date, specific plasmid- or transposon-mediated resistance to biocides has not been confirmed in mycobacteria, but it has been speculated (in consideration of other bacteria; see section 8.7.3).

8.5 INTRINSIC RESISTANCE OF OTHER GRAM-POSITIVE BACTERIA

Gram-positive, vegetative bacteria are generally found to be less resistant to biocides or biocidal processes in comparison to other microorganisms (see Fig. 8.1). Examples of some intrinsic resistance mechanisms have been described, including stationary-phase responses, stress responses, enzyme production (e.g., catalase production in *S. aureus*), efflux mechanisms, capsule and biofilm production, and spore production (in *Bacillus* spp.). In contrast to the mycobacterial cell wall structure, the typical Gram-positive bacteria cell wall does not appear to be an effective barrier to biocides. The cell wall structure has been particularly well studied in some staphylococci, but overall similar structures have been described for other bacteria with classical Gram-positive staining characteristics. The structure is composed essentially of an inner cell membrane associated with a thick coat of peptidoglycan (organized in layers) and teichoic acids (Fig. 8.25). Peptidoglycan is anchored to the cell membrane by diacylglycerol (a glyceride consisting of two fatty acid glycerol molecules). About 90% of the cell wall consists of pep-

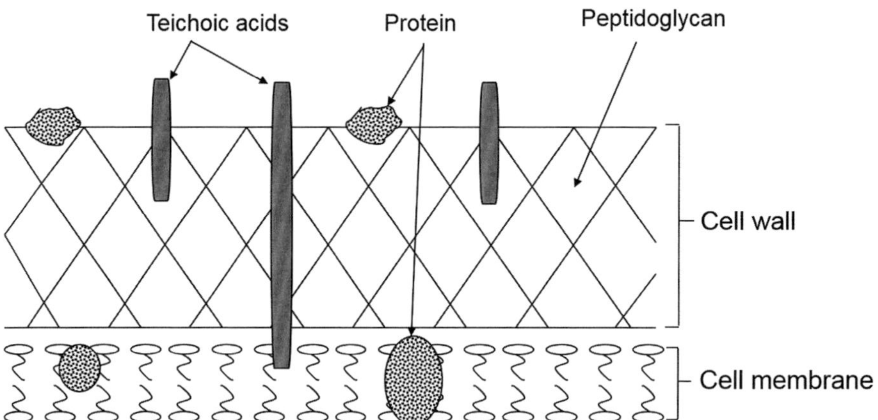

FIGURE 8.25 A representation of a typical Gram-positive bacterial cell wall structure.

tidoglycan and teichoic acids, with the remaining 10% being proteins or other materials. The teichoic acids are a major component (~30 to 50%) of the structure and consist of two types: teichoic acids coupled to the peptidoglycan and lipoteichoic acids anchored to the cell membrane. Many subtle differences from this basic structure have been described in Gram-positive bacteria to include differences in peptidoglycan cross-linking, types and extents of teichoic acids, and types of associated proteins. Many Gram-positive bacteria have branched peptides in their peptidoglycan structures, but these are not observed in *B. subtilis*. Associated proteins can include the adhesins, which are involved in attachment to surfaces (including the skin, mucous membranes, and environmental surfaces). Despite the structure and thickness of peptidoglycan, the wall has not been found to be an effective barrier to the entry of various biocides, but this can vary depending on the genus, species, strain, and stage of growth (correlating with the variable Gram staining of these and other bacteria over time). Since substances of high molecular weight can readily traverse the cell wall of staphylococci and vegetative *Bacillus* spp., this possibly explains the sensitivity of these organisms to many antibacterial agents including QACs and chlorhexidine.

The plasticity of the bacterial cell wall is a well-known phenomenon, observed as differences in size and shape during various growth phases. The growth rate and lack of any growth-limiting nutrient affect the physiological state of the cells. Under such circumstances, the thickness and degree of cross-linking of peptidoglycan are modified, and hence cellular sensitivity to various biocides may be altered. For example, the sensitivity of *Bacillus megaterium* cells to chlorhexidine and 2-phenoxyethanol is altered when changes in growth rate and nutrient limitation are made in actively multiplying cultures. However, lysozyme-induced protoplasts of these cells remained sensitive to, and were lysed by, these membrane-active agents. "Fattened" cells of *S. aureus* that are produced by repeated subculturing in glycerol-containing media also showed changes in their surface structure and were found to be more resistant to alkyl phenolics and some antibiotics such as benzylpenicillin; subculture of these cells in routine culture media resulted in reversion to biocide sensitivity. Thus, the cell wall in whole cells appears to be responsible for their modified response to biocides.

Many Gram-positive bacteria (including *Staphylococcus*, *Enterococcus*, and *Streptococcus*) produce capsules external to the cell wall, which as previously discussed can provide some level of tolerance to biocides (e.g., under preservative concentrations). The impact of cell wall changes and production of exopolysaccharides have been speculated to play a role in resistance to oxidizing agents. For example, Gram-positive bacteria were found to have persisted in washer-disinfectors using chlorine dioxide for chemical disinfection. These include *B. subtilis*, *Micrococcus luteus*, *Streptococcus* spp., and *Staphylococcus intermedius*. Laboratory investigations showed that at least two of these strains had stable tolerance mechanisms to chlorine dioxide. The *B. subtilis* isolate was tolerant to liquid chlorine dioxide, hydrogen peroxide, and peracetic acid in comparison to reference strains but was inactivated at longer exposure times and high concentrations of each biocide. The presence of endospore development was ruled out in these investigations as being responsible for tolerance. Microscopic analysis showed that this strain was heavily encapsulated with exopolysaccharide. The *M. luteus* isolate was more tolerant only to chlorine dioxide (and not other oxidizing agents), and this strain was found to be oversized (not dissimilar to the fattened *S. aureus* effects described above) and to grow in closely associated cell clumps. Despite further investigations with both strains to understand their specific mechanisms of action, the true causes of tolerance could not be identified. For example, the *B. subtilis* isolate was specifically investigated for the roles of cell aggregation, presence of exopolysaccharide, and overexpression of detoxification enzymes, but none of these were linked to the resistance profile. It is therefore likely that other mechanisms of resistance are responsible, which may include subtle changes in cell wall structure or cytoplasm-based protective mechanisms.

Enterococcus spp. have been a particular area of interest due to their known intrinsic tolerance to heat in comparison to other vegetative bacteria and their persistence in pasteurized food products. Even within this genus, the *D* values for different *Enterococcus* spp. at 72°C were found to vary from 0.3 to 5 minutes.

There is a close association between the presence of enterococci under acidic conditions (often present in fruit juices) and heat resistance. Some of the mechanisms involved have been investigated and are similar to those described for the heat shock response (see section 8.3.3). Some proteins (such as acyl carrier proteins involved in fatty acid biosynthesis) are found to be intrinsically more stable at higher temperatures (e.g., up to 80°C) in comparison to similar proteins from other bacteria (e.g., the *E. coli* homologue is inactivated at ~65°C). Thermal resistance of these proteins has been linked to differences in their secondary and tertiary structures, particularly increased hydrophobic interactions and hydroxy bonding between amino acid residues. Heat tolerance is particularly marked during the stationary phase of growth, and mechanisms have included the expression of heat shock proteins such as the chaperones GroEL and DnaK.

Listeria monocytogenes is a Gram-positive rod and, as a pathogen, is the cause of listeriosis, a foodborne illness. It has at least two distinct phases of growth: one more saprophytic, with the bacteria free-living in the general environment, and the other pathogenic, where the bacteria switch to a virulent form and develop intracellularly. Differentiation is thermoregulated, with the bacteria switching from free-living at 30°C and intracellular (or virulence) at 37°C, under gene expression regulation associated with the PrfA protein. The virulent form demonstrates greater adherence capabilities and resistance to phagocytic action. *L. monocytogenes* persistence in food-manufacturing facilities has been specifically linked to increased tolerance to QAC-based disinfectants (see chapter 3, section 3.16). Two types of resistance mechanisms were identified in isolates from these facilities. Some were found to be low-virulence types (found to be *prfA* mutants) and were more resistant to QACs such as benzalkonium chloride; these included overexpression of MFS-type efflux pumps (see section 8.3.4), presumably due to genomic mutations. Another series of isolates contained a transposon (Tn*6188*) that was found to be either associated with a plasmid or on the bacterial genome and specifically expressed a QacH transporter that increased resistance to benzalkonium chloride, some dyes, and other QACs by efflux. The impact of active efflux mechanisms for biocide tolerance in bacteria has been studied in some detail, as both intrinsic (see section 8.3.4 and below) and/or acquired phenomena (see section 8.7.3). Other potential mechanisms of resistance in *Listeria* are its ability to form or be associated with biofilms, as well as a known heat shock response (coordinated by a transcriptional sigma factor, SigB) in a process not dissimilar to that described for *B. subtilis*.

Antibiotic-resistant Gram-positive bacteria, in particular, methicillin-resistant *S. aureus* (MRSA) and vancomycin-resistant *Enterococcus*, are a significant concern in hospitals and other health care facilities. Some reports have suggested that these strains may also have increased tolerance to various antiseptic biocides, in particular, triclosan and chlorhexidine (chapter 4, section 4.6.2). Efflux (or the active pumping of the antimicrobial out of the cell) has been described as a mechanism of acquired tolerance to chlorhexidine and QACs (but not triclosan, to date) in staphylococci and has been linked to cross-resistance to antibiotics in MRSA strains (section 8.7); however, the actual MICs of these biocides have been found to vary considerably and equally in *S. aureus* environmental and clinical isolates. For example, chlorhexidine MICs range from ~0.2 to 20 mg/liter, independent of the presence of methicillin resistance (Table 8.16). These marginal differences may allow certain strains to survive the presence of biocides under residual or preservative concentrations only. There is currently no standard method of determining biocide MICs, and therefore reports in the literature can vary greatly.

The exact mechanisms of resistance in many of these strains have not been studied and may be due to various intrinsic factors as well as acquired by mutation or plasmid/transposon acquisition (section 8.7). Efflux mechanisms have been involved, considering the prevalence in the detection of efflux-associated genes that express for various MFS-type (including SMR and multidrug and toxic compound extrusion) efflux systems in clinical isolates of both MRSA and methicillin-sensitive *S. aureus* (see section 8.3.4); these include the prevalence of the chromosomal expressed *sepA*, *mepA*, and *norA* genes, but also at a lower rate plasmid-encoded *qacAB* and *qacC* genes (see section 8.7.3). Despite these mechanisms, no significant differences have been observed in the bactericidal concentrations of biocides (Table 8.16) or in the bactericidal activity of antiseptic products under in-use conditions. There is no evidence to date that vancomycin-resistant enterococci or enterococci with high-level resistance to aminoglycoside antibiotics are more resistant to biocides than are antibiotic-sensitive enterococcal strains. However, enterococci are generally less sensitive to biocides than staphylococci, and differences in inhibitory and bactericidal concentrations have also been found among enterococcal species.

Various other intrinsic mechanisms of biocide tolerance have been described in Gram-positive bacteria. The development of bacterial endospores in *Bacillus* and *Clostridium* is clearly

TABLE 8.16 Ranges of MICs and MBCs of chlorhexidine and triclosan against *S. aureus* and *Enterococcus* spp. isolates

	MIC (mg/liter)		MBC (mg/liter)	
Strain	Chlorhexidine	Triclosan	Chlorhexidine	Triclosan
S. aureus[a]	0.2–20	0.05–2	20–30	12–20
Enterococcus[b]	1–15	10–15	75	15–20

[a]Including methicillin-sensitive and -resistant (MRSA) isolates.
[b]Including vancomycin-sensitive and -resistant (vancomycin-resistant enterococci) isolates of *Enterococcus faecium* and *E. faecalis*.

an important mechanism (section 8.3.11). Similar to mycobacteria, many types of Gram-positive bacteria have been found to persist and even multiply in amoebae and other protozoa (e.g., this was first described with *L. pneumophila* and subsequently for others such as *Streptococcus* and *Staphylococcus* spp.; see section 8.4). Various staphylococci, including *S. aureus* strains, are mucoid and are surrounded by polysaccharide-rich capsules or slime layers (section 8.3.7). Nonmucoid strains are generally inactivated more rapidly than mucoid ones by some biocides, including QACs and chlorhexidine, but not significantly by others such as phenolics (depending on their concentration). Removal of the capsule or slime layer has been found to render the cell more sensitive, confirming that these layers play an important protective role either as a direct barrier to prevent penetration into the cell or by absorbing or inactivating the biocide.

8.6 INTRINSIC RESISTANCE OF GRAM-NEGATIVE BACTERIA

Gram-negative bacteria are generally more resistant to biocides than are nonsporulating, non-mycobacterial Gram-positive bacteria (Table 8.17).

Based on these data, there is a marked difference in the sensitivities of *S. aureus* and *E. coli* to certain biocides such as QACs (benzalkonium, benzethonium, cetrimide), hexachlorophene, diamidines, and triclosan but little difference in chlorhexidine susceptibility (depending on the range of bacteria tested). *P. aeruginosa* is overall more resistant to all of these agents, including chlorhexidine; other Gram-negative bacteria such as *Proteus* spp. also possess above-average resistance to cationic agents such as chlorhexidine and QACs. Overall, the tolerance varies depending on the bacteria as well as the types of biocide or biocidal process.

Similar to Gram-positive bacteria (see section 8.6), many intrinsic resistance mechanisms have also been described in Gram-negative bacteria, notably in *Pseudomonas*, *Burkholderia*, and *Methylobacterium* spp. that are commonly associated with water and environmental surface cross-contamination. These particularly include stress responses (section 8.3.3), capsule expression (section 8.3.7), biofilm development (section 8.3.8), and both intrinsic and applied efflux resistance mechanisms (sections 8.3.4 and 8.7), which have been particularly well studied in *Pseudomonas* spp. Examples of high levels of acquired biocide resistance in Gram-negative bacteria include tolerance to formaldehyde (section 8.7.3) and heavy metals (e.g., mercury; see section 8.3). Further consideration is given here to the Gram-negative cell wall structure, which acts as a barrier that limits the entry of many chemically unrelated types of antibacterial agents (Fig. 8.26 and introduced in chapter 1, section 1.3.4.1). This is at least partially due to the presence of the outer membrane, which is composed of a lipid bilayer of internal phopsholipids and external-facing glycolipids and LPS, along with associated proteins. The two major classes of proteins present are lipoproteins (with over 100 types

TABLE 8.17 MICs of various biocides (determined in test media) comparing Gram-positive and Gram-negative bacteria

Chemical agent	MIC (mg/liter) for:		
	S. aureus	*E. coli*	*P. aeruginosa*
Benzalkonium chloride	0.5	50	250
Cetrimide	4	16	64–128
Chlorhexidine	0.2–20	1	5–60
o-phenylphenol	100	500	1,000
Propamidine isethionate	2	64	256
Dibromopropamidine isethionate	1	4	32
Triclosan	0.05–2	5	>300

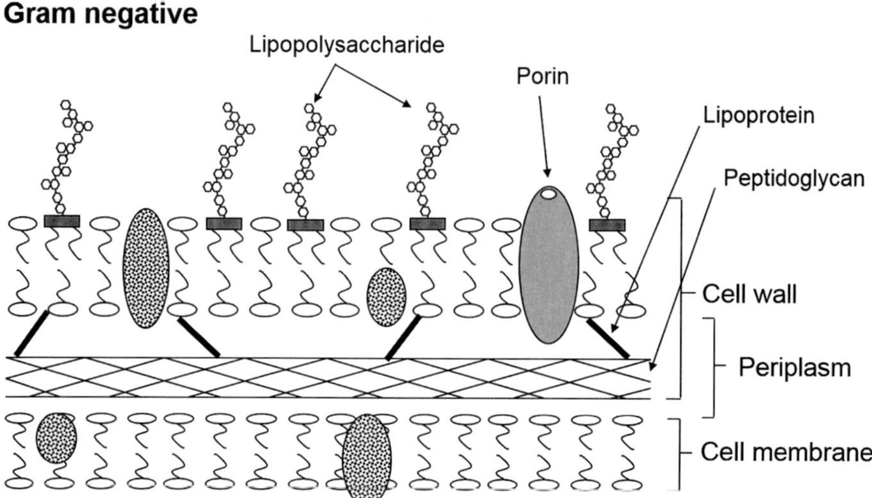

FIGURE 8.26 A representation of a typical Gram-negative bacterial cell wall structure.

identified in *E. coli* alone, generally associated with the inner surface of the membrane) and outer membrane proteins such as the porins OMpF and OmpC (transmembrane proteins) that allow for the passive diffusion of small molecules such as amino acids; other associated proteins can include enzymes (such as proteases and phospholipases).

The outer membrane is considered to provide an effective barrier to biocides, as shown by the differences in observed biocide sensitivities between Gram-positive and Gram-negative bacteria. The outer membrane has significant structural differences between these two types of bacteria; this has been verified in studies of outer membrane mutants of *E. coli*, *Salmonella enterica* serovar Typhimurium and *P. aeruginosa*. In wild-type Gram-negative bacteria, the intact LPS molecules (see chapter 1, section 1.3.7; shown in Figures 1.15 and 8.26) are a major component of the outer membrane. Low-molecular-weight hydrophilic molecules can readily pass through the outer membrane porins into the cells, but hydrophobic molecules are required to diffuse across the outer-membrane bilayer. Outer membranes are known to prevent the access of hydrophobic molecules (including antibiotics and biocides) to the periplasm, presumably due to the LPS molecules providing a highly ordered, limited fluidity structure on the cell surface (which is stabilized by the presence of divalent ions such as Mg^{+2} and Ca^{+2}). In Gram-negative deep-rough mutants, the outer membrane structure is quite distinct, essentially lacking the O-specific side-chains and most of the core polysaccharide of LPS molecules, which are replaced with phospholipid patches. These mutants, with increased surface hydrophobicity, tend to be hypersensitive to hydrophobic antibiotics and biocides, which are normally more effectively excluded from wild-type strains. Some of the possible transport mechanisms for biocides into Gram-negative bacteria are described in Table 8.18.

In addition to these hydrophilic and hydrophobic entry pathways, a third pathway has been proposed for cationic agents such as QACs, biguanides, and diamidines. It is claimed that these damage the outer membrane, thereby promoting their own uptake. Polycations have been found to disorganize the outer membrane of *E. coli*. It must be added, however, that the QACs and diamidines are considerably less active against wild-type than against deep-rough strains, whereas chlorhexidine has the same order of activity (MIC increase about 2- to 3-fold) against both types of *E. coli* strains. However, *S. enterica* serovar Typhimurium outer membrane mutants are more sensitive to chlorhexidine than are wild-

TABLE 8.18 Possible transport mechanisms of some biocides into Gram-negative bacteria

Biocide	Passage across OM[a]	Passage across IM[a]
Chlorhexidine	Self-promoted uptake due to OM damage	IM is a major target site; damage to IM enables biocide to enter cytoplasm, where further interactions occur
QACs	OM may present an important barrier Self-promoted uptake due to OM damage	IM is a major target site; damage to IM enables biocide to enter cytoplasm, where further interaction occurs
Phenolics	Hydrophobic pathway (activity increases as hydrophobicity of phenolic increases)	IM is a major target site, but high phenolic concentrations are shown to coagulate cytoplasmic constituents, suggestion penetration over time

[a]OM, outer membrane; IM, inner membrane.

type strains. External damage to allow for greater penetration of biocides can also be expected for other types of antimicrobials such as the oxidizing agents.

Gram-negative bacteria that often show particularly high levels of resistance to many biocides include *P. aeruginosa*, *B. cepacia*, *Proteus* spp., and *Providencia stuartii*. The outer membrane of *P. aeruginosa* is primarily responsible for its high resistance; in comparison with other organisms, there are notable differences in LPS composition and in the cation content of the outer membrane. The high Mg^{2+} content aids in producing strong LPS-LPS links; furthermore, because of their small size, the porins may not permit general diffusion through them. *B. cepacia* has often been shown to be considerably more resistant in the environment than in artificial culture media; the high content of phosphate-linked arabinose in its LPS decreases the affinity of the outer membrane for polymyxin antibiotics and other cationic and polycationic molecules. Not all pseudomonads are more tolerant, as is the case with *Pseudomonas stutzeri*, which is normally highly sensitive to many biocides, which implies that such agents have little difficulty crossing the outer layers of the cells of this organism. Members of the genus *Proteus* are invariably insensitive to chlorhexidine. Some strains that are highly resistant to chlorhexidine, QACs, EDTA, and diamidines have been isolated from various clinical sources. The presence of a less acidic type of outer membrane LPS could be a contributing factor in its intrinsic resistance. A particularly troublesome member of the genus *Providencia* is *P. stuartii*. Like *Proteus* spp., *P. stuartii* strains have been isolated from urinary tract infections and are intrinsically resistant to different types of biocides including chlorhexidine and QACs. Strains of *P. stuartii* that showed low-level, intermediate, and high-level resistance to chlorhexidine formed the basis of a series of studies of their resistance mechanism(s). Gross differences in the composition of the outer layers of these strains were not detected, although it was concluded that subtle changes in the structural arrangement of the cell wall could be responsible for their resistance.

The peptidoglycan content of Gram-negative bacteria has not been considered a potential barrier to the entry of biocides; this appears likely because the overall peptidoglycan content of these organisms is much less than in Gram-positive bacteria, which are inherently more sensitive to biocides. Nevertheless, there have been instances in which Gram-negative bacteria grown in subinhibitory concentrations of penicillin (which targets peptidoglycan synthesis) have been found to have deficient permeability barriers. Furthermore, penicillin-induced spheroplasts and lysozyme-EDTA-tris "protoplasts" of Gram-negative bacteria are also found to be rapidly lysed by membrane-active agents such as chlorhexidine. It is conceivable that the destabilized nature of both the outer and inner membranes in the absence of peptidoglycan and loss of cell wall integrity is responsible for increased susceptibility to biocides. The peptidoglycan is considered part of the periplasm, which is further packed with many types of proteins that have many cellular roles. The exact roles of these proteins as resistance factors are not known, but it is likely that they interact with many types of biocides (such as low concentrations of oxidizing agents) and limit further penetration into the cell; these effects may be overcome by the presence of sufficient concentrations of the biocide, as well as other factors such as formulation and temperature.

The possibility exists that the cytoplasmic (inner) membrane could be a further mechanism of intrinsic resistance. This membrane is composed of phospholipid and protein mosaic with many associated cellular roles (such as energy production and lipid synthesis) and would also be expected to prevent passive diffusion of hydrophilic molecules. It is also known that changes in the membrane lipid composition affect sensitivity to ethanol in some bacteria. Heat resistance in *Salmonella*, a concern in food-processing and pasteurization, was found to be partially due to changes in cell membrane fatty acid composition. Cultures grown at 45°C were more heat tolerant (with *D* values of ~1 minute at 58°C) than those grown at 35°C (*D* values of ~0.1 minute at 58°C); a similar effect was demonstrated by growing cultures under acidic (pH 4.5) conditions. The heat-tolerant cultures were found to have an overall decrease in membrane fluidity and in the ratio of unsaturated to saturated fatty acids, and the acid-heat-tolerant cultures demonstrated similar changes in fatty acid profiles but also an increase in cyclopropane fatty acids. However, heat tolerance in *Salmonella* is also likely to be multifactorial, to include the impact of the heat shock response (see section 8.3.3).

Chlamydia and *Rickettsia* are Gram-negative bacteria but have been shown to have similar yet distinct differences in their cell wall structures. For example, some *Chlamydia* spp. have a typical Gram-negative cell wall structure, with the exception of having any obvious peptidoglycan layer. To date, disinfection studies have shown that these bacteria are as sensitive (if not more so) as other Gram-negative bacteria, including rapid activity with halogens, alcohols, aldehydes, oxidizing agents, and moist heat at 55°C. Some newly identified strains of chlamydia-like bacteria, such as *Parachlamydia* and *Protochlamydia* spp. present with higher resistance to 55°C but not 65°C. Overall, the biocide sensitivities and any resistance mechanisms in *Chlamydia* and *Rickettsia* have not been studied in much detail, but they can persist in protozoal amoeba vegetative and cyst forms that can protect them from disinfection processes similar to other bacteria (see section 8.11).

Various other factors have been implicated in the intrinsic resistance of Gram-negative bacteria to biocides, including chlorhexidine degradation in *S. marcescens*, *P. aeruginosa*, and *A. xylosoxidans* and biofilm development. Planktonic cultures grown under conditions of nutrient limitation or reduced growth rates have cells with altered sensitivity to biocides, probably as a consequence of modifications in their outer membranes and other stress responses (see sections 8.3.1 and 8.3.3). An example of this was shown with alterations in the composition of outer membrane proteins (such as OmpA, FadL, and LamB) in *E. coli* being associated with increased phenol resistance. Similar to mycobacteria and Gram-positive bacteria, many types of Gram-negative bacteria have been found to persist and even multiply in amoebae and other protozoa (e.g., *P. aeruginosa*, *B. cepacia*, and *E. coli*; see section 8.4). Although the mechanisms of radiation (UV and γ radiation) and desiccation resistance in the Gram-negative bacterium *Methylobacterium radiotolerans* have not been published in detail, some evidence suggests that some of the resistance mechanisms described in *D. radiodurans* (see section 8.3.9) play a role. Of particular interest are proteins involved in the protection and repair of oxidation damage (to essential proteins and DNA) and the production of antioxidants (e.g., a notable pink dye and increased intracellular concentrations of manganese).

Efflux-associated mechanisms have also been well studied in Gram-negative bacteria, both as intrinsic (see section 8.3.4) and acquired (section 8.7) tolerance factors. These can include outer membrane-associated proteins (e.g., OmpA) and transmembrane efflux systems (e.g., AcrA/B-TolC). Although the impact of efflux as a mechanism of resistance to antibiotics is known to be significant, due to increased antibiotic MICs and clinical failure, the impact of cross-resistance to biocides alone is often debated. What is clear is that the presence of biocides can be associated with the upregulation of efflux mechanisms, as well as the selection of efflux resistance mutants or plasmid/transposon-acquired resistance, with immediate impacts on the efficacy of antibiotics. Further, at low (or residual) levels of biocides in various industrial or medical applications (particularly with triclosan, QACs, and antimicrobial dyes), there is mounting evidence that Gram-negative bacteria with either intrinsic or acquired efflux mechanisms are linked with their persistence in various environments. An example of this was described in dairy applications, with strains of *Escherichia* and *Enterobacter* spp. being routinely identified in the environment following the use of a QAC-based disinfectant and showing broad-spectrum resistance to biocides (QACs and triclosan) and antibiotics; resistance was particularly associated with AcrB and MdfA efflux pumps. More types of efflux pumps continue to be identified in Gram-negative bacteria such as the *Acinetobacter baumannii* AceI transporter, a new type of efflux pump known as proteobacterial antimicrobial compound efflux, which increases tolerance to chlorhexidine and certain types of QACs and antimicrobial dyes.

8.7 ACQUIRED BACTERIAL RESISTANCE MECHANISMS

8.7.1 Introduction

As introduced in section 8.3, microorganisms demonstrate intrinsic variability in their response to chemical and physical antimicrobial processes. For example, alcohols are rapidly bactericidal, fungicidal, and virucidal but demonstrate little to no effect on bacterial spores (chapter 3, section 3.5). Similarly, Gram-positive bacteria and enveloped viruses are particularly sensitive to QACs, which have less activity against Gram-negative bacteria, fungi, and mycobacteria (section 3.16). Microorganisms are expected to change in their resistance to biocides depending on various intrinsic factors discussed earlier in this chapter. But in recent years there have been growing concerns about the ability of microorganisms to stably adapt to the presence of biocides by acquiring various resistance mechanisms. This has been particularly well described in bacteria with antibiotics and other chemotherapeutic drugs, which overall demonstrate much narrower spectra of activity (see chapter 7, section 7.2).

Antibiotics are generally only effective against bacteria, due to the presence of specific targets and lack of these targets in other microorganisms. If we consider the β-lactam antibiotic penicillin, the mode of action is specific to peptidoglycan biosynthesis (Fig. 8.27).

Penicillin specifically binds to and inhibits the penicillin-binding proteins (PBPs), which are associated with the cytoplasmic membrane and specifically involved in the building and cross-linking of peptidoglycan. Most Gram-positive bacteria are sensitive to penicillin, which has generally less activity against Gram-negative bacteria, despite the presence of peptidoglycan and PBPs. The overall therapeutic effect of penicillin is to restrict the growth of sensitive bacteria at relatively low concentrations of the antibiotic by preventing cell wall biosynthesis. Intrinsic bacterial resistance to penicillin is primarily due to decreased uptake of the antibiotic and/or the presence of enzymes (β-lactamases) that degrade it. These mechanisms of resistance are not dissimilar to those that have been described for some biocides (section 8.3); however, it is clear that penicillin is not effective against microorganisms that do not contain peptidoglycan such as fungi and viruses. In addition, with the widespread use of penicillin, various bacterial acquired resistance mechanisms have been identified and investigated. These have arisen due to various mutations and acquisition of genetic material in the form of plasmids or transposons.

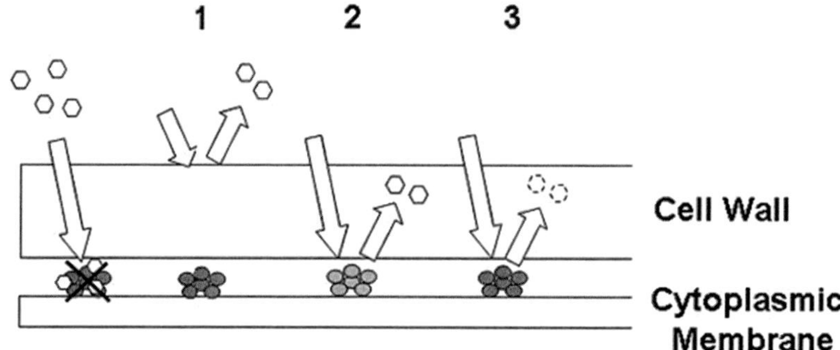

FIGURE 8.27 The primary mechanisms of action of penicillin and of bacterial resistance to it. The antibiotic normally penetrates through the cell wall to the cytoplasmic membrane-associated penicillin-binding proteins (PBPs) and disrupts their role in the synthesis of the cell wall peptidoglycan (shown on the left). The first mechanism of resistance **(1)** is exclusion from the cell, which can be intrinsic or acquired. In the second **(2)** the target PBPs have mutated to become less sensitive to penicillin binding. The third **(3)** is the presence (naturally, induced, or otherwise acquired) of β-lactamases, which hydrolyze the antibiotic.

Mutations are inherited changes in the nucleotide sequence of nucleic acids that can result in altered structures and functions within a microorganism. In the case of penicillin, an important example of the effects of genetic mutations is the direct modification of the structure of the PBPs, changing their affinity for the antibiotic. In these cases, mutations in the PBP gene lead to changes in the primary amino acid sequence of the protein and subsequent adoption of a secondary structure that is not susceptible to penicillin. Other mutational effects can include the loss of proteins (including the outer membrane porin proteins in Gram-positive bacteria, thereby restricting access to the inner cell membrane and location of the PBPs) and the overexpression of proteins due to the loss of transcriptional control. Examples of protein overexpression include the PBPs (sequestering the effect of the antibiotic) and β-lactamases (demonstrating greater degradation of the antibiotic; Fig. 8.27).

Plasmids and transposons are transmissible genetic elements that can be transferred between bacteria. They have been primarily studied in bacteria but have been identified in archaea and in eukaryotes. Plasmids are extrachromosomal DNA molecules that replicate independently within the cell and separate to the chromosomal DNA, although in some cases a plasmid can insert (or integrate) into the chromosome (so-called episomes). Plasmids have been found to encode for various functions, including their replication, virulence determinants, degradative enzymes (e.g., against toluene and salicylic acid), and other resistance mechanisms to antibiotics and biocides. They can be transferred between cells by three basic mechanisms: transformation, conjugation, and transduction. Transformation involves the ability of the cell to naturally take up plasmids from the environment (e.g., during the stationary phase of growth in *Bacillus*). Conjugation involves direct cell-to-cell contact, and this ability is encoded by the plasmid itself. Finally, transduction involves the transfer of the plasmid or genetic material by virus (in the case of bacteria, bacteriophage) transfer. Transposons (or transposable elements) are similar to plasmids because they are also mobile genetic (DNA) sequences, but they are typically not capable of autonomous replication. Transposons are capable of inserting ("transposing") into the host chromosome or plasmids, thereby replicating as part of those genetic elements. Similar to plasmids, transposons contain various sequences that encode for essential functions (e.g., enzymes involved in the transposition process), as well as antibiotic and biocide resistance mechanisms. Mechanisms of resistance to antibiotics are encoded and can be transferred between bacteria on plasmids and transposons. Using the example of the β-lactams, β-lactamases (Fig. 8.27) are plasmid or transposon-encoded and can be transferred between bacteria to confer penicillin resistance. Examples of other acquired mechanisms of resistance to antimicrobial drugs are given in Table 8.19.

Despite less specific mechanisms of action, acquired resistance to biocides has been described and is discussed in more detail in the following sections. Some of these biocide resistance mechanisms may unfortunately also demonstrate increased (or cross) resistance to antibiotics. It is important at this stage to differentiate between increased tolerance and resistance to biocides. Tolerance refers to a decreased effect of a biocide against a target microorganism, typically requiring increased concentrations or dose to be effective. Resis-

TABLE 8.19 Acquired resistance mechanisms to antimicrobial drugs

Antimicrobial agents	Resistance	Examples
Antibacterials		
Sulfonamides	Chromosomal	Mutations in dihydropteroate synthetase with lower affinity for the antibiotic
	Plasmid	Expression of antibiotic-resistant synthetases
Rifampicin	Chromosomal	Mutations in target β-subunit of bacterial RNA polymerase, which are less sensitive to the antibiotic
Aminoglycosides	Chromosomal	Mutations in the sequence of ribosomal proteins and loss of the antibiotic-binding site
	Plasmid or transposon	Expression of enzymes that modify the antibiotic, e.g., acetyltransferases
Tetracyclines	Chromosomal	Mutational loss of outer-membrane proteins and reduced penetration of the antibiotic
	Plasmid or transposon	Expression of efflux proteins
β-lactams	Chromosomal	Mutational changes in the structure of target penicillin-binding proteins and less affinity for the antibiotic
		Mutational loss of outer membrane proteins and less penetration of the antibiotic
	Chromosomal, plasmid, or transposon	β-lactamase expression which degrades the antibiotic
Antivirals		
Viral polymerase inhibitors, including reverse transcriptases (e.g., zidovudine) and DNA polymerases	Nucleic acid	Single or multiple mutations in the polymerase structure with less affinity for the antiviral
Protease inhibitors (e.g., saquinavir)	Nucleic acid	Single or multiple mutations in the polymerase structure with less affinity for the antiviral drug
Antifungals		
Flucytosine	Chromosomal	Loss or mutation in enzymes involved in the uptake, metabolism, or incorporation of the drug into RNA
Polyenes, e.g., amphotericin	Chromosomal	Membrane alterations (e.g., reduced content of ergosterol)
Azoles, e.g., ketoconazole	Chromosomal	Cell membrane changes
		Increased expression of efflux pumps
		Mutations in target enzymes in ergosterol synthesis (e.g., demethylases)

tance is the inability of the biocide or biocidal process to be effective against a target microorganism and, in the case of acquired resistance, would have been previously expected for that microorganism. An example of this difference can be explained with MIC analysis, which determines the level of an antimicrobial that inhibits the growth of a microorganism. With antibiotics (and other anti-infective drugs), an increase in MIC has significant clinical consequences, often indicating that the target microorganism is simply unaffected by its antimicrobial action. This is also practically true if the change in MIC is sufficient to allow survival of the microorganism at typical therapeutic concentrations that cannot be further increased due to toxicological concerns. Unlike antibiotics, a significant increase in MIC to a biocide (due to intrinsic or acquired mechanisms of tolerance) does not necessarily correlate with therapeutic or functional failure. In these cases, it is important to consider that microorganisms may naturally vary in their inhibitory (e.g., bacteriostatic) concentrations to biocides but not in their biocidal (e.g., bactericidal) concentrations. Also, the way that biocides are used is different from anti-infective drugs, such as their concentrations used in products, direct product application, formulation and process effects, etc.

8.7.2 Mutational Resistance

A mutation is a change in the genetic material (i.e., DNA or, in the case of some viruses, RNA) that results in a change in the nucleotide sequence of the nucleic acid. Mutations can occur for a variety of reasons and in many cases have no effect on the genes and their functions within the cell or virus. However, in other cases a mutation can have more dramatic effects and allow a microorganism to survive various environmental challenges and to pass on this beneficial change to its descendants. Mutations can range from small spontaneous changes in the nucleotide sequence to larger deletions of sections of the nucleic acid. Chromosomal mutations leading to antibiotic resistance have been recognized and studied in some detail. These investigations have provided a greater understanding of the mode of action of antibiotics and have identified a variety of mechanisms by which bacteria can circumvent the antibacterial activity of antibiotics. Examples of these mutations include specific protein targets that are no longer affected by the presence of the antibiotic or various other regulatory proteins or sequences that change the expression of target proteins, allowing the bacteria to overcome the inhibitory or lethal effects. In contrast, fewer studies have been conducted to determine whether mutations can confer resistance to biocides; however, examples have been described demonstrating similar and distinct mechanisms from those of antibiotics and other anti-infective drugs.

Many attempts have been made to induce bacterial tolerance to biocides under laboratory conditions. This is investigated by growing the microorganism at subinhibitory and/or inhibitory concentrations of the biocide over time. In some cases, stable mutants have been identified; however, more often these mutants are unstable and revert to normal sensitivity following removal of the biocide. This indicates that although the microorganism may adapt or mutate to the low concentrations of biocides, these changes may have other negative effects on microbial growth, fitness, and survival. One of the first reported examples was the identification of *S. marcescens* mutants that allowed growth in the presence of a QAC at 100 to 1,000 times the MIC of the wild-type (or parent sensitive) strain. The wild-type strain was normally inhibited at ~100 mg/liter of the QAC, in comparison to the resistant strains at up to 100,000 mg/liter; however, it should be noted that some practical problems are associated with QACs and other biocides such as chlorhexidine in that they precipitate (due to limited aqueous solubility) in liquid culture media, which can be mistaken for bacterial growth (due to observed turbidity). Similarly, these and other biocides also interact with agar components to give inaccurate MIC determinations. Despite this, these strains clearly had higher than normal resistance to the biocide.

The exact mechanism of resistance was not identified, but the resistant strains were reported to have different surface characteristics, presumably due to increased or altered lipid content on the cell surface. Although it may be speculated that the resistance mechanism may have been due to a developmental response to reduce the penetration of the biocide into the cell, the more likely conclusion is that these strains had mutated to become more resistant. The QAC-resistant strains were unstable, reverting back to QAC-sensitivity when cultured in the absence of the biocide. There have been many subsequent reports of unstable biocide-tolerant bacteria that have not been investigated in any detail due to difficulty in maintaining their tolerant phenotype under laboratory conditions. Despite this, a number of exceptions of stable resistance have been further investigated. Many of these have been associated with biocides with limited spectra of activity such as triclosan, QACs, and chlorhexidine and have been particularly well studied in recent years. Overall, these reports suggest the need for further studies into the induction of biocide resistance by mutation.

Triclosan is a bisphenol that is widely used in antiseptic formulations, including surgical scrubs, antimicrobial soaps, and deodorants (chapter 4, section 4.6). It demonstrates potent activity against Gram-positive bacteria such as staphylococci but is less active against many Gram-negative bacteria, probably by virtue of their cell wall permeability barrier (section 8.6). The mechanisms of action and resistance to triclosan have been the focus of recent research, in particular, due to the isolation of various stable triclosan mutants in bacteria. Gram-positive (e.g., *Staphylococcus*) and Gram-negative (e.g., *Escherichia*, *Pseudomonas*) bacteria mutants were found to be readily identified by serial passage in subinhibitory and inhibitory concentrations of triclosan. In contrast to the unstable *S. marcescens* mutants discussed above, stable mutational changes as a mechanism of triclosan tolerance were first reported in *E. coli* due to changes in the fatty acid composition of the cell wall. The *E. coli* mutants were developed under laboratory conditions, exhibiting a 10-fold greater triclosan MIC than a wild-type strain, but only in the presence of divalent ions. Analysis of these strains showed no significant differences in total envelope protein profiles, but did show significant differences in envelope fatty acids. Specifically, a prominent $C_{14:1}$ fatty acid was absent in the resistant strain, along with minor differences in other fatty acid species. It was proposed that in these mutants the divalent ions and fatty acids may adsorb and limit the permeability of triclosan to its site of action.

The effect of triclosan on the phospholipid membrane has been investigated in bacteria; studies have shown that the hydrophobic biocide can integrate into the upper regions of the membrane via its hydroxyl group, which causes membrane disruption and loss of various functions (including catabolic and anabolic processes) and integrity. Overall, changes in the structure of membrane-associated lipids may decrease these interactions. Minor changes in fatty acid profiles were also found in stable triclosan-tolerant Gram-positive bacteria (*S. aureus*) isolates, which had elevated triclosan MICs, but not MBCs; again, the mechanisms of resistance were not further investigated. Since these earlier reports, many investigations have identified at least four mechanisms of resistance due to mutations, many of which have also been shown with other biocides: decreased uptake (as described above due to membrane alterations), increased efflux, chromosomal mutations leading to modification of key target proteins, and overproduction of target proteins (Fig. 8.28). Some of these modes of tolerance have also been shown to be linked to the acquisition of plasmids, particularly target site modification and efflux mechanisms.

In addition to the lipid changes observed in the initial *S. aureus* and *E. coli* mutants, mutations leading to subtle changes in the bacterial cell wall-membrane structure have been described in other bacteria that appear to exclude (or sequester) the penetration of triclosan. These include increased presence of branched-chained fatty acids in staphylococcal cell membranes and changes in the outer membrane

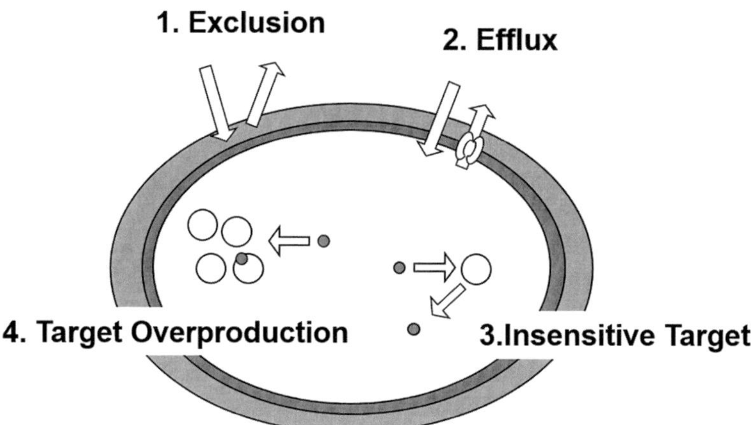

FIGURE 8.28 The modes of bacterial tolerance to triclosan due to acquired mutations. Exclusion **(1)** may be due to the loss of outer membrane porin proteins (reduced influx) or changes in the outer/inner membrane lipid structure. Efflux mechanisms **(2)** include overproduction of cell membrane/wall-associated efflux pumps due to mutation in regulator proteins. Enoyl reductases are specific targets for triclosan in the inhibition of fatty acid biosynthesis, with mutations identified that are associated with less affinity of triclosan for these enzymes **(3)**. Finally, the overproduction of enoyl reductases or other proteins provides greater tolerance of the biocide (4).

structure of *Pseudomonas* spp. Specifically, the downregulation or mutation in outer membrane proteins (porins) responsible for influx of compounds into Gram-negative bacteria has been shown to affect the MIC for triclosan by exclusion. Examples include mutations in the *ompF* porin gene of *E. coli* itself or that cause an overproduction of a protein regulator (MarA) that downregulates the expression of the OmpF porin protein (see below). These changes affect not only the tolerance to triclosan, but also cross-resistance to some antibiotics.

Efflux mechanisms of resistance, or the active transport of chemicals out of bacteria, have been particularly well described as leading to increased tolerance to triclosan and certain antibiotics. In section 8.3.4, efflux was discussed as a mechanism of intrinsic tolerance to some biocides and antibiotics. Mutations in the expression or control of these efflux systems have been shown to increase or decrease the sensitivity of biocides. The predominant efflux system in *E. coli* is the inducible AcrAB-TolC system, which plays a role in the survival of the bacteria in the gut due to the export of toxic fatty acids and bile salts. The efflux system is typical of the resistance-nodulation-division family (section 8.3.4), consisting of the inner membrane antiporter efflux protein AcrB (driven by energy from the proton motive force), the periplasmic-associated AcrA, and the outer membrane factor TolC. This efflux system has been associated with the active efflux of triclosan from the cell, but also efflux of other biocides such as antimicrobial dyes (e.g., crystal violet), detergents (e.g., SDS), organic solvents (e.g., *n*-hexane), acriflavine, QACs, chlorhexidine, pine oil, and triclosan. Similar systems have been identified in other Gram-negative bacteria such as *Salmonella* and *Pseudomonas*.

Mutations that cause the loss in expression of these efflux proteins lead to a loss of this intrinsic mechanism of tolerance; equally, mutations that allow for the overproduction of these proteins have been shown to allow for some increase (although in many cases slight) in biocide tolerance. Overproduction has been shown to be due to mutations associated with transcriptional control of efflux protein expression. The control of the expression of the AcrAB-TolC system is under various levels of control within the cell. AcrR is a protein repressor, which negatively controls the expression of the AcrAB genes in *E. coli* by binding to a DNA sequence upstream of these genes (known as an operator) and preventing their transcription. Mutations in *acr*R (leading to a loss of the protein or changes preventing its binding) or within the operator sequence that AcrR binds to have been shown to cause the overproduction of the efflux system and increased tolerance to some biocides, including triclosan. Similarly, MarA is a positive regulator of AcrAB and TolC, which when present allows for increased expression of efflux activity. The *mar* (multiple antibiotic resistance) phenotype in *E. coli* is an inducible system that can lead to tetracycline, fluoroquinolone, and β-lactam resistance; similar systems have been described in *Salmonella*, *Pseudomonas*, *Staphylococcus*, and *Mycobacterium*. MarA is a key regulator protein in *E. coli*, *Salmonella*, and other Gram-negative bacteria, which is activated under stressful environmental conditions leading to responses that allow for increased tolerance to oxidative stress, organic solvents, antibiotics, and some biocides. It itself is under negative control by a repressor, MarR. As with the AcrR repressor, removal of this control allows constitutive expression of MarA and increased expression of the efflux system. Further, MarA downregulates the outer membrane porin OmpF, which causes a decrease in the influx of various biocides including triclosan (as discussed above as an exclusion mechanism). Overexpression of MarA was found to allow a 2- to 3-fold increase in triclosan tolerance, as well as slight increases in pine oil tolerance.

Mutations or overexpression of other associated control proteins involved with stress responses (including SoxR/S and Rob) also affects the levels of AcrAB-TolC expressed in the cell by similar mechanisms (for further description of stress responses, see section 8.3.3). Mutations in these cell response systems not only affect the expression of the AcrAB-TolC efflux system but are an important part of the overall increase in stress response, which includes increased DNA repair, envelope synthesis, and biofilm generation. Other similarly chromosome-encoded efflux systems have been identified in *E. coli* (e.g., the EmrAB system), as well as in other bacteria such as *Haemophilus influenza*, *Neisseria gonorrhoeae*, *Vibrio parahaemolyticus*, and *Pseudomonas*. It should be noted that differences in the overall spectra and extent of biocides and antibiotics that are effluxed vary. Studies of the intrinsic or mutation-acquired tolerance to biocides are limited in comparison to those of antibiotics, although effects similar to those observed in *E. coli* are expected. Various inducible RND efflux pumps have been identified in *P. aeruginosa*, with variable antibiotic and biocidal resistance patterns (Table 8.20; also see section 8.3.4).

The Mex systems in *Pseudomonas* are similar to AbrAB-TolC. For example, overexpression of MexAB-OprM and MexCD-OprJ has been reported due to mutations associated with the NfxB regulatory protein, which performs a similar function as AbrR in *E. coli*. NfxB is a repressor for the expression of the MexCD-

TABLE 8.20 Examples of RND efflux pumps associated with biocide resistance in *P. aeruginosa* due to overproduction

Efflux system	Antibiotic resistance	Biocide resistance
MexAB-OprM	β-lactams, tetracycline, fluoroquinolones	Triclosan, SDS
MexXY-OprM	Fluoroquinolones	Unknown
MexCD-OprJ	β-lactams, tetracycline, fluoroquinolones	Triclosan, crystal violet, acriflavine, chlorhexidine
MexEF-OprN	Fluoroquinolones	Triclosan
MexJK-OprM	Tetracycline	Triclosan
CzrAB-OpmN	Carbapenems (e.g., imipenem)	Cadmium, zinc, copper

OprJ by binding as a tetramer upstream of the genes for these proteins and preventing its transcription. Various mutations in *nfxB* can prevent or reduce this repressor function, leading to greater expression of the efflux proteins. In these cases, increased tolerance to triclosan has been reported, as well as cross-resistance to antibiotics such as β-lactams and fluoroquinolones. Similarly, overexpression of MexEF-OprN and Mex JK-OprM has also been shown to allow for increased tolerance to triclosan. These mechanisms may play an important role in the cumulative resistance mechanisms described in *Pseudomonas* biofilms (section 8.3.8), although many of the mutations described have not been stable. Interestingly, this is not the case in the overexpression of MexXY-OprM, and indeed, limited cross-resistance has been reported with the heavy metal-associated efflux resistance with CzrAB-OpmN (Table 8.20). The overexpression of other cell wall-associated proteins has been implicated in biocide resistance in *Pseudomonas*, for example, the proportions of the outer membrane proteins OmpC and OmpF. The proportions of each outer membrane protein vary based on environmental conditions such as osmotic shock and increased temperature. They are controlled by the two-component sensory system, EnvZ-OmpR. EnvZ is an inner membrane sensory protein that, on sensing changes in osmolarity, activates the cytoplasmic OmpR, which regulates the expression of OmpC and OmpF. These changes are associated with rearrangements of the cell wall structure and can limit the penetration of biocides such as triclosan, although the exact reasons for this are unknown. In addition to chemicals, decreased levels of OmpF are found in the outer membrane in response to increased temperatures.

Overall, the increase in efflux (or exclusion) of triclosan and other antimicrobials allows survival of the cell around typical MICs of the biocide, but this has not been shown to be significant in the survival at typical in-use bactericidal concentrations. However, of greater importance is the observed cross-resistance to certain antibiotics such as tetracycline and fluoroquinolones. It is interesting to note that *E. coli* mutants with pine oil- or triclosan-induced tolerance (due to overexpression of MarA and therefore increased efflux activity) were also found to have low-level, increased antibiotic (e.g., ampicillin and tetracycline) MICs; however, when tolerance was similarly induced with the antibiotic tetracycline, much higher levels of cross-resistance were observed. It may be that efflux-mediated mechanisms allow the survival of bacteria under restrictive environmental conditions and, therefore, time to adapt further by other intrinsic or acquired resistance mechanisms. The clinical and industrial significance of these results is unclear and deserves further investigation.

A third example of modes of acquired resistance to triclosan due to mutations is target site modifications. These have been well described in antibiotic resistance mechanisms due to their more specific modes of action (see section 8.7.1) but were unexpected for biocides. Although triclosan appears to have multiple mechanisms of action, it was surprising to find that key bacterial targets for the biocide are intracellular enoyl-[acyl carrier protein] reductases (chapter 3, section 3.15); these enzymes are also specifically targeted by another bisphenol: hexachlorophene. Enoyl reductases are involved in type II fatty acid synthetic processes. Type II fatty acid synthase systems in bacteria use a dissociated group of enzymes (in contrast to mammalian type I synthases, which use a multienzymatic polypeptide complex) for the synthesis of fatty acids; this involves the cyclic addition of two carbon units to a growing fatty acid chain. Enoyl reductases catalyze the last stage in this elongation cycle, which is dependent on the presence of the cofactors NADH or NADPH. Both biocides, as well as some antibiotics such as isoniazid and the diazoborines, specifically bind to the substrate target site on this enzyme to selectively inhibit its activity (section 3.15). Specific binding of triclosan to FabI-like enoyl reductases has been observed in some Gram-positive bacteria (*S. aureus*, *Mycobacterium smegmatis*, and *M. tuberculosis*), Gram-negative bacteria (*E. coli*,

P. aeruginosa, H. influenzae), and *Plasmodium falciparum*. Triclosan preferably binds noncovalently to the enzyme and its respective cofactor, mimicking the enzyme's natural substrate.

It should be noted that not all enoyl reductases have been shown to be intrinsically sensitive to triclosan; some bacteria have single types of enoyl reductases, while others have multiple types. In the case of *E. coli*, the primary enoyl reductase, FabI, has been shown to be sensitive to triclosan, hence the ability of low concentrations of triclosan to inhibit wild-type *E. coli* strains; in contrast, the structurally different primary FabK enoyl reductase in *S. pneumoniae* and the secondary FabK enzyme in *E. faecalis* have been found to be intrinsically resistant to triclosan binding. In other bacteria, including *P. aeruginosa*, *B. atrophaeus*, *S. aureus*, *M. tuberculosis*, and *E. faecalis*, homologues of both enoyl reductase types have been identified and can be either triclosan-resistant or -sensitive forms of the enzyme. In many of these cases, triclosan tolerance is due to various intrinsic mechanisms; for example, in *P. aeruginosa* resistance is due to the presence of an effective outer membrane permeability barrier and efficient efflux systems, and in *E. faecalis* efflux (or other impermeability barriers) also plays a role.

The most studied triclosan-sensitive enoyl reductases have been *E. coli* FabI and its homologue, InhA, in *M. smegmatis* and *M. tuberculosis*. Specific genetic mutations producing amino acid changes within the active site of the enzyme have been shown to dramatically reduce the affinity of triclosan. FabI mutations were first identified *in vitro* by passaging wild-type *E. coli* strains through increasing concentrations of triclosan. Triclosan-tolerant strains were found to rapidly develop and could grow at significantly higher MICs, from approximately 1 to >75 μg/liter, depending on the specific mutation. The *Mycobacterium* enoyl reductase (InhA) was found to develop cross-resistance with triclosan to the antimycobacterial antibiotic isoniazid; isoniazid had previously been shown to target fatty acid biosynthesis, particularly inhibiting the role of InhA in mycobacteria, and resistance to the antibiotic could develop due to similar mutations. Similar mutational studies of *S. enterica* serovar Typhimurium have shown that other mutations can be responsible for high-level triclosan resistance. A collection of triclosan-mutant strains was subjected to complete genome sequence analysis, and all were found to have mutations in the FabI gene, but additional mutations were identified in other genes such as *rpoD* (encoding the primary sigma factor), *rpoS* (an alternative sigma factor involved in coordinating the stress response), and *ndh* (encoding an NADH dehydrogenase). High-level resistance was particularly associated with mutations in *fabI* and at least one sigma factor, suggesting an important role in triclosan inducing a stress response, and therefore mutations in various stress response genes may have increased bacterial tolerance to triclosan. It has been described that, on exposure to triclosan, various stress responses are activated to include changes in metabolism, cell wall adaptations, increased FabI production, and efflux pump activity. The role of Ndh in triclosan tolerance is unknown, but triclosan does bind to this protein and may play a role in inhibiting NADH recycling, and it is therefore involved in cell metabolism.

The fourth mechanism of tolerance to triclosan is due to the overproduction of certain enzymes, some of which have already been discussed above. *E. coli* mutants (initially with MICs in the range of 25 to 50 mg/liter) have been described, which did not show any mutations in the DNA sequence of *fabI* but did show overproduction of the FabI protein. Overproduction of FabI in these mutants, or when introduced to wild-type strains on plasmids, increased the overall level of triclosan required to inhibit growth. Hyper-expression of FabI in *S. aureus* mutants has also been reported to cause an increase in triclosan resistance. In another mode of resistance to triclosan, distinct *E. coli* mutants have been identified that have no mutations associated with the enoyl reductase but appeared to overexpress glucosamine-6-phosphate aminotransferase, which is involved in biosynthesis of various amino sugar-containing macromolecules. In both cases, these mutants showed increased resistance to triclosan in *E. coli*, but not to other biocides, including hexachlorophene and antibiotics. Overexpression of efflux systems as a mechanism of resistance to triclosan has been discussed above. Overproduction of other target or surface-associated proteins may allow cellular processes to proceed due to sequestration (or decreased penetration) of the available biocide. Other reports on the mode of action of triclosan have shown direct inhibition of other enzymes *in vitro*, including various transferases, suggesting that other mutations may further contribute to triclosan resistance (as described above).

The triclosan MIC for wild-type, laboratory *E. coli* strains is quite low (typically found to range between 0.1 and 2 μg/ml), but the MBC is quite high (50 to 75 μg/ml); in all investigated cases of triclosan resistance, although significant changes in MICs could be readily developed, no changes in the actual MBCs were found, suggesting that triclosan has multiple targets of action that culminate in cell toxicity. In some cases, triclosan tolerance demonstrated an MIC of >75 μg/ml, but it should be noted that triclosan is only soluble in water or growth media up to ~75 μg/ml, above which it precipitates. In an interesting link to decreased penetration as a mechanism of resistance, many of these *E. coli* triclosan-tolerant strains lose their resistant phenotype when cultured in the presence of chelating agents such as EDTA; EDTA is a permeabilizing agent that likely allows for greater penetration of triclosan to the inner cell membrane and cytoplasm. Triclosan is chemically similar in structure to triclocarban, a biocide also widely used for antiseptic applications (see chapter 3, section 3.6). It has been speculated that triclocarban has similar mechanisms of action and tolerance as triclosan, but this remains to be verified. Triclocarban has been shown to activate efflux mechanisms, but in studies with clinical strains of a variety of Gram-positive and Gram-negative bacteria, the observed MICs varied considerably for both triclosan and triclocarban and did not often correlate, suggesting differences in the mechanisms of resistance depending on the bacterial type.

In addition to triclosan, many mutational studies have focused on chlorhexidine. Chlorhexidine is a biguanide that is widely used in antiseptics (chapter 3, section 3.8, and chapter 4, section 4.6). It also demonstrates broad-spectrum bacteriostatic and bactericidal activity, in particular against Gram-positive bacteria. Increased tolerance to chlorhexidine has been induced in some organisms but has not been successful in others. In studies with the Gram-negative bacteria *Proteus mirabilis* and *S. marcescens*, mutants were developed under laboratory conditions to be up to 128 and 258 times higher than the initial chlorhexidine MIC, respectively; however, it was not possible to develop resistance to chlorhexidine in *S. enterica* serovar Enteritidis. The mutants appeared to be stable in *S. marcescens* but not in *P. mirabilis*. Some of the chlorhexidine-tolerant strains were also shown to be cross-tolerant to a QAC, benzalkonium chloride, suggesting a similar mechanism of resistance. Analysis of these strains did not show any obvious changes in their biochemical properties or in their virulence in mice. More recent studies demonstrated the development of stable chlorhexidine resistance in *P. stutzeri*; these strains showed various levels of increased tolerance to QACs, triclosan, and some antibiotics, probably by a nonspecific alteration of the cell envelope or, particularly, the outer membrane. Despite extensive experimentation using a variety of procedures, many investigators were initially unable to develop stable chlorhexidine resistance in many bacteria, but recent studies have been more successful in some Gram-positive and Gram-negative bacteria. Stable mutants have been described with *A. baumannii* and *Klebsiella pneumoniae* and appeared to be related to upregulation of efflux mechanisms. The *K. pneumoniae* mutants were developed under laboratory conditions and were also cross-resistant to the antibiotic colistin, which is considered one of the last antibiotics to be effective against multidrug-resistant forms of these bacteria. These strains were found to have mutations involved in the upregulation of capsular polysaccharide production (*phoPQ*) and efflux mechanisms (*smvR*); it is interesting to note that the specific development of colistin resistance in *K. pneumoniae* did not result in increased chlorhexidine tolerance.

In addition, stable mutants of *S. enterica* serovar Typhimurium were also developed under laboratory conditions by passage and subjected to detailed genomic and proteomic analysis. Studies included the impact of treatment of wild-type and mutant strains on exposure to chlorhexidine. Unlike similar studies with triclosan, the impact of chlorhexidine was less specific to certain cellular targets and appeared to be a more general toxic substance to the cell. Exposure of wild-type cells led to the upregulation of ~81 genes and the downregulation of ~166 genes. Upregulation included the expression of proteins involved in general energy production, SOS response, carbohydrate and cellular cofactor metabolism, and increases in cell membrane/cell wall synthesis. Processes that were downregulated included genes involved in virulence, glycolysis, and general metabolism (overall decrease in transcription and translation); interestingly, changes in efflux mechanisms were not observed in *S. enterica*. In the mutant strain, a variety of mutations (~21 altering protein structures) were identified that were particularly involved in general cellular metabolism. Others were involved in peptidoglycan crosslinking, decreased permeability, and changes in phosphate metabolism. The main mechanisms of action were concluded to be due to interruption of respiration (presumably due to effects on the cell membrane and proton motive force, consistent with previous known targets; see chapter 7, section 7.4.5) and decreased ATP production. Increased resistance in the mutant strains appeared to be associated with increased anaerobic metabolism (e.g., increased activity of pyruvate dehydrogenase and NADH dehydrogenase), but also increased SOS response (particularly DNA repair).

In contrast to mutations leading to increased tolerance to chlorhexidine, other mutations have been shown to cause hypersensitivity to the biocide. Examples include a series of outer membrane *E. coli* and *P. aeruginosa* mutants, including outer membrane protein and LPS strains, which are more sensitive to chlorhexidine and QACs, confirming the importance of the outer membrane structure in the intrinsic resistance of Gram-negative bacteria to biocides (section 8.6). Other examples of mutations leading to increased sensitivity to biocides are listed in Table 8.21.

A number of studies have investigated potential resistance mechanisms in bacterial spores. In studies with sodium hypochlorite and chlorine dioxide, no difference in biocide sensitivity was observed in spore mutants lacking the various acid-soluble spore proteins. But mutations in proteins required for the assembly of the various spore coats (section 8.3.11) produced spores that were hypersensitive, confirming the exclusion of these active agents from the spore core by the spore coats as a major mechanism of intrinsic resistance to these oxidizing agents. Other spore mutants that lack dipicolinic acid appeared to have increased water content, with a subsequent decrease in resistance to wet heat, hydrogen peroxide, iodophors, and formaldehyde; no effects were observed on resistance to dry heat and glutaraldehyde, but these mutants did demonstrate increased resistance to UV. It can be speculated that because some mutations can lead to the loss of enzymatic mechanisms of intrinsic tolerance to biocides (such as mercuric ion reductases and catalases/peroxidases, as discussed in section 8.3.5), mutations leading to overexpression of these enzymes are expected to allow some increase in tolerance to these biocides.

Efflux as a mechanism of acquired biocide resistance has been the focus of more recent investigations, as highlighted for triclosan resistance above. This was first proposed as a mechanism of resistance in proflavine (an acridine)-resistant bacteria, in which the cells had an increased ability to expel the bound dye. The more recent studies of triclosan and

TABLE 8.21 Examples of mutations causing increased sensitivity to biocides

Bacteria	Biocide sensitivity	Mechanism
E. coli, *P. aeruginosa*	Chlorhexidine, some QACs	Mutants lacking key outer membrane proteins or LPS
P. putida	Peracetic acid	Catalase overexpression mutants
B. subtilis spores	Sodium hypochlorite, chlorine dioxide, UV	Loss of spore coat structure/assembly
	Wet heat, dry heat, hydrogen peroxide, iodophors, formaldehyde	Lack of dipicolinic acid
	UV, oxidizing agents, moist and dry heat	Decreased expressions of SASPs
	Wet and dry heat	Reduced or lacking cortex
Acinetobacter calcoaceticus, *P. putida*, and *G. stearothermophilus*	Phenol and phenolics	Mutants lacking enzymes responsible for phenol degradation including phenol hydroxylases and catechol dioxygenases
Gram-positive and Gram-negative bacteria including *Pseudomonas*, *Acinetobacter*, *Bacillus*, and *Thiobacillus*	Mercury	Loss of mercuric reductase[a] activity
Mycobacterium	Glutaraldehyde and OPA	Decreased expression of cell wall-associated mycolic acids

[a]Can be plasmid-, transposon-, or chromosomally mediated.

other biocides demonstrate the significance of efflux in resistance of bacteria and cross-resistance to antibiotics. Multidrug resistance (MDR) is a particularly serious problem in enteric and other Gram-negative bacteria. MDR is a term employed to describe resistance mechanisms by genes that comprise part of the normal cell genome. These genes are activated by induction or mutation caused by some types of stress, and because they are distributed ubiquitously, genetic transfer is not considered a high risk (but transmissible efflux mechanisms of resistance may be described in bacteria; see section 8.7.3). Although such systems are most important in the context of antibiotic resistance, many examples of MDR systems in which an operon or gene is associated with changes in biocide susceptibility have been described, including:

- Mutations at an *acr* locus in the Acr system render *E. coli* more sensitive to hydrophobic antibiotics, dyes, and detergents.
- The *rob*A gene is responsible for overexpression in *E. coli* of the RobA protein that confers multiple antibiotic and heavy-metal resistance (interestingly, Ag+ may be effluxed).
- The MarA protein controls a set of genes (*mar* and *sox*RS regulons) that confer resistance, not only to several antibiotics, but also to superoxide-generating biocides (such as the oxidizing agents).

Low concentrations of pine oil (used as a disinfectant and containing pinene/terpineol as the major biocides; chapter 3, section 3.10) allowed the selection of *E. coli* mutants that overexpressed MarA and demonstrated low levels of cross-resistance to antibiotics. Deletion of the *mar* or *acr*AB locus (the latter encodes a proton motive force-dependent efflux pump) increased susceptibility to pine oil; deletion of *acr*AB, but not of *mar*, increased susceptibility of *E. coli* to chloroxylenol and to a QAC. In addition, the *E. coli* MdfA (multidrug transporter) protein confers greater tolerance to both antibiotics and a QAC (benzalkonium). The significance of these and other MDR systems in bacterial susceptibility to biocides needs to be studied further, particularly the issue of cross-resistance with antibiotics. At present, it is difficult to translate these laboratory findings to clinical use, and some studies have demonstrated that antibiotic-resistant bacteria are not significantly more resistant to the lethal (or bactericidal) effects of disinfectants than are antibiotic-sensitive strains.

The adaptation of *P. aeruginosa* to QACs and other biocides is a well-known phenomenon, but in most cases this is due to a physiological adaptation rather than to specific mutations. In many of these reports the actual mechanisms of tolerance were not specifically investigated or identified. Chloroxylenol-resistant strains of *P. aeruginosa* were isolated by repeated exposure in media containing gradually increasing concentrations of the phenolic, but resistance was also unstable. Resistance to amphoteric surfactants has also been observed and, interestingly, cross-resistance to chlorhexidine was noted. This may suggest that the mechanism(s) of such resistance is nonspecific and that it involves cellular changes that modify the response of microorganisms to unrelated biocidal agents. Outer membrane modification is an obvious factor and has indeed been found in QAC-resistant and amphoteric-resistant *P. aeruginosa* and in chlorhexidine-resistant *S. marcescens*. Such changes involve fatty acid profiles and, perhaps more importantly, outer membrane proteins. Evidence for this was shown in an analysis of *P. fluorescens* isolates that had increased tolerance to QACs, which could be reduced when EDTA was present with the QAC; similar results have been found with laboratory-generated *E. coli* mutants with increased MICs to triclosan (as discussed above). EDTA and other chelating agents have long been known to produce changes in the outer membrane of Gram-negative bacteria, especially pseudomonads. *E. coli* mutants with increased resistance to triclosan and some solvents have shown specific changes in their cell membrane lipid content; in the case of solvent resistance, a decrease in the ratio of the phospholipids (phophatidylethanolamine: phosphatidylglycerol/cardiolipin, the latter being more anionic) in the cell membrane was observed, suggesting exclusion as the mechanism of resistance. Thus, it appears that, again, the development of resistance can be associated with changes in the cell membrane/envelope, thereby limiting uptake of biocides. This is not limited to Gram-negative bacteria, as demonstrated in strains of *B. subtilis* and *M. luteus* with greater resistance to chlorine dioxide (see section 8.5). These strains appeared to be stable mutants, in comparison with reference (wild type) strains due to being heavily encapsulated with exopolysaccharide (in *B. subtilis*, demonstrating cross-tolerance to chlorine dioxide and other oxidizing agents) and increased cell size (in *M. luteus*, only demonstrating increased tolerance to chlorine dioxide).

One of the most significant reports of mutations associated with mechanisms of resistance to biocides was the isolation and analysis of glutaraldehyde- and OPA-resistant mycobacteria (see section 8.4). Water is a common source of atypical mycobacteria, which include the "rapid-growing" species such as *M. fortuitum*, *M. abscessus*, and *M. chelonae* (in relation to the "slow-growing" mycobacteria such as *M. tuberculosis*). It had been noted that *M. chelonae* strains had been isolated from flexible endoscopes and washer-disinfectors used to reprocess such temperature-sensitive medical devices. These microorganisms have been linked to nosocomial infections and "pseudo-infections," the latter due to misdiagnosis of these strains as being pathogens such as *M. tuberculosis* and *M. avium*. The identification of these isolates was initially speculated to be due to the development of biofilms over time within these machines and devices, which became intrinsically resistant to the 1 to 2% glutaraldehyde formulations that are widely used for low-temperature disinfection (chapter 3, section 3.4). Isolation and investigation of a number of these *M. chelonae* strains found that they not only showed increased MICs to glutaraldehyde but also were dramatically resistant to the biocidal effects of glutaraldehyde products (Fig. 8.29).

A range of glutaraldehyde-based products (ranging from normally effective concentrations between 0.5 and 2.5% glutaraldehyde) has been shown to be less effective against these mutant strains than expected. Testing with other aldehydes showed mixed results; 10% succinic dialdehyde/formaldehyde showed little to no change in resistance, while 0.55% OPA was also

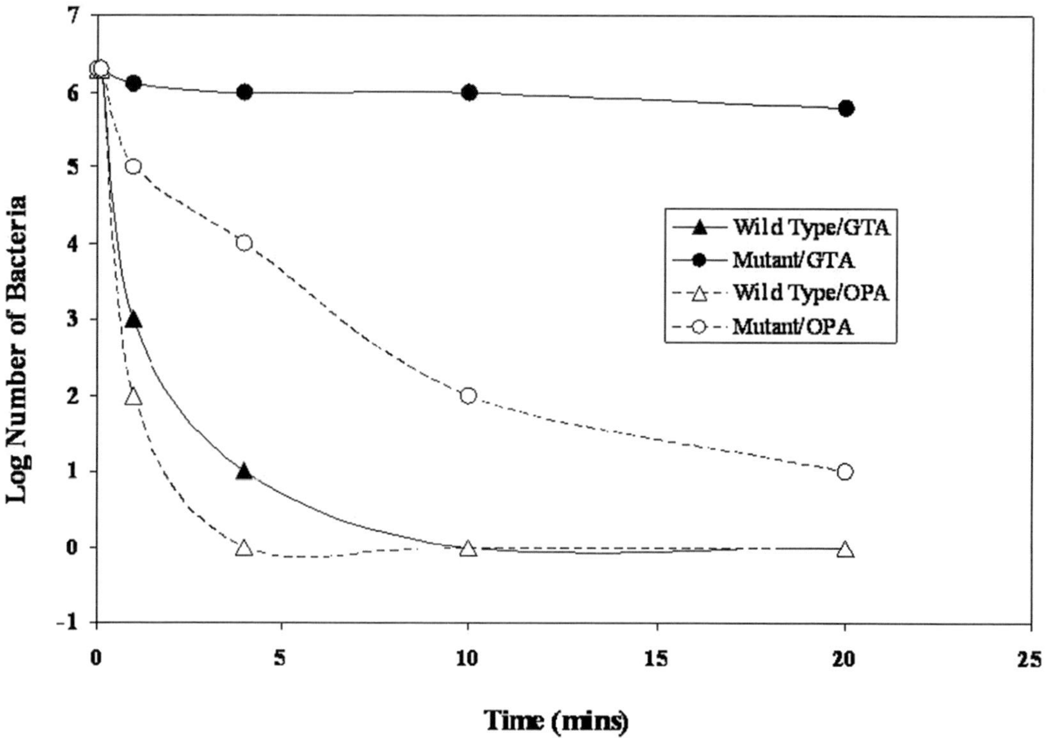

FIGURE 8.29 Demonstration of the resistance of *M. chelonae* glutaraldehyde-resistant strains. The aldehyde antimicrobial activity of a wild-type, glutaraldehyde-sensitive strain of *M. chelonae* was compared to a glutaraldehyde-resistant strain. A formulation of 2% glutaraldehyde demonstrated little to no effect against the resistant strain; another aldehyde (0.55% OPA) demonstrated efficacy but required greater exposure time than for the wild-type strain.

effective but at a slower rate than observed with wild-type *M. chelonae* strains (Fig. 8.29). Few to no differences in tolerance were observed with other biocides, including 70% ethanol, peracetic acid, and hydrogen peroxide; however, in some cases changes in MICs and MBCs have been reported and may be formulation (or product) specific. The nature of glutaraldehyde resistance in these strains has been investigated and was found to be related to cell wall/surface changes. The mutant colonies appeared to be physically drier and waxier than the wild-type strains and were found to have greater hydrophobicity. Cell wall analysis found no differences in the extractable fatty acid or mycolic acids (although there could be differences in proportions of these lipids), but there was an obvious change in the monosaccharide content of the cell wall polysaccharides arabinogalactan and arabinomannan. The exact mutation(s) in these strains were subsequently shown to be due to the lack of cell wall-associated porins (specifically, MspA and MspC). It is proposed that because these porins are major surface proteins on the cell surface, the lack of surface expression leads to an overall lack of surface proteins as a major target for aldehydes (see section 8.4). Equally, the lack of these proteins also substantially changes the surface structure of the cell wall and acts as a greater permeability barrier to glutaraldehyde. It is interesting to note that these strains remained somewhat sensitive to other aldehydes, including OPA, presumably due to greater penetration of these aldehydes into the cell wall (chapter 7, section 7.4.3).

Following on these reports, subsequent isolation and testing of *M. chelonae* and *M. gordonae* strains from washer-disinfectors that use glutaraldehyde found a prevalence of glutaraldehyde-resistant strains (up to 50% of isolates); in one study efflux pumps were confirmed not to be involved as a resistance mechanism. It has also been demonstrated that some strains have increased tolerance to 70% ethanol in comparison to other mycobacteria. Overall, the mechanism of resistance in these strains appears to be due to exclusion of the biocide from the cell or inaccessibility of key cell wall targets. These mutation-related resistance mechanisms cannot be assumed to occur in other bacteria, although glutaraldehyde-resistant strains of *Pseudomonas* have also been identified but appear to have distinct mechanisms of resistance. Two *P. aeruginosa* isolates with high-level resistance to glutaraldehyde under clinically used conditions were identified from endoscope reprocessing machines used for aldehyde-based chemical disinfection; although the mechanisms of resistance in these strains have not been investigated to date, transcriptional studies of *Pseudomonas* on exposure to glutaraldehyde have shown a variety of genes between repressed (~22 genes) and induced (~79 genes). Overall analysis of these has shown that processes that are induced include lipid and polyamine biosynthesis, phosphonate degradation, and efflux mechanisms. Mutations in these processes are also likely to be associated with acquired tolerance to glutaraldehyde in these bacteria. Although it has been speculated that efflux systems may be involved with the active transport of aldehydes out of the cell, this hypothesis is in conflict with the mechanism of aldehydes as protein cross-linking agents (see chapter 7, section 7.4.3, and section 8.4).

It is generally accepted that environmental isolates of bacteria are invariably less sensitive to biocides than are laboratory strains. Although it is expected that in many cases this is primarily due to physiological adaptation of bacteria within their environments (section 8.3), various challenges in these situations may also play an important role in the mutational adaptation of these isolates. These mutations may directly affect key biocide targets within cells or otherwise provide the cell with greater resistance to the biocide. In addition, other subtle mutations or adaptations can afford further benefits to allow the bacteria to survive in the presence of biocides. For example, subinhibitory antibiotic concentrations have been speculated to cause subtle changes in bacterial outer structure, thereby stimulating cell-to-cell contact and other responses or survival mechanisms; it remains to be tested if residual concentrations of biocides in clinical or industrial situations could produce the same subtle effects, although some studies have suggested such adaptations.

8.7.3 Plasmids and Transmissible Elements

Plasmid- and/or transposon-mediated mechanisms of resistance in bacteria were first described with heavy metals such as silver- and mercury-based biocides. Despite these earlier examples, for many years plasmids and transposons were not generally considered responsible for the biocide tolerance observed across bacterial species or strains, unlike many reports of transmissible element-associated resistance to antibiotics. However, further investigations have described increasing numbers of examples of biocide resistance determinants that are encoded on plasmids and/or transposons in bacteria. These have included biocides such as chlorhexidine, QACs, and triclosan, as well as diamidines, acridines, and other dyes such as ethidium bromide. In many cases, the exact mechanisms of tolerance are unknown and are often linked to changes in the cell membrane or cell wall (e.g., by general exclusion). In others, specific examples of plasmid-encoded tolerance to various biocides by enzymatic degradation and efflux have been identified and investigated in some detail (Table 8.22).

Plasmid-encoded resistance to biocides has been extensively investigated with mercurials (both inorganic and organic), silver compounds, and other cations and anions. Mercurials have been less used as disinfectants in recent years, but inorganic salts (e.g., $HgCl_2$) and organomercurial compounds (e.g., merbromin and

TABLE 8.22 Identified and possible mechanisms of plasmid-encoded resistance to biocides

Biocide	Mechanism
Chlorhexidine	Inactivation: Speculated to be plasmid-mediated and known to be chromosomally mediated
	Efflux in *S. aureus* and other staphylococci, as well as some Gram-negative bacteria such as *Burkholderia*
	Decreased uptake
QACs	Efflux in *S. aureus* and other staphylococci
	Efflux in *L. monocytogenes*, *E. coli*, *Klebsiella*, and other Gram-negative bacteria
	Decreased uptake
Triclosan	Target modification in *Staphylococcus*
	Efflux in *Pseudomonas* and *Staphylococcus*
Silver compounds	Efflux in *Salmonella*, *E. coli*, *Pseudomonas*, and other Gram-negative bacteria
	Extracellular accumulation by sequestration and reduction in *Enterobacteriaceae*
	Efflux in *Staphylococcus*
Formaldehyde	Inactivation by formaldehyde dehydrogenase
	Cell surface alterations (outer membrane proteins)
Glutaraldehyde	Potential plasmid-encoded resistance in *Mycobacterium*
Acridines[a]	Efflux in *S. aureus*, *S. epidermidis*, and other bacteria
Diamidines	Efflux in *S. aureus*, *S. epidermidis*, and other bacteria
Crystal violet[a]	Efflux in *S. aureus*, *S. epidermidis*, and other bacteria
Mercurials[b]	Inactivation (reductases, lyases) in Gram-positive and Gram-negative bacteria
Ethidium bromide	Efflux in *S. aureus*, *S. epidermidis*, and other bacteria

[a]Now rarely used for antiseptic or disinfectant purposes (chapter 3, section 3.7).
[b]Organomercurials are still used as preservatives, e.g., in paints (chapter 3, section 3.12).

thiomersal) are still employed as preservatives in some types of industrial products (chapter 3, section 3.12). Mercury resistance in bacteria can be intrinsic (chromosomally encoded) in some cases, including strains of *Pseudomonas* and *Thiobacillus*, but is more often described as being acquired through the acquisition of plasmids or transposons (Table 8.23).

These plasmids and transposons are found to be particularly widespread within Gram-negative bacteria (particularly well described in *Pseudomonas* and *E. coli*), although a number of Gram-positive chromosome-associated (e.g., in *Bacillus*) and plasmid-based (e.g., *S. aureus* pI258) mechanisms have been described. They can be transferred between bacteria by conjugation, transduction, and transformation (as discussed in section 8.7.1). Mercury itself is an antimicrobial metal (chapter 3, section 3.12). It is a potent intracellular toxin, linked especially to binding to the sulfhydryl groups of proteins and enzymes. The mechanisms of mercury tolerance have been particularly well studied due to their potential use for bioremediation of mercury-contaminated wastewater. As described in section 8.3.6, the mechanism of resistance is based on the expression of mercuric reductases, irrespective of being intrinsic or acquired, that cause the enzymatic conversion of the mercury ion (Hg^{+2}) to mercury vapor (Hg^0), which then vaporizes from the cell. Mercuric reductases are encoded by *mer*A genes that demonstrate significant similarities in their amino acid sequences, suggesting a common original source,

TABLE 8.23 Examples of acquired (plasmid or transposon) resistance to mercury in bacteria

Bacteria	Plasmid or transposon[a]
Pseudomonas fluorescens	pMER327
P. putida	Group G and H plasmids, Tn*5041D*
Xanthomonas sp.	Tn*5053*
E. coli	pR100, pNR1, Tn*5057*
Acinetobacter sp.	pKLH102, pKLH104, pKLH1
S. marcescens	pDI1358
S. aureus	pI258
S. enterica serovar Typhimurium	pMG101

[a]Plasmids are generally designated as pXXX (p for "plasmid") and transposons as Tn*XXX* (Tn for "transposon").

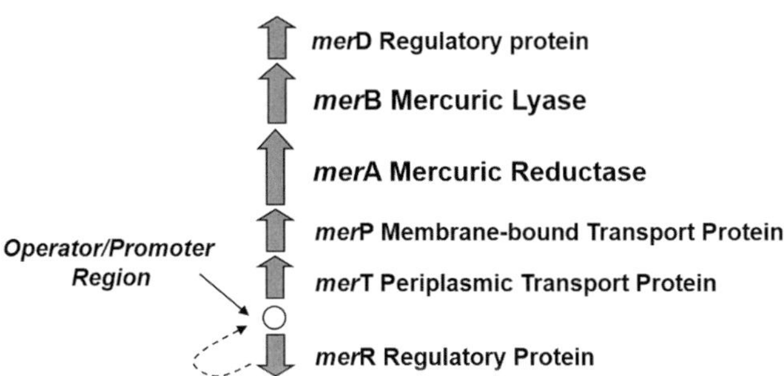

FIGURE 8.30 The simplified structure of a typical mercury-resistance operon in Gram-negative bacteria. The numbers, types, and control of expression of proteins from the operon can vary from isolate to isolate. In all cases a mercuric reductase (MerA) is expressed; however, only broad-spectrum resistance-associated plasmids and transposons are found to have MerB homologues (which are enzymes that hydrolyze organomercurial compounds to release the mercuric ion for subsequent reduction). The other proteins expressed are involved in mercury transport and control of the expression of the operon.

with the exception of the Gram-positive reductases, which appear to be more distinct and diverse. In some cases, the plasmids can also carry antibiotic resistance genes; for example, inorganic (Hg^{2+}) and organomercury resistance is a common property of clinical isolates of *S. aureus* containing plasmids that also express penicillinases (which break down penicillin). MerA is expressed from an operon that is also relatively conserved within Gram-negative bacteria (Fig. 8.30).

Expression of the genes involved with mercury resistance is inducible in the presence in mercury, under control of the MerR activator/repressor protein. MerA allows for the expression of the resistance proteins in the presence of Hg^{2+} and their repression in its absence. The mechanisms involved in the neutralization of mercury are summarized in Fig. 8.31.

In Gram-negative bacteria, Hg^{2+} binds to the periplasmic encoded MerP protein that transfers the toxic ions to the cytoplasmic membrane protein MerT and from there to the cytoplasmic MerA enzyme. MerA is an NADPH-dependent flavoprotein that causes the reduction of Hg^{2+} to Hg^0; due to the high vapor pressure of Hg^0, it rapidly volatilizes out of the cell. In some plasmids, an additional enzyme, MerB, is also expressed and is an organomercuric lyase; this enzyme catalyzes the separation of Hg^{2+} from various organomercury compounds (such as phenylmercury),

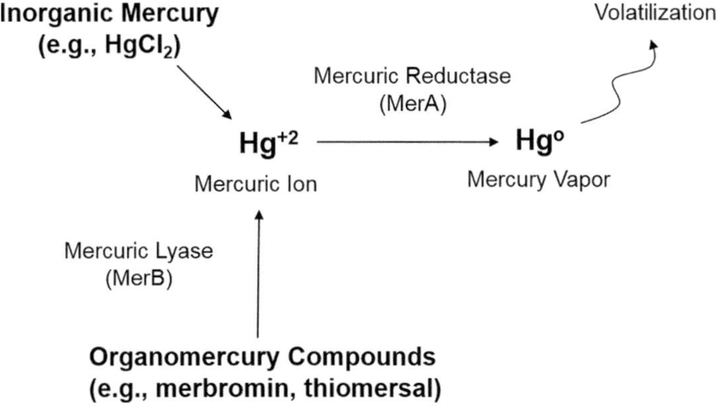

FIGURE 8.31 Mechanisms of resistance to mercury.

thereby allowing broad-spectrum resistance to these compounds. Plasmids and transposons that confer resistance to mercurials may therefore be further considered as either (i) "narrow spectrum," specifying resistance to Hg^{2+} and to some organomercurials (such as merbromin), or (ii) "broad spectrum," with resistance to the same compounds as the narrow-spectrum biocides and to additional organomercurials. In the case of the narrow-spectrum mechanisms described, the resistance may be simply due to exclusion from the cell, suggesting that other resistance mechanisms may also be present. Hg^{2+} is known to be transported out of the cell by the transporter proteins MerP and MerT, by association with cysteine residues in their structures.

Unlike mercury, silver and copper are still widely employed as biocides, and acquired resistance mechanisms may have greater risks, particularly on clinical applications (chapter 3, section 3.12). In both cases, plasmid-mediated resistance in bacteria has been described (Table 8.24).

Plasmid-encoded resistance to silver has been described in *Salmonella*, *Pseudomonas*, *Serratia*, *Klebsiella*, *Enterobacter*, *Acinetobacter*, and *Citrobacter* spp. Resistance to silver can be a significant concern in the treatment of wounds with silver nitrate and silver sulfadiazine. In the investigations of specific outbreaks, such as with *S. enterica* serovar Typhimurium and *Enterobacter cloacae* wound infections, resistance to therapeutic concentrations of silver appeared to be associated with the presence of a plasmid, although in other cases the resistance mechanism may also be attributable to chromosome-encoded mechanisms (particularly intrinsic mechanisms such as stress responses, enzymatic/chemical neutralization, capsule production, and cell wall structural changes). The mechanisms of resistance have been described in some detail for *Salmonella* tolerance to silver and cross-resistance with silver and copper in *E. coli*, with both associated with decreased heavy metal accumulation. At least two main mechanisms, efflux systems and sequestration, have been identified. The *Salmonella* pMG101 plasmid is a large 180-kB plasmid that encodes cross-resistance to heavy metals (silver and mercury ions) and antibiotics (such as ampicillin, chloramphenicol, tetracycline, and streptomycin). The silver-associated mechanisms are encoded in an ~14-kB section known as the *sil* operon (Fig. 8.32). The genes are encoded in three transcriptional units under separate promoter controls: *silCFBAGP*, *silRS*, and *silE*. Under stressed conditions, with the presence of increased external concentrations of silver ions, the inner membrane SilS detects the presence of silver and causes phosphorylation of the response regulator SilR. SilR normally represses the expression of the *silCFBAGP* transcriptional unit, and its phosphorylation derepresses this control, leading to the expression of the Sil efflux protein mechanisms. SilCBA is an RND-type efflux transporter (see sections 8.3.4 and 8.3.6) that pumps

TABLE 8.24 Examples of plasmid-mediated resistance to silver and copper in bacteria

Bacteria	Resistance	Mechanism
E. coli	Copper, silver	Chromosomal and plasmid-mediated resistance; an example is the plasmid pRJ1004, which encodes the *pco* genes (e.g., including for the protein PcoE) and SilE, which have been shown to detoxify copper and silver in the periplasm by sequestration
K. pneumoniae	Copper, silver	pLVPK expresses periplasmic proteins, which are thought to sequester copper and silver ions
Salmonella spp.	Silver	Plasmids (e.g., pMB101) encoding P-type ATPase and cation/protein antiporter efflux proteins, as well as SilE that sequesters silver in the periplasm by binding
A. baumannii	Silver	Plasmid (pUPI199) associated with efflux proteins and can be transferred to *E. coli* by conjugation
P. syringae	Copper	Plasmid (e.g., pPT23D) encoding Cop extracellular and periplasmic proteins that sequester copper ions

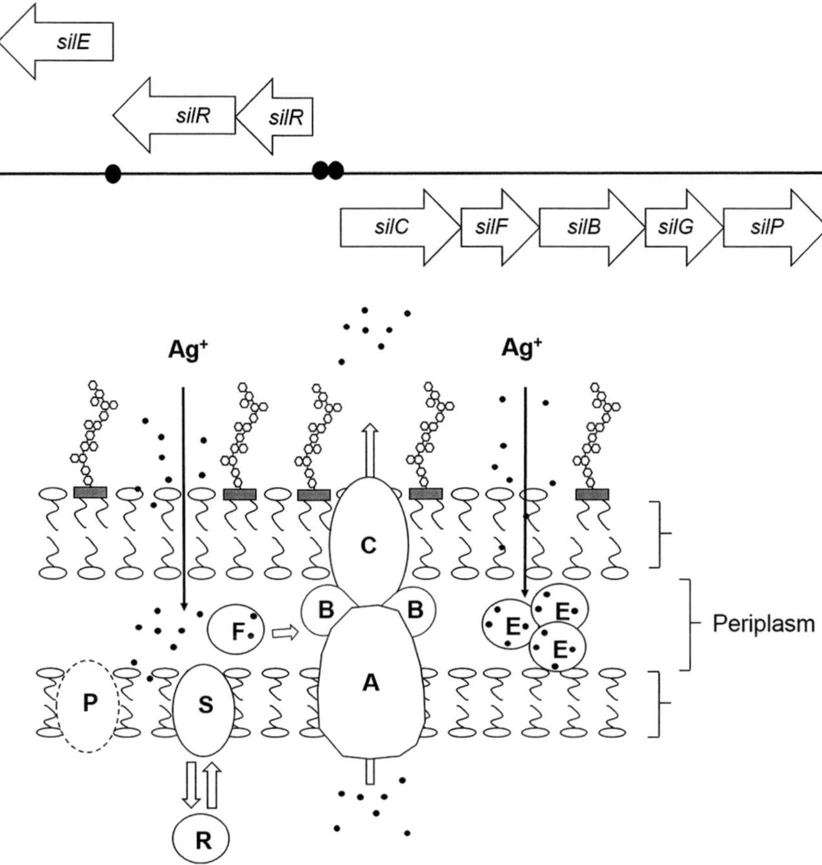

FIGURE 8.32 Acquired silver resistance in *Salmonella* associated with the pMG101 plasmid. pMG101 is a 180-kb plasmid that encodes the *sil* tolerance genes in an ~14-kb section (above). The genes are encoded in three operons: *silCFBAGP*, *silRS*, and *silE*. Central to the mechanism of resistance are the SilR and SilS proteins (below). SilS is a sensor protein that detects the increased levels of silver ions and causes the derepression of SilR that represses the expression of *silCFBAGP*. SilA, B, and C are components of an RND-type efflux system that pumps silver ions out of the cell. SilF is an accessory protein that transports ions to the efflux mechanism, and SilE is a silver-binding protein that sequesters the heavy metal availability. The action of SilP remains to be further defined.

silver ions out of the periplasm; SilF is involved in this mechanism by binding and transporting silver to the efflux proteins. The role of SilP has not been specifically described, but it appears to act as a silver transporter protein. SilE, a small (143-amino acid) periplasmic protein, acts by a different mechanism by binding silver (about six Ag^+ ions) to form a compact, nanoparticle-type structure that appears to be linked to specific methionine and histidine amino acid residues. This sponge-like mechanism alone affords some tolerance to silver, but at low levels. Similar mechanisms of tolerance have been well described in the *E. coli cus* operon and protein functions (which are chromosome-based) but expresses cross-resistance to silver and copper. The CusCBA proteins make up the RND-type efflux system, and CusF acts as a periplasmic transporter; CusS is an inner membrane sensor, and CusR is a cytoplasmic sensor.

An additional copper and silver sequestration protein has been identified on the large copper-tolerance plasmid pRJ1004. pRJ1004 encodes a series of Pco proteins similar to those described above for the Sil proteins in *Salmonella*, although their roles in resistance remain to be fully understood. PcoE has been shown to bind and sequester up to nine copper ions and seven silver ions, leading to protein dimerization in the periplasm. Similar mechanisms of resistance have been shown in other bacteria, such as with *Pseudomonas* peptides and proteins (e.g., the Cop proteins expressed from pPT23D) that sequester copper and other heavy metals. Overall, plasmid-mediated resistance to heavy metals is widespread in Gram-negative bacteria, with *sil* and *cop* often colocalized on plasmids and/or associated with transposons (e.g., transposons R478 and Tn7). Attempts to develop or identify similar (mutation- or transmissible element) acquired resistance mechanisms in Gram-positive bacterial pathogens, particularly in *S. aureus*, have not been as successful to date. They may be expected to potentially occur due to similar reprocessor-efflux-metallochaperone systems that are chromosomally based in Gram-positive bacteria such as the *Enterococcus hirae* CopYZBA and *B. subtilis* CopZA/CsoR systems for copper homostatis. An example of a plasmid-mediated efflux system has been described in *S. aureus*; plasmid pI258 expresses the regulator protein CadC that controls the expression of an ATPase-type system that is specific to lead and cadmium efflux.

Plasmid-encoded resistance to a variety of toxic metals including arsenic, cadmium, lead, and zinc have also been described (Table 8.25). The mechanisms of tolerance to heavy metals are similar to those described for copper and silver above, although in many cases further investigations of these mechanisms are warranted.

Many of these systems have also been investigated for their potential use in bioremediation of metal contamination in various industrial applications. Examples include the plasmid-encoded arsenic resistance mechanisms described in *E. coli* (pR773) and *S. aureus* (pI258), which encode efflux systems. In the *E. coli* plasmid pR773, resistance is mediated by the expression of the *arsRDABC* operon. When arsenate enters the cytoplasm, it is first reduced (by ArsC) to arsenite and then pumped out of the cell by the arsenite-specific ArsAB ATPase efflux system. The expression of the *ars* operon is controlled by the two regulator proteins ArsR and ArsD. ArsR has been shown to repress the transcription of the operon, which is relieved in the presence of arsenite. The *S. aureus* mechanism is similar yet distinct;

TABLE 8.25 Plasmid-mediated resistance to various toxic metals in bacteria

Bacteria	Plasmid/transposon	Resistance	Mechanism
Gram-positive			
S. aureus	pI258	Cadmium, zinc	Efflux-ATPase (CadA)
		Arsenic	Efflux-antiporter (ArsB)
	pII147	Cadmium	Membrane-associated sequestration
Staphylococcus xylosus	pSX267	Arsenic	Efflux-membrane potential (ArsB)
Gram-negative			
Ralstonia eutropha	pMOL28, pMOL30 (which includes transposons)	Cadmium, zinc, copper, mercury, chromium, nickel	Efflux systems, e.g., the Czc system on pMOL30 for copper, cadmium, and zinc, and the Cnr system on pMOL28 for copper and nickel; mechanisms include proton antiporters, chaperone transporters, ATPase efflux systems, and sequestration proteins/peptides
L. monocytogenes	pLm74/Tn*5422*	Cadmium	Efflux similar to pI258 in *S. aureus* but specific to cadmium (CadAC); also encoded on a transposon but found to be plasmid- rather than chromosome-associated
E. coli	pR773	Arsenic	Efflux-ATPase (ArsAB)

the simpler operon *arsRBC* encodes for an efflux protein which is driven by energy from the membrane potential, with similar action of the ArsR and ArsC proteins in *E. coli*.

Other examples are strains of *R. eutropha*, which have a remarkable capability to survive in the presence of a variety of toxic metals. They appear to have multiple resistance mechanisms that include those encoded on the bacterial chromosome, on transposons, and on two large plasmids (or megaplasmids; pMOL28 and pMOL30). pMOL28 expresses tolerance to cobalt, chromium, and mercury; pMOL30, to a wider range of metals such as silver, cadmium, copper, mercury, and lead. Both plasmids encode for efflux pumps, which have specificity to various metals (Table 8.25), including proton antiporters and ATPases, as well as proteins and peptides that include chaperones (metals transport systems) and sequestering peptides. As with copper and silver, multiple acquired resistance mechanisms have been confirmed, which include (i) efflux mechanisms; (ii) the expression of cell surface proteins that transport and/or bind the metal ions; (iii) metal detoxifying proteins expressed in the cytoplasm, including those described in bacteria, yeast, and fungi such as metallothioneins and other metal-binding proteins; and (iv) specific mutations or overexpression of key target enzymes or other proteins. A number of these resistance mechanisms have also been described in yeasts (section 8.10) and other eukaryotes.

Studies have examined the possible role of plasmids in the resistance of Gram-negative bacteria to other biocides. More than 30 groups of broad-host-range plasmids have been identified in *Enterobacteriaceae* and *Pseudomonas*. Examples are the IncP group, which are widely distributed between these bacteria and can include multiple mechanisms of resistance to antibiotics (e.g., aminoglycosides and β-lactams), including enzymatic modification or hydrolysis, efflux, and target modifications. They can include simple or multiple transposons that are linked to these mechanisms. Initial studies with one such plasmid, RP1 (which encodes resistance to the antibiotics carbenicillin, tetracycline, and neomycin/kanamycin), did not significantly alter the resistance of *P. aeruginosa* to QACs, chlorhexidine, iodine, or chlorinated phenols, although an increased resistance to hexachlorophene was observed. Hexachlorophene has a much greater effect on Gram-positive than Gram-negative bacteria, so it is difficult to assess the significance of this finding. Transformation of this plasmid into *E. coli* and *P. aeruginosa* did not increase sensitivity to a range of biocides tested. Despite this, other plasmids in the IncP group have been shown to express resistance to QACs, such as pB2/B3, pB5, pKJK5, and pBRSB222. These are mostly linked to efflux mechanisms by QacE proteins (expressed by *qacE* or, particularly, its mutant form, *qacEΔ1*), or other small drug export efflux proteins driven by the proton motive force (see section 8.3.4).

The Qac efflux mechanisms were first described in detail in staphylococci (discussed later in this section), and plasmid-associated *qac* genes are widely described in Gram-positive bacteria, such as *qacA*, *qacE*, and *qacF*, which express SMR systems. These systems can efflux various QACs, antimicrobial dyes, and chlorhexidine, depending on the specific pump (see Table 8.26). In contrast, a limited number of similar Qac proteins (particularly those expressed by *qacEΔ1*) have been described to be plasmid-based in Gram-negative bacteria. In *Acinetobacter*, for example, *qacEΔ1* is linked to resistance mechanisms for the antibiotic sulfonamide encoded on a mobile integron that is transferred by a transposon associated with plasmids. Integrons are genetic elements that can become associated with chromosomes and mobile elements such as plasmids and transposons; they are transferred from one DNA source to another by site-specific recombination. They have a minimum structure composed of a recombinase, a recombination site, and a promoter that drives the expression of the integron genes, but they can also include various other genes including efflux mechanisms. A strong link has been shown between these QAC tolerance mechanisms and

TABLE 8.26 Examples of *qac* genes and susceptibility of *S. aureus* strains to some antiseptics and disinfectants

qac gene[a]	MIC ratios[b]						
	PF	CHG	Pt	Pi	CTAB	BZK	CPC
A	>16	2.5	>16	>16	4	>3	>4
B	8	1	>4	2	2	>3	>2
C/D	1	1	1	1	6	>3	>4
MIC (μg/ml)	40	0.8	<50	50	1	<2	<1

[a]*qac* genes were previously known as nucleic acid-binding compound-resistance genes, because many of the biocides demonstrating increased tolerance have modes of action related to nucleic acid binding.

[b]For comparison, the ratios shown are the MICs for strains of *S. aureus* carrying the various *qac* genes divided by the MIC value for a strain carrying no gene or plasmid. The actual MIC of the sensitive strain that did not carry the gene or plasmid is shown in the last row. PF, proflavine; CHG, chlorhexidine diacetate; Pt, pentamidine isethionate; Pi, propamidime isethionate; CTAB, cetyltrimethylammonium bromide; BZK, benzalkonium chloride; CPC, cetylpyridinium chloride.

broad-spectrum antibiotic resistance in *E. coli*, *Acinetobacter*, and *Pseudomonas*, but not in *Klebsiella*. Overall, the plasmid (and transposon)-associated *qacE* and *qacE*Δ*1* tolerance mechanisms have been found to be widely distributed among the *Enterobacteriaceae* and *Pseudomonas* spp.

Other plasmid-mediated biocide tolerance mechanisms, separate from efflux, are likely to be involved in changing the surface permeability of Gram-negative bacteria. One example is associated with increased tolerance to biocides by stress responses. *Burkholderia* spp. have been found to have multiple, larger genomes, and one (the megaplasmid pC3, or "chromosome 3") has been shown to confer greater tolerance to heat, some oxidizing agents, and chlorhexidine in comparison to plasmid-cured strains. The heat tolerance was tested and shown only up to 42°C, but the chlorhexidine tolerance was more significant. Some of these strains have been shown to survive in 0.5% chlorhexidine antiseptic products, leading to failure (associated infections) in clinical use. The specific mechanism of resistance has not been described to date but has been associated with efflux and other cell-wall-associated modifications; *Burkholderia* spp. are also efficient biofilm-forming bacteria. Another example is the plasmid pR124, which alters the OmpF outer membrane porin protein in *E. coli*; cells containing this plasmid are more resistant to at least one QAC (cetrimide) and to other agents. Changes in the presence, structure, or proportion of various cell envelope porins or LPS in Gram-negative bacteria may indirectly allow for increased or decreased sensitivity to biocides by altering biocide penetration (as previously discussed in section 8.6). Similar mechanisms are proposed to be involved in the increased resistance to glutaraldehyde and OPA in mycobacteria.

Bacterial resistance mechanisms to formaldehyde and industrial biocides can be plasmid encoded in Gram-negative bacteria such as *Enterobacteriaceae* and *Pseudomonas* spp. Structural alterations at the cell surface (including outer membrane proteins) and enzymatic degradation (formaldehyde dehydrogenase; see section 8.3.5) have been described. Plasmid-based formaldehyde dehydrogenases are found to be widespread and highly conserved in *E. coli* (e.g., on pVU3695) and other *Enterobacteriaceae*; they have also been described in *Pseudomonas* spp. and in eukaryotes such as yeast (*Saccharomyces cerevisiae*). Enzyme activity is localized at the cell wall surface and is due to oxidation of formaldehyde by glutathione- and NAD-dependent dehydrogenase activity. Formaldehyde-resistance plasmids in *S. marcescens* and *E. coli* have been reported to change the expression of some outer membrane proteins and therefore cell surface hydrophobicity, presumably rendering the bacterial surface less reactive with the aldehyde. The variety of membrane proteins normally associated with the cell wall were found to be identical; however, the expression of a number of these proteins appeared to be reduced in the plasmid-containing strains. Other reports on formaldehyde resistance in Gram-negative bacteria have been associated with changes in the composition and structure of the outer membrane, which were also cross-resistant to glutaraldehyde and independent of the expression of formaldehyde dehydrogenase.

Subtle changes in protein expression at the cell wall surface of other bacteria such as mycobacteria are thought to play a role in resistance to aldehydes, including glutaraldehyde and OPA. Toluene resistance in pseudomonads due to degradation by oxygenase-catalyzed hydroxylation has been shown to be chromosomal and plasmid encoded. Examples are the *Pseudomonas* TOL plasmids for toluene resistance and the TOM (toluene ortho-monoxygenase) plasmid, which encodes enzymes for toluene and phenol degradation in *B. cepacia*. In both cases, they allow phenols and/or toluene to be used as single sources of carbon and energy. The TOM pathway is a three-component enzyme system consisting of a hydroxylase, an oxidoreductase, and a protein involved in the electron transfer between these enzymes. Its significance as a mechanism of resistance to phenol- and cresol-based disinfectants or preserved products is not known.

Staphylococci, particularly antibiotic-resistant isolates such as MRSA strains, are major causes of health care-acquired infection throughout the world. MRSA strains demonstrate marked resistance to various antibiotics, including methicillin, penicillin, and gentamycin, that can be both chromosomally and/or plasmid encoded. Many of these mechanisms are due to active efflux systems in staphylococci, including the prevalent chromosome-based efflux proteins SepA, NorA, and MepA in *S. aureus*. Other plasmid-based efflux systems are further discussed in this section. The analysis of plasmids from these strains found that *S. aureus* and coagulase-negative staphylococci (such as *S. epidermidis*) can have one or more plasmids, which can vary in size and copy number. These plasmids were initially subdivided into three different types:

1. Large β-lactamase-heavy metal resistance plasmids, which carry transposons (e.g., TN*552*) that confer penicillin resistance (penicillinase expression) but also tolerance to heavy metals (including mercury and arsenic, as discussed for the plasmid pI258 above)
2. The pSK41 family of conjugative plasmids
3. The pSK1 plasmid family, which can confer both increased tolerance to aminoglycoside antibiotics (including kanamycin and gentamycin) and cross-tolerance to various cationic biocides

Based on MICs, *S. aureus* strains carrying these latter plasmids (with various *qac* genes) were found to have less sensitivity to the inhibitory effects on biocides, including QACs, chlorhexidine, and diamidines, together with intercalating dyes such as ethidium bromide and acridines (Table 8.26). No decrease in susceptibility of antibiotic-resistant strains to phenolics (phenol, cresol, chlorocresol), povidone-iodine, or tested preservatives (parabens) were shown. These plasmids have been the focus of research to identify the genetic aspects of plasmid-mediated biocide-resistant mechanisms. In *S. aureus* and other staphylococci, these mechanisms have been found to be encoded by at least three major efflux (or multidrug) tolerance determinants that can be widely distributed (Table 8.26). These particularly include QacA, QacB, and QacC.

These determinants were all found to encode for efflux proteins driven by energy from the proton motive force (section 8.3.4), and in staphylococci they have been described as two gene families (*qac*A/B and *qac*C/D or similar types) that show sequence similarities. The *qac*A/B family of genes (Table 8.27) encode larger, proton-dependent export proteins (of the major facilitator superfamily; section 8.3.4) that have significant homology to other energy-dependent transporters such as the tetracycline transporters found in various strains of tetracycline-resistant bacteria. QacA and B were two of the first bacterial multidrug-resistant transporters identified. QacA, for example, is an induced 514-amino-acids-long protein located in the cell membrane, consisting

TABLE 8.27 *qac* genes and resistance to QACs and other biocides[a]

Multidrug resistance determinant	Gene location	Resistance encoded to[b]
*qac*A	pSK1 family of multiresistant plasmids, also β-lactamase and heavy metal resistance families	QACs, CHX, diamidines, acridines, EB, triclosan?
*qac*B	β-lactamase and heavy metal resistance plasmids (e.g., pSK23)	QACs, acridines, EB
*qac*C[c]	Small plasmids (<3 kb) or large, conjugative or nonconjugative plasmids, such as pSK41, pSM52, and pSH4126	Some QACs, EB, triclosan?
qacE	Commonly described in Gram-negative bacteria (e.g., *E. coli, A. baumannii*, and *Klebsiella* spp.); associated with integrons and plasmids such as the IncP-1 plasmids	Some QACs, EB
qacF	First described in Gram-negative bacteria (e.g., *Enterobacter aerogenes*) as mobile elements (integrons), and subsequently in Gram-positive bacteria (e.g., enterococci and staphylococci)	Some QACs, EB
qacG	pST94 in *Staphylococcus* spp.	Some QACs, EB
qacH	p2H6 in *Staphylococcus saprophyticus*; also linked to transposons such as Tn*6188*, which can be plasmid- or chromosome-based	Some QACs, EB, proflavine

[a]Although the Qac efflux mechanisms were first identified in *S. aureus*, they have since been identified in other staphylococci and other Gram-positive bacteria. Some Qac mechanisms have subsequently been identified in Gram-negative bacteria. Not all Qac genes are shown.

[b]CHX, chlorhexidine salts; EB, ethidium bromide.

[c]Originally called *ebr, smr*, and *qacD*.

of 14 transmembrane domains. The *qac*A gene is present predominantly on the pSK1 family of multiresistance plasmids but is also likely to be present on the chromosome of clinical *S. aureus* strains as an integrated family plasmid or part thereof. pSK1 is an ~28-kB plasmid which can carry the transposon Tn*4001* (which confers resistance to the aminoglycosides gentamycin, kanamycin, and tobramycin) and may also carry a gene that confers resistance to trimethoprim. Efflux of >30 toxic substances has been described, including cationic and lipophilic biocidal compounds, with transcription of *qac*A under control of the QacR repressor, which is derepressed in the presence of QacA substrates (such as the QACs). In addition to staphylococci, QacA has been identified in *E. faecalis*. The *qac*B gene is detected on large, heavy metal-associated resistance plasmids such as pSK23, but despite conserved similarities to *qac*A appears to have a narrower range of biocide efflux activity (more specific to intercalating dyes such as ethidium bromide and QACs, and not cross-resistant to chlorhexidine or the diamidines).

The *qac*C (previously known as *ebr, smr*, or *qac*D) genes (e.g., encoded on pSK89 and pSK41) are smaller proteins (~107 amino acid residues) with four transmembrane domains and have similar phenotypes and sequence homologies. Within this group are the QacE, F, H, G, J, and Z efflux proteins. These encode a group of SMR-type proton motive force-dependent efflux proteins (section 8.3.4). QacE and QacF were identified in Gram-negative bacteria, but QacF-like proteins have also been identified in Gram-positive bacteria (e.g., in *Enterococcus* and *Staphylococcus* spp.). The QacF gene (e.g., in *Enterobacter aerogenes*) is present on a mobile element (an integron) that can transfer between plasmids by site-specific recombination, which is probably responsible for its more widespread occurrence. QacH, G, and J have been described to date only in staphylococci, and QacZ in *E. faecalis*.

pSK41 (Fig. 8.33) is a 46.4-kB conjugative plasmid that is a typical example of the evolution of plasmids in staphylococci. The plasmid consists of multiple resistance mechanisms on a single plasmid that have evolved from the insertion of transposons and integration of other plasmids. The transposon Tn*4001* confers aminoglycoside resistance and neomycin/bleomycin antibiotic resistance from genes

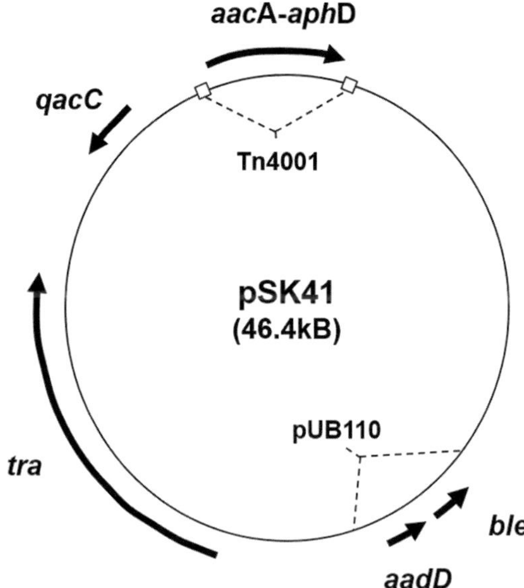

FIGURE 8.33 pSK41, an example of a multidrug resistance plasmid in staphylococci (not drawn to scale). pSK41 is a 46.4-kB plasmid encoding various genes for its transfer by conjugation (*tra*), resistance to antibiotics (gentamycin, tobramycin, and kanamycin by *aac*A-*aph*D; neomycin by *aad*D; and bleomycin by *ble*), and a biocide efflux pump (*qacC*). The plasmid contains sequences from a transposon (Tn*4001*) and an integrated plasmid (pUB110).

provided by the integration of a plasmid (pUB110), and the *qacC* gene encodes a QAC efflux pump. Other members of the pSK41 family of plasmids can also confer trimethoprim resistance. Other genes encoded on pSK41 include those required for the conjugation of the plasmid from one strain to another (*tra* genes). The difference in tolerance between clinical isolates with these plasmids to QACs has been proposed to be due to the different copy number of plasmids that may be present in each strain.

Overall, plasmid-encoded tolerance determinants are considered widespread among *S. aureus* and other staphylococci. In clinical and industrial isolates, 10 to 80% of *S. aureus* and *S. epidermidis* strains are reported to have *qacA*/*B*-based plasmids, depending on the geographical area (e.g., they are at the higher end of this range in various Asian countries). There is some concern over their demonstrated relationship between the increased MICs to biocides (often used as antiseptics and disinfectants, such as chlorhexidine and benzalkonium chloride) and antibiotics such as the β-lactams. Based on DNA homology, it has been proposed that *qac*A and related genes carrying resistance determinants evolved from preexisting genes responsible for normal cellular transport systems and that the biocide-resistance genes evolved prior to the introduction and use of topical antimicrobial products and other antiseptics and disinfectants. In the case of antibiotics, the presence of a specific resistance mechanism frequently contributes to the long-term selection of resistant variants under *in vivo* conditions. Whether low-level resistance to cationic antiseptics, e.g., chlorhexidine and QACs, can likewise provide a selective advantage on staphylococci carrying *qac* genes remains controversial.

Other Gram-positive bacteria have also been found to encode for similar efflux pumps. For example, *Lactococcus lactis* strains have been identified with efflux pumps driven by both proton pumps (LmrP) and ATP hydrolysis (QacA-like), although the spectrum of biocides effluxed appeared to be restricted to certain intercalating dyes such as ethidium bromide, which are not generally used as biocides. QacA-type plasmids (and associated transposons such as Tn*6188*) have been identified in *Listeria* spp. Plasmid-mediated efflux pumps are therefore important mechanisms of resistance to many antibiotics, metals, and cationic biocides such as QACs, chlorhexidine, diamidines, and acridines, as well as to dyes such as ethidium bromide.

There is some evidence of plasmid-associated tolerance to biocides by different mechanisms in staphylococci. A notable example is the acquisition of transposons and transposon-associated plasmids with increased tolerance to triclosan. The mechanism of tolerance is due to transfer of additional copies of *fabI*, the gene expressing an enoyl reductase known to be a primary target for triclosan in many bacteria (see section 8.7.2), from *Staphylococcus haemolyticus*. The *sh-fabI* gene has been found to be carried by an ~3-kB transposon known as Tn*ShaI*, containing a single insertion sequence, IS*1272*, which can also be transmitted by an integrating plasmid carrying the transposon (known as Tn*Sha2*). Tn*Sha2* is more prevalent in *S. haemolyticus* and *S. epidermidis* (where the plasmid integrates into the chromosome), and Tn*ShaI* is more common in *S. aureus*, due to acquisition. These elements are widespread in staphylococci and lead to the presence of at least duplicate copies of the target gene, with increased tolerance to the biocide.

Similar to Gram-negative bacteria, other mechanisms of biocide resistance in Gram-positive bacteria are likely, although few studies have shown specific links to transmissible element-associated resistance. Examples are antibiotic-resistant corynebacteria that have been implicated in human infections, especially in the immunocompromised. *Corynebacterium jeikeium*, for example, was found to be more tolerant than other coryneforms to cationic disinfectants, ethidium bromide, and hexachlorophene, but studies with plasmid-containing and plasmid-cured derivatives produced no evidence of plasmid-associated resistance. The mechanisms of tolerance appeared to be due to chromosome-based factors, particularly related to efflux and cell wall permeability. Complete sequence analysis of a *C. jeikeium* isolate has shown acquired efflux mechanisms linked to transposons on the chromosome that may be partially associated with resistance in this and other *Corynebacterium* spp. Similarly, *Enterococcus faecium* strains showing high-level resistance to vancomycin, gentamicin, or both antibiotics are not more resistant to chlorhexidine or other investigated biocides. Stable chromosomal mutants of *E. faecium* to chlorhexidine but not QACs have been described, which appeared to be due to increased protein expression and cell wall surface changes. The transfer of plasmids and transposons (such as Tn*5384*) between staphylococci and enterococci has been shown and linked to antibiotic and mercury resistance, suggesting that other biocide tolerance acquisition is likely.

Despite the extensive dental use of chlorhexidine as an oral antiseptic, strains of *Streptococcus mutans* and other cariogenic microorganisms have been found to remain sensitive. Increased chlorhexidine tolerance is observed in *S. mutans* under stressed conditions (e.g., in response to starvation) as an intrinsic physiological response; however, plasmid transfer between *S. mutans* and other Gram-positive bacteria (such as *L. monocytogenes*) has been described. The ability of *S. mutans* to generate and interact with biofilms may also increase the opportunity for genetic transfer with other bacteria. Transformation involves the ability of the cell to naturally take up plasmids or other genetic material from the environment (e.g., in the Gram-positive bacteria *Bacillus* and *Streptococcus*). Transformation has not been naturally described as a mechanism of acquisition of biocide tolerance genes but is likely to occur. Under experimental conditions, chlorhexidine-tolerant strains of *Streptococcus sanguis* were isolated, and the DNA was extracted and directly mixed with chlorhexidine-sensitive strains. Subsequent recovery at normally inhibitory concentrations of chlorhexidine allowed for the isolation of tolerant-transformants, with resistance profiles similar to the original mutants. The nature of resistance in these strains was not identified, and further investigations are warranted to verify transformation as a mechanism of biocide resistance exchange.

It is of some interest to note that the transfer of genetic material by conjugation, transformation, or transduction can be inhibited by the presence of biocides. Subinhibitory concentrations of biocides such as chlorhexidine, PVPI, phenols, and QACs have been shown to reduce the conjugation of plasmids between Gram-positive and Gram-negative bacteria. Similar results have been reported for phage transduction.

8.8 MECHANISMS OF VIRAL RESISTANCE

Viruses are nonmetabolizing and dependent on host cells for their survival and multiplication (chapter 1, section 1.3.5). This may be expected to limit their adaptability to the antimicrobial mechanisms of action of biocides and biocidal processes. The major modes of resistance of viruses to biocides have been shown to be directly related to virus structure. Other associated, and often indirect, factors have been shown to provide some protection to virucidal agents (Fig. 8.34).

Like other microorganisms, viruses are normally associated with extraneous materials, including cell debris, proteins, carbohydrates, lipids, and various inorganic salts. The presence of these materials affects the biocide penetration to and activity at the individual viral particles, providing a protective mechanism of resistance. These materials are often directly associated with viruses, because they require host cells for multiplication and can be found within or closely associated with cells or cellular debris. This mechanism is an important consideration for the safe disinfection of viruses associated with various organic and inorganic materials, including body fluids such as blood, serum, and saliva, or when associated with liquids or foods. The presence of these materials also aids the virus to survive on surfaces for extended periods of time, presumably by preventing drying; this is particularly true of the enveloped viruses, which generally do not survive long on surfaces but can survive for several days in the presence of blood (as observed with the hepatitis B virus in blood). In contrast, some nonenveloped viruses, including parvoviruses and poliovirus, can survive for up to several years.

Although viruses cannot form biofilms on their own (section 8.3.8), they are found to be associated with or entrapped within existing bacterial biofilms. For example, some studies of polioviruses and other enteroviruses in water have shown that they have affinity to and can accumulate within biofilms as an indirect mechanism of resistance to biocides. Recent evidence has also suggested that bacteriophages can play an important role in the assembly and architecture of bacterial biofilms (e.g., with *Pseudomonas* spp.), leading to increased resistance to desiccation and biocide penetration. Finally, the presence of viruses in biofilms is also expected to increase the opportunity for uptake into protozoa, which in vegetative and dormant (e.g., cyst) form can protect viruses (and other microorganisms) against the attack of biocides (particularly chemical biocides; see section 8.11). Waterborne viruses such as the enteroviruses (e.g., polioviruses, echoviruses, and coxsackieviruses), have been shown to be

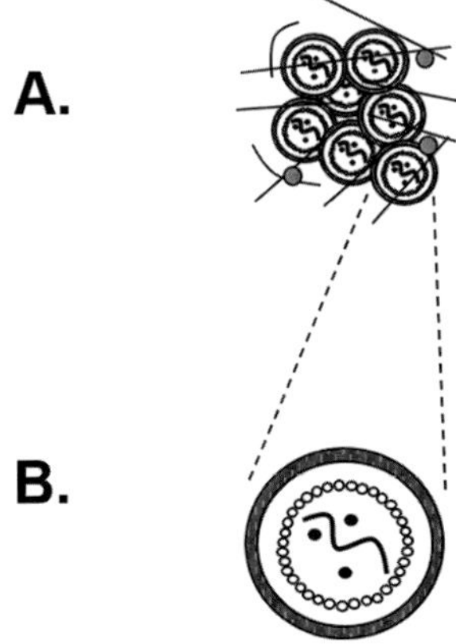

FIGURE 8.34 Mechanisms of viral resistance to biocides. The typical structure of an enveloped virus is shown as an example (chapter 1, section 1.3.5). Resistance can be due to indirect factors such as **(A)** viral clumping and protection (e.g., due to the presence of associated soils) or **(B)** directly to the structure of the virus particles, including the presence of an envelope, capsid structure, and access to damage the internal nucleic acid.

taken up and survive in *Acanthameoba* spp. (such as *A. castellanii* and *A. polyphaga*). Coxsackievirus b3 was specifically shown to survive multiple cycles of protozoa cyst formation and excystation over 6 months. Adenoviruses have been shown to be protected from water disinfection by sodium hypochlorite when taken up by *A. polyphaga*, confirming this protection mechanism of tolerance.

Another indirect mechanism involves viral aggregation, or clumping. Viral clumping has been implicated in various outbreaks of viral disease. A notable example was studied with the preparation of poliovirus vaccines. Polio vaccines are produced from either live attenuated (less virulent) strains or as inactivated poliovirus (IPV or enhanced IPV) preparations. IPV vaccines were first introduced in the 1950s by treatment of live, infectious poliovirus preparations with formaldehyde (typically mixed with 37% liquid formaldehyde for up to 12 days). The surface structure of the virus is directly affected by formaldehyde, dramatically reducing its infectious nature; however, the virus particles retain most of their immunogenic properties and therefore their potential as a vaccine. In the investigation of an outbreak of poliovirus associated with IPV preparations, it was found that viral clumping allowed the protection of individual virus particles from contact with formaldehyde; these preparations subsequently retained their infectivity when introduced into sensitive hosts. Various techniques are now used to ensure adequate contact with the biocide, including prefiltering of virus pools through 0.2-μm filters to remove viral aggregates prior to inactivation. The direct effects of formaldehyde on the surface structure of the virus are unknown but are believed to be due to cross-linking of the capsid proteins. Studies of poliovirus and similarly nonenveloped foot-and-mouth virus have found that formaldehyde-treated preparations become more resistant to acid pH (at which they normally disintegrate), and it was difficult to extract the viral nucleic acid (RNA) from them. It is not known if the viral RNA was directly affected by formaldehyde; it seems likely that both of these effects are due to cross-linking of the viral capsid to give a more rigid structure.

Another example of viral persistence to biocides by clumping has been described with outbreaks of Norwalk virus in drinking water and tolerance to chlorination. Laboratory investigations of the virucidal effects of peracetic acid on enteroviruses and rotaviruses showed a biphasic survival curve, which in these cases may also be interpreted as evidence of a more sensitive population of viruses that are rapidly killed by the biocide and a more resistant population of viral aggregates that require a longer time for penetration.

Following penetration of the biocide through any extraneous material to the virus particles, the major viral targets are the viral envelope (when present), the capsid, and the viral genome. The viral envelope is characteristic of the enveloped viruses (chapter 1, section 1.3.5) and contains various lipids and proteins typical of a cell membrane. This envelope, being derived from eukaryotic host cell membranes, may be considered to offer minor protection to the inner viral core from initial biocide damage. But these envelopes play important roles in the infectivity of the virus (including virus attachment and entry into target cells), and damage to the envelope can therefore dramatically reduce the virus's ability to infect cells. Enveloped viruses are therefore less resistant than nonenveloped viruses to biocides (see Fig. 8.1).

The presence or absence of an envelope was the basis of the original classification of viruses proposed in the 1960s based on their relative susceptibilities to disinfectants and their chemical nature. This classification is based on whether the viruses are "lipophilic" in nature, because they possess a lipid envelope (e.g., herpes simplex virus and HIV) or "hydrophilic" because they do not (e.g., poliovirus and parvoviruses). Lipid-enveloped viruses were found to be sensitive to lipophilic-type biocides, such as 2-phenylphenol, cationic surfactants (QACs), chlorhexidine, and isopropanol, as well as to solvents such as ether and chloroform. The initial classification was further refined into three groups (Table 8.28):

TABLE 8.28 Viral classification and response to biocides[a]

Viral group	Lipid envelope[b]	Examples of viruses	Effects of disinfectants[c]: Lipophilic	Effects of disinfectants[c]: Broad spectrum
A	+	Herpes simplex virus, HIV, Newcastle disease virus, rabies virus, influenza virus	S	S
B	–	Nonlipid picornaviruses (poliovirus, coxsackievirus, echovirus), parvoviruses	R	S
C	–	Other larger nonlipid viruses (adenovirus, reovirus)	R	S

[a]This is often referred to as the Klein and Deforest classification.
[b]Present (+) or absent (–).
[c]Lipophilic disinfectants include QACs and chlorhexidine; S, sensitive; R, resistant.

(i) lipid-containing (enveloped) viruses, (ii) small, nonlipid (nonenveloped) viruses, and (iii) a group of some larger nonlipid viruses with moderate resistance to some biocides. In general, larger viruses are more sensitive to biocides than smaller viruses, although this varies depending on the virus family, type, and strain. Adenovirus serovars, for example, have been found to vary in their intrinsic tolerance to disinfectants, presumably due to differences in their various capsid proteins. Disinfectants were also traditionally classified into two groups based on virus resistance: broad-spectrum disinfectants that inactivated a broad range of viruses and lipophilic disinfectants that failed to inactivate small, nonlipid viruses such as picornaviruses and parvoviruses. These classifications are widely used today as the basis for testing and verifying the virucidal efficacies of disinfectants in Europe, Australia, the United States, and other countries. Indicator viruses of each type, such as poliovirus (small, nonenveloped), adenovirus (large, nonenveloped), and herpes simplex virus (enveloped), are used to establish the virucidal activity of the disinfectant under recommended use conditions. The use of certain viruses is discouraged due to their potential pathogenicity or, in the case of polioviruses, due to eradication schemes.

The viral capsid is proteinaceous in nature. Therefore, biocides that disrupt the structure and function of these proteins (including glutaraldehyde, hypochlorite, ethylene oxide, hydrogen peroxide, and heat) have broad-spectrum virucidal activity. This is presumably due to the loss of infectivity associated with damage to the capsid in the case of the nonenveloped viruses. Chlorine dioxide or iodine treatment of polioviruses has been shown to interact directly with the capsid proteins, leading to disintegration and release of the viral RNA. Separation of the nucleic acid was proposed as being important for total viral inactivation; however, chlorine dioxide alone was also shown to damage the viral RNA and prevent subsequent viral replication in the host cell. Other virucidal effects can include damage to or loss of capsid-associated proteins that are required for viral infectivity (e.g., reverse transcriptase is carried by retroviruses and is required for release into the cell with the nucleic acid for replication). It is important to note that the destruction of the viral capsid can result in the release of a potentially infectious nucleic acid and that viral inactivation may not be complete unless accompanied by damage or destruction of the viral nucleic acid.

Viruses are either RNA- or DNA-based and can be single-stranded or double-stranded (see chapter 1, section 1.3.5). The infectivity of poliovirus RNA genomes and the effects of biocides have been particularly well studied. Poliovirus RNA retains its infectivity when isolated from the viral capsid. The nucleic acid is less infectious than the whole virus, but in some studies similar infectivity could not be shown with other RNA viruses such as hepatitis A and feline calicivirus. Free nucleic acids are more sensitive to biocides with known activity against RNA/DNA (chapter 7). The effects of radiation treatment, for example, with UV light, is dose dependent, with lower doses directly affecting the nucleic acid and forming photoproducts (such as dimers) typical of their mode of action (chapter 7, section 7.4.4). Higher doses of UV also affect the structure and function of capsid and other associated proteins. Oxidizing agents, such as chlorine and peracetic acid, can cause viral disintegration, with specific effects on viral proteins, lipids, and nucleic acids. Polioviruses are relatively sensitive to the effects of heat, with loss of capsid structure observed at 45 to 55°C; the effects of heat can vary depending on the virus and capsid type, with parvoviruses, for example, demonstrating greater resistance to heat than other viruses. These effects are related to the secondary and tertiary structures of the capsid proteins, with varying degrees of protein denaturation (section 7.4.4). Clearly, at higher temperatures general denaturation of macromolecules (including nucleic acids) leads to a general loss of viral structure and infectivity when heat penetration has been successful. Some parvoviruses have been shown to be highly resistant to the effects of dry- and even wet-heat processes, as well as to a range of chemical biocides. Resistance was shown to vary depending on the specific virus. Of the parvoviruses, porcine parvovirus and minute virus of mice demonstrated the highest level of tolerance to a variety of chemicals (including alkali, oxidizing agents, and aldehydes) at concentrations and contact times that were readily effective against poliovirus and other nonenveloped viruses. Both viruses were resistant to dry-heat conditions up to 90°C, with some studies showing a resistance profile equivalent to bacterial spores such as *B. atrophaeus* spores, which are considered the most resistant to dry-heat inactivation (see chapter 5, section 5.3); these viruses also showed resistance to moist-heat (boiling) inactivation up to ~80°C.

Other nonenveloped viruses such as rotaviruses, coxsackieviruses, and human papillomaviruses have shown particular resistance to chemical inactivation and persistence (due to drying) in various environments. Resistance appears to be due to the small, compact structures of these viruses and the overall lack of reactive amino acid residues at their surfaces. The capsids of parvoviruses, for example, are composed of ~60 proteins of two to four proteins (known as VP1 to VP4) depending on the virus types. They form tightly knit β-barrel structures interconnected by protein loops that are interlocked to form a stable protein shell around the nucleic acid; they vary in the numbers and types of exposed amino acids and can be further stabilized by binding Ca^{2+} ions. Although these structures are often resistant to the effects of many chemical biocides such as alcohols and QACs, they are inactivated by increased concentrations or exposure conditions (e.g., temperature, pH, and formulation effects) by other biocides such as the aldehydes and oxidizing agents. Reports of the complete lack of virucidal activity of aldehydes (such as glutaraldehyde and OPA) against certain strains of human papillomaviruses do not appear to correlate with the known structures of these viruses or studies with other highly resistant nonenveloped viruses (such as the parvoviruses). Access to certain amino acids such as lysine is an important factor in protein susceptibility to cross-linking by aldehydes (see chapter 7, section 7.4.3), and these appear to be present on the surface of human papillomaviruses (which are known to play a role in virus infectivity). The number and accessibility of lysine residues (or other reactive amino acid residues) within a given surface protein type are therefore an important consideration in the sensitivity of nonenveloped viruses to glutaraldehyde and other aldehydes. Likewise, the limited availability of reactive sites on protein amino acid side chains or peptide bonds in capsid structures due to their topology at the surface of nonenveloped viruses may limit the activity of other biocides such as phenolics and oxidizing agents, as well as limiting heat penetration.

As discussed above, the direct effects of the biocide or biocidal process on the viral nucleic acid are important to ensure the complete inactivation of the virus, particularly nonenveloped viruses. Therefore, biocides with known mechanisms of action against nucleic acids, such as oxidizing agents, radiation, heat, and aldehydes, are considered more effective than others (e.g., chlorhexidine and the QACs). This is particularly important in consideration of viroid disinfection. Viroids are naked, infectious, single-stranded RNA molecules but are relatively stable in structure and have been reported to be easily transmitted between plants. Their inactivation has not been studied in any detail, and they were originally considered to be relatively sensitive to hard-surface disinfectants; however, some studies have found that viroids were not affected by some detergents (including QACs) and phenolics but were inactivated by a propanol-benzoic acid formulation. It may be expected that biocides that target nucleic acids should be effective against viroids, but further testing is required to test the sensitivity of viroids to disinfectants.

Unfortunately, the penetration of various biocides into different types of viruses and their interactions with viral components have not been well studied. Some insights into these effects have been provided by investigations with bacteriophages (chapter 1, section 1.3.5). Bacteriophages (or phages) are bacterial viruses and are proposed as potential surrogates for assessing the virucidal activity of disinfectants due to their relative resistance in comparison to eukaryotic viruses. Morphological changes in the structure of the *P. aeruginosa* phage F116 on exposure to biocides have been studied under electron microscopy. Various effects were noted, including changes in the head and tail structure, leading to loss of phage infectivity and release of head DNA, which were dependent on the biocide concentration and exposure time. These effects were particularly observed with biocides that disrupt protein structure, including phenol, alcohol, peracetic acid, and glutaraldehyde; in contrast, chlorhexidine had little effect on phage structure and infectivity. Some studies have found that phage preparations have varying tolerances to the effects of sodium hypochlorite, with more resistant fractions being isolated at increased concentrations of available chlorine. These effects did not seem to be due to phage aggregation or obvious morphological differences in their structures. It is likely that this may be due to differences in the intrinsic structure of the various phage proteins and their sensitivity to biocides.

Overall, there are many conflicting results on the action of biocides on different virus types. This is primarily due to the different test systems used to study virus inactivation. An important example is virus preparation, in which viral suspensions are generally associated with cellular debris, and attempts to prepare purified fractions can lead to loss of infectivity. Other variables include the specific virus strain, cell culture method (which is often not available for specific viruses), and the disinfectant tested, including the neutralization method used (see chapter 1, section 1.4.2). Liquid biocide formulation can play an important role in virucidal activity. For example, clumping has already been discussed as a mechanism of viral resistance to disinfection. Because cross-linking biocides can entrap viruses within clumps, the effects of various detergents on some biocides can allow for their dispersion but not necessarily their inactivation. Further, some reports have suggested that the structural integrity of a virus could be altered by an agent that reacted with viral capsids to cause increased viral permeability to other biocides. Process effects such as temperature and phase of biocide exposure (e.g., liquid or gaseous hydrogen peroxide; see chapter 3, section 3.13) can also be important. For example, in bacteriophage and virus studies with hydrogen peroxide, low levels of virus persistence have been observed on exposure to liquid (or condensed) hydrogen peroxide, but not with gaseous peroxide (which may be due to clumping or overall limited penetration of liquid hydrogen peroxide over time). An interesting phenomenon described for bacteriophages and other viruses is referred to as "multiplicity reactivation," which has been observed under laboratory conditions. In these cases, it was envisaged that the viral particles were damaged due to the effects of the biocide under study to render them noninfectious but that complementary reconstruction of infectious particles can occur by reassociation of various virus components. In the case of UV- or alkylating agent-treated double-stranded DNA viruses (such as herpes simplex virus), this may be due to various virus components cooperating to allow for virus infectivity or to damaged DNA sections being repaired within the host cell.

It has often been considered unlikely that viruses will be found to have acquired resistance to biocides, but they have shown the ability to become resistant to various antiviral agents by genetic changes in various viral targets on exposures to biocidal treatments over time. A proposed mechanism is the mutation of key capsid proteins with increased resistance to the effects of biocides and biocidal processes by secondary or tertiary structural changes. With this is mind there remains the possibility of viral adaptation to new environmental conditions. A number of reports have suggested that this can occur. Laboratory poliovirus preparations were selected with increased tolerance to chlorine inactivation by gradual passage through increasing sublethal concentrations of chlorine; a similar development was described with *Pseudomonas* bacteriophages. In these cases, the mechanisms of resistance were not identified. More recent studies of the MS2 bacteriophage, with chlorine dioxide disinfection, have shown the ability of biocide exposure to select for more tolerant virus strains over time. Chlorine dioxide is an oxidizing agent (see chapter 3, section 3.13) distinct from chlorine, a halogen (see section 3.11), which is known to react with and degrade viral structural proteins. Exposure of bacteriophage preparations to chlorine dioxide over time was shown to select for mutations in the expression of amino acids in phage proteins that were more tolerant to biocide reactivity (particularly phage coat proteins). These structural changes included uncharged asparagine residues to the negatively charged aspartic acid residues. Specific changes to a certain coat protein, known as protein A, were important due to its role in cell infectivity, where mutants also had increased infectivity profiles. The development of the tolerant profile appeared to be unique to chlorine dioxide, and similar attempts to generate chlorine-tolerant forms in parallel were unsuccessful in these studies. As new methods of virus cultivation and investigation are developed, these will likely allow for a greater understanding of the unique mechanisms of viral inactivation by, and viral resistance to, biocides.

8.9 MECHANISMS OF PRION RESISTANCE

Transmissible spongiform encephalopathies are a group of fatal neurological diseases of humans and other animals. They are caused by prions, abnormal proteinaceous agents that contain no agent-specific nucleic acid (chapter 1, section 1.3.6). An abnormal protease-resistant form (PrP^{res}) of a normal host protein is implicated in the pathological process, although other factors have been proposed to be involved. Prions are considered highly resistant to most physical and chemical agents, with even greater resistance than bacterial spores in many cases (Table 8.29).

It is important to note that in earlier experiments with prion inactivation, crude preparations (brain homogenates from infected animals) were used to investigate the efficacy of various biocides and biocidal processes. The presence of extraneous materials (in particular, a high concentration of lipid associated with brain tissue) could, at least to some extent, mask the true efficacy or optimization of these processes against the infectious agent. Such experiments were important in the consideration of laboratory or animal carcass/material decontamination procedures but may not apply to all potentially contaminated situations. For example, for surface disinfection or sterilization applications (such as those performed during blood fractionation, on environmental surfaces, or with reusable medical devices), cleaning is typically performed prior to biocidal treatment, and the cleaning process is likely to affect any subsequent priocidal method. Considering the proteinaceous nature of prions,

TABLE 8.29 The effects of various disinfection and sterilization methods against prions

Effective	Partial or possible effectiveness[b]	Ineffective
Steam sterilization (121°C ≥1 hour)[a]	Liquid hydrogen peroxide	Formaldehyde
1–2 N NaOH ≥1 hour	Peracetic acid (in formulation at ≥50°C)	Glutaraldehyde
Steam sterilization (132–136°C ≥18 mins)[a]	Ozone	Alcohols
≥2% available chlorine for ≥1 hour[a]	Some acids, depending on concentration, formulation, and temperature exposure	Radiation (ionizing or nonionizing)
Incineration[a]		Dry heat
Hydrogen peroxide gas[c]		Ethylene oxide
Certain types of gas plasma (e.g., based on argon/oxygen and oxygen)[c]		Most phenolic disinfectants
Some phenolic disinfectant formulations[c]		QACs
Some alkaline cleaning formulations (pH ≥10.5)[c]		Pasteurization or boiling
Prolonged boiling in SDS or 1 N NaOH		
4 M guanidinium hydrochloride (≥1 hour)		
Prolonged protease digestion[c]		

[a]Some reports have shown incomplete inactivation, depending on the contaminated material and exposure to the process.
[b]The effectiveness of these methods has not been fully confirmed or investigated.
[c]Efficacy is variable depending on the specific process and/or formulation used.

it was not surprising to find that cleaning alone could remove or inactivate prions from surfaces; however, the efficacy of cleaning processes can vary significantly. For example, washing with water alone was infective, presumably due to the hydrophobic (lipid) nature of the contaminated brain material used in these investigations and the hydrophobicity of prion proteins. Washing with various types of detergent-based cleaning formulations in the neutral pH range (e.g., pH 5 to 9), in the presence or absence of proteases (enzymatic cleaners), can show some physical removal but little impact on degrading the prion protein itself. Cleaning with some of these formulations did appear to render the remaining infectious material more sensitive to subsequent steam sterilization, but in other cases the remaining material was more resistant to inactivation. The exact mechanisms associated with these results are unknown (but are considered in Fig. 8.35), but they do highlight that the impact of surface cleaning varies considerably depending on the cleaning formulation and process.

Finally, efficient physical removal and prion degradation (or fragmentation) has been shown with a variety of alkaline cleaning formulations, typically at pH >9. The efficiency of these processes varies considerably depending on the formulation, cleaning process conditions (in particular, temperature), and pH. Some of these cleaning processes alone were sufficient to completely remove and/or inactivate prion infectivity from highly contaminated surfaces, while others were only partially effective depending on the process conditions tested. These cleaning formulations would not typically be considered as effective broad-spectrum antimicrobial agents (e.g., against certain viruses, mycobacteria, or bacterial spores), highlighting that prions may be more resistant to many biocidal agents that are widely tested and used against microorganisms (such as radiation and heat-based processes) but may be more sensitive to other biocides due to their unique proteinaceous nature. An example could be the use of proteases as a method of prion inactivation. Although prions are considered resistant to proteases (hence their designation as PrP for "protease-resistant-protein"), various proteases, including proteinase K and keratinases, have been shown to degrade prions over time, depending on their concentration and exposure conditions. Despite these studies, the development of specific protease formulations that reduce the infectivity (or transmissibility) of prions have not proved successful

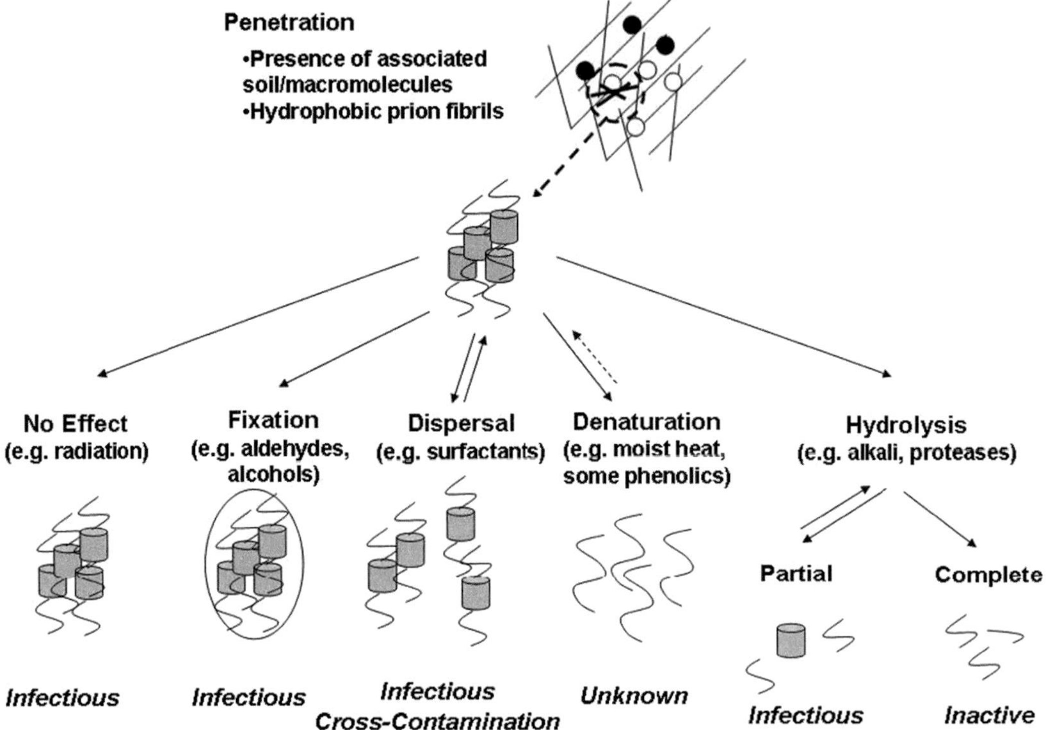

FIGURE 8.35 Mechanisms of resistance and modes of action of biocides against prions. Prions (as hydrophobic protein fibrils) are present in associated macromolecules (including lipids, carbohydrates, and proteins), through which the biocidal process needs to penetrate. Following penetration, ineffective processes include those that have no effect on proteins, that fix proteins, or that cause prion protein dispersal (potentially leading to cross-contamination). Biocidal processes that denature and/or hydrolyze (or degrade) proteins have been shown to be effective against prions; however, with denaturation alone, renaturation of the protein could occur to give the reassociated infectious protein form. Further, protein hydrolysis may be partial or complete. In some cases, partial hydrolysis of the protein is ineffective, because smaller components of the protein retain an infectious nature.

to date. This may be because only part of the prion protein (the protease-resistant hydrophobic core) is known to be responsible for the disease infectivity, and proteases may or may not specifically degrade this area of the protein to inactivate its disease induction capability.

In general, most physical and chemical disinfection or sterilization methods have been shown to have little to no impact on prion inactivation (particularly when present in crude extracts such as prion-infected tissues) (Table 8.29). These include broad-spectrum antimicrobial methods such as radiation, aldehydes, and ethylene oxide. The most effective process is boiling (or superheating under pressure) over time in concentrated solutions of alkali such as sodium hydroxide (at 1 to 2 N). Lower concentrations of hydroxides (NaOH and KOH) have been shown to be effective against surface prion contamination in combination with surfactants and other formulation effects. An example is a disinfectant formulation of 0.2% SDS, 0.3% NaOH, and 20% *n*-propanol, which has been shown to be effective against prions, bacteria, and viruses. The effects of alkali on prions have been studied and shown to cause protein and peptide fragmentation over time; these effects can be enhanced at increased concentrations and/or temperatures. Such methods have been used for whole-carcass dissolution. In contrast, prions can survive harsh acid treatment, such as at 1 M hydrochloric acid at room temperature for periods of up to 150 hours (but some activity has been shown at higher temperatures, at 65°C). Formaldehyde, unbuffered glutaraldehyde (acidic pH), and ethylene oxide have little effect on infectivity, although chlorine-releasing agents (especially hypochlorites), sodium hydroxide, some phenols, and guanidine thiocyanate are more effective.

It is not surprising to find that biocides with cross-linking mechanisms of action (see chapter 7, section 7.4.3) are not effective against prions, including the aldehydes, alcohols, and phenolic disinfectants. Although formaldehyde was often cited as an effective method, these effects appear to be due to the cross-linking activity preventing the availability of the prion molecules due to entrapment within extraneous materials; clinical and laboratory studies with prion-infected tissues fixed onto reusable neurosurgical instruments following formaldehyde treatment have shown disease transmission on subsequent patient use, suggesting that the prion material remained infectious and transmissible over an extended period (in some cases years). An exception within this group of biocides has been described with one particular phenolic formulation and was due to a unique mixture of phenolic compounds in the product formulation. Similar yet distinct formulations were not effective. The mechanism of action is unknown, but the formulation showed no obvious effects on the prion protein structure. Extended (in comparison to normal) steam sterilization processes are effective, although hydration of the prion-infected material appears to be important for optimal inactivation of prions. For example, steam sterilization processes appeared to be more effective when contaminated tissues were immersed in water and then exposed to the steam process, in comparison to direct exposure to dried materials.

Gaseous hydrogen peroxide has also been shown to be effective under atmospheric and vacuum conditions, which has been linked to degradation of the prion protein by peptide bond breakage. The priocidal effects vary considerably depending on the specific hydrogen peroxide gas process, and this variability may be due to the presence or absence of peroxide condensation during gas exposure (see chapter 3, section 3.13). Liquid peroxide, in contrast, did not seem to be effective at concentrations up to 60%, which may be due to the differences in mechanisms of action of liquid and gaseous peroxide (see section 3.13 and chapter 7, section 7.4.2). Priocidal activity has also been reported for other gaseous oxidizing agents such as ozone and gas plasmas (particularly those that include a portion of oxygen as the source gas), depending on the specific process tested. In these processes, fragmentation of the prion protein has been demonstrated. Sodium hypochlorites (and other chlorine-releasing agents) have been widely reported to be effective against prions, including 1.5 to 2% (15,000 to 20,000 ppm) available chlorine at ~20°C and 30 minutes of exposure time or a lower concentration of chlorine in formulation with detergents at 20 to 45°C; other halogens such as iodine have been reported to be dramatically less effective. Chlorine has also been shown to cause fragmentation of the prion protein. Considering the results from these investigations, the proposed mechanisms of prion resistance are summarized in Fig. 8.35.

Prions aggregate to form protein particles (or fibrils) within various tissues but are predominantly observed within neural tissues (such as the brain and spinal cord). These particles are hydrophobic and are associated with various cellular materials present within the contaminated tissue; for example, brain tissue contains a high concentration of lipid materials. These effects create a penetration challenge to the biocidal process. Various biocides and biocidal processes have been shown to be ineffective against prions. With the information presently available, it is difficult to explain the extremely high resistance of prions, save to comment that the protease-resistant protein (or, specifically, the hydrophobic core of the protein) is abnormally stable to degradative processes due to its unique β-sheet folded structure. In the case of radiation methods, the mechanism of resistance is proposed as evidence for the lack of any specific nucleic acid associated with prion infectivity; however, the effects of various radiation sources have not been studied in any detail, and radiation can damage other macromolecules including proteins (chapter 7, section 7.4.4). Biocides that have a cross-linking or fixing mode of action, including alcohols and aldehydes, have also been shown to be ineffective against prions, presumably due to the lack of any degradative effect on the target protein but actual cross-linking within other associated extraneous materials. Biocides or biocidal processes that denature or cause the fragmentation of proteins have been shown to be effective against prions. Moist heat and certain phenolic formulations are proposed to inactivate prions by denaturation. It has been speculated that renaturation of the denatured protein under some conditions could occur, although this has not been observed experimentally. Biocides such as sodium hypochlorite, sodium hydroxide, and hydrogen peroxide gas appear to cause fragmentation or other structural changes to prions, rendering them noninfectious. It is still possible (but considered unlikely) that other, as yet unidentified, factors are involved in prion infectivity and need to be similarly degraded to ensure complete inactivation.

8.10 MECHANISMS OF FUNGAL RESISTANCE

Compared to bacteria, less is known about the ways fungi can circumvent the action of biocides and biocidal processes. Despite this, two general mechanisms of resistance have been identified or are expected to occur: intrinsic resistance, a natural property or development of the organism during normal growth, and acquired resistance (Table 8.30).

Filamentous fungi (molds) grow by cell division but do not separate to form long lines and branches of cells known as hyphae, which further develop to form a mass of hyphae known as a mycelium (plural “mycelia”). As mycelial growth enters into stationary phase, a variety of fruiting bodies or other structures, which contain spores, develop. Fungal spores are found in a variety of shapes and sizes and can be asexual and/or sexual. A variety of unicellular fungi grow in a similar way to bacteria, for example, yeasts; they can also produce spores during their life cycles. The vegetative forms of fungi (yeasts and molds) are generally found to be more resistant to biocides than most nonsporulating bacteria (Table 8.30). It is tempting to speculate that the cell wall composition in fungi (chapter 1, section 1.3.3.2) confers a higher level of intrinsic resistance on these organisms. Vegetative molds are also typically found to be more resistant than yeasts (Tables 8.31 and 8.32). This is likely due to the overall coprotection of molds by mycelial growth. The various types of molds vary considerably in sensitivity to biocides, with *Asper-*

TABLE 8.30 Possible mechanisms of fungal resistance to biocides

Type of resistance	Possible mechanism	Example(s)
Intrinsic	Sporulation	Phenolics, QACs, desiccation, radiation, UV, ethylene oxide
	Hyphal clumping	UV, ethylene oxide, aldehydes
	Exclusion	Chlorhexidine, QACs, ethylene oxide
	Enzymatic inactivation	Formaldehyde, hydrogen peroxide and other oxidants, chlorine
	Phenotypic adaptation	Ethanol, oxidizing agents, halogens, copper, radiation
	Biofilm development	Oxidizing agents, halogens, copper, ethanol
	Efflux	Not widely demonstrated to date[a]
Acquired	Mutation	Some preservatives, biguanides, chlorine
	Plasmid-mediated responses	Not demonstrated to date

[a]Efflux, including inducible, systems are known to be a mechanism of fungal resistance to antibiotics.

TABLE 8.31 Comparison of the relative resistance of bacteria and fungi to biocides

			D value (minutes)[a,b]				
Antimicrobial agent	pH	Conc. (% [wt/vol])	*A. niger*	*C. albicans*	*E. coli*	*P. aeruginosa*	*S. aureus*
Phenol	5.1	0.5	20	13.5	0.94	<0.1	0.66
	6.1	0.5	32.4	18.9	1.72	0.17	1.9
Benzalkonium chloride	5.1	0.001	–	9.66	0.06	3.01	3.12
	6.1	0.002	–	5.5	<0.1	0.05	0.67

[a]D values were estimated at 20°C on exposure to phenol and benzalkonium chloride. The D value is defined as the time to kill 1 log (or 90%) of the microbial population under stated test conditions.
[b]–, no inactivation: fungistatic effect only.

gillus spp. often considered to be the most resistant to inactivation by multiple mechanisms of intrinsic resistance. The different types of fungal spores and the various structures they may be contained within also present a wide range of sensitivities to biocides. Fungal spores are more resistant than vegetative fungi but considerably less resistant than bacterial endospores to most biocides or biocidal processes.

The overall tolerance of fungi to biocides is primarily due to various mechanisms of intrinsic resistance. The predominantly polysaccharide-based (glycan) cell wall presents a protective barrier to reduce or exclude the entry of an antimicrobial agent such as QACs, triclosan, oxidizing agents (at lower concentrations), and chlorhexidine. The cell wall structures of fungi are varied and differ from those of bacteria (chapter 1, section 1.3.3.2). A typical fungal cell wall consists of fibrils of chitin or cellulose embedded within a matrix of various cross-linked glycans and associated proteins and lipids. These structures are considered effective barriers against the penetration of biocides. The cell walls of a number of yeasts have been described in some detail, although less is known about the specific structure of other fungi (Table 8.33). In general, mold cell walls predominantly consist of glucans, with specific linked outer cell wall glucans and inner polysaccharides, such as chitin or cellulose and/or proteins.

The role of the cell envelope or wall in intrinsic resistance is primarily due to exclusion from the cell. Of the various fungi tested, strains of *Aspergillus* are generally considered to be the most resistant to biocides and biocidal processes. This may be due to the higher proportion of linked β-glucans in the cell wall, but it is more likely that biocide tolerance is due to other factors such as hyphal clumping (preventing biocide penetration) and the development of spores (for *Aspergillus* spp., these can include conidiospores and ascospores, which are discussed in more detail below). Further, the fungal cell wall structures are known to be dynamic, with changes in the composition and proportions of components observed in response to different nutritional and environmental factors, not dissimilar to the phenotypic changes observed in bacteria (section 8.3.1). An example of phenotypic adaptation to antifungals has been described in *Aspergillus*, where an accumulation of cell

TABLE 8.32 Fungicidal concentrations of biocides for yeasts and molds

	Yeast	Molds	
Antimicrobial agent	*C. albicans*	*Penicillium chrysogenum*	*A. niger*
	QACs		
Benzalkonium chloride	10	100–200	100–200
Cetrimide/CTAB[a]	25	100	250
Chlorhexidine	20–40	400	200

[a]CTAB, cetyltrimethylammonium bromide, a type of QAC.

TABLE 8.33 Examples of the components of cell walls in fungi

Species	Cell wall components[a]			
	β-glucans	α-glucans	Mannoproteins	Chitin
S. cerevisiae	+ (~50–60%)	–	+ (~40%)	+ (~2%)
C. albicans	+ (~40–60%)	–	+ (~40%)	+ (~2%)
C. neoformans	+ (~15%)	+ (~35%)	+	+
A. fumigatus	+ (~80%)	+	+ (~3%)	+
Histoplasma capsulatum	+	+	?	?

[a]+, present; –, absent.

membrane ergosterol may be partially responsible for increased tolerance to azoles and may also be expected to increase tolerance to certain biocides that target the cell membrane. Yeasts grown under different conditions have variable levels of sensitivity to ethanol. For example, yeast cells with linoleic acid-enriched plasma membranes appeared to be slightly more tolerant to ethanol than cells with enriched oleic acid, from which it has been inferred that a more fluid membrane enhances ethanol resistance. The role of various fungal cell membrane sterols in the activity and penetration of biocides is not known but may play similar roles. Further, active response mechanisms have been described in yeasts that salvage and repair damage to the cell wall, which may provide some protection to the cell at subfungicidal concentrations of biocides. An example has been described in *S. cerevisiae*, in which cell wall maintenance genes are upregulated in response to biguanides (and may also be similarly affected by mutations in associated regulation genes). The impact of other growth phase adaptations on biocide tolerance, including enzyme expression, capsule production, and biofilm development, will be discussed later in this section. Overall, the impact of these and other phenotypic changes during normal growth do lead to variations in biocide sensitivity.

The cell wall structures of yeasts are similar to yet distinct from molds, with differences in the types of glucans and linked proteins identified (Table 8.33). Although yeast cell wall mutants have been described, their respective sensitivities to biocides have not been investigated. Overall, the yeast cell wall appears relatively flexible, which allows a yeast cell to be dimorphic, changing from single-celled to hyphal growth. In some limited studies with chlorhexidine susceptibility in the yeast *S. cerevisiae*, the penetration of the biocide was inhibited by the cell wall glucan, the wall thickness, and relative porosity (Table 8.34).

These findings can provide a tentative picture of the cellular factors that modify the response of *S. cerevisiae* to chlorhexidine. Cell wall-free protoplasts of *S. cerevisiae* were prepared by glucuronidase in the presence of β-mercaptoethanol and were found to be readily lysed by chlorhexidine concentrations well below those effective against normal

TABLE 8.34 Parameters affecting the response of *S. cerevisiae* to chlorhexidine

Parameter	Role in susceptibility of cells to chlorhexidine[a]
Cell wall composition	
Mannan	No role reported to date
Glucan	Possible significance: at lower concentrations and with cell wall-free forms, CHG can cause cell lysis
Cell wall thickness	Increases in cells of older cultures: expected reduced CHG uptake
Relative porosity	Decreases in cells of older cultures: expected reduced CHG uptake
Plasma membrane	Seems to be as sensitive as bacterial membranes, but alterations in lipids/proteins could change chlorhexidine susceptibility

[a]CHG, chlorhexidine diacetate.

(whole) cells. Furthermore, culture age influences the response of *S. cerevisiae* to chlorhexidine and other biocides; cells walls are much less sensitive at stationary phase than those in the logarithmic growth phase, where the uptake of chlorhexidine was much less during stationary phase. Studies with the antifungal antibiotic amphotericin B demonstrated a phenotypic increase in the resistance of *C. albicans* as the organisms entered the stationary growth phase, which was attributed to cell wall changes involving tighter cross-linking. These reports suggest that a similar increase in biocide resistance may occur, but this has not been investigated in any further detail.

The porosity of the yeast cell wall is affected by its chemical composition, with the wall acting as a barrier or modulator to the entry and exit of various agents. Assays have been developed to study the porosity of the yeast cell under normal growth conditions, including the uptake of fluorescein isothiocyanurate dextrans and the periplasmic enzyme invertase or polycation-induced leakage of UV-absorbing compounds as indicators of yeast cell wall porosity. Studies conducted with these assays have found that the relative porosity of cells decreases with increasing culture age. As the age of the *S. cerevisiae* culture increased, there was a significant increase in the cell wall thickness. In parallel, biocide permeability was reduced as the culture aged, as indicated by the uptake of radiolabeled chlorhexidine. Mannan mutants of *S. cerevisiae* show an order of sensitivity to chlorhexidine similar to the parent strain, suggesting that mannan does not play a significant role in cell wall tolerance to biocides. The yeast wall mannoprotein consists of two fractions: SDS-soluble mannoproteins and SDS-insoluble, glucanase-soluble mannoproteins; the latter appear to limit cell wall porosity. Thus, glucan and possibly some mannoproteins play a key role in determining uptake, and hence activity, of chlorhexidine in *S. cerevisiae*. *C. albicans* is less sensitive and takes up less chlorhexidine in comparison, but studies with this organism and with molds are few.

Various enzymes that are involved in the degradation and metabolism of formaldehyde in fungi and other eukaryotes have been identified. These mechanisms can be a particular concern in the use of formaldehyde or formaldehyde-releasing agents as preservatives (chapter 3, section 3.4). These include glutathione-dependent formaldehyde dehydrogenases and alcohol dehydrogenases in *Candida* and *Saccharomyces* spp. Glutathione reductases have also been described in *Rhodoturula* spp. that play a role in intrinsic tolerance to mercury. The expression of these enzymes can be considered an intrinsic mechanism of resistance similar to those described in bacteria (section 8.3.5) and may also be potentially linked to acquired resistance mechanisms. Another example is the expression of formate oxidase in *Aspergillus* spp., which can grow and metabolize in the presence of formaldehyde up to 0.45%. In addition to intrinsic expression of the enzymes, specific acquired mechanisms due to enzyme production have been described. *Saccharomyces* mutants have been described that have increased sensitivity to formaldehyde due to the loss of enzyme activity and increased tolerance due to overexpression of the associated enzyme(s). Similar hypersensitive yeast mutants have been described with alkylating agents such as ethylene oxide. Some strains of yeast have also been found to produce catalase and cytochrome *c* peroxidases that degrade hydrogen peroxide.

A limited number of fungi have been shown to produce capsules, or capsule-like structures, external to the cell wall that can present a further intrinsic barrier to biocide penetration. These include species of *Tremella*, *Trichosporon*, and *Sporothrix*, but the most studied is the *Cryptococcus neoformans* capsule (Fig. 8.36).

C. neoformans is an opportunistic human pathogen, particularly identified from immunocompromised patients. This basidiomycete fungus presents with various intrinsic mechanisms of resistance to biocides, including capsule formation on vegetative cells, the production of asexual fruiting bodies, which consist of desiccated clumps of cells, and the sexual

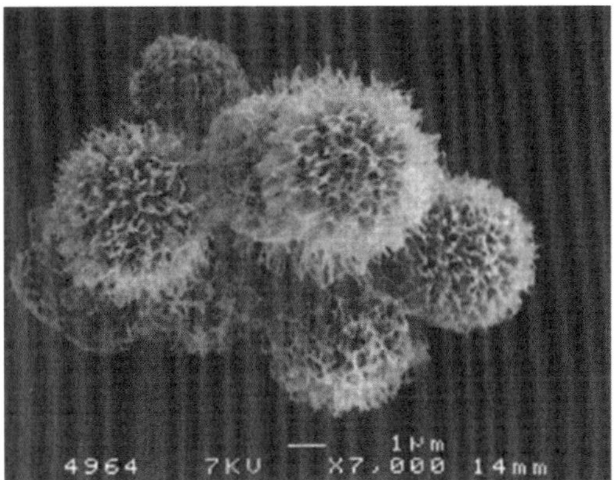

FIGURE 8.36 Scanning electron micrograph of an encapsulated *C. neoformans* strain. The capsule appears as a loose fibrillar network. (Reprinted from A. Casadevall and J.R. Perfect, *Cryptococcus neoformans* [ASM Press, Washington, DC, 1998].)

production of spores (basidiospores). The latter two mechanisms develop on nutrient starvation, suggesting stress response mechanisms similar to those of bacteria (section 8.3.3). Vegetative cells produce an exopolysaccharide capsule, which is tightly associated with the cell wall and plays an important role in the pathogenic nature of the microorganism in evading the immune response to infection and persistence. The capsule consists of two major polysaccharides: glucuronoxylomannan and galactoxylomannan. Approximately 90% of the capsule consists of glucuronoxylomannan, which is a mannose polymer with various sugar side chains; galactoxylomannan, which is a similar galactose polymer, is a much smaller component (~5%). Various other associated polysaccharides and proteins have also been described in capsules. Capsule formation is induced during asexual budding and changing growth conditions, suggesting a protection mechanism for the capsule similar to that described for bacteria as a stationary-phase phenomenon (section 8.3.1). Capsule synthesis is mediated by the *CAP* and *CAS* genes; various mutants that lack capsules or capsule components have been isolated and are more sensitive to some biocides at typical inhibitory or fungicidal concentrations. The relative tolerance of capsulated compared to noncapsulated cells has not been studied in detail.

As with bacteria, the presence of a capsule allows for greater affinity to surfaces that may also protect the fungal cells from inactivation. In studies with clinical isolates of *C. albicans*, *C. neoformans*, and *Rhodotorula rubra* the activity of various biocides (including iodine, chlorhexidine, hydrogen peroxide, alcohol, and sodium hypochlorite) and UV radiation resulted in dramatic differences in susceptibility between planktonic and surface-bound cells (possibly linked to biofilm development). *Cryptococcus*, *Candida*, and *Saccharomyces* spp. display gross morphological changes in response to stress (particularly oxidative stress) that are likely to be associated with increased tolerance to biocides. These are referred to as titan, polyploid cells. They can range in size from 5 to 10 times larger than normal cells and have multiple copies of their genomes ("polyploid"). Their polyploid nature is proposed to allow greater diversity or persistence by allowing chromosomal rearrangements and translocations in response to environmental stresses. Although studies describing increased tolerance to biocides have not been reported to date, it is tempting to describe these mechanisms as similar to various stress responses in bacteria (e.g., increased resistance to QACs, chlorhexidine diacetate, oxidizing agents, and even radiation) (see sections 8.3.3 and 8.3.9). Some of these modes of resistance may be growth-phase related, but others may be stable phenotypes, because many fungal environmental isolates are found to display greater tolerance levels to biocides than strains widely used in laboratory investigations.

Fungi, in particular molds, grow within tangled webs of individual hyphae and as part of a larger mass of mycelia forming mat- or mass-like structures (Fig. 8.37); this provides a penetration challenge to biocidal processes. An example has been described with UV radiation (chapter 2, section 2.4), against which fungi demonstrate high resistance, presumably due to a lack of penetration into the mycelium structure. At the level of individual hyphae, it should be noted that some studies have suggested that "lower" fungi hyphae are more

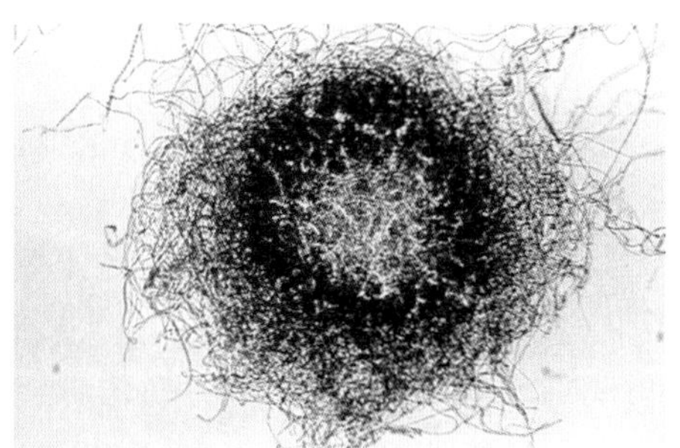

FIGURE 8.37 Example of a mass of fungal mycelial growth. Image courtesy of CDC-PHIL/Dr. Lucile K. Georg, 1971 (ID#15693), with permission.

sensitive to biocides than "higher" fungi due to the presence of septation (or separation between cells) in the latter. The septa may provide some protection to neighboring cells in the presence of a biocide, although these effects are considered minor. In addition, the cells at the ends of hyphae are actively dividing ("apical growth"), whereas other cells may be in a more dormant form. It is also expected, although it has not been investigated in any detail, that actively growing and multiplying cells are more sensitive to biocides than the are dormant cells, suggesting that within a given fungal mycelium, cells will display various levels of tolerance to antimicrobials.

Resistance mechanisms resulting from limited biocide penetration have been described with isolates of *Pyronema domesticum* and their intrinsic resistance to ethylene oxide. Ethylene oxide is a broad-spectrum biocide that is widely used for low-temperature sterilization of devices and other materials (chapter 6, section 6.2). Isolates of *P. domesticum* have been found to survive typical ethylene oxide sterilization processes associated with devices using cotton (e.g., in sponges and gauzes), particularly those sourced from China. Other *Pyronema* strains have since been identified in cotton from other countries, including the United States. Studies with these strains showed that they were sensitive to steam sterilization but exhibited significantly increased tolerance to radiation (E-beam and γ irradiation). In the case of ethylene oxide, resistance has been described as being up to 10 times higher than that typically described for *B. atrophaeus* spores, which are often cited as the most resistant to ethylene oxide sterilization (see section 6.2). *P. domesticum* is an ascomycete mold that appears to have at least two significant mechanisms of tolerance for ethylene oxide inactivation. First, and typical of many ascomycetes, it produces sexual spores (known as ascospores) within bodies known as ascocarps, specifically, bowl-shaped apothecia. Apothecia consist of tightly interwoven hyphae with many asci that contain four to eight ascospores. Second, they produce hardened (or desiccated) clumps of fungal hyphae known as sclerotia, which appear to be dormant and can also include asexual and sexual spores (a more detailed discussion on the various types of spores found in fungi is provided later in this section). The desiccated nature of the sclerotia is presumed to reduce the penetration of ethylene oxide, which requires humidity for optimal antimicrobial activity (see section 6.2). Both the sclerotia and, particularly, the ascopsores have also been shown to be highly cross-resistant to γ and E-beam radiation.

Similar, yet not as extreme, mechanisms of resistance have been described in other ascomycetes such as *Aspergillus* spp. They are often reported to have high resistance to UV light, gaseous biocides, and liquid disinfectants, particularly related to the types of spores produced. Many species can produce walled ascocarps known as cleistothecia, which are spherical and provide multiple layers of protection to internal ascopsores. In addition, they produce asexual conidiospores in abundance that can demonstrate high persistence in the environment (being some of the most common environmental contaminants found in the air and associated surfaces). Conidiospores often present with thickened wall structures and photoprotective, black pigments, which have been shown to contribute to increased biocide tolerance including UV light and heat (up to 56°C in comparison to nonpigmented forms). Tolerance can be induced, for example, by exposure to light during growth (in comparison to culturing in the dark). The production of thickened-walled ascospores in *Chaetomium* spp. as a tolerance mechanism to peracetic has been described.

Various fungi have been associated with biofilm formation. Biofilms are communities of microorganisms that are attached to surfaces and can include various microorganisms including bacteria, protozoa, and fungi (section 8.3.8). Various molds and yeasts have been described as being biofilm-formers by binding to surfaces and proliferating within a protective exopolymeric structure. These include *Aspergillus*, *Candida*, *Rhodotorula*, *Cladosporium*, and *Cryptococcus* spp. They have been identified in water systems and associated with implantable or indwelling devices, as well as with "dry" biofilms similar to bacteria identified on various environmental surfaces (see section 8.3.8). *C. albicans* biofilms are a particular concern on implantable devices and have been shown to be highly resistant to various antimicrobial agents. Tolerance in these cases is not only due to the complex, polysaccharide structures of biocides but also to the increased production of antioxidants and enzymes (e.g., superoxide dismutase and catalase), as shown in studies with chlorine and hydrogen peroxide. In addition, various fungi can become associated with preexisting bacterial biofilms, along with miscellaneous debris, where they proliferate and cooperate within the biofilm. These complex associations offer protection against the effects of biocides. Similar to bacteria and viruses, certain fungi (for example, *C. neoformans*) have been shown to survive and grow in *Acanthamoeba castellanii* as a further protective mechanism. Interestingly, the passage of *C. neoformans* or *Histoplasma capsulatum* through amoeba has been associated with increased virulence, which may be linked to greater tolerance to enzymes and oxidizing agents that are present in amoeba and other host cells as cellular responses to pathogen invasion.

The typical life cycle of a fungus is shown in Fig. 8.38. In many cases fungi reproduce by both asexual and sexual reproduction. Asexual reproduction can occur by budding or binary fission in yeast (where one cell produces a bud to form another cell) but also by fragmentation of the fungal hyphae allowing the fragment to disperse and multiply. However, the

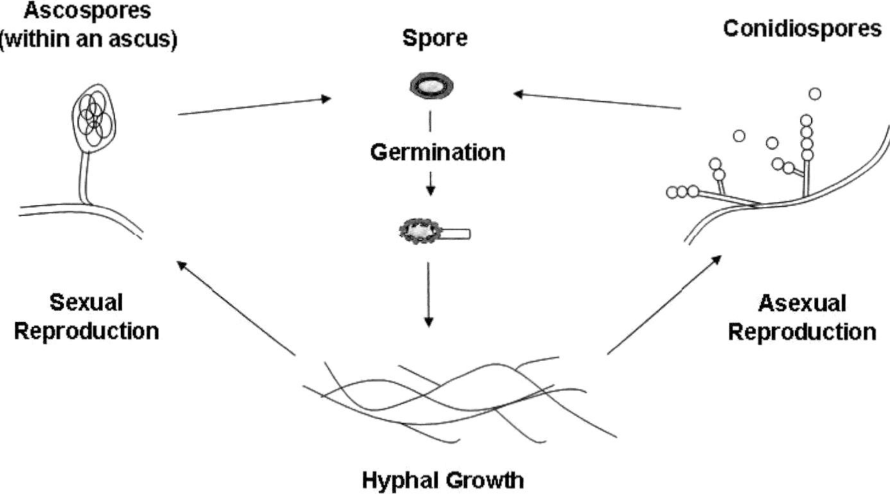

FIGURE 8.38 Fungal (ascomycota) life cycle. The life cycle shown is typical of ascomycota such as *Neurospora*. In the case of yeasts such as *Saccharomycetes*, the single cells reproduce asexually by binary fission or budding and sexually by two cells uniting to lead to the development of ascospores. Asexual and sexual spores (which are different in structure) are formed in other fungi, although in some cases only asexual conidiospores have been described (Table 8.34).

most common form of asexual reproduction is by the production of asexual spores in response to various environmental factors, including nutrient limitations.

Fungi are traditionally classified based on their microscopic morphology, including the presence of septation between individual cells within the hyphae structure and the various types of spores or spore-forming ("fruiting") bodies developed. The various types of fungal asexual and sexual spores are summarized in Fig. 8.39 and classified in Table 8.35. Genetically, asexual spores are produced by mitosis, and sexual spores by the fusion of the protoplasts and nuclei of two cells, followed by meiosis.

Similar to some bacteria, fungi form spores in response to various environmental stimuli including nutrient restrictions, competition, and low concentrations of fungistatic/fungicidal biocides. Spores therefore have fundamentally two major functions: survival and dispersal. The main types of asexual spores are conidiospores (or conidia) and sporangiospores. Conidiospores are developed from specialized, aerial hyphae known as conidiophores that bud spores and are borne naked on the hyphae structure. In contrast, sporangiospores are formed within fruiting bodies known as sporangia, which are also mounted on specialized hyphae (sporangiospores). Asexual spores develop by nutrient accumulation within a specific vegetative cell, where they swell in size, convert available nutrients into lipid or carbohydrate reserves, and develop a specialized external spore wall. In some cases, spongiospores are considered more tolerant to various biocides in comparison to conidia, because they develop a double spore wall, in contrast to the conidial single spore wall. The different types of sexual spores are also developed within specialized structures (including oospores, zygospores, and ascospores, the latter within an ascus; Fig. 8.39) or naked on specialized hyphae (e.g., basidiospores). There are different mechanisms of sexual spore development, which generally involve the development and maturation of a spore wall around a cell nucleus and cytoplasm. In the case of development within a fruiting body such as an ascus, the spores can be further protected from attack by materials that surround and support the spore within these structures (and within clumps of mycelia, as described for *Pyronema* and *Aspergillus* earlier in this section). These structures can act as a multiprotective layer to the individual viable spores. Another class of fungi, the deuteromycota, or "imperfect" fungi, do not (or are not known to) produce sexual spores.

The molecular structures of fungal spores have not been described in detail. In general, they are known to be surrounded by a rigid wall of various thicknesses, primarily made of polysaccharides but also containing proteins, lipids, and pigments. The spore wall is distinct in structure from the normal vegetative cell wall, being less fibrous and more multilayered.

TABLE 8.35 Examples of various spores produced by fungi

Groups[a]	Examples	Septation[b]	Asexual spores	Sexual spores
Low				
Zygomycota	*Rhizopus*, *Mucor*	–	Sporangiospores	Zygospores
Oomycota	*Phythophthora*, *Pythium*	–	Zoospores	Oospores
High				
Ascomycota	*Saccharomyces*, *Aspergillus*, *Candida*, *Neurospora*	+	Conidia (conidiospores)	Ascospores
Basidiomycota	*Cryptococcus*, mushrooms, puffballs	+	Uncommon	Basidospores
Deuteromycota ("imperfect" fungi)	*Thermomyces*, *Nattrassia*	+	Conidiospores	–

[a]The classification of fungi often shows discrepancies, but in this case, fungi can be grouped into a "low" class that do not have true septa between individual cells, and a "high" class whose members are septate, as well as the types of spores they produce.

[b]+, present; –, absent.

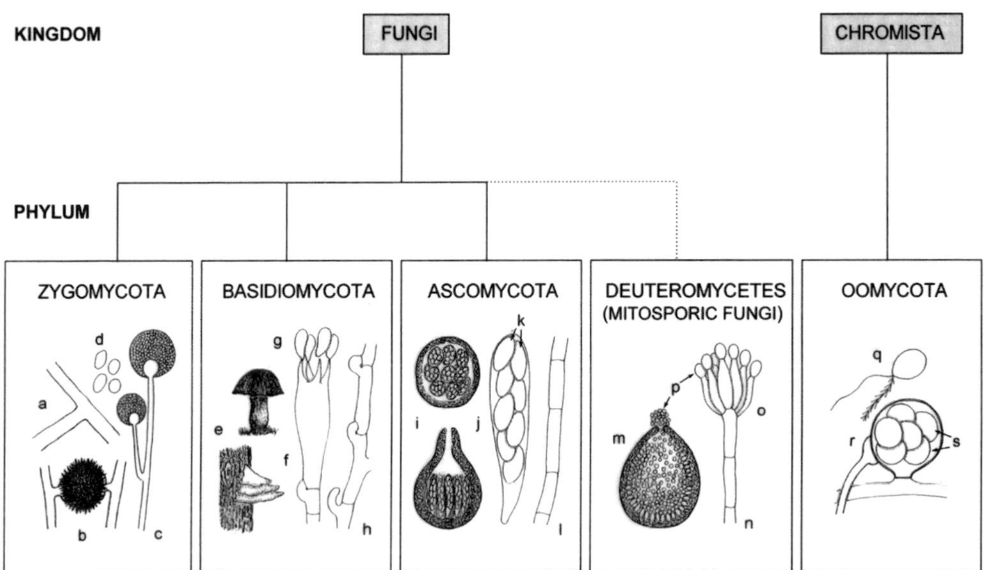

FIGURE 8.39 Examples of various types of fungal spores and spore-bearing structures. Zygomycota: a, aseptate hypha; b, zygospore; c, sporangiophore (with spores within sporangia); d, sporangiospores. Basidiomycota: e, basidiomata; f, basidium; g, naked basidiospores; h, hypha with clamp connections. Ascomycota: i, ascomata; j, ascus, containing spores; k, ascospores; l, septate hypha. Deuteromycetes: m, pycnidium; n, conidiophore; o, conidiogenous cells; p, conidia. Oomycota: q, zoospore (motile); r, gametangia; s, oospores. (Reprinted from J. Guarro et al., *Clin Microbiol Rev* 12:454-500, 1999.)

Internally, fungal spores contain nutrient reserves (carbohydrates and fats) and have low water content (normally as low as 1% in vegetative mycelia) and low metabolic activity. The thickness of the spore wall appears to be related to the extent of dormancy. Some spores (generally asexual spores such as conidia and sporangiospores) have thin walls and low nutrient reserves, which can be easily disseminated and germinate rapidly under suitable conditions. These spores also contain typical vegetative cell organelles and are actively metabolizing, but at a much lower rate than vegetative cells. Some asexual zoospores are motile due to the expression of flagella. In contrast, other spores develop thicker cell walls and higher reserves, which are more suitable for survival under adverse conditions. Fungal spores are generally more resistant than vegetative fungal cells or hyphae, but not to the same extent as bacterial spores. Sexual spores are particularly more resistant to drying, heating, and some biocides.

Typically, most fungal vegetative forms and spores are heat sensitive at 50 to 60°C. Despite this, some fungi that produce ascospores with a higher resistance to heat and radiation than normally observed for fungi have been identified. These include heat-resistant species of *Byssochlamys*, *Talaromyces*, and *Eurotrium*. These have been identified as frequent contaminants in thermally processed foods (in particular, fruit juices) and have been implicated in food spoilage. Pasteurization (chapter 2, section 2.2) is a heat disinfection process generally applied to solid or liquid foods to reduce the risk of the presence of pathogens and/or food spoilage organisms. It is widely used for the treatment of milk and milk products, beer, and juices to extend their shelf life. Typical pasteurization can range from 63 to 66°C for ≥30 minutes and 71 to 72°C for ≥15 to 16 seconds. Many fungal heat-resistant isolates survive these processes and require higher temperatures to be fungicidal (in the 80 to 95°C range). The mode of resistance is unknown but is clearly related to the structure of the ascospores. As described above in the case of *Pyronema*, ascospores and related structures have been identified with higher resistance to other biocidal processes such as radiation and EO. It is expected that the nature of resistance of these spores is due to both protection within masses of hyphae and to the intrinsic resistance of the developed spores, including having desiccated protoplasm and multiple spore wall layers. Studies with *Aspergillus* have shown that conidia and vegetative cells are relatively sensitive to QAC and alcohols, but ascospores demonstrate greater tolerance. The overall resistance of ascospores also increased with age and varied from species to species. The level of desiccation of *Aspergillus* ascospores has been linked with intrinsic resistance to UV light, ethylene oxide gas, and likely other gaseous biocides.

The germination of fungal spores is similar to that described for bacterial endospores (section 8.3.11). This includes germination of the spore, followed by water uptake with an increase in spore size and development of a germ tube, which grows into a vegetative cell or actively growing hyphae. The initiation of germination has been shown to vary in the different spore types. In some cases, there are factors that prevent the germination of the spore and need to be relieved prior to continuing. These include inhibitory factors within the spore (for example, spore phosphate levels) or, in the case of *Microsporum* spores, an external protein layer which needs to be degraded by an intrinsic spore enzyme before germination can proceed. Other germination mechanisms are similar to endospores, with the spore sensing the environment for the presence of nutrients and water or the absence of inhibiting factors, including biocides. These mechanisms play a role in the survival of fungi at fungistatic concentrations of biocides.

As in bacteria, heavy metal resistance in *C. albicans* and, to a lesser extent, *S. cerevisiae* has been described. Two major mechanisms of resistance have been described in eukaryotes: the expression of metal-binding proteins (e.g., metallothioneins) and efflux mechanisms. In the case of *C. albicans* both mechanisms occur in response to toxic levels of copper. These include the expression of copper metallothioneins that bind copper via thiol groups of exposed cysteine residues within the protein (e.g., CUP1) and copper efflux by P-type ATPases (e.g., CRP1 and CRD1p, the latter extruding both copper and silver ions). The difference in tolerance between *C. albicans* and *S. cerevisiae* has been proposed to be due to the lack of specific copper efflux in *S. cerevisiae*, where both strains examined produced metallothioneins. Overall, there is little evidence of efflux as a mechanism of biocide tolerance in fungi. In some yeasts (e.g., *Candida boidinii*), the extrusion of formic acid has been proposed to provide a greater level of tolerance to formaldehyde; increased tolerance is at least partially due to the expression of a nuclear membrane-associated exporter that has been shown to be overexpressed in the presence of formaldehyde. Other efflux mechanisms have been described in *C. albicans*, which are expressed early in biofilm development; these have been linked to antifungal (azole) resistance and include two types of efflux mechanisms, ABC and MFS pumps (see section 8.3.4); the significance of these pumps in the tolerance to biocides remains to be investigated.

Similarly, there is little evidence of acquired resistance by mutation (except to some preservatives) or by plasmid-mediated mechanisms, although these mechanisms are likely to exist, considering investigations in and similarities to bacteria (see section 8.7.3). In one example, the mutational loss of a cytoplasmic membrane pump in *S. cerevisiae* was shown to cause an increase in resistance to QACs such as benzalkonium chloride; this pump was involved in the transport of leucine into yeast cells, suggesting a similar mechanism of transport and tolerance due to expulsion from the cell cytoplasm. *Schizosaccharomyces* mutants with stable tolerance to various heavy metals have been isolated. Resistance linked to plasmid acquisition has not been studied, but increased tolerance to various antifungal agents has been artificially constructed under laboratory conditions; the significance of these results in the environment for biocidal resistance is not known. Overall, it may be expected that mechanisms of acquired biocide tolerance similar to those described in bacteria remain to be identified in yeasts and molds.

In conclusion, relatively few rigorous studies have been conducted to understand intrinsic and extrinsic resistance mechanisms to biocides in yeasts and molds. As vegetative microorganisms, various fungi have demonstrated mechanisms of resistance similar to those described in more detail for bacteria, including excluding cell wall structures, stationary-phase phenomena, biofilm development, degradative enzyme production, and sporulation. Less is known about acquired mechanisms of resistance, but it may be expected that similar mechanisms remain to be identified and further described in fungi.

8.11 MECHANISMS OF RESISTANCE IN OTHER EUKARYOTIC MICROORGANISMS

Protozoa are single-celled eukaryotes, but they do not contain a true cell wall (chapter 1, section 1.3.3.4). Their vegetative forms (including trophozoites and sporozoites) do not present a significant challenge to most biocides, even at low-level concentrations or doses. The exception to this has been described in one study with the unexpected resistance of trophozoites (particularly amoeba) to glutaraldehyde (even at 2% glutaraldehyde in formulation for 30 minutes exposure); this high level of resistance varies depending on the particular protozoal strain, with clinical and environmental isolates demonstrating greater resistance than reference laboratory strains of the same genus. The modes of action of the various biocides and biocidal processes are not considered to be different from those described in bacteria. For example, chlorhexidine and other biguanides have been shown to primarily affect the structure and function of the plasma membrane, as observed by electron microscopy analysis of treated protozoa. Various intrinsic mechanisms of resistance have been described in protozoa that appear to be similar to those identified in bacteria and fungi, but they have not been well described. Vegetative forms survive various hostile environments, including the presence of host resistance mechanisms such as the production of superoxide ions and hydroxyl radicals. As in bacteria and fungi, these mechanisms can be linked to increased tolerance to oxidizing agents and some halogens. One example that has been described in *Leishmania* is the production of superoxide dismutase, which neutralizes the presence of superoxide ions (section 8.3.5). This may be part of an overall stress response, as described in *A. castellanii* trophozoites with the expression of various shock proteins on exposure to heat, oxidizing agents, and pH changes; the exact functions of these proteins have not been defined but are likely to be similar to those described in bacteria. They may include DNA repair mechanisms, which have been specifically described in UV-irradiated *Cryptosporidium* spp. Other physiological adaptations include the overproduction of surface glycoproteins or other proteins or carbohydrates, which may act to sequester the presence of the biocide and alterations in protozoal permeability. Efflux and/or decreased influx mechanisms have also been described and have been implicated in antiprotozoal drug (e.g., chloroquine) resistance. Multidrug-resistance ABC efflux pumps have been identified in *P. falciparum* and may also allow for increased tolerance to biocides (including triclosan), as described in bacteria (section 8.3.4).

Many protozoa grow and multiply within host cells, including *Plasmodium* in hepatocytes and red blood cells and *Leishmania* in white blood cells; the ability for intracellular persistence of these protozoa may provide protective mechanisms against the effects of biocides. *Acanthamoeba* spp. have also been shown to express many factors associated with stress responses similar to those described in bacteria, such as chaperones (which allow protein refolding), DNA repair mechanisms, and efflux protein systems (see section 8.3.3). Further, many amoeba (particularly *A. castellanii*, other *Acanthamoeba* spp., *Hartmannella*, and *Naegleria*) have been associated with bacterial biofilms and can become an integral part of a mature biofilm community. A variety of bacteria (e.g., *Legionella*, *Enterobacteriaceae*, *Pseudomonas*, *Staphylococcus*, and *Mycobacterium* spp.), viruses (coxsackieviruses, enteroviruses), and fungi (e.g., *Cryptococcus*) have been found to survive, and in some cases multiply, within *Acanthamoeba* and other amoebae. These microorganisms have been identified in vegetative and cyst forms of amoebae, allowing for their protection against biocides and biocidal processes. For this reason, amoebae are often referred to as the Trojan horses of microbiology. In some studies, bacteria that have been injured by chemical disinfection (e.g., *Legionella* treated with sodium hypochlorite) were found to be unculturable by normal laboratory growth techniques but were subsequently shown to be resuscitated in *Acanthamoeba*. This finding is an example of viable but nonculturable forms of microorganisms that can present on suboptimal treatment with biocides and biocidal processes (see section 8.3.12).

Acquired mechanisms of resistance have not been identified or investigated in any detail in protozoa, but it may be expected that various mutations could develop to increase tolerance to biocides. An example is the demonstration that triclosan inhibits protozoa such as *Plasmodium*, *Toxoplasma*, and *Babesia* by interacting with enoyl acyl carrier protein reductases involved in fatty acid synthesis and similar to specific targets identified in bacteria (section 8.7.2); it is likely, considering identified mutations that allow for resistance to antiprotozoal drugs, that similar mechanisms of tolerance to triclosan and other biocides, as described in bacteria, may also occur in protozoa. Other mutations could also increase tolerance to many biocides by increasing expression of various stress responses in protozoa, similar to those described in bacteria (including potential efflux mechanisms). Gene transfer has been reported in protozoa, but no links to biocide resistance have been identified to date.

Protozoa produce dormant forms during their life cycles, such as cysts or oocysts (chapter 1, section 1.3.3.4). Intestinal protozoa such as *Cryptosporidium*, *Entamoeba*, and *Giardia* are all known pathogens in humans and animals and produce resistant, transmissible cysts (or oocysts for *Cryptosporidium*) that can be transmitted in water or associated with contaminated surfaces. Although the intrinsic resistance of oocysts and cysts varies, these dormant protozoal forms are considered more resistant to biocides than viruses, vegetative bacteria, and fungi but less resistant than *Ascaris* eggs and bacterial spores. *Giardia* cysts and *Cryptosporidium* oocysts have been isolated from chlorinated water and have been implicated in disease outbreaks due to inadequate disinfection. *Cryptosporidium parvum* is an obligate intracellular pathogen that can cause severe gastrointestinal disease, in particular, in immunocompromised individuals. In response to environmental stress, it develops oocysts, which consist of a double layer of a protein-lipid-carbohydrate matrix that is produced within the oocyst itself during maturation (Fig. 8.40). *C. parvum* oocysts have been shown to be the most resistant to chemical disinfection in comparison to other protozoal cysts, such as those of *Giardia lamblia*. Of the biocides widely used for water disinfection, oxidizing agents such as ozone and hydrogen peroxide are considered the most effective protozoan cysticides, followed by chlorine dioxide, iodine, and free chlorine, all of which are more effective than the chloramines.

The thicknesses of the *C. parvum* oocyst walls vary, and thinner-walled oocysts are considered less resistant to biocides and other environmental factors than the thicker-walled types. The ultrastructure of the oocyst wall can vary from species to species, but in general it consists of a four-layered structure: an outer

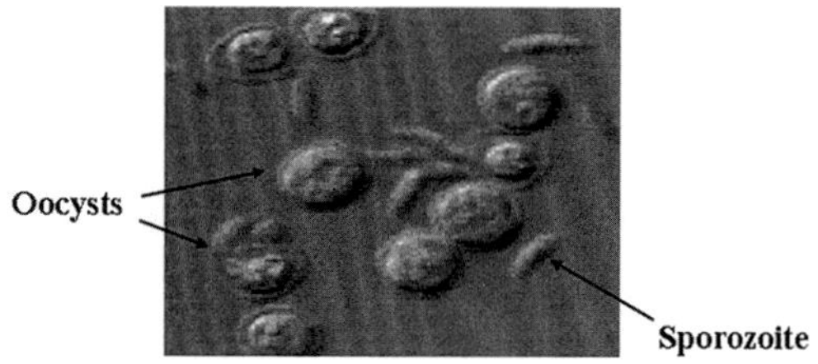

FIGURE 8.40 *C. parvum* oocysts and sporozoites.

glycocalyx, a lipid layer, a protein layer, and an inner polysaccharide layer. The glycocalyx (~8 nm) consists of glucose and other sugars and is easily removed from the structure and is therefore not thought to play a significant role in biocide resistance. But the other three layers provide a formidable barrier to chemical biocides due to a mixture of hydrophobic and hydrophilic structures. The outer, thinner lipid layer (~4 nm) is composed of fatty acids and phospholipids, and the larger protein layer (~13 nm) is thought to consist of ~12 types of proteins (although some of these may be associated with other layers). The innermost polysaccharide is the larger and more variable-sized layer (ranging from 25 to 40 nm); the types of polysaccharides have not been fully identified but may include polymers such as *N*-acetyl-D-galactosamine.

In studies of various surface sterilization and disinfection methods, steam, ethylene oxide, methyl bromide, and hydrogen peroxide gas sterilization processes were confirmed to be effective against *C. parvum* oocysts. In contrast, formaldehyde gas treatment was found to be less effective, even over extended exposure conditions. Liquid hydrogen peroxide formulations (at 6 to 7.5%) were also effective, but oocysts have been described as being resistant to normal, in-use concentrations of peracetic acid-, sodium hypochlorite-, phenolic acid-, QAC-, iodophor-, glutaraldehyde-, and OPA-based disinfectants. As with other microorganisms, the presence of soils limited the activity of the disinfectants tested due to reduced penetration. Peracetic acid-based formulations were effective at higher exposure temperatures (>40°C), but oocysts were also found to be relatively sensitive to temperatures in the 50 to 60°C range, therefore presenting little resistance to heat in comparison to chemical biocides. Oocysts were also inactivated by UV radiation, γ radiation (but required higher doses at ~1 kGy), freeze-thawing cycles, and on drying or desiccation, unlike bacterial spores. The mechanisms of chemical biocide resistance are unknown, but it would be reasonable to assume that cysts are similar to spores, and restrict the access of chemical disinfectants in comparison to vegetative forms. In some studies, resistance appeared to be primarily due to interaction with the protein components of the cyst wall layers.

The cysts of the amoeba *A. castellanii* have also been studied in some detail (Fig. 8.41).

These cysts are significantly more resistant than vegetative trophozoites (Table 8.36).

Several studies have compared the responses of cysts and trophozoites of *A. castellanii* to disinfectants employed in contact lens solutions and followed the development of resistance during encystation and the loss of resistance during excystation. Similar to the development of bacterial spores (section 8.3.11), as *A. castellanii* trophozoites developed and matured into cysts, tolerance to various biocides could be detected; early in development, tolerance to hydrochloric acid was observed, followed by benzalkonium chloride, hydrogen peroxide, and moist heat, with resistance to chlorhexidine observed in the later stages of cyst maturation. The lethal effects of chlorhexidine and of a polymeric biguanide were found to be time- and biocide concentration-dependent, and mature cysts were clearly more resistant than pre-encysted trophozoites or postexcysted cysts. The cyst wall, and overall dense cyst structure, appears to act as a barrier to the uptake of these biocides, presenting classical mechanisms of intrinsic resistance. Amoebal cysts are resistant to heat at 55°C, but not at 65°C, but demonstrate a greater tolerance profile to chemical disinfectants. Chlorine

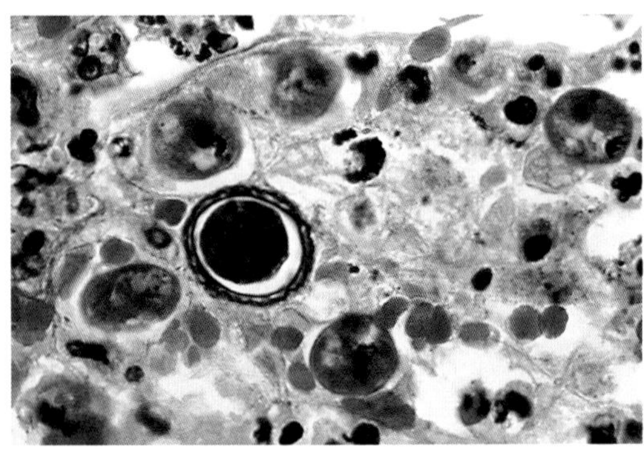

FIGURE 8.41 *Acanthamoeba* cyst.

TABLE 8.36 The minimum amoebicidal concentrations of *Acanthamoeba* trophozoites and cysts

Biocide[a]	Minimum amoebicidal concentration (mg/liter)	
	Trophozoites	Cysts
Chlorine	2	>50
Peracetic acid	15	150
BNPD	250	>5,000
BKC	60	>5,000

[a]BNPD, bromonitropropanediol, a bromine-releasing agent; BKC, benzalkonium chloride, a QAC.

(or sodium hypochlorite) has been particularly well studied, due to the persistence of cysts in water, and higher concentrations and/or contact times (e.g., 0.25% for 10 minutes) are required for effectiveness, depending on the particular strain. Similar results were reported for other oxidizing agents (e.g., hydrogen peroxide and peracetic acid), but the efficacy against cysts was dramatically increased by formulation effects (e.g., hydrogen peroxide in acidic formulation). Individual isolates of *A. castellanii* and *A. polyphaga* were found to range considerably in their tolerance profiles to these and other (e.g., OPA) disinfectants, again with environmental isolates demonstrating greater tolerance than laboratory strains. Interestingly, amoebal cysts were very sensitive to alcohol disinfection, but glutaraldehyde was relatively ineffective (similar to resistance profiles described for amoebal trophozoites, discussed above).

The mechanisms of tolerance in these isolates were not investigated in detail, but those with thicker cyst walls were generally more resistant to the biocides tested; the high level of resistance to glutaraldehyde may be linked to the lack of exposed or available proteins at cyst or trophozoite surfaces, limiting the surface cross-linking activity of the biocide (see chapter 7, section 7.4.3, and similar mechanisms of resistance described in *Mycobacterium*, section 8.4). The amoebal cyst wall structure is different from that described in *Cryptosporidium*, consisting of two main layers: an outer exocyst (a fibrous matrix composed predominantly of proteins and polysaccharides) and the inner endocyst layer (a more granular structure, composed mostly of cellulose). The main cyst layers are separated by a space that appears to consist of interconnecting filaments. Note that the cell walls of other protozoa have been found to contain chitin, highlighting the diversity in this group of microorganisms. A typical *A. castellanii* cyst is composed of an inner cyst core surrounded by a cell membrane, a thinner endocyst, the interlayer space, and a thicker, outer endocyst. The multilayered walls of *A. castellanii* cysts have been shown to develop with the initial deposition of inner cellulose-based wall layers and subsequent maturation of external protein/polysaccharide wall coats; in some cases, the endocyst appears to be less prevalent in mature cysts. Some studies have suggested that the development of the inner cellulose-based layers appears to play a major role in the resistance to biocides, although the outer protein layers seem to present a greater barrier to biocide penetration. *Acanthamoeba* is capable of forming (or associating with preexisting bacterial) biofilms on surfaces such as contact lenses. Although protozoal biofilms have yet to be studied extensively in terms of their response to disinfectants, it is apparent that they could play a significant part in modulating the effects of chemical agents.

Algae are also often associated with poor or nutrient-rich water conditions (chapter 1, section 1.3.3.3). They are a diverse group of single-celled eukaryotes that can grow as free-living cells or as associated filaments. Some algae are known fish and human pathogens, including *Gonyaulax* and *Pfiesteria*. Similar to those in fungi, their cell wall structures vary significantly to include different polysaccharides such as cellulose and chitin, but in some cases (e.g., *Euglena*) they lack a cell wall. In limited investigations, algae have been found to be relatively sensitive to most biocides that are used for water disinfection, including chlorine, chlorine dioxide, ozone, bromine, and UV radiation. The most widely used biocides for algae control (generally algistatic rather than algicidal applications) are copper compounds, including copper sulfate, QACs, chlorine, bromochlorodimethyl hydantoin, and hydrogen peroxide. These are used to reduce algae growth in pools, water baths, tanks, and other water applications. Since many algae can grow as associated filaments, their close association within a biofilm either on or in water or associated with a surface can provide a mechanism of limited resistance to biocidal activity. Algae can be associated with bacterial biofilms, but they have also been found to produce their own extracellular polysaccharides, which can protect the cells within an algal biofilm. There is some evidence to suggest that algae have active stress responses similar to bacteria (section 8.3.3) that can allow for greater tolerance to sublethal concentrations of biocides. Increased tolerance to copper and other heavy metals have been described. Algae are capable of accumulating heavy metals; physiological adaptations to the presence of copper include thickening of cell walls (when present) and an increase in the presence of vacuoles which contain copper precipitates. In some strains, the presence of heavy metals also causes an increase in lipid and starch deposits within the cell. Active efflux as a mechanism of biocide resistance has been described in *Euglena* and cadmium tolerance; other algae have shown evidence of heavy metal efflux, which is activated on exposure to such biocides. The extent of cross-resistance to other biocides has not been investigated. As another example, algae have been shown to mount a two-phased response to the presence of increased silver ions. At lower concentrations of silver, the major mechanism of resistance is due to the production of antioxidants, typical or similar to mechanisms in bacteria; at higher concentrations, active efflux protein expression is observed to pump silver out of the cell.

In addition to physiological adaptations, there is also evidence of acquired mechanisms of biocide tolerance in algae. Stable *Chlamydomonas reinhardtii* mutants were developed in the laboratory with increased tolerance to heavy metals. In some of the mutants, tolerance was restricted only to increased concentrations of cadmium, but other mutants were cross-resistant to cadmium, copper, hydrogen peroxide, and UV light. Although the exact mechanism(s) of resistance were not identified, it was proposed to be due to a specific chromosomal mutation event and associated with a change in stress response. There are many reports of the isolation of copper-tolerant algae strains following exposure to sublethal concentrations of copper; in some cases, these mutant strains appeared to be smaller than the parent strains and had reduced metabolic activity. Other mechanisms are associated with limiting the transportation of copper into the cell, by transporter mutations (non- or reduced-expression). Finally, algae reproduce both asexually (by mitosis) and sexually (by the production of zygospores or zoospores). In the case of *Chlamydomonas*, sexual reproduction leads to the formation of a zygote, which then excretes a thick wall to form a zygospore. Similar to other sporulation processes, sexual reproduction is initiated under unfavorable environmental conditions. The zygospore consists of food (starch and lipid) reserves, surrounded by a multilayered wall and is a resistant, dormant structure. Many zygospore development (maturation) mutants have been identified but have yet to be used to study biocide resistance mechanisms. The intrinsic tolerance of zygospores or other algal spores against biocides has not been studied in detail but is clearly an important intrinsic mechanism of resistance to drying, starvation, and other environmental stresses.

The helminths (generally known as worms) are a diverse group of multicellular eukaryotic microorganisms (chapter 1, section 1.3.3). They can be further subclassified into the nematodes (roundworms) and flatworms (including trematodes and cestodes). Although many helminths are pathogenic and frequently identified, their responses to various biocides and biocidal processes have not been studied in any detail. Many are described as important animal and/or human pathogens, which can be difficult to control environmentally, and others are often associated with contaminated water and indicative of poor sanitation conditions. The adult worms and larval forms vary in shapes and sizes, with the former protected externally by a rigid proteinaceous cuticle; these forms are relatively sensitive to exposure conditions outside their hosts, including the presence of biocides. Stress responses (heat and oxidative stress) have been reported, similar to those in bacteria and protozoa, to include the transcriptional control of antioxidants and detoxifying enzymes (e.g., thioredoxin, as oxidoreductase). Efflux mechanisms have also been shown to be induced under certain conditions, but the impacts on biocide resistance are unknown. Similar to the protective mechanisms discussed with bacteria in protozoa (see above), bacteria such as *E. coli* and *Pseudomonas* spp. have been shown to be taken up by *Caenorhabditis elegans*, survive over time, and increase the tolerance of the bacteria to biocides. A greater concern is the production of dormant eggs or cysts (Fig. 8.42 and Fig. 8.43), which demonstrate marked resistance to biocides during their life cycles.

The structure of *Ascaris* eggs has been investigated in some detail as a frequent contaminant of wastewater (see Fig. 8.43). They consist of an inner core (oocyte), which is enclosed within a lipid membrane and surrounded by three main layers: an inner layer of lipoprotein, middle layers of the polysaccharide chitin, and an external proteinaceous layer. Other helminth eggs are morphologically similar but vary in their shapes (generally oval), sizes (ranging from ~30 to 150 μm in length),

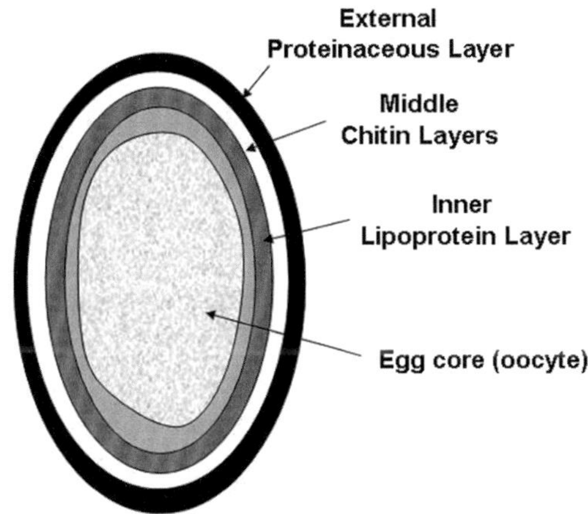

FIGURE 8.43 Representation of the structure of a helminth (*Ascaris*) egg.

and the chemical constituents of various egg layers. Helminth eggs are generally found in water at low concentrations but have a low infectious dose and can survive typical bactericidal concentrations of chlorine and ozone; studies on the effects of other biocides have been limited, but efficacy has been observed with other oxidizing agents. The biocidal resistance of helminth eggs is presumably due to reduced uptake of chemical biocides through the various egg layers to the sensitive core. Further, helminth eggs also demonstrate tolerance to radiation (UV disinfection) and heat, although temperatures of >70°C are found to be effective over time. Chlorine, ozone, UV radiation, and heat have all been shown to be

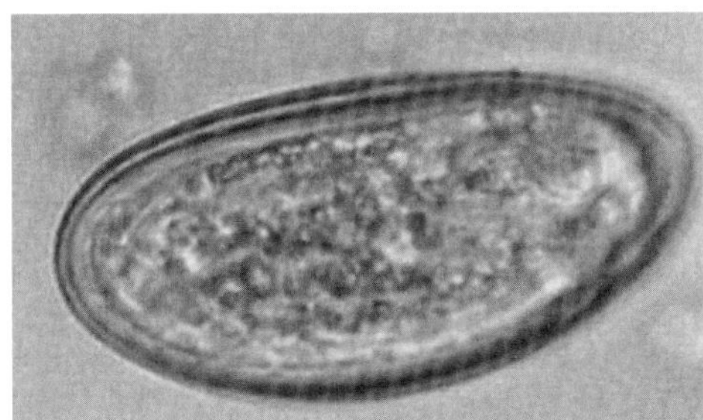
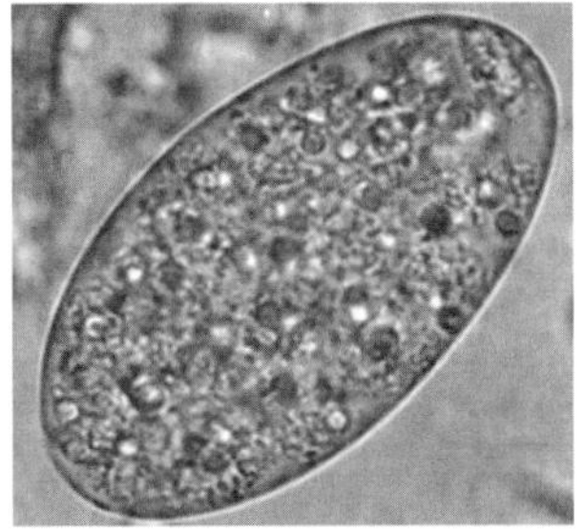

FIGURE 8.42 Micrograph examples of helminth eggs from *Enterobius* (left) and *Fasciola* (right). Enterobius image: Image courtesy of CDC-PHIL/B.G. Partin; Dr. Moore, 1978 (ID#14617), with permission. Fasciola image: Image courtesy of CDC-PHIL/Dr. Mae Melvin, 1973, with permission.

effective in a dose-dependent manner, requiring high concentrations or temperatures or long exposure times to be efficient in comparison to those tested and used to control bacteria and virus levels in water. Ozone treatment appears to cause the disintegration of the various shell walls and loss of viability. In some cases, strong acids or alkali are also used, which are believed to hydrolyze the various egg layers. Overall, the multiple-layer structure of helminth eggs is the main intrinsic mechanism of resistance to biocides and biocidal processes. Other resistance determinants, including acquired mechanisms, have not been described, although they are possible, considering the development of resistance to specific antihelminthic drugs.

INDEX